# Routledge Handbook on the Politics of Global Health

In the early twenty-first century, key public health issues and challenges have taken centre stage on the global scene, and health has been placed at the heart of our collective aspirations for human development and well-being. But significant debate exists not only about the causes, but also about the possible solutions for nearly all of the most important global health challenges.

Competing visions of the values and perspectives that should underlie global health policies have emerged, ranging from an emphasis on cost effectiveness and resource constraints on one extreme, to new calls for health and human rights, and renewed calls for health and social justice on the other. The role of different intergovernmental agencies, bilateral or unilateral donors, public or private institutions and initiatives, has increasingly been called into question, whilst the spread of neoliberal policies and programmes, and existing international trade regimes and intellectual property rights, are deeply implicated in relation to global health responses.

This volume critically evaluates how the global health industry has evolved and how the interests of diverse political and economic stakeholders are shaping the context of a rapidly changing institutional landscape. Bringing together leading authors from across the world, the Handbook's eight sections explore:

- Critical perspectives on global health
- Globalisation, neoliberalism, and health systems
- The changing shape of global health governance
- Development assistance and the politics of global health
- Scale-up, scale-down, and the sustainability of global health programmes
- Intellectual property rights, trade relations, and global health
- Humanitarian emergencies and global health politics
- Human rights, social justice, and global health

The *Routledge Handbook on the Politics of Global Health* addresses both the emerging issues and conceptualisations of the political strategies, policy-making processes, and global governance of global health, along with expanding upon and highlighting the critical priorities in this rapidly evolving field. It provides an authoritative overview for students, practitioners, researchers, and policymakers working in or concerned with the politics of public health around the globe.

**Richard Parker** is Senior Visiting Professor in the Institute for the Study of Collective Health (IESC) at the Federal University of Rio de Janeiro and Executive Director of the Brazilian Interdisciplinary AIDS Association (ABIA), as well as Editor-in-Chief of the journal *Global Public Health*, published by Routledge.

**Jonathan García** is Assistant Professor in Global Health at Oregon State University, where he directs the graduate programme in Global Health. His research on global health disparities is carried out in partnership with community-based organisations in Brazil, Peru, and India.

# Routledge Handbook on the Politics of Global Health

*Edited by Richard Parker and Jonathan García*

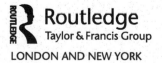

LONDON AND NEW YORK

First published 2019
by Routledge
4 Park Square, Milton Park, Abingdon, Oxon OX14 4RN
605 Third Avenue, New York, NY 10017

First issued in paperback 2023

*Routledge is an imprint of the Taylor & Francis Group, an informa business*

*British Library Cataloguing-in-Publication Data*
A catalogue record for this book is available from the British Library

*Library of Congress Cataloging-in-Publication Data*
Names: Parker, Richard G. (Richard Guy), 1956– editor. | García, Jonathan, editor.
Title: Routledge handbook on the politics of global health /
edited by Richard Parker and Jonathan García.
Description: Milton Park, Abingdon, Oxon ; New York, NY : Routledge, 2019. |
Includes bibliographical references and index.
Identifiers: LCCN 2018036939 | ISBN 9781138238596 (hardback) |
ISBN 9781315297255 (ebook)
Subjects: LCSH: Medical policy–International cooperation. |
World health. | Globalization–Health aspects.
Classification: LCC RA394 .R68 2019 | DDC 362.1–dc23
LC record available at https://lccn.loc.gov/2018036939

ISBN: 978-1-03-256996-3 (pbk)
ISBN: 978-1-138-23859-6 (hbk)
ISBN: 978-1-315-29725-5 (ebk)

DOI: 10.4324/9781315297255

Typeset in Bembo
by Out of House Publishing

Publisher's Note
The publisher has gone to great lengths to ensure the quality of this reprint but points out that some imperfections in the original copies may be apparent.

# Contents

# Figures

# Tables

# Contributing authors

**César Abadía-Barrero** is a medical anthropologist whose research integrates different critical perspectives in the study of how for-profit interests transform access, continuity, and quality of health care. He has conducted action-oriented ethnographic and mixed-method research on health care policies and programmes, human rights judicialisation and advocacy, and social movements in health in Brazil and Colombia.

**Neil Krishan Aggarwal** is a cultural psychiatrist and Assistant Professor at Columbia University. His books include *Mental Health in the War on Terror* (2015), *The Taliban's Virtual Emirate* (2016), and a forthcoming book on the Islamic State's media, slated for publication in 2018.

**Peter Aggleton** is Emeritus Professor of Education and Health at UNSW Sydney and an honorary distinguished professor at The Australian National University in Canberra, Australia. He is Editor-in-Chief of several international journals and has worked internationally in HIV and sexual health for over 25 years.

**Luis L.M. Aguiar** is Associate Professor of Sociology at the University of British Columbia, Canada. He researches the regional identity and economy of the Okanagan Valley in British Columbia and has numerous publications stemming for this work. *Hinterland of Whiteness* details the functioning and reproduction of whiteness in the valley, and will be published by the University of British Columbia Press in 2019. Professor Aguiar also researches low wage workers, organising and labour movements. He is an avid soccer player, and writer completing a manuscript of the sociology of Cristiano Ronaldo. With colleagues in Lisbon and Barcelona, he is developing a research programme on malfeasant celebrities.

**Adriana Ardila-Sierra** is a public health researcher at the Fundación Universitaria de Ciencias de la Salud FUCS in Bogotá, Colombia, who has studied and conceptualised the transformation of medical labour under neoliberalism. Currently, she uses ethnographic methods to investigate the unfolding of a new governmental health care model for indigenous communities in the eastern province of Guainía.

**David Bangsberg** is currently the Founding Dean of the OHSU-PSU School of Public Health. He was former Director of Mass General Hospital Global Health as well as Professor at Harvard Medical School and Harvard School of Public Health.

**Irene Andia Biraro** is Senior Lecturer in the department of Internal Medicine, School of Medicine, College of Health Sciences, Makerere University, Kampala, Uganda.

**João Biehl** is Susan Dod Brown Professor of Anthropology and Co-Director of the Global Health Programme at Princeton University. He is the author of the award-winning books *Vita: Life in a Zone of Social Abandonment* and *Will to Live: AIDS Therapies and the Politics of Survival*. He has also co-edited *Unfinished: The Anthropology of Becoming* and *When People Come First: Critical Studies in Global Health*.

**Yap Boum II** is the Regional Representative in Africa for Epicentre, the research arm of MSF, Professor of Faculty of Medicine, and the Co-Founder of Kmerpad.

**Carlos Correa** is Director of the Center for Interdisciplinary Studies on Industrial Property and Economics at the Law Faculty, University of Buenos Aires, and Special Advisor on Intellectual Property and Trade of the South Centre (Geneva). He has been Visiting Professor in post-graduate courses of several universities and consultant to various regional and international organisations. He has advised several governments on intellectual property, innovation policy, and public health. He was a member of the UK Commission on Intellectual Property, of the Commission on Intellectual Property, Innovation and Public Health established by the World Health Assembly and of the FAO Panel of Eminent Experts on Ethics in Food and Agriculture. He is the author of several books and numerous articles.

**Johanna T. Crane** is currently Associate Professor of Science, Technology, and Society at the University of Washington-Bothell and the author of the recent book *Scrambling for Africa: AIDS, Expertise, and the Rise of American Global Health Science*.

**Marcos Cueto** received his doctoral degree in History from Columbia University in 1988. He is a full professor of the Casa de Oswaldo Cruz a unit of Fiocruz, the main Brazilian biomedical insti-tute, and co-editor of the journal *História, Ciências Saúde – Manguinhos* published by Fiocruz in Rio de Janeiro. During the past years he has been a visiting professor at NYU, Sanford, Princeton, the Graduate Institute (Geneva) and Shanghai universities. He has also been a fellow at the Woodrow Wilson International Center for Scholar, and a visiting researcher at the Department of Sociomedical Sciences of Columbia University Mailman School of Public Health. In Spring 2018, he is the Robert F. Kennedy Visiting Professor at the Department of History of Science at Harvard University. His more recent book, co-authored with Steven Palmer, *Medicine and Public Health in Latin America: a History* (2016) won the George Rosen award of the American Association for the History of Medicine. He is also author of: *Cold War and Deadly Fevers: Malaria Eradication in Mexico, 1955–1970* (2007) and *The Value of Health: A History of the Pan American Health Organization* (2007). Presently he is doing research on the history of AIDS in Brazil and completing a book on the history of the World Health Organization and the Cold War.

**Lorena Di Giano** is Executive Director of Fundación Grupo Efecto Positivo (FGEP) in Argentina and General Coordinator of RedLAM – FGEP is the leading organisation of RedLAM, the Latin American Network for the Access to Medicines. Currently, she is coordinating a regional programme focused on improving access to antiretrovirals (ARVs) by addressing intellectual property barriers in countries of Latin American region. She is a lawyer who specialised in Human Rights and HIV and AIDS. She is an experienced advocate who has dedicated her professional background to defending the human rights of people living with HIV (PLHIV), especially women living with HIV/AIDS. She has offered legal support and representation for PLHIV in local and national courts in Argentina, as well as at the Inter-American Commission on Human Rights, in cases of human rights violations. In the past she has worked for the Argentinean Network of Women Living with HIV/AIDS, as the Project Manager and Campaigner, and also undertaken facilitation and training activities in topics such as human rights, gender, leadership, and advocacy. From 2004 and 2007 she has served as a member of UNAIDS Theme Group in Argentina, representing people living with HIV. She has a law degree from Universidad Nacional de Mar del Plata in Argentina. Lorena Di Giano served from December 2015 to September 2016 as a member of the Expert Advisory Group of the United Nations Secretary General's High-Level Panel on Access to Medicines and Innovation.

**Monika Doshi** has been working on HIV research with sex workers in Asia and Africa over the last 15 years. She began her work in public health and human rights with Avahan, the Gates-funded India AIDS Initiative, through the American India Foundation's William J. Clinton Fellowship for Service. She holds a Master of Public Health degree and a Certificate in Health and Human Rights from the Johns Hopkins Bloomberg School of Public Health.

**Debolina Dutta**, originally from India, is a doctoral researcher at the Institute for International Law and the Humanities, Melbourne Law School in Melbourne, Australia. Her PhD research looks into the forms, practices, and politics of legal knowledge production in post-colonial India, including by sex worker movements. She has collaborated with the sex workers' movement in India, particularly with the Kolkata-based DMSC, for over a decade. In 2011, she co-directed *We Are Foot Soldiers*, a documentary film which tells the story of the collectivisation of children of sex workers in Sonagachi, Kolkata. The film received the third prize at Jeevika: Asia Livelihood Documentary Film Festival in 2012. She is currently putting together a collaborative book project with sex workers of DMSC, VAMP, the Maharashtra-based sex workers' collective, and a graphic artist. This illustrated book titled *The Rule of Laughter* tells the stories of how sex workers in India use laughter and humor in their activism to counter the criminalisation of their daily lives and livelihood. She was a recipient of the Audrey Rapoport Prize for Scholarship on Gender and Human Rights in 2017 for an article on sex workers' activism in India and post-colonial feminisms.

**Daniel E. Esser** is Associate Professor of International Development at American University in Washington, DC. His research investigates political and procedural determinants of aid effectiveness. He has published on global health finance, the political economy of development assistance for health, and accountability in bilateral and multilateral aid relations.

**Eduardo Faerstein** has MD (UERJ 1976) and MHS (UERJ 1987) degrees, and a PhD in Epidemiology (Johns Hopkins University 1995). He is Associate Professor of Epidemiology, Institute of Social Medicine, State University of Rio de Janeiro, Brazil, where he has been on the faculty since 1983, and coordinator of the Brazil Center for Global Health. He is currently Vice-President of the Brazilian Association of Collective Health (ABRASCO) and of the Alliance of Public Health Associations of the Americas.

**Tamer M. Fouad** is an oncologist at the National Cancer Institute, Cairo University and an Adjunct Assistant Professor at the University of Texas, MD Anderson Cancer Center. He is a member of the Editorial Board of the *Journal of Global Oncology*.

**Jonathan García** is Assistant Professor in Global Health at Oregon State University, where he directs the graduate programme in Global Health. He has a doctoral degree in Sociomedical Sciences from Columbia University. His research on global health disparities is carried out in partnership with community-based organisations in Brazil, Peru, and India.

**Vivette García-Deister** is Associate Professor in Science and Technology Studies at the School of Sciences of Mexico's National Autonomous University, in Mexico City.

**Radhika Gore** is a postdoctoral fellow in primary care research at the NYU School of Medicine. Her research focuses on the social and institutional challenges that health care providers and organisations confront in addressing the social determinants of health in primary care settings, with an emphasis on the design and implementation of chronic disease programmes in urban, low-income, minority communities.

**Anand Grover** is Senior Advocate, Supreme Court of India and Director, Lawyers Collective, India. He is the former (2008 to 2014) United Nations Special Rapporteur on the right of everyone to the enjoyment of the highest attainable standard of physical and mental health.

**Yanzhong Huang** is Professor and Director of Global Health Studies at Seton Hall University's School of Diplomacy and International Relations. He is also a senior fellow for global health at the Council on Foreign Relations and the founding editor of *Global Health Governance: The Scholarly Journal for the New Health Security Paradigm*.

**Albrecht Jahn** is a consultant for obstetrics, and global health specialist. He worked for the European Union's Directorate General for Research covering international health research and with WHO on Research and Development policies. Since 2010, he covers Global Health Policies and Systems at Heidelberg University.

**Nora Kenworthy** is Assistant Professor in the School of Nursing and Health Studies at the University of Washington Bothell, and an Adjunct Assistant Professor of Anthropology at the University of Washington Seattle. She is the author of *Mistreated: The Political Consequences of the Fight Against AIDS in Lesotho*.

**Salmaan Keshavjee** is the Director of Harvard Medical School's Center for Global Health Delivery-Dubai and Associate Professor of Global Health and Social Medicine in the Department of Global Health and Social Medicine. Keshavjee has played a key role over the last two decades in international efforts to treat drug-resistant tuberculosis.

**Shamshad Khan** is an Assistant Professor in the Department of Communication, University of Texas, San Antonio. In his international health and communications research, he collaborates with researchers in India, Kenya, China, and Canada and has published in *Social Science & Medicine*; *Health Communication*; *Global Public Health*; *Culture, Health and Sexuality*; *Critical Public Health*; and *PLoS ONE*.

**Elizabeth J. King** is Assistant Professor in the School of Public Health and Associate Director of the Weiser Center for Europe and Eurasia at the University of Michigan. She has extensive academic and research experience in the field of global public health, with special focus on Eastern Europe.

**Neda Milevska Kostova** is Executive Director of Studiorum, a research think-tank working on health and well-being policies in South Eastern Europe. She has extensive academic and consultancy experience in health policy and contributed to the development of a number of national health policies in countries of South Eastern Europe.

**Heidi J. Larson** is Director of the Vaccine Confidence Project at the London School of Hygiene & Tropical Medicine, where she is Professor of Anthropology, Risk and Decision Science. Her particular research interest is the impact of rumors and risk perceptions on health programmes, particularly vaccines and immunisation.

**Jacob Levich** is an administrator at Stony Brook University and an independent researcher in the field of public health. He has written extensively about the Gates Foundation, most recently in the *American Journal of Economics and Sociology*.

**Rene Loewenson** is Director of the Training and Research Support Centre (TARSC) in Zimbabwe. She is an epidemiologist with a 30-year history of research, technical, and policy advice on health systems, primary health care, and health equity internationally. She has coordinated numerous international research networks, including as a founder of and cluster lead in EQUINET.

**Robert Lorway** holds the Canada Research Chair in Global Intervention Politics and Social Transformation in the Centre for Global Public Health, University of Manitoba. His anthropological research is concerned with health interventions that target marginalised people and has written on the subject in *Namibia's Rainbow Project: Gay Rights in an African Nation* and *AIDS Activism, Science and Community across three Continents*.

**Purnima Mane** is a visiting professor at UNSW Sydney. She has worked on HIV and sexual and reproductive health internationally and in India for over 25 years and is a board member of several organisations working in these fields. She is a founding editor of the journal, *Culture, Health and Sexuality*.

**Katherine Marsi** holds master's degrees in social work and public health and has worked both domestically and abroad on HIV and hepatitis C prevention and surveillance. She has particular interest in global challenges in effective epidemic control, and the interconnectivity between public health and social justice.

**Mandisa Mbali** is Senior Lecturer in Historical Studies at the University of Cape Town (UCT). She has published work on AIDS activism, gender and sexuality and health and the race politics of international health and humanitarianism. She is the author of *South African AIDS Activism and Global Health Politics*.

**Arima Mishra** is Professor in Medical Anthropology and Public Health in School of Development, Azim Prmji University, Bangalore, India. Her research interests span from examining the interface between global health discourses and local realities pertaining to maternal and child health, revitalisation of local health traditions and health equity and is based on extensive field work in different states in India.

**Gabriella Meltzer** is a doctoral student at New York University's College of Global Public Health and a former global health research associate at the Council on Foreign Relations.

**Bente Molenaar-Neufeld** is a senior research associate at the Centre for Trade Policy and Law (CTPL) at Carleton University in Ontario, Canada. She works on a broad range of trade related issues, has a strong interest in trade and gender as well as global health. Previously, she worked at the North-South Institute.

**Laura Murray** is a post-doctoral fellow at the Institute of Social Medicine at the State University of Rio de Janeiro and affiliated with the Federal University of Rio de Janeiro through the research and advocacy collaborative, Prostitution Policy Watch (*Observatório de Prostituição*). She is a member of Davida – a sex workers' rights collective founded by Gabriela Leite, a collaborator of the Brazilian Network of Prostitutes, and the director of the 2013 documentary film, *A Kiss for Gabriela*. Her ethnographic research focuses on the intersections between sexuality, gender, politics, activism, and the State.

**Devynne Nelons** graduated in 2010 from Temple University with a B.A. in Health Sociology and in 2018 with an MPH in Global Health at Oregon State University. Her work lies at the intersection of critical global health and nursing practice. ORCID ID:0000-0001-5456-0749

**Kari Marie Norgaard** is Associate Professor of Sociology and Environmental Studies at University of Oregon where she thinks and writes about the intersections of climate change, emotions, tribal environmental justice, gender, colonialism, health, race, and climate denial.

**João Nunes** is Lecturer in International Relations at the University of York, UK. Previously he was a research fellow at the University of Warwick and at the Gothenburg Centre for Globalization and Development. He is the author of the book *Security, Emancipation and the Politics of Health*, and of articles published in the journals *Review of International Studies*, *Third World Quarterly*, and *Security Dialogue*, among others.

**Elsa Oliveira** is a researcher at the African Centre for Migration & Society (ACMS), Wits University, Johannesburg. Since 2010, she has worked with migrant sex workers on a range of projects. In 2013, she launched the MoVE with Dr. Jo Vearey, a project that works with civil society partners, including the Sisonke Sex Worker Movement. A central aim of MoVE is to facilitate the co-production of knowledge through participant involvement and engagement public audiences.

**Yi-Ching Ong** is Associate Research Scholar and Lecturer in Princeton University's Global Health Programme. She holds a PhD in Microbiology and Immunology from Stanford University and an MPhil in Development Studies from Oxford University. She trained in Social Epidemiology while a Robert Wood Johnson Foundation Health & Society Scholar at Columbia University. Her work focuses on interdisciplinary conceptual frameworks for infectious disease disparities.

**Gorik Ooms** is a human rights lawyer and a global health scholar, Professor of Global Health Law & Governance at the London School of Hygiene & Tropical Medicine, Adjunct Professor at the Law Faculty of Georgetown University, and Visiting Professor at the Faculty of Medicine and Health Sciences of Ghent University.

**Richard Parker** is Senior Visiting Professor in the Institute for the Study of Collective Health (IESC) at the Federal University of Rio de Janeiro and Executive Director of the Brazilian Interdisciplinary AIDS Association (ABIA) (http://abiaids.org.br/), as well as Editor-in-Chief of the journal *Global Public Health*, published by Routledge. He also is founder and chair of the Global AIDS Policy Watch (http://gapwatch. org/), founder and co-chair of Sexuality Policy Watch (http://sxpolitics.org/), as well as Professor Emeritus of Sociomedical Sciences and Anthropology and a member of the Committee on Global Thought at Columbia University in New York City.

**Biraj Patnaik** is Amnesty International's South Asia Director. He was previously the Principal Adviser to the Supreme Court of India Commissioners on the Right to Food case, and he has been part of the right to food campaign in India since its inception. All views expressed in his chapter are personal.

**Sushena-Reza Paul** is a behavioural scientist, physician, and sexual health specialist with extensive experience in supporting community-led HIV/STI and violence prevention programmes in Asia and Africa. She has served as Director of the HIV prevention programme in Mysore for key populations under Avahan, and she is the technical support director for the sex worker collective, Ashodaya Samithi. She has published in journals such as *AIDS*, *The Lancet*, and *STI*.

**Ruth J. Prince** is a social anthropologist with interests in east Africa, critical global health, development, and citizenship. She is Associate Professor in Medical Anthropology at University of Oslo and principle investigator of the project, 'Universal Health Coverage and the Public Good in Africa', a 5-year anthropological study funded by the European Research Council. Publications include *Making and Unmaking Public Health in Africa: Ethnographic and Historical Perspectives*, edited with Rebecca Marsland (Ohio University Press, 2013) and a special issue in *Medical Anthropology Quarterly* titled 'What is Life Worth? Exploring biomedical interventions, survival, and the politics of life' (2012).

**Nana Poku** is the Executive Director of the Health Economics and AIDS Research Division (HEARD) at the University of Kwazulu Natal. He was formerly Executive Director, United Nations Commission on HIV/AIDS and Governance in Africa (2003–5) and Director of Operational Research, World Bank AIDS Treatment Acceleration Programme (2004–6).

**Sabina Faiz Rashid** is Dean of BRAC James P Grant School of Public Health at BRAC University, in Dhaka, Bangladesh. She has a PhD in Medical Anthropology and Public Health from The Australian National University, Canberra, Australia. She has been working in Bangladesh since 1993 and joined the School in 2004. She teaches: *Introduction to Public Health, Anthropology and Reproductive and Sexual Health and Rights and Qualitative Research Methods* in the international Master of Public Health programme, which has had students from 29 countries enrolled. She has 23 years of experience in ethnographic and qualitative research, focusing on gender, sexual and reproductive health and well-being of adolescents, adult women and men living in urban slums settlements, sexuality and well-being of young people and excluded groups, and the health service delivery needs of vulnerable communities. She established the Center for Gender, Sexual and Reproductive Health and Rights (CGSRHR) in 2008 and co-manages the Center for Urban Equity and Health (CUEH), with both centres undertaking training, research, and advocacy activities in Bangladesh.

**Ron Reed** is a traditional Karuk dipnet fisherman who served for over a decade as the Cultural Biologist for the Karuk Tribe. Ron Reed comes from a long and prominent family of traditional spiritual leaders and cultural practitioners, and he is the father of six children. He has long been an important tribal spokesperson communicating the cultural and health impacts of river and forest mismanagement to audiences around the world. At home he works to restore Karuk culture and society through reconnecting people, especially tribal youth, to the natural world. His work has been featured in prominent news outlets around the world including National Geographic, National Public Radio, and High Country News.

**William S. Schulz** is a PhD student in the department of Politics at Princeton University, and an Affiliated Researcher of the Vaccine Confidence Project at the London School of Hygiene & Tropical Medicine. His research interests include political behaviour, social psychology, public health, science communication, and data visualisation.

**Gita Sen** is Distinguished Professor at the Public Health Foundation of India, and Adjunct Professor at the Harvard School of Public Health. She is an advocate and activist for social and economic justice, gender equality and women's human rights. She is a founding member and currently General Co-coordinator of the South feminist network, Development Alternatives with Women for a New Era (DAWN).

**Aaron Shakow** is Director of the Initiative on Healing and Humanity at Harvard Medical School's Center for Global Health Delivery-Dubai. Shakow's historical research addresses sociopolitical constructions of disease and their impact on health care systems and international relations. He has taught at Harvard, MIT, and Brandeis University.

**Ron Smith** is a professor of International Relations at Bucknell University. He is trained as a political geographer and has conducted extensive fieldwork in the Middle East and Latin America. He examines the impacts of geopolitics, siege, and occupation on targeted populations related to health, sovereignty, and development.

**Cindy Sousa** is Assistant Professor at Bryn Mawr College Graduate School of Social Work and Social Research. Dr. Sousa's work highlights the relationships between and particular effects of distinct types of violence; the protective role of culture, place, and community; and professional responsibility in the face of collective suffering.

**Kristefer Stojanovski** is a doctoral student in health behaviour and health education at the University of Michigan. He has extensive experience in public and mental health research in South Eastern Europe. He is an Associate Member of the European Academic Network on Roma Studies and a former Fulbright grantee to Macedonia.

**Katerini T. Storeng** is Associate Professor at the Centre for Development and the Environment, University of Oslo and honorary lecturer at the London School of Hygiene and Tropical Medicine. Her research spans the interface of medical anthropology and global public health, engaging both global policy and the local social and economic realities of health.

**Sundar Sundararaman** has been part of the HIV response in India from the time HIV was detected in 1986 in Madras. With a background in Psychiatry, he has been associated with the Indian National Programme on HIV/AIDS for three decades and has been involved in the WHO Global Programme on AIDS in South Asia and the Far East. He has also served on the Technical Panel that advised the Avahan Programme.

**Matthew Thomann** is Assistant Professor of Anthropology at the University of Memphis. His work has appeared in *Culture, Health, and Sexuality*; *Global Public Health*; *Critical African Studies*; and *Journal of Homosexuality*.

**Håkan Thörn** is Full Professor of Sociology, and a member of the steering group for the Centre of Globalization and Development (GCGD) at the University of Gothenburg. His research focuses on globalisation, social movements, and civil society, and he has published a number of books and articles in international journals on these topics.

**Dr. Anne Marie Thow** is Senior Lecturer in Health Policy at the University of Sydney. Her research uses theories of public policy making to explore facilitators and barriers to best practice public health nutrition policy globally, with a particular focus on the interface between economic policy and nutrition.

**Tayler Tobey** graduated Suma Cum Laude from Oregon State University with degrees in Kinesiology and International Studies. After completing a medical internship in Ecuador, she has continued to participate in domestic and international medical programmes.

**Oyewale Tomori** is the immediate past president of the Nigerian Academy of Science. As the virologist with WHO-AFRO, from 1994–2004, he set up the Polio Laboratory Network, providing diagnostic support for the global polio eradication initiative. He is a member of the US National Academy of Medicine.

**Anete Trajman** has MD, Msc., and PhD degrees from the Federal University of Rio de Janeiro. She is currently a visiting professor at the State University of Rio de Janeiro, Brazil and at the McGill Univeristy, Canada, and has been engaged in both universities in global health-related research, teaching, and activism.

**Karen van Rompaey** has more than ten years of experience in international development, working for academic, non-profit, international, and public organisations. She currently works as Knowledge Manager at the Uruguayan Agency for International Cooperation. She holds a master's degree in International Politics from Warwick University, UK.

**Emily E. Vasquez** is a doctoral candidate in the Department of Sociomedical Sciences at the Mailman School of Public Health, Columbia University, in the US.

**Marcela Fogaça Vieira** is graduated in Law (2006), specialised in Intellectual Property Law (2010), and holds a master's degree in Health Policy (2015). She has been working with access to medicines and intellectual property issues at civil society organisations in Brazil since 2005 and has provided consultancy for several international organisations.

**Alan Whiteside** is the Chair in Global Health Policy at the Balsillie School of International Affairs and Wilfrid Laurier University and Professor Emeritus at the University of KwaZulu-Natal. He established the Health Economics and HIV/AIDS Research Division (HEARD) in Durban in 1998.

**Jim Whitman** is Professorial Fellow and Co-Director of the HEARD PhD Programme, University of Kwazulu Natal and general editor of the Palgrave *Global Issues* series.

**Jeremy Youde** is Associate Professor in the Department of International Relations at the Australian National University. He previously held appointments at San Diego State University, Grinnell College, and the University of Minnesota Duluth. He has written four books and more than 30 articles on global health politics. He received his PhD in Political Science from the University of Iowa.

# Introduction

## Routledge Handbook on the Politics of Global Health

*Jonathan García and Richard Parker*

During the first three decades of the twenty-first century, the political dimensions of global health challenges have become a central focus for attention. First in the Millennium Development Goals, and more recently in the Sustainable Development Goals, health has been placed at the heart of our collective aspirations for human development and well-being. Some argue these goals are necessary fictions – unrealistic and utopian by nature. Visions of what global health could and should be, and of how it might be achieved, have varied significantly. While there may be widespread agreement about the importance of addressing poverty, inequality, and environmental degradation in order to achieve greater population health through human development, understandings of how these factors translate into health and illness vary widely, as do policies and political strategies designed to address them. Significant debate exists not only about the causes, but also about the possible solutions for nearly all of the most important global health challenges, ranging from newly emerging or re-emerging infectious diseases such as HIV and AIDS, hepatitis, malaria, and drug-resistant tuberculosis; the spread of chronic conditions such as diabetes, hypertension, and heart-disease; the shape of humanitarian and public health emergencies in the wake of catastrophic storms, earthquakes or tsunamis; the crises and health consequences faced by displaced populations and refugees; to the growing spectre of emerging global pandemics as different as Ebola or Zika viruses.

Diverse and often polarised views now characterise the response to what have been seen as new global health issues, such as reproductive and sexual health and rights, or the geopolitics of violence against ethnic and sexual minorities. Heated debates have increasingly taken shape in relation to human rights and social justice as they relate to access to essential medicines, or research, innovation and development of vaccines and technologies. Equally important, the role of different intergovernmental agencies, bilateral or unilateral donors, public or private institutions and initiatives, has increasingly been called into question. Their hegemonic role in seeking to determine how best to utilise rapidly increasing resources with the goal of scaling-up key global health initiatives has received increasing attention. More recently, critical analysis has focused on the ways in which donors have confronted an extended global financial crisis or crises, and the reality of diminishing budgets, at least in real terms. While much has been made of the scale-up of major global health programmes, such as the global response to HIV and AIDS (and other long-term challenges such as tuberculosis and malaria), now nearly three decades into the new world of large-scale Global Health Initiatives (GHIs) in the twenty-first century, there are important signs that we are witnessing the actual scale-down of previously grander policies and programmes.

Although the expansion of serious public health problems, increasingly taking shape on a global scale, has been one of the defining features of recent history, both the political determinants of many of these problems, and contested political visions about how best to confront them, have been equally important. Like most aspects of contemporary life, the range of key global health problems has been impacted in profoundly important ways by political and policy processes and tensions associated with globalisation. Political and policy processes are driven by the spread of neoliberal policies and programmes that have affected health, education, and welfare programmes in countries around the world. Structural adjustment projects, and policy-based lending of international development aid have extended neoliberal reforms across the global South. These key structural determinants of health emerging in recent decades have gone hand in hand with globalisation. If global capitalism has produced unprecedented wealth and significant levels of development, which may be associated with increasing health status, it has also created new forms of economic polarisation and increasing marginalisation of the poor, both in the North and in the South. Polarisation has been linked in important ways to newly emerging and re-emerging infectious diseases – as well as to changes in lifestyle that have exacerbated chronic disease around the world. At the same time, the globalisation of neoliberal policies and programmes has weakened the institutional architecture needed to respond to these growing health challenges at precisely the time when responses are most needed, just as it has created a new class of global political and policy elites who often impose their presumably well-intended 'solutions' on marginalised and disempowered populations.

The discourse of inclusion of global perspectives in the politics of health has sought to advance the field of global health towards greater equity. From more democratic policy formation processes to an emphasis on continuous community engagement in the implementation of health policy, perspectives from the global South are paramount to addressing neglected diseases that affect highly marginalised groups living in pockets of deep social exclusion. While this movement for global inclusion has been mostly positive, it also feeds into the rise in populism throughout the world. Throughout Latin America, the surge of ideological populism has slowly shifted countries like Venezuela into dictatorship. At the same time, populist movements in the United States and Europe mobilised masses of socio-economically excluded people against migrants coming from war-torn regions. These tensions between structural 'othering' and inclusion have shaped global health governance, frameworks based on equity, and resource mobilisation.

These factors, in turn, have been associated with sharply divergent visions not only about the causes of global health problems, but about how best to respond to global health challenges. Whether to emphasise primary health care and to build health systems from the ground up, or to opt instead for vertical health programmes and more technical or technological solutions to disease control, are the kinds of questions that have divided approaches to global health for decades. But as we have moved more fully into an era of global health since the late-1990s, such debates have increasingly been linked to deeply divided visions of the values and perspectives that should underlie global health policies, ranging from an emphasis on cost effectiveness and resource constraints on one extreme, to new calls for health and human rights, and renewed calls for health and social justice on the other. The appropriate roles for states and intergovernmental agencies, for private enterprise, for civil society – ranging from grassroots activists, community-based organisations and non-governmental groups to private philanthropy, foundations and private–public partnerships – have all been hotly debated. Existing international trade regimes and intellectual property rights have increasingly come to be understood as deeply implicated in relation to global health responses, and the politics of research, development, and innovation have come to be seen as directly relevant to equitable access to essential medicines. Perhaps most important, all such issues have come to be hotly debated in the early twenty-first century in forums as sharply opposed as those of the World Economic Forum and the World Social Forum, making global health one of the most highly politicised fields in contemporary public debate, and underlining the stakes involved in opting for different visions of the 'global health industry' that has taken shape in recent decades.

Nearly two decades have passed now since the field of global health began to announce itself, roughly at the turn of the century in 2000, as a fundamentally new approach, or even paradigm, as opposed to earlier approaches known as international health or, before that, tropical medicine. But as this time has passed, much of the optimism that initially greeted this supposed paradigm shift has unfortunately proven to be somewhat exaggerated. Many observers hoped that the idea of a truly 'global' system would be taken seriously, and we would better understand the health issues both in the global North and the global South as profoundly interrelated and mutually implicated. In reality, we have found that the 'global' has often been little more than a new label for what was previously the primary focus of both tropical medicine and international health: the health challenges of the so-called developing world, found primarily in poor countries largely located in the global South. This failure to fully transform our understanding of the spatial and social dimensions of global health has also been accompanied by an even greater failure to transform the fundamental power relations that have long operated in earlier approaches: the inequities between North and South that have so consistently produced and reproduced relations of colonialism and imperialism in ways that have established the global North as the centre of power, development assistance, scientific expertise, decision-making, and general domination in relation to global health policies and programmes. While global health problems have continued to be seen as somehow 'out there' in the distant global South, solutions all too often are supposedly invented in the global North and exported to the locations where they are perceived to be needed, with all-too-little involvement of those supposedly in need in terms of participating as anything even remotely resembling equal partners in the decision-making process.

With these issues in mind, this volume seeks to push back against these tendencies in a number of significant ways. It includes analyses of important global health issues that in fact affect the global North as well as the global South (and that recognise that in the contemporary global capitalist system, the 'fourth world' can often be found as much inside the 'first world' as it is inside the 'third world'). It also includes chapters that directly analyse and critique these existing relations of power and inequality, unmasking both the large-scale political economic processes as well as the more mundane administrative, accounting, and evaluation practices that reproduce these ongoing inequities. Perhaps most important, this *Handbook* explicitly seeks to give equal representation to Southern voices and visions, understanding them as every bit as important as their Northern counterparts for building the kinds of analysis and interpretations of the field of global health and the responses that are needed to address the challenges facing this field now and in the future.

Building on these understandings, the chapters in this *Handbook* thus take on a critical evaluation of how the global health industry has evolved and of the interests of diverse political and economic stakeholders shaping the context of a rapidly changing institutional landscape. Unlike most of the work available on global health, they provide a serious engagement with perspectives from the global South that call into question the dominance of political perspectives and policies elaborated in the global North, and that grapple with some of the limitations of technocratic approaches (promoted by many international agencies and key donor countries) when faced with challenges that are fundamentally political. Many of the most serious health threats facing the world community today reach beyond the sovereign borders of nation-states and require the attention not only of governments but also of a range of non-state institutions and actors. Yet precisely because this is the case, they also open up possibilities for political tensions, conflicting interests, and contested visions in ways that have only begun to be explored through critical research and analysis. This volume brings together many of the most important authors who have begun to pioneer research on these issues from across a range of disciplinary perspectives, providing an important overview of the political challenges currently facing this rapidly emerging field.

The *Handbook* is organised in eight main sections (Parts I to VIII). Part I, *Critical perspectives on global health*, seeks to provide a range of analyses that engage critically with the current state of the field and point towards possible alternative futures. Although the early roots of global health can be found both in tropical medicine, as it emerged in the colonial era of the late-nineteenth century, and in international health, as it took shape following World War II, the field that since roughly the start of the new millennium has come to describe itself as global health has been seen as ushering in a bold new era of development and innovation. Yet many continuities in existing power relations and inequalities were silently reproduced in the development of this emerging field, just as new forms of domination and control were created through the evolving conceptual and institutional architecture global health. It is not surprising, therefore, that a growing critique has emerged of many of the dominant tendencies and trends in the field of global health. This section of the *Handbook* highlights some of the perspectives advanced through what has increasingly been described as 'critical global health'. It includes a focus on issues ranging from the politics of knowledge in global health to the geopolitics of global health policies and programmes.

The first chapter in Part I, 'Fault-lines in global health: intersecting inequalities, human rights, and the SDGs', by Gita Sen, examines the transformations in global political economy, as well as in the environment and institutions affecting the health of people in both the South and the North, during the decades between the Alma Ata Declaration in 1978 of 'Health for All by the Year 2000' and the enunciation in 2015 of Sustainable Development Goal 3 (SDG3) to 'Ensure healthy lives and promote well-being for all at all ages'. She focuses on both agreements and disagreements between the global South and the North in relation to development agendas, human rights challenges, and health inequalities, and analyses how to advance a truly universal agenda in relation to health for all people. The second chapter, 'The right to health under capitalism: threats, confrontations, and possibilities', by César Abadía-Barrero and Adriana Ardila-Sierra, develops a critical analysis of the two interrelated perspectives of the right to health – the right to medical care and the right to be healthy – as they have evolved together with the development of the capitalist system during the nineteenth and twentieth centuries. It analyses the ways in which global capitalism has silenced comprehensive notions of the right to health, such as those included in the Alma Ata Declaration and in social medicine proposals that advocate for primary health care through participatory mechanisms, and argues that human rights proposals must develop a critical political economy framework and collaborate with other social justice struggles in order to advance an emancipatory agenda in relation to the right to health. The third chapter, 'South African AIDS activism: lessons for high-impact global health advocacy', by Mandisa Mbali, focuses on the recent history of HIV and AIDS to illuminate the ways in which committed activism can successfully challenge global capitalist structures and neoliberalism's intensification of health inequalities. It examines the ways in which South Africa's Treatment Action Campaign (TAC) used human rights advocacy and built ties to an emerging transnational HIV treatment access movement to overcome the AIDS denialism of the South African government and successfully demanded increases in international aid to support HIV treatment access in developing countries.

While the response to HIV in South Africa and elsewhere may have offered important lessons, as well as reasons for optimism in relation to the politics of global health, there are also significant reasons for continued concern. In the fourth chapter, 'Neglect in global health', João Nunes focuses on the question of agenda-setting in global health by exploring the politics of why certain questions become neglected in global health. He argues that neglect is linked not only to specific diseases but also determinants and groups, and that the quality of attention is crucial to determining if and how an issue is neglected – and it illustrates using the examples of water and sanitation, and the 2014 Ebola outbreak in West Africa. The fifth chapter, 'The politics of funding research in global health partnerships', by Johanna T. Crane, Irene Andia Biraro, Tamer M. Fouad, Yap Boum II, and David Bangsberg, examines the inequities that exist in much global health research. Even though the rhetoric of the field of global health emphasises the importance of 'partnerships' between wealthy and poor nations, the funding mechanisms and administrative practices used by key funding agencies such as the US National Institutes of Health (NIH) continue to create barriers for equitable collaboration between North and South. This analysis highlights the ways in which funding arrangements undercut true partnership between Northern and Southern institutions, often undermining rather than building capacity in the global South. The last chapter in this section, 'From global health to planetary and micro global health: theorising global health's present remodeling and scaling', by João Biehl and Yi-Ching Ong, examines diverse critiques of the contemporary field of global health (embodied in notions of neo-colonialism, neoliberalism, governmentality, and humanitarianism), and explores the ways in which this field is being remodelled through new movements such as planetary health and design thinking. It argues for the urgent need for critical analysis, for a fuller integration of theory, method, and praxis, and for greater attention to people's life-worlds as essential for reinventing the field of global health in the future.

Taken together, the chapters in Part I of the *Handbook* provide an important critique of the current status quo in the field of global health. They highlight the ways in which critical social science thinking has called into question the epistemological assumptions and intellectual dominance of biomedicine and public health in determining the most important challenges facing the field. They show us how science travels across borders, how technical solutions to global health challenges often fail to comprehend political barriers, and what kinds of solutions might be created if people's needs were actually the primary focus of concern. They provide a key point of departure for the *Handbook* and articulate many of the most important themes that will be addressed in the other sections of the volume.

Part II of the *Handbook*, on *Globalisation, neoliberalism, and health systems*, examines health outcomes and health inequities at multiple levels produced by the political economic structures resulting from globalisation. Globalisation is characterised by a more open flow of economic goods and services, as well as movement in people, ideas, and cultures. Global health politics get negotiated at the intersection of these 'flows' – as a necessary attempt to address the health of populations affected by social, cultural, and economic processes. Political economic structures that facilitate the free global exchange of financial goods and services have been strategically 'bundled' with the regulation of local commodities, natural resources, and the means of production. Open economic policies, currency pegging, and production out-sourcing have had deep global health implications. The health effects of neoliberalism have ranged from structural vulnerabilities created by weakened health systems to local occupational hazards in labour camps and sweatshops. Global health outcomes are thus negotiated among stakeholders that very meaningfully include private industry and multinational corporations, although economic externalities at the international level have not been addressed properly.

The first chapter in Part II, 'Boundaries of global health politics in the 'fourth world': determinants of political will for hepatitis C treatment', by Jonathan García, Devynne Nelons, Tayler Tobey, and Katherine Marsi, describes the striking global health disparities that exist within pockets of deep social and economic exclusion in the 'fourth world', which require a political solution based on global solidarity. This chapter advances the concept of the fourth world as a useful framework for identifying and addressing health disparities that affect the most marginalised populations across societies. The authors discuss the rise in chronic hepatitis C virus (HCV) infection among people who inject drugs (PWID) in settings such as the United States, Canada, Australia, and the United Kingdom as a product of political, economic, social, and cultural marginalisation. The cost of treating HCV in these countries (i.e., due to their overall economic standing) doubly excludes the most vulnerable PWID from access to highly effective, life-saving treatment. This chapter highlights the importance of social mobilisation to generate political will to address HCV treatment access. The second chapter, 'Sabotaged bodies, sacrifice, and lost youth under punitive neoliberalism', by Luis L. M. Aguiar, describes the embodied and psychosocial experience of young men going north to earn a wage in the rugged landscapes of the interior of Canada. In this location, promises are made of economic development feeding into the future economic well-being of those willing to work hard in a reinvigorated capitalism extracting 'black gold' from complex land ecologies. Aguiar embeds this discussion in an argument of primitive accumulation processes disposing workers in one geography to make them available in another.

The third chapter, '"Willingness to pay": how health care user fees spread around the world, 1965–2015', by Aaron Shakow and Salmaan Keshavjee, examines the impact of financing models on the rise of global health over the last half-century and their implications for population health in poor countries.

They stress the interconnected history of key ideas and policies, showing how debates over cost-control associated with the US Medicare legislation of 1965 were exported after the global price inflation of the following decade, driven by development institutions that were increasingly well-positioned to impose the same policies worldwide. The chapter illustrates how models such as the 'revolving drug fund' and dogmas about limiting recurrent expenditures and the 'price inelasticity of demand' for health care helped create global health as a coherent discipline. Neoliberal approaches to health, the chapter concludes, were marked both by naked self-interest and by longstanding features of imperial liberalism. In the fourth chapter in this section, 'The politics of health systems strengthening', Katerini T. Storeng, Ruth J. Prince, and Arima Mishra describe how the most powerful global health donors – from the Bill & Melinda Gates Foundation, to the Rockefeller Foundation, and USAID – have belatedly joined the World Health Organization in espousing commitment to health systems strengthening for future epidemic preparedness and to achieve 'Universal Health Coverage'. In practice, however, different global health actors imbue the notion with vastly different meanings and propose a range of potentially contradictory approaches. This reflects not just technical disagreement about policies and programmes, but also deep fault lines in public health ideologies. Drawing on examples from Kenya, India, and other countries, this chapter discusses how debates about health systems and initiatives to strengthen them cut to the core of the politics of global health. The fifth chapter, 'National and subnational politics of health systems' origins and change' by Radhika Gore, explores the deeper role of these global political forces in defining national sovereignty in health services provision. Each state addresses health threats based in part on its institutional capacity, history, political priorities, and relations within society. Understanding global health politics therefore requires understanding of how public health challenges and debates are refracted not only through the governing structures and machinations of the *global* health community, but also through health system institutions and actors *within states*. This chapter discusses the state's inattention to primary care in urban India in the context of urbanisation.

The chapters in Part II of the *Handbook* thus present the consequences of social, economic, and cultural globalisation for the health of marginalised people in both the global North and South. The section highlights how neoliberalism has driven marginalisation and exploitation, and how political responses have evolved at the international as well as national and sub-national levels.

Part III, *The changing shape of global health governance*, addresses the core dimension of organising supranational systems in response to processes, such as globalisation and neoliberalism, which have highlighted the need for nations to collectively address challenges resulting from our increasing interconnectedness. Chapters in this section of the *Handbook* examine how governance can be organised and enforced through agreements and development goals. Ranging from environmental movements to mitigate the health effects of climate change to transnational coalitions working to address refugee crises resulting from political unrest, there are a wide variety of public health problems that require governance at the international level. In this section, chapters document political challenges to creating treaties, governing bodies, and adherence to international agreements drawing from examples from a variety of contemporary global public health issues.

In the first chapter of Part III, 'Reforming the World Health Organization', Yanzhong Huang and Gabriella Meltzer analyse the WHO's years-long reform process, describing its successes and failures to adapt to the shifting global health landscape. It begins with an overview of the organisation's history since its establishment in 1948. Despite key achievements such as the eradication of smallpox, and response to the 2003 SARS outbreak, the organisation faces tremendous governance challenges in sustaining its leadership in global health in the twenty-first century. The chapter then examines the reform process by discussing how the reform was conceived, what measures were pursued, and their effectiveness. Particular attention is paid to the role of the global South in pushing for these reforms. The 2014 Ebola outbreak in West Africa epitomised the aforementioned governance challenges and signalled the lack of progress in the WHO reform. Unfortunately, the Ebola crisis thus far has not spurred fundamental change in WHO management, governance, or financing structures.

The chapters that follow describe regional health governance and highlight the role of perspectives from stakeholders in the global South. The second chapter in Part III, 'Health governance: a neglected and an uncharted path of governance in Africa' by Oyewale Tomori, explores 'good governance' as the foundation for economic development, political stability, orderly development, health, and social well-being. Despite strenuous efforts, good governance has eluded many African countries, while health governance remains a neglected and uncharted arm of governance. Establishing good governance, which enhances health governance, is a reliable tool for improving health and especially for preventing and controlling emerging and re-emerging disease outbreaks. In the third chapter, 'Learning from research on experiences of health diplomacy in Africa', Rene Loewenson and Bente Molenaar-Neufeld examine the role of African agencies in global and south-south health diplomacy in addressing selected key challenges to health and health systems in east and southern Africa (ESA). The chapter explores four key areas of health diplomacy: agenda setting, policy development, policy selection, and negotiation and implementation. The evidence highlights the complex political nature of global health diplomacy, with effective engagement enabled by political leadership and champions, with clearly articulated policy positions, regional interaction, unified platforms across African countries and good communication within countries, with embassies and with allies in the international community. The case studies suggest, however, that framing health diplomacy in the region within a 'development aid' paradigm carries an opportunity cost if it weakens attention to structural determinants. The fourth chapter, 'China's role in global health governance', by Jeremy Youde, examines China's growing economic and political clout in global health governance as both a donor *and* recipient of official development assistance for health. The chapter argues that China has concentrated on using health as part of its larger diplomatic strategy, supporting national health programmes in particular states through bilateral means. In particular, over the past 25 years, China has significantly boosted its health diplomacy engagement with sub-Saharan Africa. This chapter discusses the history of China's health diplomacy efforts in Africa, its connection to global health governance institutions, and the lingering questions about China's role in global health governance engagement.

The next chapters zoom out to explore frameworks that advance our understanding of global health governance. In the fifth chapter, 'Aiming for synergies between global health security and global health equity, with help from a Framework Convention on Global Health', Gorik Ooms and Albrecht Jahn argue that a substantial part of the global resources for health are probably being mobilised out of concerns about shared risks (i.e., for the sake of health security), rather than out of concerns about fairness. The chapter presents the Framework Convention on Global Health to identify and address issues of global security and equity. The sixth chapter in Part III, 'Health and global governance: the case of development cooperation on' by Håkan Thörn, argues that global health governance is defined by unequal power relations and involves rationalities and techniques that harmonise policy interventions and standardise their design, implementation, and evaluation. Addressing the debate on the extent to which 'advanced liberal' forms of governance can be deployed effectively in 'developing countries' in the global South, the chapter demonstrates how global health governance involves new forms of power operating at the scale of transnational populations through strategies of governance that particularly target civil society. The analysis demonstrates how the introduction of a 'package of responsibilisation', involving a cluster of techniques defined by the rationalities of marketisation, scientisation, and standardisation, shapes civil society organisations' activities in order that they become competitive service providers, use evidence-based methods, and produce measurable results.

Taken together, Part III of the *Handbook* lays out existing challenges for global and regional health governance systems and presents frameworks to evaluate equity and effectiveness in these systems. These chapters give special attention to the role of various political stakeholders in areas of global health (e.g., health development, human rights, national security, evidence-based medicine) in responding to crises (e.g., Ebola, SARS, HIV) with profound mental and physical health implications. Equally important, this section discusses a variety of power dynamics and institutional configurations that draw on unique social, cultural, and economic resources.

Part IV of the *Handbook* focuses on *Development assistance and the politics of global health*.

Development assistance is an essential dimension of how political strategies are negotiated on the global level and is often centred on improving health outcomes and the context of vulnerability. Global health efforts have been developed with funding from multilateral agencies (e.g., World Bank, IMF, UNDP, UNAIDS), bilateral agreements (e.g., PEPFAR), charitable organisations such as private foundations (e.g., the Rockefeller Foundation, the Ford Foundation, and, especially in recent years, the Bill & Melinda Gates Foundation), and transnational non-governmental organisations. The power dynamics between funders and aid recipients has been criticised for mirroring colonisation and for promoting ideological conflicts. Chapters in this section of the *Handbook* explore a range of funding structures and aid recipients, identifying the factors that promote dependence and political economic inefficiency.

In the first chapter in Part IV, 'Global health challenges in the era of the Sustainable Development Goals', Nana Poku and Jim Whitman examine the relative success of the health-related outcomes achieved as a result of the Millennium Development Goals (MDGs) and explore the degree to which the Sustainable Development Goals (SDGs) from 2015 may be able to consolidate and extend those achievements. They note the ways in which the SDGs reflect a rapidly changing world in which health is now focused much more broadly than was in the case during the period of the MDGs (which were focused primarily on HIV and AIDS) – and a time when rapidly rising costs contrast with diminished resources. They argue that continuing the forward momentum of the MDGs is by no means guaranteed in the new development climate of the SDGs, and question whether the area of global health will be able to achieve the status and support that it had prior to 2015. The second chapter in this Part of the *Handbook*, 'Disrupting global health: the Gates Foundation and the vaccine business', by Jacob Levich, focuses on the dominant private development agency operating in the contemporary field of global health, the Bill & Melinda Gates Foundation, and develops a sharp critique of the ways in which what has come to be described as 'philanthrocapitalism' impacts on the people's health. It questions the extent to which such organisations like the Gates Foundation can be understood as fundamentally benevolent, and suggests that the Foundation's emphasis on the practices and organisational norms of corporate capitalism is central to a strategy for bringing 'disruptive innovation' to the field of global health. In the third chapter in this Part of the *Handbook*, 'National influence in global health governance: the case of the United Kingdom's Department for International Development', Daniel E. Esser focuses on the continued importance – even in an age of philantrocapitalism – of bilateral development aid agencies such as the United Kingdom's Department for International Development (DFID). Esser shows how DFID succeeded, under the direction of a number of progressive leaders, in building a track-record of evidence-based aid allocation as well as a coherent approach to international multilateralism, while managing to maintain a productive relationship with a financially powerful but publicly unaccountable partner organisation such as the Gates Foundation.

The final two chapters in Part IV of the *Handbook* offer detailed case studies of the politics of development assistance as they play out in different national and local settings. In the fourth chapter of Part IV, 'The crossroads of development assistance and national development agendas in the countries of South Eastern Europe', Neda Milevska Kostova, Elizabeth J. King, and Kristefer Stojanovski examine the role of foreign development assistance for South Eastern Europe (SEE) countries as they embarked on a series of political and economic transformations after gaining independence in the 1990s. They argue that most SEE governments failed to see health as an investment in economic growth and lacked clear visions for their health sectors, which opened the way for donor-driven agendas focused on privatisation, health technology investments and the medicalisation of health. While this situation began to change as SEE countries joined the European Union, nearly two decades after gaining independence, there continues to be a serious misalignment between development assistance and the health-related needs of these nations. In the final chapter in Part IV, 'On the life history of HIV interventions in India: Avahan, organic intellectuals, and the fate of community mobilisation', Robert Lorway, Shamshad Khan, Monika Doshi, Sundar Sundararaman, and Sushena-Reza Paul examine the Avahan initiative for HIV prevention in India, funded by the Bill & Melinda Gates Foundation. They focus on HIV prevention interventions for sex workers and critique the standardised measurement practices and the neoliberal logics of efficiency and accountability that have guided these programmes. But they also highlight the ways in which sex workers adapt donor-imposed approaches to the purposes of their own social justice advocacy in struggling to transform the social conditions that create oppression and vulnerability.

Issues of scale and sustainability are central to Part V of the *Handbook*, which focuses on *Scale-up, scale-down, and the sustainability of global health programmes*. Scaling-up global health responses, particularly through large GHIs, has emerged as especially important. But visions of how best to achieve scale-up – whether through bilateral or multilateral initiatives, as the result of governmental or intergovernmental initiatives or based on 'public–private partnerships' (PPPs), and so on – have varied greatly, often revealing significant political tensions and even conflicts. The sustainability of scale-up has proven to be a major challenge, as the goal of scale-up has frequently turned into the reality of scale-down as donors withdraw their support, often in unplanned ways and with serious unintended consequences. The chapters in this section explore the politics of agenda setting and shifting priorities, and the complex ways in which the scale-up and scale-down of global health programmes affect both the field of global health and the lives of those that global health programmes are intended to serve.

The first three chapters in Part V all examine different dimensions of the global response to HIV and AIDS, which has in many ways been at the forefront of constructing the field of global health. In the first chapter, 'Scaling-up and losing the signal: the global HIV and AIDS epidemic', Alan Whiteside examines the impressive successes that were achieved in the response to HIV through the creation of new agencies and initiatives such as UNAIDS, PEPFAR, and the Global Fund to Fight AIDS, Tuberculosis, and Malaria. He argues that AIDS showed us that global resources can be mobilised for urgent health issues, but also just how hard it can be to maintain momentum over time as global attention shifts to new issues. The second chapter in Part V, 'Brazil and the changing meanings of "universal access" to antiretrovirals during the early twenty-first century', by Marcos Cueto, echoes many of these issues through a detailed case study of the Brazilian response to HIV, which is often considered to be one of the most important success stories in the global response to epidemic. It looks at Brazil's pioneering antiretroviral treatment access programme that was put in place in the late 1990s, providing a model for the global scale-up of HIV treatment in the 2000s. But it also highlights recent challenges that Brazil has faced in sustaining its successful programme, emphasising just how much sustainability depends on broader political commitment – and how vulnerable sustainability can be when such political commitment falters. In the third chapter in Part V, '"Ending AIDS" or scaling down the HIV response?', Nora Kenworthy, Matthew Thomann, and Richard Parker extend this analysis through a critique of recent discourses about the imminent end of AIDS on the part of many of the leading agencies charged with coordinating the global response to the epidemic. They suggest that the 'end of AIDS' narrative has increasingly become a kind of smoke screen that may actually cover up the ways in which the scale-up is increasingly being transformed into scale-down in many parts of the world.

The fourth and fifth chapters in Part V both seek to assess some of the key lessons that have been learned in seeking to implement and sustain major global health programmes. In the fourth chapter, 'Enabling positive change: learning from progress and setback in HIV and sexual and reproductive health', Purnima Mane and Peter Aggleton argue that even though major challenges still exist in the fields of HIV and sexual and reproductive health internationally, remarkable progress has nonetheless been made in recent years. Their chapter reflects on key lessons learned in HIV policy and practice in India, in abortion legislation in Mozambique, and with respect to age at marriage and contraceptive access in Bihar State in India. They argue that evidence, grassroots action, and political leadership are all critical factors contributing to success in global health initiatives, and they emphasise that it is through the combination of these components that progress is made possible. In the last chapter in Part V, 'The global politics of polio eradication', William S. Schulz and Heidi J. Larson look at an even longer struggle than the fight against HIV and AIDS as they examine the political dimensions of the World Health Assembly's 1988 resolution to eradicate polio, and the long-term history of the Global Polio Eradication Initiative. Using examples drawn from Latin America, Nigeria, Afghanistan, and Pakistan, they explore the delicate balance of sometimes conflicting interests and political influence – and they examine the Polio Eradication Initiative's lasting legacy as it closes in on the last reservoirs of the disease, and they consider whether eradication will manage to keep the promises of benefits beyond polio that helped secure approval of the 1988 resolution in the first place.

Part VI of the *Handbook* explores the area of *Intellectual property rights, trade relations and global health*. Chapters in this section describe how trade agreements, governing bodies (e.g., World Trade Organization, World Social Forum), and intellectual property rights have shaped the politics of global health. In the first chapter, 'Politics of access to medicines and human rights', Anand Grover provides a kind of overview of the politics of access to medications in the early twenty-first century. He argues that access to essential medicines is an integral part of the right to health, which has been explicitly enunciated in a number of international instruments, and he recounts the ways in which struggles for treatment access, initially focused on antiretroviral treatment for HIV infection, have increasingly broadened to a wide range of health conditions as part of ongoing attempts to achieve greater health equity.

The second chapter in this section, 'Trading away global health? Unravelling the intellectual property, trade and investment nexus, and the impact on the right to health', by Karen van Rompaey, elaborates in greater detail on many of the themes introduced by Grover, emphasising that the realisation of health as a fundamental human right requires equitable access to medicines. Although multilateral agreements give developing countries some room to manoeuvre to address serious public health emergencies, they have often faced retaliation and litigation from developed countries and patent holders, and the right to health for the most vulnerable is therefore threatened by existing profit-driven intellectual property, trade and investment regimes. Van Rompaey argues that it is only by mainstreaming the right to health in national and international policy that it will be possible for developing countries to enhance the physical accessibility and affordability of medicines in order to improve global health. In the third chapter in this section, 'Will the amendment to the TRIPS Agreement enhance access to medicines?', Carlos Correa explores how the implementation of intellectual property protections as prescribed by WTO rules and included in free trade agreements has changed the scenario for access to medicines in developing countries. Correa argues that serious inequities in access to medicines have increased as a result, with no evidence that the adoption of these standards has led to greater pharmaceutical innovation. He emphasises that although the reform of the TRIPS Agreement that entered into force in January 2017 was negotiated with the aim of facilitating access to patented medicines in countries without manufacturing capacity in pharmaceuticals, it has not constituted an effective tool to address inequalities of access in these countries, and points to possible revisions that should be considered to address this ongoing challenge.

In the fourth chapter in Part VI, 'Taking on the challenge of implementing public health safeguards on the ground: the experience of Argentina and Brazil from a civil society perspective', Marcela Fogaça Vieira and Lorena Di Giano look at the ways in which communities, civil society organisations, and governments from the global South have questioned the private appropriation of common social goods through intellectual property protections. Although international organisations have produced numerous recommendations for countries to adopt measures against the negative impact of intellectual property protections on human rights – including the United Nations Secretary-General's High-Level Panel on Access to Medicines in 2016 – actually using those measures can be difficult. The chapter analyses the experience of civil society organisations and governments in Argentina and Brazil as they have sought to implement measures available in the current intellectual property system in order to impact health and well-being. Finally, in the fifth chapter of this section of the *Handbook*, 'The politics of malnutrition: achieving policy coherence in a globalised world', Anne Marie Thow and Biraj Patnaik focus on the challenges that existing trade regimes and practices pose in relation to the global burden of malnutrition. They point to the power differentials that characterise the key global institutions that govern food – in particular, the World Health Organization, the World Trade Organization and the World Food Program – and that determine whose voices are heard, and the frames that underpin understandings of the best solutions for food insecurity and malnutrition. They argue that creating more coherent global food policy will require engaging with the politics of trade, creating alternative visions for how competing policy agendas can be managed, and renegotiating global governance structures in order to protect those affected by malnutrition.

Taken together, the chapters in this section of the *Handbook* describe the various ways in which the field of global health has been shaped by the political economy of patents, trade, and unequal access. They point to the need to address many of the most deeply rooted features of the contemporary global capitalist system if we are to address the most pressing barriers to greater health equity. Most importantly, they recognise that without confronting political economic interests and the commodification of health created by current intellectual property and trade regimes, the possibility of achieving health as a global public good will remain little more than an aspirational goal.

Part VII of the *Handbook*, *Humanitarian emergencies and global health politics*, focuses on political strategies to provide aid during natural disasters, armed conflict, and other situations that result in mass migration – all of which represent among the most important global health responses in contemporary history. Humanitarian responses have rallied support and contestation from a variety of stakeholders, including faith-based organisations and multilateral coalitions. This section explores how the politics of humanitarian responses are framed globally and how relief efforts affect broader political agendas.

In the first chapter of Part VII, 'Forced migration and health: problems and responses', Eduardo Faerstein and Anete Trajman present a broad overview of the scale of forced migration as a humanitarian crisis requiring a political solution. The chapter explores drivers of mass migration, including climate change, highlighting the heightened health problems faced by forced migrants, depending on the stage and circumstances of migration. In refugee camps, overcrowding poses the danger of transmission of infectious diseases such as hepatitis, infectious diarrhoea, tuberculosis, and other oral-faecal and respiratory infection outbreaks, in addition to food insecurity and infant-maternal health-related problems. Once settled in cities, forced migrant workers often have poor health associated with employment in low-skill and insecure jobs, with long working hours. Mental health problems, particularly post-traumatic stress syndrome, are very prevalent in both settings. The chapter argues that global governance on this growing problem is needed, but also points out that the current international political climate precludes optimistic predictions about the fate of forced migrants in the near future. In the second chapter in this section, 'Geopolitics, political violence, and global health: ethical obligations for professionals acting within wars and conflict settings', Cindy Sousa explores the health consequences of political violence, which further weakens vulnerable public health infrastructure. This chapter contends that political violence creates conditions that are favourable to the neoliberal agenda, particularly the priorities of privatisation and increased dependence on outside 'expert' assistance. Humanitarian global health efforts may be complicit with and may benefit from the destabilised state to insert the private sector, to support 'disaster capitalism'. Sousa examines the relationships between political violence, neoliberalism, and global public health. She calls for a need to support sovereignty and public health infrastructure in conflict and post-conflict settings by emphasising advocacy, collective self-determination, and social justice.

The third chapter in this section, 'Sovereignty, development, and health: humanitarianism and health care provision in the Gaza Strip' by Ron Smith describes the political challenges to organising and offering health services in regions affected by conflict and war. The chapter discusses the complex politics of humanitarianism and the effects of neoliberal economic policy on humanitarian aid provision, which complicate efforts to provide care for the most vulnerable. Much of the frustration with humanitarian aid revolves around questions of agency and control of aid budgets and donor priorities. Smith examines the impacts of health care provision in sites where sovereignty is denied. Using the Gaza Strip as a case study with references to Iraq, Yemen and other sites of under- and de-development, he explores the impossibility of creating comprehensive, effective systems of care and prevention in societies where sovereignty and the right to life are denied.

The political complexities of understanding and addressing the mental health consequences of humanitarian emergencies are explored in the fourth chapter in Part VII, 'Drone operators, terrorists, and the biopolitics of public health in the War on Terror' by Neil Krishan Aggarwal. This chapter presents a critical discourse analysis of mental health scholarship in the War on Terror that constructs drone operators and terrorists as new targets of intervention. It reviews the work of theorists who have criticised public health for prioritising national security interests over the treatment of individuals. These theories are extended to articles in psychiatry and psychology identifying drone operators and terrorists, termed 'violent extremists', as recipients of public health interventions. Even though drone operators kill violent extremists by piloting unstaffed, weaponised aircraft, mental health scholarship represents drone operators as victims and extremists as victimisers. The chapter examines how psychiatric knowledge and practices construct new definitions of normal and abnormal behaviour and how public health acts as a technology of biopolitical population surveillance.

The final section of the *Handbook*, Part VIII, *Human rights, social justice, and global health*, lays out a range of ethical frameworks for international development, for global health politics, and for understanding human dignity and justice on the global scale. This section includes chapters that identify and describe the globalisation of ideologies (e.g., gender equality, sexual rights, and geopolitics of sexuality; democratic political ideology and meaningful community-engagement; sovereignty and genomic justice) that define fundamental human rights and global social justice. These discourses have gained strong recognition in global health governance through the World Health Organization and the United Nations. Chapters in this section describe the development of these ethical frameworks and focus on political decisions weighing public health and human rights.

In the first chapter of this section, 'The invisible reality of "chintar rog" (a life of chronic worry): the illness of poverty in Dhaka's urban slum settlements', Sabina Faiz Rashid provides an ethnographic account of social suffering shaped by social and political processes. Rashid explores the biomedical 'disease' model that dominates much of public health theory and practice is missing the important connection people make between their bodies and their everyday life worlds. In many parts of the world, health is experienced and embodied in the emotional, mental, spiritual, physical, social, and political-economic worlds people inhabit. Chintar rog ('worry illness') as expressed by the impoverished living in Dhaka slum settlements, humanises the medical domain by paying attention to people, not just disease-specific worlds to which human beings peripherally belong. For residents, life is one of exhausting and relentless uncertainty, unstable jobs, insecurity and crime, difficult living conditions, fragile relationships and networks. Chintar rog speaks of their endless pain, worry, and suffering.

As the human rights framework links structural inequities and health, it also emphasises the role of community-engagement in resolving these inequities and local conflicts that affect health. The second chapter of this section, 'Salmon, fire, and the environmental and political contexts of tribal health' by Kari Marie Norgaard and Ron Reed, presents a case study of long-term collaborations between academics and the Karuk Tribe to show how both policy and academic debates can be meaningfully reframed by including the environmental dimensions of human health. In the US, no other tribe had made such a claim that dams were giving them an artificially high rate of diabetes in a dam relicensing process. This chapter highlights how collaborative partnerships, which are essential in the politics of global health, lead to the formation of innovative policies linking environmental and human health.

In the third chapter of this section, 'Research and sex work: how neo-colonialism and biomedicalisation impact struggles for sex workers' rights', Laura Murray, Elsa Oliveira, and Debolina Dutta identify large gaps between what activists are demanding, what research is finding, and the types of policies made regulating sex work. They map the production of knowledge about 'sex work', 'sex workers' or 'prostitution' in articles published between 2006–2016. They found that the majority of academic research is funded and led by authors in the global North, and that research on sex work-related policies is primarily about countries in the global North, while research on sex work in relation to HIV and AIDS is overwhelmingly about global South contexts. The chapter problematises the disparities within these articles, taking a critical perspective of the power imbalances that crosscut these various fields of research and their possible implications in relation to the human rights of sex works.

The final chapter of this section, 'In pursuit of genomic justice: sovereignty, inclusion, and innovation in Mexico' by Emily E. Vasquez and Vivette García-Deister, extends this conversation even further to describe the links between genomic justice and broader struggles for justice in the domains of health and development, arguing that investments in this field would fortify national sovereignty in Mexico, promote inclusive anti-racist science, and transform care. The chapter describes Mexico's position as a model for how developing countries might confront the new field of genomic science and its high-tech possibilities. In Mexico, policymakers, scientific entrepreneurs, and one of Latin America's most powerful health philanthropies, the Carlos Slim Foundation, have seen in genomic science the potential to improve public health outcomes and reduce health care costs. To better understand the implications of mobilising this kind of high-cost technoscience as a justice tool in the arena of global health, the authors analyse these justice claims, tracking who they empower and the assumptions they reinforce, to offer new insight into the field's stakes for both health and social progress.

The *Routledge Handbook on the Politics of Global Health* seeks to address both the emerging issues and conceptualisations of the political strategies, policy-making processes, and governance of global health, along with expanding upon and highlighting the critical priorities in this rapidly evolving field. We have organised and edited this *Handbook* with a diverse readership in mind. Fundamentally, it aims to describe and inform about the changing nature of global health politics, along with advocating for new approaches to researching and addressing population health within the global health governance system. It should therefore appeal to a wide range of people working in health, human rights, political science, social policy and development. This will include trainee health professionals (including medical and nursing students in all fields of public health); graduates and undergraduates in political science, sociology, history, economics, anthropology and psychology of health; students working in the fields of human rights and development; as well as public health practitioners, researchers, and policymakers.

Beyond these traditional audiences, our hope is that the book will appeal to activists, advocates, and practitioners around the globe who are working in the diverse fields of global civil society, emerging infectious disease control, environmental health politics, gender, sexual and reproductive health, health systems, capacity building, social work, and globalisation. Ideally this *Handbook* will stand as a key reference work in relation to the politics of global health. But we think that readers will see that it also differs from other such texts in a number of important ways. Most significantly, in a field which has often tended to reproduce many of the patterns and power relations that characterised earlier periods in the history, it brings together leading authors from across the world to reflect on past, present, and future approaches to analysing and understanding and the politics of global health – and it explicitly seeks to include Southern voices and visions as equally (if not more) important as Northern views for understanding the politics of global health and defining the key priorities and approaches that offer the greatest potential for successful development of this field.

# Part I
# Critical perspectives on global health

# 1

# Fault-lines in global health

## Intersecting inequalities, human rights, and the SDGs

*Gita Sen*

At the heart of struggles over the modern day political economy of health is the public budget. Health protection and promotion policies would have the status of the proverbial 'motherhood and apple pie', absent any concern over financial resources! Such status has, however, been missing for over three and a half decades, ever since financialised globalisation put down deep roots in national and global economies and polities. The decades between the Declaration of 'Health for All by the Year 2000' in 1978 at Alma Ata, and the enunciation in 2015 of Sustainable Development Goal 3 (SDG3) to 'Ensure healthy lives and promote well-being for all at all ages' have seen many ups and downs in the resources, environment, and institutions affecting the health of people in both the global South and North. It is not an exaggeration to say that global health has been on a roller coaster. Periods of optimism have been followed by sharp downswings and backlashes belying the fragile consensus about 'health for all', only to be followed by new panaceas.

Synergies and contradictions between three factors have impacted this health roller coaster: (i) poorly regulated financialised globalisation and the consequent explosion in global and national economic inequality; (ii) South–North disagreements and fissures about development resources, *inter alia* trade, taxation, official development assistance (ODA), investment flows; and (iii) the growing potential for human rights versus backlashes against them.

In the period since Alma Ata, the rise and rise of the neoliberal financial agenda has led to sharp increases in economic inequality (Stiglitz, 2012; Piketty, 2014; Seguino, 2014), matched by the growth of private corporate power at multiple levels, national and multinational. Pitched battles between South and North have enlivened multinational forums such as the World Trade Organization, the UN Conference on Trade and Development, and the UN Economic and Social Council's bodies. Rising public concern and knowledge about their implications for health outcomes and health policies (Benatar, et al., 2011) have been paralleled by a surge in popular mobilisation for human rights (Yamin, 2016). But such mobilisation has been countered by conservative, religion-referent organisations making common cause with a growing number of illiberal democracies (Rodrik and Mukand, 2015). This has fomented extra-judicial and state-sanctioned backlashes to the expanding potential of health and human rights for all (Corrêa, et al., 2016). It is clearly essential to locate health politics and agendas, global and national, in this larger political economy. Within this context, forces pushing for increases in health resources and budgets (aggregate and sector specific) co-exist with pressures to hold the line, if not to cut back.

The pressure for more resources is fuelled by the global epidemic of non-communicable diseases (NCDs) combined with untamed, resurgent, and new infectious diseases (Garrett, 1994; Osterholm, 2005).

Large-scale public mobilisation, such as through the People's Health Movement, has taken the primary health care agenda of Alma Ata forward to the concerns and language of universal health care (UHC), arguing for budgetary increases and expanded public services to ensure coverage and access for poor people. Intertwined, but often independent of this health movement, other social movements – of women, youth, disabled people, indigenous, LGBTQI, Dalit, ethnic/racial minorities to name only some – have come into their own, demanding access, affordability, quality, and accountability in health services as necessary to the fulfilment of their human rights (Sen, 2017).

On the other side of the debates over resources stand the forces of neoliberalism, calling for fiscal austerity, a shrinking state, and privatisation (Stuckler, et al., 2009) leading to reduced real resources for health, education, and social services generally, in both South and North (Ortiz, et al., 2015; Rowden, 2009). These forces operate in uneasy juxtaposition to the backlash against human rights, not only against basic civil and political freedoms, but also against feminist, youth, and LGBTQI demands for greater attention and resources for gender equality, and the fulfilment of sexual and reproductive health and rights.

What may these fault-lines imply for forward movement from the Millennium Development Goals (MDGs) to the Sustainable Development Goals (SDGs), in particular SDG3 on health, and towards a genuinely universal agenda of health for all people? A feminist lens provides some promise but also raises troubling questions.

## Exploding and intersecting inequalities

There is ample evidence of the increase in economic inequality during the last two to three decades of financialisation (Piketty, 2014; Stiglitz, 2012; OECD, 2008; Vázquez Pimentel, et al., 2018). What has been its impact on health? While there are some direct answers (Benatar, 1998; Navarro, 2007) to this question, pathbreaking work by Wilkinson and Pickett (2009) brought together evidence on the importance of economic inequality for health and well-being. While disparate research linking health access and outcomes to inequality in household incomes (Subramanian and Kawachi, 2004; Arcaya, et al., 2015) has existed for many contexts and different aspects of health, Wilkinson and Pickett's work argued strongly that inequality per se was more important than average levels. Economic inequality within countries belonging to a high-income cross-section appeared to have significantly greater impact on a range of health and well-being outcomes than average national per capita incomes. These national level comparisons complement evidence from within-country studies about the importance of economic differentials for specific health issues.

Multiple pathways may work separately or together to link socio-economic status inequalities to health:

- *Financial burdens*: Shrinking public resources and rising out of pocket health expenditures are known to be regressive in their impact. The growing incidence of NCDs in many countries (high-, low-, or middle-income) affects both rich and poor but exacerbates the greater real burdens on the poor and marginalised. The resulting need for longer-duration and more expensive care implies higher costs over longer time-spans which can mean higher burdens on the poor in terms of opportunity costs including foregone income, larger proportions of health to non-health expenditure in household budgets, and higher debt-burdens due to borrowing for health care.
- *Capacity to care*: An important contributor to rising economic inequality is the global increase in the share of precarious work (Standing, 2011; Vázquez Pimentel, et al., 2018) in total employment. Such jobs are not only poorly paid but also lack stability and have minimal health or other benefits. They are often under working conditions that fall below the minimal International Labour Organisation (ILO) standards for decent work. The burden of health care, in terms of both financial costs and human labour, falls disproportionately on those at the lower ends of the spectrum who have the least financial and physical capacity to provide for care. It particularly affects those responsible for unpaid caring labour within households, usually women and girls.

- *Policy voice and attention*: The higher the extent of inequality, the greater the distance separating those above from those below, and the lower the levels of empathy or solidarity across groups (Benatar, et al., 2003; Sen, 2007). The greater this separation of the powerful from those with less economic and social power, the greater the substantive disenfranchisement of the latter; and the lower the voice of the latter in policy decisions, or even in being able to draw policy attention to their concerns.
- *Public resources*: The above impacts the volume and stability of commitment of public financial resources to the health needs of those at the lower ends of the socio-economic order.

A closer examination of these pathways points to the importance of *intersecting* inequalities (Sen, et al., 2009; Krieger, 2011; Sen and Iyer, 2012; Walby, et al., 2012; van Deurzen, et al., 2014). Health is affected not only by economic inequality, but also by the ways in which economic income/wealth differentials interact with other drivers of social inequality such as gender, ethnicity, caste, race, disability, sexual orientation, and gender identity or expression, to name some. The rapidly growing literature on such intersections makes it clear that it is insufficient to focus on the impact of economic inequality alone as did earlier work on social determinants of health. In fact, such a narrow focus can both exclude and distort the effects of other drivers of inequality, masking the true impacts of social (as opposed to economic) inequality. Attention to horizontal inequality, as the inequality across social groups has been called, has grown but much of it still does not tackle intersectionality, per se.

What health policies need to account for better is the challenge posed by what may be called 'deep poverty' (Sen and Iyer, forthcoming). When economic poverty is intertwined with other social drivers (such as those mentioned earlier), this can make its impacts more obdurate and resistant to change. Economic poverty is not randomly distributed across a population, but inheres in groups distinguished by social, geographic, physical, or other characteristics (Sen, 1997; Sen, et al., 2009). Recent work by UN Women (2018) builds on these ideas, referring to this as the phenomenon of 'clustering'. The economically impoverished are often female, disabled, indigenous, Dalit, members of religious or ethnic minorities, non-heterosexual, and so on.

In addition, members of socially oppressed or marginalised groups may have specific health concerns or needs that affect them regardless of income level. For instance, even if access to income may provide some cushioning for some, trans or lesbian women may fear violence in a homophobic society. All people with disability may face stigma, and Dalits, indigenous people, or racial/ethnic minorities may be excluded from access to health services or oppressed in health facilities.

Overall it can be argued that the explosion of global inequality in recent decades has very likely had deleterious effects on health. Its impacts on the health of specific sub-groups such as children may have been somewhat ameliorated by targeted programmes. But continuing weakness in health system capacities, the sharp increase in the prevalence of NCDs, growing reliance on the unpaid care work of women within households that are increasingly reliant on precarious incomes, and non-recognition of the health needs of vulnerable groups and geographies mean that the pathways of voice and choice may continue to deepen the grooves of exclusion and marginalisation.

This context of growing inequality makes the volume and stability of public resources an important predictor of future trajectories. Global debates and agendas have played a key role in this.

## South versus North

The target of 0.7 per cent for the ratio of ODA to Gross National Income (GNI) was adopted by the OECD/DAC countries (except for the US and Switzerland) in the early 1970s, following on the report of the Pearson Commission on International Development, and the need estimates worked out by the Nobel winning economist, Jan Tinbergen. Some donors, mainly from Nordic countries, were able over the next decade to actually meet this target or to make significant progress towards it, amplifying thereby the resources available for development assistance, including for health and other aspects of human development. The climate for development resources in the 1970s was largely an expansive one, with the World Bank following the ILO's lead in prioritising basic needs, anchoring its lending policies on 'redistribution with growth'. It provided the larger platform for the Alma Ata Declaration of 'health for all' in 1978, and for an emerging global policy response to the rising social movements of this decade. While these movements were largely led by feminists demanding gender equality and minorities calling for racial/ethnic justice, other groupings emerged and grew in the following decades.

By the early 1980s, this climate had changed drastically. A sharp turn towards fiscal austerity and shrinking national budgets was integral to the so-called Reagan–Thatcher revolution, marking the rise to policy dominance of the forces of neoliberal globalisation and financialisation. The impacts on health outcomes and budgets of the ensuing decades of hard and then more moderated structural adjustment programmes have been well documented. While the World Bank did increase its resources for the social sectors in the 1990s, together with the IMF it continued its pressure on government spending, and in support of increased reliance on the private sector.

Needless to say, the Alma Ata goal of health for all did not make much progress in such a climate. Selective primary care replaced the goal of full primary health care, which was overshadowed in time by specific concerns such as child, infant, and maternal mortality rates, the growth of the HIV pandemic, shortages in human and financial resources, and the weakening of health system capacities.

Globally, the 1980s and 1990s witnessed the emergence of sharp clashes over resources and policy autonomy between high- and low- to middle-income countries under the auspices of the UN, as real ODA stagnated, and national spending was brought under fiscal austerity programmes. The World Trade Organization (WTO), which came into existence in 1995, became the principal multilateral site for trade regulation, negotiation of trade agreements, and enforceable dispute resolution. The WTO has been criticised for becoming the third leg of the global neoliberal framework (along with the IMF and the World Bank), for being less than transparent, and for serving the North's interests. At the same time, thanks to strong mobilisation by HIV/AIDS activists and Southern governments, it is the site of both the Agreement on Trade-Related Aspects of Intellectual Property Rights (TRIPs) and later the Doha Declaration on the TRIPS Agreement and Public Health, with flexibilities to protect public health and provide access to medicines for all.

Sadly, this advance is an exception, and the fault-line between South and North has never been adequately bridged (Petchesky, 2003), even though the following years saw shifts in position through the rise of important low-income countries to middle-income status, and the creation of the G20, the BRICS (i.e., the growing regional role of Brazil, Russia, India, China, and South Africa), and the meteoric rise of China to the position of the world's second largest economy.

The South versus North fault-line carried through into the formulation of the MDGs. The actual goals, targets, and indicators of the MDGs belied the soaring aims of the Millennium Declaration. They have been critiqued as having been written in the UN's basement by a group of international bureaucrats, heavily influenced by OECD/DAC pressure and ideas (Fukuda-Parr and Hulme, 2009). Partly as a reaction to this, the processes for the discussion and finalisation of the SDGs (including their targets and indicators) were much more open, inclusive, and drawn out. As a result, the implications for health are more robust. They not only affirm a life-cycle concern for all ages, but also go beyond traditional maternal and infant/child deaths to include NCDs, substance abuse, road traffic accidents, pollution, sexual and reproductive health services, and universal health coverage (financial risk protection, access to quality essential health care services, and essential medicines and vaccines). They recognise the Framework Convention on Tobacco Control, and the Doha Declaration on the TRIPS Agreement and access to medicines.

Despite these undoubted achievements, the question of financial resources for the implementation of the SDGs remains contested and inadequately addressed. It is a continuing source of deep tensions between South and North. While the agreed ODA commitment of 0.7 per cent of GNI has remained largely unmet by Northern governments, tax havens and illicit financial flows have grown in numbers and volume (Palan, 2009). By around 2010, it was estimated by the Bank of International Settlements that around half of all international banking assets and liabilities were routed through offshore financial centres, and one-third of all multinational corporations' Foreign Direct Investment (FDI) goes through tax havens (Sen, 2017).

Against this backdrop, and the pressure on resources due to a limping economic recovery after the financial crisis of 2008, the third UN International Conference on Financing for Development, held in Addis Ababa in July 2015, was viewed as the space where the financing mechanisms and volumes for the SDGs would be worked out. Held in the middle of the SDGs process, the conference was the site of great South versus North tension (DAWN, 2015). The South's attempt to promote an independent global tax body, which would close loopholes that allow tax avoidance, illicit financial flows, and the bleeding of resources from vulnerable South countries, failed. Fairer and more transparent global and national tax systems can mobilise more than enough resources for the SDGs, but this was opposed by powerful countries that themselves promote and serve as tax havens.

Of equal concern as the financing issue is the status of human rights in the implementation of the SDGs. As a whole, the SDGs (including SDG3) are weak on explicit affirmation of human rights, with only ad hoc references in a few targets and indicators across the 17 goals. They avoid, thereby, the legally binding nature of accountability that is intrinsic to human rights conventions and standards (Sen, 2017; McInerney-Lankford, 2017). Despite this, it is important to note that the SDGs go much farther than the MDGs in drawing on the broad framework of international human rights and their specific conventions and agreements.

## Human rights and its discontents

Social mobilising by the excluded and oppressed has been a force in bringing concerns for human rights to the centre of health debates from the 1970s on. This has arguably been most powerful in the context of HIV-linked advocacy by gay activists and of feminist mobilisation for sexual and reproductive health and rights (SRHR). The discussion in this section focuses on the latter.

Major UN conferences of the 1990s in Vienna (1993), Cairo (1994), and Beijing (1995) saw feminist mobilisation on a significant scale (Corrêa, et al., 2016). The feminist movement was able to grow and mature into a powerful global force through the strength of its commitment to the cause of gender equality and women's human rights. Important advances with significant implications for health and human rights were made, including the official recognition in Vienna of women's rights as human rights, and of violence against women as a violation of those rights; the paradigm change of Cairo that shifted population-related policy towards SRHR; and a broad consensus in Beijing on advancing gender equality, women's empowerment, and human rights across 12 broad areas.

It is worth emphasising that much of this mobilisation was happening in the face of surging neoliberal agendas, including weakening multilateralism, as detailed earlier. Continuing crises shaped resources and policies. The ability of the national state to respond to feminist demands was eroding in both the South and the North, as its institutions fragmented under the neoliberal onslaught. The challenge of growing global inequality, the deepening chasm between South and North, and diminished national policy space meant that the implementation of the agreements reached in the 1990s conferences was always going to be a challenge.

But worse was to come. The spill-over effects of a rising tide of global conservatism and religious fundamentalism in many parts of the world fuelled the growing strength of conservative forces in UN spaces, opposing gender equality and women's human rights in the name of culture, tradition, and religion. Many UN spaces witnessed this, becoming increasingly and bitterly contested between feminists and forces attempting to turn back the clock on the achievements of the conferences of the 1990s in terms of gender equality and women's human rights. Increasingly, and especially during the SDGs processes and the parallel 20th year reviews of Cairo and Beijing, a growing number of national governments in the South were being pressured by US evangelical forces. Together with the rising group of 'illiberal' democracies, they joined in this backlash. This added a further twist to South versus North battles, one that had been successfully overcome by feminists before through the creation of strong cross-regional negotiating groups in support of SRHR and gender equality. This approach became more and more challenging to implement in the fraught environment of UN negotiations.

It did not help that feminist, youth, LGBTQI, and other groups still tended to be outside mainstream advocacy for universal health coverage. They were largely viewed as separate silos during the long months of SDG negotiations during 2013 to 2015. The final crafting of SDG3 on health uses careful language on 'health for all at all ages' which is inclusive, but it is certainly not explicit about the needs of the most oppressed. There is no wording on human rights at all in relation to health, barring the bitterly contested reference to reproductive rights in target 5.6 of SDG5 on gender equality.

## Which way forward?

Progressive health movements have at times been slow to recognise that political distance between movements for universal health coverage on the one side, and those for the health and human rights of social groups with distinct health concerns on the other, has tended to weaken both sides. Some of this distance may be due to differences in backgrounds and epistemic communities. Those who support a broad right to health through UHC are more likely to come from biomedical backgrounds, while those mobilising for the rights of socially oppressed groups such as women or indigenous people are over-whelmingly from those groups themselves, and likely to have social science credentials. Differences in backgrounds, histories, languages, and experiences feed lack of understanding and poor communication, despite attempts to bridge the gaps.

It has made it difficult to confront either the rigors of fiscal austerity or the backlashes against human rights in a sustained way. Clearly, more systematic attempts need to be made to incorporate human rights and intersectionality into UHC discussions and agendas. This has to take the form of not simply a narrow, sanitised, or siloed engagement with issues, but the inclusion of both sets of activists in each other's gatherings and debates. Bringing in and engaging with the lived experiences of people is the best and often the only way to build empathy and solidarity.

When it comes to financial resources for health, the neoliberal approach is to push towards privatisation – the private sector, public–private partnerships, and private foundations. What is downplayed is the possibility of reducing drug costs and out of pocket expenditures through active use of the WTO's TRIPs flexibilities, the tackling of tax havens and illicit flows in order to improve national budgets and policy space, and strengthening public sector provisioning of health services to become a robust competitor to well-regulated private providers.

A common front between UHC and human rights activists across a diverse, intersectional, and plural spectrum can strengthen support for increased public resources for health, better access to services, stronger financial protection, and consistent fulfilment of the human rights and health needs of all, including of the most oppressed.

## References

Arcaya, M.C., Arcaya, A.L., and Subramanian, S.V. (2015) 'Inequalities in health: definitions, concepts, and theories', *Global Health Action*, 8: 27106.

Benatar, S.R. (1998) 'Global disparities in health and human rights', *American Journal of Public Health*, 88(2): 295–300.

Benatar, S.R., Daar, A.S., and Singer, P.A. (2003) 'Global health ethics: a rationale for mutual caring', *International Affairs*, 79(1): 107–38.

Benatar, S.R., Gill, S., and Bakker, I. (2011) 'Global health and the global economic crisis' *American Journal of Public Health*, 101(4): 646–53.

Corrêa, S., Germain, A., and Sen, G. (2016) 'Feminist mobilizing for global commitments to the sexual and reproductive health and rights of women and girls', In: E. Chesler and T. McGovern (Eds.) *Women and Girls Rising: Progress and resistance around the world*, London and New York: Routledge, pp. 51–68.

DAWN. (2015) 'DAWN informs: special issue on FfD3', available at http://dawnnet.org/publication/dawn-informs-august-2015/ (accessed on 8 April 2018).

Fukuda-Parr, S. and Hulme, D. (2009) 'International norm dynamics and "the end of poverty": understanding the Millennium Development Goals (MDGs)', BWPI Working Paper 96, University of Manchester.

Garrett, L. (1994) *The Coming Plague: Newly emerging diseases in a world out of balance*, New York: Farrar, Strauss and Giroux.

Krieger, N. (2011) *Epidemiology and the People's Health: Theory and context*, New York: Oxford University Press.

McInerney-Lankford, S. (2017) 'Human rights and the SDGs: progress or a missed opportunity?', OxHRH Blog, available at http://ohrh.law.ox.ac.uk/human-rights-and-the-sdgs-progress-or-a-missed-opportunity/ (accessed on 8 April 2018).

Navarro, V. (2007) *Neoliberalism, Globalization and Inequalities: Consequences for health and quality of life*, Amityville, NY: Baywood.

OECD. (2008) *Growing Unequal: Income distribution and poverty in OECD countries*, Paris: OECD.

Ortiz, I., Cummins, M., Capaldo, J., and Karunanethy, K. (2015) 'The decade of adjustment: a review of austerity trends 2010-2010 in 187 countries', ESS Working Paper No. 53, Geneva: ILO, Columbia University and South Centre.

Osterholm, M.T. (2005) 'Preparing for the next pandemic', *New England Journal of Medicine*, 352(18): 1839–42.

Palan, R. (2009) 'The history of tax havens', available at www.historyandpolicy.org/policy-papers/papers/history-of-tax-havens (accessed on 8 April 2018).

Petchesky, R. (2003) *Global Prescription: Gendering health and human rights*, London: Zed Books.

Piketty, T. (2014) *Capital in the 21st Century*, Cambridge: Harvard University Press.

Rodrik, D. and Mukand, S. (2015) 'The puzzle of liberal democracy' Project Syndicate, available at www.project-syndicate.org/commentary/liberal-regimes-democracy-puzzle-by-dani-rodrik-and-sharun-mukand-2015-05 (accessed on 8 April 2018).

Rowden, R. (2009) *The Deadly Ideas of Neoliberalism: How the IMF has undermined public health and the fight against AIDS*, London: Zed Books.

Seguino, S. (2014) 'Financialization, distribution and inequality', In: G. Sen and M. Durano (Eds.) *The Remaking of Social Contracts: Feminists in a fierce new world*, London: Zed Books, pp. 33–48.

Sen, G. (1997) 'Empowerment as an approach to poverty', in *Human Development Papers 1997 – Poverty and Human Development*, New York: UNDP.

Sen, G. (2007) 'The role of solidarity in institutions of governance', In: B. Hettne (Ed.) *Studies in Development, Security and Culture, Volume II: Human values and global governance*, Basingstoke: Palgrave Macmillan, pp. 177–87.

Sen, G. (2017) 'The SDGs and feminist movement building', background paper for UN Women (2018) *Turning Promises Into Action: Gender equality in the 2030 agenda for sustainable development*, New York: UN Women.

Sen, G. and Iyer, A. (2012) 'Who gains, who loses, and how: leveraging gender and class intersections to secure health entitlements', *Social Science and Medicine*, 74(11): 1802–11.

Sen, G. and Iyer, A. (forthcoming) 'Why is intersectionality important for health policy in LMIC contexts?' In: O. Hankivsky and J. Jordan-Zachery (Eds.) *Palgrave Handbook on Intersectionality and Public Policy*, Palgrave MacMillan.

Sen, G., Iyer, A., and Mukherjee, C. (2009) 'A methodology to analyse the intersections of social inequalities in health', *Journal of Human Development and Capabilities*, 10(3): 397–415.

Standing, G. (2011) *The Precariat: The new dangerous class*, London: Bloomsbury.

Stiglitz, J.E. (2012) *The Price of Inequality*, London: Allen Lane/Penguin.

Stuckler, D., King, L., and McKee, M. (2009) 'Mass privatisation and the post-communist mortality crisis: a cross-national analysis', *The Lancet*, 373(9661): 399–407.

Subramanian, S.V. and Kawachi, I. (2004) 'Income inequality and health: what have we learned so far?' *Epidemiologic Reviews*, 26(1): 78–91.

UN Women. (2018) *Turning Promises Into Action: Gender equality in the 2030 agenda for sustainable development*, New York: UN Women.

van Deurzen, I., van Oorschot, W., and van Ingen, E. (2014) 'The link between inequality and population health in low and middle income countries: policy myth or social reality?', *PLoS ONE*, 9(12): e115109.

Vázquez Pimentel, D.A., Aymar, I. M., and Lawson, M. (2018) *Reward Work, Not Wealth*, Oxford: OXFAM GB.

Walby, S., Armstrong, J., and Strid, S. (2012) 'Intersectionality: multiple inequalities in social theory', *Sociology*, 46(2): 224–40.

Wilkinson, R. and Pickett, K. (2009) *The Spirit Level: Why more equal societies almost always do better*, London: Allen Lane.

Yamin, A. (2016) *Power, Suffering and the Struggle for Dignity: Human rights frameworks for health and why they matter*, Philadelphia: University of Pennsylvania Press.

# 2

# The right to health under capitalism
## Threats, confrontations, and possibilities

*César Abadía-Barrero and Adriana Ardila-Sierra*

The widespread knowledge of atrocities committed during the Second World War, specifically the violations of human rights in territories controlled by the Nazis, elevated human rights as the most important moral idea concerning social justice, with significant discursive roles and practical implications (Beitz, 2009; Moyn, 2010). The aftermath of the war also saw the reconfiguration of the world economy and the emergence of the United States as the world's foremost economic and military power. In this chapter, we establish a dialogue between critical political economy and critical human rights scholarship to show how, since they were first recognised, human rights have been challenged and transformed by the profit needs of the capitalist system. We will argue that market and popular demands for justice are repeatedly co-produced (Abadía-Barrero, 2015; Iriart, et al., 2011) and that pushing forward an *emancipatory* human rights agenda entails a confrontation with core capitalist interests.

Following Charles Beitz (2009), we propose to engage with the human right to health from two interrelated perspectives:

- The '*right to medical care*', entailing access to quality biomedical health services. It includes the four key measures for assessing the compliance of health care systems with the human right to health included in the general comment No 14 of the United Nations Committee on Economic, Social and Cultural Rights (2000): Availability, Accessibility, Acceptability, and Quality.
- The '*right to be healthy*', which is contingent on favourable social, economic, and political conditions. It includes states' three types of obligations: Respect, Protect, and Fulfil, included in the same general comment.

We will demonstrate that confrontations in the nineteenth and twentieth centuries between a social and an individual/biological understanding of health moved the international health agenda towards the pre-eminence of the right to medical care over the right to be healthy. Furthermore, we will show how the individual/biological understanding of health facilitated the expansion of for-profit health industries, and more recently of the health insurance sector. The result is a constant increase in health care costs to the point that the right to health is being reduced to a minimal package of 'essential' services covered by insurance. We argue that the attack on the comprehensive and decommodified understanding of the right to health is another contradiction of the capitalist system. Although the system requires the social reproduction of classes for its continued existence, which means that individuals must have access to health care

services and populations must flourish, the drive for accumulation threatens the viability of social reproduction (Fraser, 2016).

At stake, then, is the tension between human rights and capitalism, characterised by threats, confrontations,
and possibilities.

## Threats

The Declaration of Alma Ata (1978) was perhaps the broadest official recognition of the right to health. It
called for urgent and effective national and international action to support Primary Health Care (PHC)
(Beitz, 2009; Chapman, 2011; Yamin, 1996). Besides promoting high levels of community participation in
the planning and operation of PHC, it assumed that community-based care was the first level of integrated,
progressive, comprehensive, and universal health care systems. Alma Ata's bottom-up proposal for PHC
intended more than anything to transform the power dynamics that affect health priorities, by empowering
communities and neutralising the primacy of technology-driven medical interventions. With its call to
improve living conditions, Alma Ata reaffirmed the importance of coordinated actions by social, political,
and economic sectors in promoting health and well-being. Hence, disease prevention and health promotion became cornerstone elements of PHC (Breilh, 2007).

While Alma Ata has been seen as a starting point for the history of PHC (Yamin, 1996), it was in fact
the culmination of larger historical debates between proponents of a social understanding of the right to
be healthy and an individualistic understanding of the right to medical care. Representative landmarks of
those historical debates included:

- The triumph of Pasteur's microbiology over Virchow's social medicine at the end of the nineteenth
century, which signalled an important shift in intellectual hegemony regarding health and medicine
(Waitzkin, 2011). Advocates of microbiology, disease control programmes, and pharmaceuticals, infused
with an imperialist perspective and a developmentalist morality, heavily influenced international debates
around tropical medicine and international health, which culminated in the creation of the WHO (Birn
and Fee, 2013; Cueto and Palmer, 2015). As a consequence, the Social Medicine perspective, which
conceived of ill health as resulting from social deprivation and poor living conditions, was relegated to
a secondary status (Allende, 2005; Waitzkin, et al., 2001).
- After the Bretton Woods Conference (the 1944 United Nations Monetary and Financial Conference
that regulated the international monetary system and set a system of fixed exchange rates centred on the
US dollar and gold) the mixing of liberal economics and human rights became evident in the language
used to promote the agreements that were reached at the conference: 'international development', 'economic stability', 'prosperity', and 'international peace'. The US delegation convinced other participating
countries that the common good could be achieved only in the context of free trade, international loans
to underdeveloped countries,[1] and the protection of Intellectual Property (IP), which included medical
products, among other things (Waitzkin, 2011).
- After the Second World War, the world powers were not very enthusiastic about an international human
rights agreement (Wolff, 2012), and the ground-breaking 1948 declaration on human rights was only
agreed upon after much debate in a post-war context characterised by the reconfiguration of political, military, and economic power. While civil and political rights were widely ratified for immediate
implementation, social, economic and cultural rights faced more resistance, especially from the US
(Wolff, 2012).
- Since it was first drafted in 1954, the International Covenant on Economic, Social and Cultural Rights
extended the right to health 'to the enjoyment of the highest attainable standard of physical and mental
health'. This meant that the conception of health as a human right implied ensuring that the population lived in conditions of well-being. In the context of the Covenant, political stability and economic

development came to be considered preconditions for the right to health, which was inseparable from the fulfilment of other civil, political, economic, social, and cultural rights (Yamin, 2016, pp. 53–64).

- The welfare state, applied with some variations in Europe and then extended precariously to the rest of the world, became a hegemonic project to compensate for the destructive moments of the accumulation of capital by guaranteeing workers social security protections and benefits (Fraser, 2016; Smith, 2011). Improvements in living standards and increased access to health-related services seemed to reflect a harmonious relationship between capitalist development and health as a human right. The maintenance of this model, however, was threatened by the international expansion of capitalist dynamics (Harvey, 2005).
- In the mid-twentieth century, authoritarian 'stable democracies' and dictatorial regimes backed by the US government targeted key defenders of social medicine, leading to Ramón Carrillo's exile from Argentina to Brazil, Ernesto Guevara's murder in Bolivia and Salvador Allende's death on the day of the military coup in Chile (Cárdenas, 2010; Klein, 2007).

Later, representatives of Alma Ata signatories described most of the population as continuing to live in precarious conditions where health networks never reached them. The proposals agreed upon at Alma Ata, including a focus on PHC and 'health for all by the year 2000', were actively resisted by representatives of imperialism. While US policymakers promoted market-based programmes, large philanthropic organisations, most prominent among them the Rockefeller Foundation, sponsored a 'selective primary health care' (SPHC) approach that reduced PHC to targeted short-term health programmes, obfuscating the idea of a comprehensive right to health comprising both access to medical care and the right to be healthy (Birn and Fee, 2013; Palmer, 1998).

The SPHC was supported by governments dominated by US interests through economic and political ties (Birn, et al., 2016, p. 739). In addition, US imperial prerogatives 'facilitated the return of earlier neoclassical economic models' that de-emphasised state protection (Birn, et al., 2016, p. 739; Smith-Nonini, 2010).

The twentieth century was characterised by intense ideological conflicts as described earlier, and the right to health suffered conceptual, political, and practical delimitations that transformed the human rights framework from the right to be healthy to a reduced notion of access to forms of medical care deemed to be cost-effective. In addition, as we will explain in the next section, specific inter-capitalist disputes between the medical industrial complex and financial sectors at the end of the century further commodified the population's right to health care. This commodification depended on different countries' political struggles and each individual's capacity to purchase services.

## Confrontations

The medical-industrial complex (MIC) includes the industries that exert outsized influence over policy making to assure an ever-expanding market for their products. One example of policies affected by the MIC is patent protection. After Bretton Woods, pharmaceutical and biotechnology products became subject to patent protection laws, and the right to health implied an expansion of MIC power and profits (Dumit, 2012; Waitzkin, 2011).

The medical-financial complex (MFC) refers to groups that base their business model on private insurance against human misfortune. When financial groups that administered individual insurance plans in the US became interested in expanding their business globally, they helped to shape international financial institutions' structural adjustment policies (SAP) to pressure countries into shifting their health and welfare policies from public and social to individual and private (Basilico, et al., 2013; Gershman and Irwing, 2000). This required the dismantling and privatisation of pension and health care systems, initially in Latin America and then rapidly across the globe (Armada, et al., 2001; Stocker, et al., 1999). These neoliberal adjustments aggressively confronted global aspirations for consolidating the right to health (Chapman, 2016).

In keeping with their profit-driven priorities, health insurers 'realize more profits by cutting access to services and treatments, especially the more costly ones' (Iriart, et al., 2011, p. 2). For this reason, they undertook cost control by 'using administrative procedures to limit physicians' prescriptions and referrals' (Iriart, et al., 2011, p. 2). Nonetheless, the pharmaceutical industry – the most powerful sector of the MIC – began a 'silent reform' in order to reposition itself within the ever-expanding health markets (Iriart, et al., 2011). Silent reforms meant faster approval and expedited marketing of patented products and altered clinical parameters to increase the number of 'sick' people or to create new 'pathologies', thereby increasing demand for their products (Dumit, 2012; Iriart, et al., 2011; Iriart and Merhy, 2017). These silent reforms were enthusiastically promoted by providers and hospital networks, leading to increased billing, allowing insurance companies to renegotiate the prices of their policies.

As health care costs keep rising, the profits of financial, industrial, and professional sectors increase. Iriart and Merhy (2017) explain that what we are witnessing is a new inter-capitalist alliance between the medical industrial complex and the financial sectors in the health industry, thus conforming a medical-industrial-financial complex (MIFC). As a consequence, countries can continue increasing their spending on health in order to show their commitment to the 'right to health', but the majority of resources will serve only to increase the profits of the MIFC.

The 2015 United Nations Sustainable Development Goals (SDG) transformed the framework of the debate from Universal Health *Care* (UH*Care*) to Universal Health *Coverage* (UH*Coverage*). This change was the latest expression of the capitalist interests that sustain the MIFC. Indeed, UH*Care* proposes unified, solidarity-oriented, single-tiered systems in which comprehensive and universal benefits are paid out of a collective pool. Perhaps more importantly, UH*Care* is based on PHC/Social Medicine/Community Participation principles, which, as we have seen, threaten MIFC profits. UH*Coverage*, in contrast, posits coverage as the individual's capacity to pay an administrator to manage his or her insurance plan, in a context where market competition, supposedly, promotes quality and controls costs (Birn, et al., 2016; Iriart and Merhy, 2017; Titelman and Uthoff, 2005).

UH*Coverage* shifts the conversation to how well or poorly private insurance markets 'cover' the population and keep health costs down. In addition, the technical elements of affordability are presented as each individual's capacity to purchase health insurance. Hence, individual health plan contracts are unequal, depending on the purchasing power of different people, companies and countries. However, the large majority of people in the global South as well as the poor in the global North are unable to afford policies at the prices imposed by the MIFC. As a result, current 'global health' debates promoted by the World Bank revolve around state subsidies for a reduced 'right to health' package, which implies defining a supposedly adequate clinical package that offers only the 'essential' or 'vital' medicines and interventions that people and countries can afford, based on anti-democratic assessments of cost-effectiveness (Birn, et al., 2016, p. 746). As the experiences of Mexico and Colombia illustrate, the intention behind UH*Coverage* is to defund and privatise public health systems and transfer public resources and private family wealth to the MIFC (Abadía-Barrero, 2015; Laurell, 2015). The right to health of poor population sectors is cynically invoked by promoters of neoliberal health reform as a moral imperative reflecting the importance of dismantling public approaches so as to cover the poor, who had previously been excluded from insurance (Abadía-Barrero, 2015; Londoño and Frenk, 1997). In its contemporary version, the language of human rights has been further co-opted by SDGs' UH*Coverage* proposal (Birn, et al., 2016).

What we are starting to witness with the UH*Coverage* agenda is the consolidation of MIFC hegemony over global health. As this agenda advances, several consequences come to light:

• Because they are considered financial risks for insurance companies, women, the sick, and the elderly are charged more for their plans and used as examples to legitimate increases in the overall cost of the system.

- Uncovered or insufficiently covered populations are forced to take on debt, and people and societies with 'comprehensive' insurance coverage are forced to increase the proportion of their resources allocated to 'health care'.
- As steadily rising health care costs increase MIFC profits, societies are compelled to discuss how best to restrict access to medical technology, reducing the scope of the right to health care.
- Defending comprehensive coverage to advance the right to health means having to advocate for several technological 'innovations' produced by the MIC's silent reforms, though their benefits to health are unproven. In fact, not only do different health care products and protocols lack impartial scientific support, but many have proven to be harmful (Dumit, 2012).
- Sequential speculative practices involving relations between the MIC and the MFC create vicious cycles that increase the cost of care to the point that ever more diseases become catastrophic in terms of risk coverage.
- Focalised governmental subsidies and philanthro-capitalism allow the poorest sectors access only to minimal health coverage at the rates they can afford, which nonetheless allows the MIFC to profit from even these sectors of the population.

As we see, a shift to neoliberal policies is further dismantling social welfare in the name of health justice and the right to health, thereby transferring resources from the state and from private income and wealth to the fictitious or speculative capital of the MIFC, commodifying the right to health.

## Possibilities

Human rights discourse has been critiqued as instrumental to the needs of those who prioritise capital accumulation. In the stories we have presented thus far, we can see this instrumentality: the human right to health has been invoked to advance a commercial understanding of health. The principle of progressiveness in the realisation of human rights, congruent with the resources available (a process called priority setting), can also be critiqued as reflecting a human rights analysis subsumed by the logic of capital. Nonetheless, several experiences illustrate the possibility of confronting capitalist interests and favouring human rights at the local, national, and global levels.

The establishment of the WHO Commission on the Social Determinants of Health (CSDH), and its 2008 report, are considered landmarks in repositioning critical discussions of global health. The way that the report shifted the technical and practical discussions around health and political discussions around how to achieve health justice are important to discussions of human rights within the context of capitalism. The WHO report was critiqued, however, for missing an opportunity to incorporate a human rights framework into the strategies for accomplishing its intended objective of reducing health inequalities (Chapman, 2011). Furthermore, the CSDH report borrowed,

> [T]he principles of empowerment and participation from human rights without incorporating the conceptual foundation of a human rights approach or offering a compelling alternative rationale. What results is an uncomfortable hybrid in which advocacy of community empowerment is grafted onto a report that focuses primarily on top-down initiatives through changes in government policy. This results in a weak conception of empowerment.
>
> *Chapman, 2011, p. 142*

If the WHO had previously been accused of partnering with leading financial institutions in pushing forward a neoliberal agenda for health policy (Armada, et al., 2001; Navarro, 2004), the CSDH report was criticised for depoliticising the understanding of power, given its lack of a critical understanding of the social, political, and economic context over the past 30 years. The limited use of the concept of power, both a central piece of human rights debates and of critical understanding of the capitalist system, prevented the commission from clearly identifying the underlying causes of health inequalities in the world. Vicente Navarro critiques the report's conclusions by saying that it is not inequalities that kill people, 'it is those who are responsible for these inequalities that kill people' (Navarro, 2009, p. 423). By 'those who are responsible', Navarro means members of the new class alliance between elite groups in developed and developing nations that promoted neoliberal ideology and remained unmentioned in the report.

Meanwhile, a global network of activists and organisations was working hard to build upon a productive dialogue between advocates of the human right to health and its agenda for equity, and the transformative agenda of social medicine, to put 'primary health care back on the agenda of development organizations and multilateral institutions' (Chapman, 2011, p. 146). This network, the People's Health Movement, launched a global Right to Health and Healthcare Campaign in 2005 to:

> [U]nite the efforts of activists subscribing to a human rights approach at the local, national and international levels to promote equitable access to quality health services. The global campaign consists of three phases: (1) grassroots organizations carrying out rights-based assessments of national health policies; (2) participants in the national assessments being linked in global mobilization around the right to health; and (3) mobilization for the implementation of plans for universal recognition of the right to health and legitimating of the actions to respect, to protect and to fulfil it.
>
> *Turiano and Smith, 2008, cited in Chapman, 2011, p. 146*

Other experiences illustrating how human rights language has been effectively leveraged in confronting capitalist interests exemplify interesting possibilities for articulating a critical human rights agenda with other emancipatory and anti-capitalist social justice struggles:

- In the 1990s, the Brazilian state partnered with a coalition of HIV civil society organisations and managed to alter the World Trade Organization's patent-protection laws, arguing its need to protect the right of Brazilian citizens to access anti-retroviral medications (Galvão, 2002). Human rights language and access to generic or significantly less expensive medications indeed transformed the lives of many Brazilians, at the same time reducing HIV-related stigma and discrimination (Abadía Barrero, 2011). Other 'cutting-edge human rights arguments against hegemonic interpretations of IP are offered by Oxfam, Doctors Without Borders and others, though Amnesty, Human Rights Watch, and even some committees of the UN system have also issued statements endorsing counter hegemonic visions' (Godoy, 2013, p. 39).
- In other cases, PHC/Social Medicine proposals have been part of social and political platforms that have proposed larger structural and anti-capitalist reforms. During the 1980s in El Salvador, for example, community health workers managed to provide health care through popular clinics. As members of the communities where they worked, these health workers were deeply trusted. Interestingly, El Salvador's 'popular health' was part of a broader effort to break free from the legacies of colonialism and imperialism. Unfortunately, a 1992 peace agreement came hand in hand with neoliberal policies disrupting the work of popular clinics. Nonetheless, physicians mobilised popular support and advocated for the Human Right to Health. Eventually, privatisation efforts led by the World Bank were reversed (Smith-Nonini, 2010).
- The legacy of social medicine in Latin America is experiencing a new revival with an interesting and promising integration of PHC, harmonious relationships with nature, and anti-capitalist human rights agendas. Here we are witnessing a historical update of the main thesis of the Social Medicine tradition, which is that the right to health is more dependent on social conditions than on medical interventions (Tajer, 2003; Waitzkin, 2011).

Proposals for social medicine are not necessarily antagonistic to expanding health care services and improving access to necessary medical care, as demonstrated through the experience of the Chilean national health service during the presidency of Salvador Allende (Tedeschi, et al., 2003, p. 2015), in Ramón Carrillo's 1947 proposals for Argentina (Cueto and Palmer, 2015, p. 138), and in policies and programmes proposed by Dr Ernesto (Che) Guevara to expand medical care after the 1959 Cuban revolution. If these proposals and policies were antagonistic to alternatives, those alternatives were the commodification of medical care and for-profit initiatives advanced in the name of the right to health.

## Conclusions

In this chapter, we have presented a historical understanding of human rights discourse as one of the means by which the capitalist system implicitly threatens and challenges the possibilities for building an emancipatory agenda. We illustrated how a comprehensive understanding of the right to be healthy (derived from Social Medicine and PHC traditions) has been actively opposed by a reduced and commodified approach entailing a right to medical care. With current proposals such as UH*Coverage* intended to further commodify health, the comprehensive right to health is increasingly compromised with a co-optation of human rights discourse. We summarised a longer process within which military, economic, and ideological violence has been used in an attempt to silence proposals for a right to health that challenge MIFC hegemony. The economic, political, and social changes needed to guarantee people's right to be healthy are increasingly disregarded, and profit-making mechanisms are promoted as the only reasonable approach to accomplish a commodified version of the right to health.

Despite the danger of co-optation, several communities and social groups have found that the legal and practical frameworks for human rights serve them well in their revolutionary struggles for social justice and emancipation. Importantly, scholars of human rights have joined forces with other critical scholars in pointing out the problems presented by a commodified version of the human right to health (Chapman, 2016). To remain aligned with bottom-up and critical approaches that can effectively transform the underlying social determinants of health, however, advocates for human rights as an academic and political strategy need to protect themselves from efforts by the MIFC to co-opt and misappropriate human rights discourse. One strategy could be to integrate the human rights agenda with other emancipatory proposals and incorporate other important conceptual elements. In this chapter, we have highlighted two such elements: 1) The need to advocate for PHC and universal health care as strategies to promote the right to be healthy, and 2) The need to denounce MIFC profits as the most important underlying determinant impeding people's right to medical care. In short, one of the ways in which a human rights approach can shield itself from the destructive influence of capital is by assuming a clear anti-capitalist agenda.

Advancing an *emancipatory* health as a human rights agenda will require an understanding of how capitalist forces shape social realities around the world, constituting the underlying determinant of human rights. Furthermore, advocates of this agenda must propose a historicised understanding of the right to health as the right to medical care and the right to be healthy, which has evolved within the logic of the capitalist system. We have argued that this agenda would benefit from establishing fruitful and committed discussions with critical political economy and collaboration with other anti-capitalist movements and social justice struggles.

## Note

1   When the US increased interest rates to combat inflation in 1979, Latin America's foreign debt more than doubled to US$327 billion in three years. By the early 1980s, a full-blown 'debt crisis' had materialised, with massive transfers of very large sums of money to international banks as debt repayment (Birn et al., 2016; and Graeber, 2014).

## References

Abadía Barrero, C.E. (2011) *I Have AIDS but I am Happy: Children's subjectivities, AIDS, and social responses in Brazil*, Bogotá: Universidad Nacional de Colombia.

Abadía-Barrero, C.E. (2015) 'Neoliberal justice and the transformation of the moral: the privatization of the right to health care in Colombia', *Medical Anthropology Quarterly*, 30(1): 62–79.

Allende, S. (2005) 'Medical and social reality in Chile', *International Journal of Epidemiology*, 34(4): 732–36.

Armada, F., Muntaner, C., and Navarro, V. (2001) 'Health and social security reforms in Latin America: the convergence of the World Health Organization, the World Bank and transnational corporations', *International Journal of Health Services*, 31: 729–68.

Basilico, M., Wigel, J., Motgi, A., Bor, J., and Keshavjee, S. (2013) 'Health for all?: competing theories and geopolitics', In: P. Farmer, J.Y. Kim, A. Kleinman, and M. Basilico (Eds.) *Reimagining Global Health: An introduction*, Berkeley and Los Angeles: University of California Press, pp. 74–110.

Beitz, C.R. (2009) *The Idea of Human Rights*, Oxford and New York: Oxford University Press.

Birn, A.E. and Fee, E. (2013) 'The art of medicine: the Rockefeller Foundation and the international health agenda', *The Lancet*, 381(9878): 1618–19.

Birn, A.E., Nervi, L., and Siqueira, E. (2016) 'Neoliberalism redux: the global health policy agenda and the politics of cooptation in Latin America and beyond', *Development and Change*, 47(4): 734–59.

Breilh, J. (2007) 'Pour une épidémiologie responsable'. In *La Santé pour tous! Se réapproprier Alma Ata*. Ginebra: Cetim, pp. 179–93.

Cárdenas, S. (2010). *Human Rights in Latin America: A politics of terror and hope*, Philadelphia: University of Pennsylvania Press.

Chapman, A.R. (2011) 'Missed opportunities: the human rights gap in the Report of the Commission on Social Determinants of Health', *Journal of Human Rights*, 10(2): 132–50.

Chapman, A.R. (2016) *Global Health, Human Rights and the Challenge of Neoliberal Policies*, Cambridge and New York: Cambridge University Press.

Cueto, M. and Palmer, S.P. (2015) *Medicine and Public Health in Latin America: A history*, New York: Cambridge University Press.

Dumit, J. (2012) *Drugs for Life: How pharmaceutical companies define our health*, Durham and London: Duke University Press.

Fraser, N. (2016) 'Contradictions of capital and care', *New Left Review*, 100(July–Aug): 99–117.

Galvão, J. (2002) 'Brazilian policy for the distribution and production of antiretroviral drugs: a privilege or a right?' *Cadernos de Saúde Publica*, 18: 213–19.

Gershman, J. and Irwing, A. (2000) 'Getting a grip on the global economy', In J.Y. Kim, J.V. Millen, A. Irwin, and J. Gershman (Eds.) *Dying for Growth: Global inequality and the health of the poor*, Monroe (Maine): Common Courage Press, pp. 11–43.

Godoy, A.S. (2013). Of Medicines and Markets: Intellectual property and human rights in the free trade era. Stanford, CA: Stanford University Press.

Graeber, D. (2014) *Debt: The first 5,000 years*, Brooklyn: Melville House.

Harvey, D. (2005) *A Brief History of Neoliberalism*, Oxford: Oxford University Press.

Iriart, C., Franco, T., and Merhy, E.E. (2011) 'The creation of the health consumer: challenges on health sector regulation after managed care era', *Globalization and Health*, 7: https://doi.org/10.1186/1744-8603-7-2.

Iriart, C. and Merhy, E.E. (2017). 'Disputas inter-capitalistas, biomedicalización y modelo médico hegemónico', *Interface – Comunicação, Saúde, Educação*, (ahead), 0–0. https://doi.org/10.1590/1807-57622016.0808

Klein, N. (2007) *The Shock Doctrine: The rise of disaster capitalism*, New York: Picador.

Laurell, A.C. (2015) 'The Mexican popular health insurance: myths and realities', *International Journal of Health Services*, 45(1): 105–25.

Londoño, J.L. and Frenk, J. (1997) 'Structured pluralism: towards an innovative model for health system reform in Latin America', *Health Policy*, 41: 1–36.

Moyn, S. (2010) *The Last Utopia: Human rights in history*, Cambridge, MA: Belknap Press of Harvard University Press.

Navarro, V. (2004) 'The world situation and the WHO', *The Lancet*, 363: 1321–23.

Navarro, V. (2009) 'What we mean by social determinants of health', *International Journal of Health Services*, 39(3): 423–41.

Palmer, S. (1998) 'Central American encounters with Rockefeller public health, 1914–1921', In: G. Joseph, C. Legrand, and R. Salvatore (Eds.) *Close Encounters of Empire: Writing the cultural history of U.S.-Latin American relations*, Durham, NC: Duke University Press, pp. 311–32.

Smith, G.A. (2011) 'Selective hegemony and beyond populations with "no productive function": a framework for enquiry', *Identities-Global Studies in Culture and Power*, 18: 2–38.

Smith-Nonini, S.C. (2010) *Healing the Body Politic: El Salvador's popular struggle for health rights – from civil war to neoliberal peace*, New Brunswick, NJ: Rutgers University Press.

Stocker, K., Waitzkin, H., and Iriart, C. (1999) 'The exportation of managed care to Latin America', *New England Journal of Medicine*, 340: 1131–36.

Tajer, D. (2003) 'Latin American social medicine: roots, development during the 1990s, and current challenges', *American Journal of Public Health*, 93(12): 2023–27.

Tedeschi, S.K., Brown, T., and Fee, E. (2003) 'Considerations on human capital', *American Journal of Public Health*, 93(12): 2012–15.

Titelman, D. and Uthoff, A. (2005) 'The role of insurance in social protection in Latin America', *International Social Security Review*, 58(2–3): 43–69.

Waitzkin, H. (2011) *Medicine and Public Health at the End of Empire*, Boulder, CO: Paradigm Publishers.

Waitzkin, H., Iriart, C., Estrada, A., and Lamadrid, S. (2001) 'Social medicine then and now: lessons from Latin America', *American Journal of Public Health*, 91: 1592–601.

Wolff, J. (2012) *The Human Right to Health*, New York: W.W. Norton and Co.

Yamin, A.E. (1996) 'Defining questions: situating issues of power in the formulation of a right to health under international law', *Human Rights Quarterly*, 18: 398–438.

Yamin, A.E. (2016) *Power, Suffering, and the Struggle for Dignity: Human rights frameworks for health and why they matter*, Philadelphia, Pennsylvania: University of Pennsylvania Press.

# 3

# South African AIDS activism

## Lessons for high-impact global health advocacy

*Mandisa Mbali*

Transnational AIDS activists have referred to the 'Durban effect', which occurred at and immediately following the 2000 International AIDS Conference held in the South African city. This was a moment where the first international march for HIV treatment was held. It was also one where AIDS activists demanding universal access to antiretrovirals (ARVs) from the global South and North met for the first time. The period was also singular in that several clinical and social science researchers started to support the civil society advocates in their call. In relation to these events, it can be noted that South African AIDS activists in the Treatment Action Campaign (TAC) were absolutely pivotal in catalysing this phenomenon: one which was a clear case of Africans (with their allies abroad) democratising knowledge to push for the internationally powerful to be morally and politically accountable for global health injustice.

Given the relative effectiveness of such transnational HIV treatment activism, it is hardly surprising that it is often cited by global health scholars and practitioners as an example to be emulated in relation to increasing access to medicines for other epidemic diseases such as Hepatitis C (HCV) and Tuberculosis (TB) in developing countries (Heydari, et al., 2015; Stop TB Partnership and UN Office for Project Services, 2015). Beyond common issues of relatively limited access to medicines to treat these conditions, these three examples are not merely socio-economically, and culturally, disparate: people living with HIV, or vulnerable to acquiring the infection, are often afflicted by either/both HCV and TB.

The socio-economic and political factors rendering people vulnerable to HIV infection also determine risk of contracting HCV: a noteworthy number of people who inject drugs and men who have sex with men living with HIV are also at high risk for HCV. People who live with TB or HCV face similar levels of societal stigma as people living with HIV, and frequently also lack access to the latest, and most effective, medicines. In this context, it can be asserted that the transnational AIDS activism of the Durban moment, and its aftermath, remain relevant to the politics of global health today.

The history of transnational activism recounted in this chapter remains relevant at the time of writing; a time where fiscal austerity, 'donor fatigue', and excessive drug pricing remain barriers to universal access to HIV prevention and treatment around the world. This chapter makes the case that transnational civil society mobilisation is still required to address neoliberalism's exacerbation of health inequalities in relation to AIDS. In a deeper sense, such activism is still required to tackle global health injustices related to the global AIDS pandemic. The chapter begins with a discussion of the South African movement's critical contribution of moral legitimacy to the transnational HIV treatment access movement in its early years. It contends that domestically generated components thereof – the TAC's success in popularising and defending the science behind HIV treatment; its effective socio-economic rights litigation and its use of 'struggle symbolism' – were critical in bolstering its legitimacy both in South Africa and internationally. Then the bulk of the chapter describes the early global achievements of the TAC and its allies: i.e., increased funding to fight global AIDS and for intellectual property (IP) arrangements enabling access to cheaper generic medicines. Finally, it ends with a brief description of ongoing AIDS activist campaigns in relation to these two facets of neoliberalism listed previously.

## The TAC's use of rhetoric, symbols, and rights-based arguments[1]

In order to understand the TAC as a *South African* social movement, we need to recognise that its emergence was highly relevant and noteworthy in the South African context of President Thabo Mbeki's AIDS denialism, a set of discourses influenced by the history of racism and its intersection with essentialised African sexuality. The TAC combatted this denialism by using human rights-focused, anti-apartheid-derived, and scientifically accessible framings of the disease.

From the mid-1990s, there was an international revolution in HIV medicine in relation to the prevention and treatment of HIV infection: the effective use of antiretrovirals, or ARVs, for prevention of mother-to-child transmission (PMTCT) and for the chronic treatment of HIV. South African AIDS activists responded to these developments by beginning to campaign for Zidovudine (AZT) for PMTCT; they only later shifted to arguing for universal access to ARVs for chronic use.

In relation to the former president's AIDS denialism we can note that he believed the scientific consensus concerning AIDS was racist and this related to his reassertion of African nationalism as part of his vision of generating an 'African Renaissance'. More specifically, Mbeki made a steady succession of strange remarks around AIDS, with a dramatic crescendo during his July 2000 address at Durban International AIDS Conference (Mbeki, 2000). Most controversial was his failure in this address to explicitly mention HIV as the cause of both AIDS, as a syndrome, and the local and global epidemics of the disease. The government's lack of political will to introduce ARVs for PMTCT into the public sector of the health system cannot be understood in the absence of Mbeki's AIDS denialist views.

The then minister of health eventually decided to introduce Nevirapine for PMTCT to a limited number of 'pilot' sites, but it was not enough for the activists. On 21 August 2001, the TAC launched a constitutional challenge to the government's policy of limiting PMTCT to the pilot sites in the Pretoria High Court. They asked the court to determine the policy unconstitutional and that the government be ordered to make the drug available to all pregnant women living with HIV who went into labour at public health facilities. The TAC's resort to this constitutional litigation in South Africa must be viewed against the backdrop of the failure of efforts to secure the policy change through other means, such as meeting with the two ministers of health and obtaining relevant media coverage.

In early July 2002, the Constitutional Court ordered the national and provincial governments to remove restrictions to Nevirapine being prescribed outside pilot sites and to permit and facilitate its use where medically indicated, by developing a comprehensive and coordinated plan for its provision. This judgement hinged around the right to access to health care services in South Africa's Constitution.

The TAC's use of a 'right to health' line of legal argument in this case and the 'Pharma v. Mandela' case discussed later was a turning-point in the history of South African AIDS activism. Prior AIDS-related human rights litigation focused on defending the right to privacy. South Africa's new constitution and the medical breakthrough of combination ARV therapy catalysed a change in the role activists saw for the state in designing and implementing AIDS policy. I want to argue here that they drew on a thick definition of freedom (Mbali, 2013).

Previously, activists had drawn upon a classical liberal conception of the state's human rights obligations in relation to people living with HIV, emphasising what Isaiah Berlin termed 'negative' freedom – freedom from unwelcome governmental intrusion into their privacy (2002). In the post-apartheid period, activists were now also supportive of state intervention in drug pricing and the development of ARV rollout policies to enable it to provide medicines to all of its citizens. By making their case through constitutionally enshrined socio-economic rights, they were asserting a new vision for South African AIDS activism which was grounded in what Sen has termed 'substantive freedom', or society-wide poverty reduction (1999).

In the international system, socio-economic rights, including the right to health, were (and are) enshrined in the International Convention on Economic, Social and Cultural Rights and that the Committee on Economic, Social and Cultural Rights which aimed (and aims) to ensure compliance with this treaty. Countries which had ratified the treaty (including South Africa in later period) had to submit regular reports to the UN Committee on Economic, Social and Cultural Rights (CESCR). But the Committee could only make *recommendations* to relevant governments on ways in which they could improve their work to progressively realise the right to health. In this context, activism was one of the only accountability mechanisms to ensure reasonable progress towards global health justice.

In relation to the TAC's 'treatment literacy' programme, what we can note is that it was vital in generating public support for the litigation, and the TAC more generally (Robins, 2008; Geffen, 2010; Mbali, 2013; Hodes, 2014). As part of this programme, activists gave several talks and workshops and media interviews, many of which were in African languages and which used locally intelligible metaphors and explanations for things such as what HIV was, how PMTCT occurred, and the mechanisms through which ARVs could reduce MTCT. In a context where most South African public schools did not teach about ARVs, these workshops generated public support for an otherwise poorly understood intervention.

In terms of the TAC's marshalling of anti-apartheid symbolism, Nelson Mandela's critical support for the movement in this period also facilitated the TAC's efforts at social mobilisation around the issue. In late June 2002, the former president very publicly visited and offered his support to the movement's leader, Zackie Achmat, who was living with AIDS and whose illness was exacerbated by his 'drug fast', in his Muizenburg home. In December of that year, he also visited the TAC/MSF's Khayelitsha-based ARV pilot site set-up to demonstrate that combination ARV drug therapy was possible in 'resource-poor' settings in South Africa. Mandela famously put on one of the movement's characteristic HIV-POSITIVE t-shirts, which was a gift given to him by Matthew Damane, the first patient at the clinic. The MSF/TAC pilot site was extremely important in convincing both international and national policymakers that universal provision of ARVs was feasible.

The next edition of these t-shirts with Mandela's image on the back were worn by activists who participated in the movement's second civil disobedience campaign in January 2003 – the image of one of the leaders of the Defiance campaign in the 1950s was being invoked to support a new civil disobedience campaign for ARV drug access. Shortly after this campaign the government developed an operational plan for the roll-out of ARVs. The TAC, however, went on to face numerous struggles in the second five years of its history to push the government to optimally implement this roll-out plan.

It can be noted that the AIDS policies of the Zuma administration were extremely different in relation to those of the Mbeki government, most notably in their not being informed by AIDS denialism, consisting of a much more concerted drive for an ARV roll-out and novel proposals to address inequality in the distribution of resources within the health system – the National Health Insurance (NHI) scheme (Mbali, 2016).

## The TAC and the transnational HIV treatment access movement[2]

This transnational movement successfully demanded an increase in foreign aid for HIV treatment in developing countries and international measures to widen access to cheaper generic drugs and limit the harm caused by inflexible free trade agreements promoted by the multinational pharmaceutical companies. In its discussion of the TAC's – and its international allies' – influence on global health diplomacy and governance, this section of the chapter describes their campaigns around the need for increased foreign aid to fund ARVs.

Donor states and intergovernmental health organisations were, generally, against ARV provision in developing countries in the late 1990s and early 2000s. This was on the grounds that they did not deem them to be 'cost-effective'. In a different vein, USAID-chief Andrew Natsios made racist remarks before the International Relations Committee of the US House of Representatives on AIDS in Africa; here he claimed that Africans supposed failure to understand 'Western time' was a barrier to their ability to adhere to ARV treatment (US Congress Proceedings and Debates, 2001).

Donor agencies of governments such as those of Norway and the UK frequently made sweeping generalisations about the limited capacity of health systems on the African continent to roll-out ARVs. Instead, there was a focus on individuals' responsibilities to change their sexual behaviour, which often excluded a substantial analysis of the impact of structural factors such as gender inequality in the growth of the HIV epidemic. Similarly, while the UNAIDS epidemic updates in the period under discussion were relatively exhaustive on the demographic and economic impacts of AIDS in sub-Saharan Africa, they omitted to suggest that these could be ameliorated by universal access to HIV treatment or to highlight the pharmaceutical industry's role in constraining access. The World Bank – a constituent part of UNAIDS – barely discussed the issue of the provision of ARVs in Africa in its AIDS policy documents, a measure which was, again, presented as unaffordable in contrast with primary prevention, which was viewed as having been more cost-effective.

On 9 October 2002, the TAC held protests at US consulates in Johannesburg and Durban calling for substantial increases in American foreign aid for the Global Fund. In the same period, Health Global Access Project (Health GAP) – one of the TAC's American allies – began to call for the creation of a US 'Presidential AIDS Initiative', which they envisaged would provide dramatically increased levels of foreign aid to combat global AIDS. Late November 2002 saw the American activists demonstrate in front of the White House. Thirty-one of them chained themselves together for a die-in, and they were subsequently arrested.

Outside of the public eye and inside the White House, critical conversations on these issues were also taking place. African and American HIV specialists were meeting with representatives of the Bush administration to develop a detailed plan for steep increases in American foreign aid for global AIDS. The resultant President's Emergency Plan for AIDS Relief (PEPFAR) dramatically scaled-up the number of people living with the disease who were taking combination ARV therapy in African and Caribbean countries. While pressure for the plan had also emerged from influential Evangelical figures such as Franklin Graham, the public pressure generated by the AIDS activists in Durban and DC played a consequential role in this turn of events (Messac, 2011; Mbali, 2013).

In relation to the TAC's advocacy on drug pricing, it can be noted that TAC intervened in important ways in a high-profile court case between the government and several high-profile multinational pharmaceutical companies. The court case which has been called Pharma v. Mandela challenged a 1997 bill which President Mandela signed into law: the Medicines and Related Substances Ammendment Act (hereafter, the Medicines Act). Section 15c of the Medicines Act enabled parallel importation and compulsory licensing (Heywood, 2001). Compulsory licensing can be defined as involving a government forcing a patent-holder to allow another entity (either the state or a private company) to use its patent. In many cases, the patent-holding company will be paid a royalty which is either negotiated with, or legislatively enforced by, the state. The generic competition it facilitates is an effective way to enable a reduction in the prices of medicines. Parallel importation entails a government capitalising on the fact that pharmaceutical companies often charge diverse prices for patented drugs in different countries. A government which has parallel-imported a brand name drug has bought it in another country where it is cheaper.

In February 1998, the Pharmaceutical Manufacturers' Association of South Africa (or PMA), which represented 40 major multinational corporations, obtained an urgent high court interdict which prevented the 1997 Medicines Act from becoming the law. This industry association tried to argue that Section 15c of the Medicines Act was unconstitutional. The TAC decided to apply for leave to intervene as an *amicus curiae* in the PMA's court case in January 2001, after being informed of the dates of the hearing. It argued that measures in the act dealing with parallel importation, generic substitution, and the establishment of a pricing committee were both 'necessary and justifiable' given the need for HIV medicines in the context of South Africa's epidemic (Heywood, 2001, p. 12).

The TAC argued that none of the clauses were unconstitutional, and that they were instead necessitated by the government's positive duty to 'progressively realize' the rights to access to health care services and to protect rights such as those to dignity, life, equality, and the duty to act in the best interests of the child (Heywood, 2001, p. 12). It also argued that the poor were directly dependent upon the state's ability to progressively realise these rights. TAC activists also drew attention to the fact that under South African constitutional law the state could limit certain rights (such as that to private property) as long as the infringements were 'reasonable and justifiable in an open and democratic society based on human dignity, equality and freedom' (Heywood, 2001, p. 13).

In a deeper sense, the TAC was contending that in some instances corporate persons' legal rights to IP could be limited in order to progressively realise individuals' human rights to dignity and access to health care. Ronen Shamir has offered the analysis that,

> [t]he ultimate purpose of the [TAC's] brief ... was to re-frame the dispute as a 'right to health' case and, within this context, to establish a direct link between South Africa's AIDS crisis and the high cost of drugs incurred on the needy due to the pharmaceutical industry's economic leverage.
>
> *Shamir, 2005, p. 46*

In its papers, the TAC also contended that the industry's research and development costs for several AIDS drugs had already been recouped and that in any event some of them, such as Pfizer and Glaxo, had failed to provide these costs to the TAC (Mbali, 2013). James Love from the Consumer Project on Technology's supporting affidavit was critical in undermining the industry association's case that high revenues were required to finance innovation. Love alleged that the industry had overstated its research and development costs and downplayed the extent to which the American government had co-financed such costs.

The PMA's opposition to the TAC's amicus application partly rested on the grounds that whether or not medicines were cheap or expensive was irrelevant to the main application. It also argued that the TAC's amicus application had not mentioned the state's role in addressing the AIDS epidemic. Deeb complained to *The Guardian* that 'This law is arbitrary and gives the health minister too many powers ... There is a lack of due process. The minister can make a decision that a drug is too expensive and the drug companies have no right to defend themselves' (McGreal, 2001, n.p.). Ayanda Ntsaluba, the South African Director-General of Health, replied that even with steep price reductions the government could not afford to buy many brand-name drugs.

On 6 March, Judge President Bernard Ngoepe ruled in the TAC's favour: it was admitted as an amicus for the duration of the case. This meant that even though the TAC was not a party in the case, they could submit arguments to the court in relation to it. The case was then adjourned to 18 April, when the pharmaceutical industry eventually settled with the South African government.

One crucial development almost certainly influenced by the media-glare caused by the case was that the WTO published its Doha Declaration on the Trade-Related Aspects of Intellectual Property Rights (TRIPS) Agreement and public health on 14 November 2001. The Declaration clarified 'flexibilities' under the TRIPS Agreement: member states now had the right to obtain compulsory licences in the event of a self-defined national health emergency, such as those related to HIV/AIDS, TB, and malaria (World Trade Organization, 2001).

As described in Chapter 31 by Vieira and Di Giano and Chapter 24 by Cueto in this volume, Brazil, a middle-income country, whose leaders had adequate political will and which had the industrial capacity to manufacture generic HIV medicines, capitalised on this clarification of TRIPS to gain leverage in negotiations with pharmaceutical companies (Nunn, 2009). Unlike its middle-income counterpart Brazil, South Africa tragically failed to take advantage of these even clearer TRIPS flexibilities to produce ARVs because of its government's AIDS denialist policies.

Trade policy and legal scholar Ellen 't Hoen has framed the Doha Declaration as having 'signalled a sea change in thinking about patents and medicines' and having been at 'the root of a cascade of activities aimed at reformulating IP [intellectual property] protection as a social policy tool for the benefit of society as a whole' (2009, p. xvi). In the post-Doha period, between 2001 and 2007, 52 developing and less-developed countries issued compulsory licences to produce generics, took advantage of government-use provisions or did not enforce pharmaceutical patents ('t Hoen, 2009, p. xvi).

## Lessons for contemporary global AIDS activism

At the time of writing this chapter, transnational health activists continue to demand new, and more just, approaches to global health diplomacy and governance and they could certainly derive lessons from the first few joint campaigns of the TAC and transnational HIV treatment access movements. There are two ongoing areas of focus for TAC and its allies' global advocacy: the issue of global AIDS funding and the issue of IP-related barriers to a widening of access to HIV treatment (including that for TB).

It has become common for intergovernmental organisations and scientists to refer to an 'end to AIDS' (Economist, 2011; Lancet Editor, 2015; UNAIDS, 2014). There is, however, a real risk that the accomplishment of an admirable and conceivable future goal could be seen by key actors to be closer than it actually is. This rhetorical and conceptual slippage could – intentionally or otherwise – create the impression among politicians and general publics that the ongoing AIDS pandemic is already consigned to the past-tense. Policymakers, donors, scientists, and activists' energy and attention could be dissipated and expended elsewhere, when AIDS remains a global public health crisis (see, also, Chapter 25, by Kenworthy, Thomann and Parker, in this volume).

Some global health scholars have critiqued what they view being 'AIDS exceptionalism', which asserts that too much global health funding is allocated to the disease (Denny and Emanuel, 2008; England, 2008). Critics have framed this as consisting of a misperception, owing to the ongoing new HIV infections and AIDS-related morbidity and mortality, especially in heavily affected populations and countries, such as South Africa (El-Sadr, et al., 2011; Nattrass and Gonsalves, 2010; Smith and Whiteside, 2010). They have also pointed to the ways in which HIV treatment provision can, and should, be part of effective primary health care services (Yu, et al., 2008). Differently put, in addressing other diseases of global inequality, there is merit in drawing on, and learning from, the successes of AIDS activism and global and national health programmes generated due to its effectiveness; not to pitting patients with different diseases of inequality against each other.

AIDS remains a major global health issue, citing the UNAIDS 2016 global AIDS update, we can note that it is estimated that:

- Since 2003 when the first global treatment target was developed there has been a 43 per cent reduction in AIDS deaths, internationally (2016, p. 1).
- In 2015 there were 2.1 million new infections worldwide and 36.7 million people living with HIV/AIDS, of whom only 17 million were on AIDS treatment (2016, p. 1). Fifty-four per cent of people living with HIV globally lacked access to treatment, many of whom did not know their HIV status (2016, p. 11).

UNAIDS has set the 90-90-90 target for 2020, that is that 90 per cent of all people should know their HIV status, 90 per cent of HIV-positive people should be able to access treatment and 90 per cent of these people should have suppressed viral loads (2016, p. 5). To reach this target, they have called for increased investment and innovation, internationally.

The foreign aid issue remains a key focus for transnational AIDS advocacy: during the first few months of the Trump administration in the US, in March 2017, AIDS activists expressed fears that there would be swingeing cuts to both domestic and foreign aid budgets to address the disease. In the US, TAC ally, Health GAP, condemned what they referred to as 'status quo austerity budgeting' in relation to early Trump-era budget proposals on foreign aid to address the pandemic (2017). At issue is the need for additional yearly US contributions to PEPFAR and the Global Fund to meet the UNAIDS 90-90-90 target. Health GAP has called for an extra US$2 billion to prevent avoidable AIDS deaths (2017). While neither PEPFAR nor the Global Fund eventually received funding cuts in Trump's budget blueprint, the American AIDS activists have remained unsatisfied with consistently flat US funding to address the global pandemic (AIDSpan, 2017). In addition, at the time of writing in November 2017, funding cuts to PEPFAR had, once more, been proposed by Trump and rejected by activists (Devex, 2017).

As we have seen, the TAC and its international allies successfully campaigned for a reduction in the prices of ARV drugs. High drug prices remain a significant barrier to access to HIV treatment in developing countries. Amy Kapczynski has demonstrated the persistent issue of long and inflexible patents as a key underlying driver of inflated drug prices (2009). Since the early 2000s, academics and student activists at US universities such as Yale have highlighted their universities' roles in ensuring affordable access to medicines in developing countries. It is frequently the case that US universities licence drugs they have developed to multinational pharmaceutical and biotechnology ('biotech') companies who most often fail to take steps to ensure access to affordable generic drugs in developing countries. This movement is called Universities Allied for Essential Medicine (UAEM) and now has branches in Europe, Canada, Brazil, and South Africa (UAEM, 2017).

In relation to universities' roles in determining pharmaceutical pricing, we can also note that they play a large role in drug development, the laboratory-based early stages of which are largely funded by the US taxpayers via the National Institutes of Health (NIH), which disburses a total of nearly US$32.3 billion in research money per annum, 80 per cent of which goes to researchers based at 2,500 universities, medical schools, and research institutes in the US and globally (NIH, 2017). UAEM has argued that the NIH has the mandate to force universities to ensure that drug prices are reasonable in developing countries (Basey, 2017). UAEM has advocated that the NIH require universities to only licence their essential drugs to pharmaceutical or biotech companies on the condition that they allow more affordable generic medicines or biosimilars to be produced.

In the TAC's campaigning on drug pricing, they argued that long and/or inflexible types of patents inhibit generic competition, which can be linked to a reduction in the cost of medicines, especially in developing countries. The TAC, and its international allies such as MSF, has recently tried to press for reform of South Africa's IP legislation, drawing on TRIP's flexibilities and experiences from other middle-income developing countries. It is illustrative to place this campaigning in the context of TB – a common co-morbidity with HIV infection – in South Africa and many other low- and middle-income countries.

In South Africa, where TB is the leading cause of death, its incidence has declined too slowly and there are significant and growing epidemics of multi-drug resistant (MDR) and extremely drug resistant (X-DR) TB (Churchyard, et al., 2014; Department of Health, 2017). When discussing AIDS activists' increasing TB advocacy in recent years, we must note that it was far from an inevitable development. American AIDS activist Mark Harrington wrote an article in 2010 arguing that in comparison with HIV/AIDS there had been 'weak advocacy and anaemic research funding' in relation to TB (2010, p. S260).

Many extant treatment regimens for X-DR and M-DR TB are excessively long, complicated, and frequently extremely suboptimal, in terms of patient outcomes. In the case of X-DR TB, it remains very difficult to cure and is often fatal. Activists, policymakers, and physicians have, therefore, made a strong case for further research into TB treatment, especially in the instances of drug resistant strains of the virus (Stop TB Partnership and UN Office for Project Services, 2015, p. 84; MSF, 2016b, p. 2).

In this context, civil society and the government have made growing calls for a widening of access to delamanid, a promising new treatment for MDR-TB. The MSF and South African health minister Aaron Motsoaledi have argued for Otsuka, the Japanese manufacturer of delamanid, to widen access to the drug (MSF, 2016a; Motsoaledi, 2017). While the international concern and Department of Health have reached an agreement that the drug will be made available to 200 patients in four provinces, the government has still asked for Otsuka to reduce the cost of the drug to widen access to it in heavily affected developing countries such as South Africa (Motsoaledi, 2017).

Such drug donation programmes are inherently problematic from a bioethical standpoint, in relation to day-to-day questions and dilemmas they pose for physicians and public health administrators, such as:

- What are the guidelines when there aren't enough of the donated drugs?
- Which patients should receive them?
- What happens when they run out?
- How can a health authority plan a sustainable intervention with an uncertain drug supply?

While the company had registered the drug with the Medicines Control Council (MCC) at the time of writing, questions over the drug's pricing and patent licensing remain unresolved.

In this context, it is important to note that Fix the Patent Laws (FTPL), a coalition of NGOs including TAC and MSF, have lobbied for reforms to South Africa's patent law to incorporate the TRIPS flexibilities referred to earlier (FTPL, 2017). Activists and scholars who have called for the Department of Trade and Industry (DTI) to create more opportunities for third parties such as NGOs to oppose patents through a substantive search and examination (SSE) system similar to that of India (Vawda, et al., 2016). India's Patent Act has been used by NGOs to challenge patents at the pre- and post-grant phases of the approval process (Kapczynski, et al., 2016). The most famous legal case around these issues was Novartis's unsuccessful 2007 challenge to the rejection of a patent application in India. This was an attempt on the company's part to 'evergreen' the drug, that is, to extend the life of its patent on a frivolous basis where no evidence had been obtained that it was more effective or fundamentally different to its predecessor (for more on evergreening, see also Chapter 31, by Vieira and Di Giano, in this volume). As a result of the ruling in this case, in India, enhanced therapeutic effectiveness must be proven before a patent is granted (Kapczynski, 2009).

In comparison to India's IP policies, South Africa's depository system (where patents are granted based on 'formalities' of an application) is underdeveloped to widen access to medicines. In general, South Africa is granting patents at a higher rate when compared to other middle-income countries. What has proven frustrating for the activists is that the proposed reforms have yet to make it into law.

## Concluding remarks

South African activists' important contributions to the international HIV treatment access movement can be viewed as a result of the 'Durban effect'. Transnational AIDS activism remains central to keeping the pandemic on the agenda of global health policymakers. The transnational history of the TAC recounted in this chapter contains vital lessons for global health activists, in general.

Activists' creativity in rendering scientific knowledge into their own local idioms is central to increasing popular support for campaigns for access to new medicines and, when provided, their patient-uptake. Global health activists can also draw on the symbolism of prior transnational social movements which have had moral legitimacy and political support (as in the case of South African AIDS activists' use of anti-apartheid metaphors). Transnational AIDS activism has in its own right reached this point of being a well of moral symbols and repertoires for other global health movements.

Contemporary global health injustice is epitomised by shortages in the foreign aid required to consistently implement effective AIDS policies around the world. Patients living with, and affected by, different diseases of inequality should not be placed at a disadvantage relative to each other in terms of foreign aid allocations. HIV treatment and prevention programmes can, and have, been used to strengthen primary health care provision.

South-South and North-South activist/scholar/practitioner alliances are critical in challenging global health injustice. For example, it has been effective for South African activists (in the TAC) to form strategic alliances with human rights and IP lawyers from the global North (such as those at Yale University) and South (such as the Indian Lawyers' Collective in Mumbai) to challenge unjust IP laws and trade agreements. New ideas on legal and diplomatic means to reduce the prices of medicines can, and should, flow multi-directionally around the globe.

The socio-economic right to health is the most philosophically substantive articulation of health as freedom. Some countries, such as South Africa, have these sorts of rights enshrined in their constitutions at a national level enabling activists to effectively use litigation around them to advance health justice. Yet, international law enshrining socio-economic rights has weak accountability mechanisms, which fail to directly alter the geographies of global health disparity. A long-term challenge global health activists may well grasp, in future, would be to systematically draw attention to this flaw in global governance.

Transnational AIDS activism – as exhibited in the collaborations between the TAC and its international allies – is an example and a resource for other types of global health activism and interventions. It remains premature to phrase the present moment as characterised by the 'end of AIDS'. Instead, there is a great deal of scope for further thought, and action, on transnational AIDS activism as a conceptual, strategic, and human treasure chest to improve the health of the world's population, considered as a whole.

## Notes

1   This section of the chapter is heavily derived from chapters four and six of Mbali (2013); readers are advised to consult these for further citations in relation to the events described.
2   This section of the chapter is also derivative of material discussed in chapters five and seven of Mbali (2013); again, readers are encouraged to read these chapters for further citations in relation to the narrative of events offered.

## References

AIDSpan. (2017) 'Global Fund untouched by Trump's proposed budget cuts', available at www.aidspan.org/node/4153 (accessed on 30 July 2017).

Basey, M. (2017) 'Universities and IP: address at The Berkman Klein Center for Internet & Society, Harvard Law School', available at www.youtube.com/watch?v=UvIsyWtjfoI&t=118s (accessed on 31 July 2017).

Berlin, I. (2002) 'Two concepts of liberty', In: H. Hardy (Ed.) *Liberty*, Oxford: Oxford University Press, pp. 166–217.

Churchyard, G.J., Mametja, L.D., Mvusi, L., Ndjeka, Hesseling A.C., Reid, A., Babatunde, S., and Pillay, Y. (2014) 'Tuberculosis control in South Africa: successes, challenges and recommendations', *South African Medical Journal*, 104(3) (Suppl. 1): 244–8.

Denny, C.C. and Emanuel, E. (2008) 'US health aid beyond PEPFAR: the mother & child campaign', *Journal of the American Medical Association*, 300(17): 2048–51.

Department of Health. (2017) 'South Africa's National Strategic Plan for HIV, TB and STIs', available at www.gov.za/sites/www.gov.za/files/nsp%20hiv%20tb%20sti_a.pdf (accessed on 30 July 2017).

Devex. (2017) 'PEPFAR to "accelerate" implementation in 13 countries under new strategy', available at www.devex.com/news/pepfar-to-accelerate-implementation-in-13-countries-under-new-strategy-91064 (accessed on 20 November 2017).

Economist. (2011) 'Thirty years of a disease: the end of AIDS?', available at www.economist.com/node/18774722/ (accessed on 31 July 2017).

El-Sadr, W., Gonsalves, G., and Mugyenyi. (2011) 'No need for apologies', *JAIDS*, 57 (Suppl. 2): S68–S71.

England, R. (2008) 'The writing is on the wall for UNAIDS', *British Medical Journal*, 336: 1072.

FTPL. (2017) 'Open letter to Hon. Minister Rob Davies, re: urgent finalisation of the draft intellectual property policy', available at www.fixthepatentlaws.org/ (accessed on 29 July 2017).

Geffen, N. (2010) *Debunking Delusions: The inside story of the TAC*, Sunnyside: Jacana.

Harrington, M. (2010) 'From HIV to tuberculosis and back again: a tale of activism in 2 pandemics', *Clinical Infectious Diseases*, 50 (S3): S260–6.

Health GAP. (2017) 'Re: skinny on Trump's austerity budget', e-mail (16 March).

Heydari, S., Kembabazi, A., Monahan, C., and Ragins, K. (2015) 'Ending an epidemic: overcoming the barriers to and HCV-free future', available at www.yaleghjp.org/global-hcv (accessed on 30 July 2017).

Heywood, M. (2001) 'Debunking "conglomo-talk": a case study of the Amicus Curiae as an instrument for advocacy, investigation and mobilisation', available at www.ldd.org.za/index.php?option=com_zine&view=article&id= 179%3Adebunking-conglomotalk-a-case-study-of-the-amicus-curiae-as-an-instrum&Itemid=14 (accessed on 13 February 2012).

Hodes, R. (2014) *Broadcasting the Pandemic: A history of HIV on South African television*, Cape Town: HSRC Press.

Kapczynski, A. (2009) 'Harmonization and its discontents: a case study of TRIPS implementation in India's pharmaceutical sector', *California Law Review*, 97: 1571–651.

Kapczynski, A., Kesselheim, A.S., and Ezer, T. (2016) 'Submission to the Department of Trade and Industry on the intellectual property consultative framework', available at www.tac.org.za (accessed on 4 May 2017).

Lancet Editor. (2015) 'The end of AIDS?', available at www.thelancet.com/journals/lanhiv/article/PIIS2352-3018(15)00029-6/fulltext (accessed on 20 July 2017).

Mbali, M. (2013) *South African AIDS Activism and Global Health Politics*, Houndmills and New York: Palgrave Macmillan.

Mbali, M. (2016) 'AIDS activism and the state in post-apartheid South Africa at twenty', In: A. Pallotti and U. Engel (Eds.) *South Africa After Apartheid: Politics and challenges of the democratic transition*, Leiden: Brill.

Mbeki, T. (2000) '13th International AIDS Conference Durban, speech of the president of South Africa at the opening session of the conference', available at www.virusmyth.com/aids/news/durbspmbeki.htm (accessed on 13 February 2012).

McGreal, C. (2001) 'Dying for drugs: South Africa's sick wait for judgment day: multinationals go to court today over a law aimed at cutting the cost of medicines', The Guardian.

Messac, L. (2011) 'Lazarus at America's doorstep: elites and framing in federal appropriations for global AIDS relief', unpublished paper.

Motsoaledi, A. (2017) 'Launch of delamanid clinical access research project speech', available at www.health.gpg.gov.za/ News/Pages/LAUNCH-OF-DELAMANID-CLINICAL-ACCESS-RESEARCH-PROGRAMME-SPEECH-BY-DR-AARON-MOTSOALEDI,-MINISTER-OF-HEALTH.aspx (accessed on 29 July 2017).

MSF. (2016a) 'MSF urges Japanese pharmaceutical giant to widen access to key drug for drug-resistant TB in South Africa', available at www.msf.org.za/stories-news/press-releases/msf-urges-japanese-pharmaceutical-giant-widen-access-key-drug-drug (accessed on 30 July 2017).

MSF. (2016b) 'TB briefing paper: An overview of MSF's programmatic use and clinical research with new TB treatment regimens', available at www.msfaccess.org/content/briefing-paper-tb-overview-msf%E2%80%99s-programmatic-use-and-clinical-research-new-tb-treatment (accessed on 30 July 2017).

Nattrass, N. and Gonsalves, G. (2010) 'AIDS funds undervalued', *Science*, 300: 600.

NIH. (2017) 'What we do: Budget', available at www.nih.gov/about-nih/what-we-do/budget (accessed on 20 November 2017).

Nunn, A. (2009) *The Politics and History of AIDS Treatment in Brazil*, New York: Springer.

Robins, S.L. (2008) *From Revolution to Rights in South Africa: Social movements, NGOs and popular politics after Apartheid*, Oxford: James Currey.

Sen, A. (1999) *Development as Freedom*, Oxford: Oxford University Press.

Shamir, R. (2005) 'Corporate responsibility and the South African drug wars: outline of a new frontier for cause lawyers', In: A. Sarat and S.A Scheingold (Eds.) *The Worlds That Cause Lawyers Make: Structure and agency in legal practice*, Stanford: Stanford University Press.

Smith, J. and Whiteside, A. (2010) 'The history of AIDS exceptionalism', *Journal of the International AIDS Society*, 13(47): 1–8.

Stop TB Partnership and UN Office for Project Services. (2015) 'The paradigm shift 2016–2010: global plan to end TB', available at www.stoptb.org/global/plan/ (accessed on 29 July 2017).

't Hoen, E. (2009) *The Global Politics of Pharmaceutical Monopoly Power*, Diemen: AMB.

UAEM. (2017) 'Who we are', available at www.devex.com/news/pepfar-to-accelerate-implementation-in-13-countries-under-new-strategy-91064 (accessed on 20 November 2017).

UNAIDS. (2014) 'Fast-track: ending the AIDS epidemic by 2030', available at www.unaids.org/sites/default/files/ media_asset/JC2686_WAD2014report_en.pdf (accessed on 31 July 2017).

UNAIDS. (2016) 'Global AIDS Update 2016', available at www.unaids.org/sites/default/files/media_asset/global-AIDS-update-2016_en.pdf (accessed on 20 November 2017)

US Congress Proceedings and Debates. (2001) 'Shame on Mr. Natsios, Hon. Janice D. Shakowsky of Illinois in the House of Representatives', Wednesday 20 June, United States of America Congressional record: proceedings and debates of the 107th Congress, volume 147, part 8 (Washington, DC: United States Government Printing Office), 11275, available at www.schakowsky.house.gov/index.php?option=com_content&view=article&id=196&catid=17:2001-press-releases&Itemid=35 (accessed on 1 September 2010).

Vawda, Y., Baker, B., Rens, A., Schonwetter, T., Ncube, C., and Prabhala, A. (2016) 'Submission by academics, experts, scholars and pro-access advocates on the Department of Trade and Industry's intellectual property consultative framework', available at http://infojustice.org/wp-content/uploads/2016/10/Academics-etc-Submission-on-IP-Consultative-Framework-Final-30-Sept-2016-yv.pdf (accessed on 30 July 2017).

World Trade Organization. (2001) 'Doha Declaration on the TRIPS agreement and public health', available at www.wto.org/english/thewto_e/min01_e/minded_trips_e.htm (accessed on 22 July 2011).

Yu, D., Soteyrand, Y., Banda, M.A., Kaufman, J., and Perriëns, J.H. (2008) *Globalisation and Health*, 4:8.

# 4

# Neglect in global health

*João Nunes*

One of the perennial questions in the study of global health politics pertains to how priorities are defined. What makes issues rise in – and fall out of – the agenda? Which actors are determinant in this process? What motivations – political, economic, security, or other – motivate global health actors to privilege certain diseases? And is the emergence of new and powerful global health actors – such as philanthropic organisations or transnational corporations – likely to change existing priorities? These questions are bound to become more important as the world is faced with a mixture of longstanding problems (e.g., infectious diseases like tuberculosis), growing concerns (e.g., chronic diseases), and emerging issues (e.g., antimicrobial resistance). Investigating the processes of agenda-setting is crucial if we are to mobilise and use our limited resources to reduce health risks and alleviate suffering.

Instead of considering issue-prioritisation from the standpoint of high-profile cases and how they became important, this chapter takes a different route and explores how certain questions become neglected in global health. This is not merely about taking a different perspective on the same problem. The standpoint of neglect raises radically different questions about the nature of visibility and invisibility in global health, and how they are reproduced. This chapter presents a novel interpretation of the meaning of neglect based on two core ideas: first, that neglect encompasses not only specific diseases but also determinants and groups; second, that neglect is not simply about lack of visibility, since quality of attention matters when determining if and how an issue is being neglected. The chapter then uses this reconceptualisation of neglect to enquire into the mechanisms of its reproduction, before illustrating with the examples of water and sanitation, and the 2014 Ebola outbreak in West Africa.

## The politics of agenda-setting

How do health issues become matters of international political concern? Inversely, how do they fail to emerge as significant? In order to answer this question, it is worth considering how health has been defined as something to be governed at the global level. Ideas about global health governance – what it means and what it entails – provide a good entry-point into the processes of agenda-setting. Since at least the nineteenth century, the world has witnessed the development of rules, regimes, and institutions seeking to govern health at the international level (Howard-Jones, 1950; Fidler, 2001; Huber, 2006). More recently, scholars and policymakers have begun to speak of 'global health governance', defined as the set of 'collaborative activities among states, IGOs, and NGOs that seek to influence the character of particular international problems' (Zacher and Keefe, 2008, p. 15). The term global health governance denotes an approach to the management of global health that emphasises the combined impact of a variety of state and non-state actors in the absence of a single authority, as well as the ability of these actors to recognise and tackle issues through increased cooperation, coordination, and consensus. According to this approach, problems of insufficient coordination, inadequate allocation of resources, or new demands can be addressed by governance mechanisms adapting and transforming in response to external shocks – what some authors have described as a model of 'punctuated equilibrium' (Price-Smith and Huang, 2009).

Many narratives surrounding global health governance share a belief in the incremental development of cooperative mechanisms, supported by enhanced regulation, standardisation of procedures, scientific and technological progress. This optimistic view has clashed with glaring failures: acute inequalities in health provision, groups excluded from access to health care, and huge discrepancies in health indicators (Farmer, 1999; Marmot, 2015). One of the ways in which these failures reveal themselves is through the persistence of issue-areas that are given less attention (by policymakers, funders, the media, or the public) than would be expected given their burden on individuals and societies. In other words, the inability to adequately overcome the neglect of certain issues is one of the most important shortcomings of the governance of health. This neglect pertains not simply to particular diseases – for example, the so-called neglected tropical diseases (Fenwick, 2012; Hotez, 2013). Neglect also encompasses the systematic exclusion of certain groups from the highest standards of health care available. Neglect shows that global health governance is still unable to identify and tackle the problems faced by a significant percentage of the world's population – particularly the problems of those who are disadvantaged because of their class, gender, race, or sexual orientation.

Neglect reveals inefficient resource allocation and inadequate agenda-setting in global health politics. One common explanation for neglect assumes it to be a mere epiphenomenon of the interests of powerful actors and donors. These interests would shape incentives to commit funding and resources, thus helping to determine what is present (and absent) in the agenda. In this sense, neglect happens because the problems of less powerful states, regions, or groups are marginal to the interests of those with the ability to decisively influence outcomes in global health. Whilst this explanation can be helpful when seeking to identify the circumstances that make neglect possible, it does not tell us much about how interests are being formed. What are the political, social, and cultural processes that enable the interests of powerful actors to be defined in such a narrow way? Why is the plight of disadvantaged others – impossible to dismiss in an era of social media and 24/7 news channels – not enough to spur a solidarity-based response? As Simon Rushton and Owain Williams (2012, p. 152) have put it, the literature has tended to focus on the '"end product" of a policy process without really addressing what structures and determines the policy process'. It is not enough to say that neglect happens because of the interests of powerful actors. Rather, one needs to probe into the practices of mis-recognition, silencing, and moral indifference that enable interests to be shaped in particular ways.

Understanding neglect requires one to consider the politics of problem-definition in global health, that is, the processes through which certain issues become problems whilst others do not. Global health problems are not self-evident realities but the result of (ambiguous and contested) claims and demands put forward by actors. These claims are underpinned by narratives that structure reality in certain ways. Schön and Rein (1994, p. 23) have used the term 'frame' to refer to these narratives, conceiving policy debates as 'disputes in which the contending parties hold conflicting frames', the latter determining 'what counts as a fact and what arguments are taken to be relevant and compelling'. Frames are determinant in shaping interests, insofar as actors' 'problem formulations and preferred solutions are grounded in different problem-setting stories rooted in different frames' (Schön and Rein, 1994, p. 29). Therefore, problem-definition should not be seen as a value-neutral process of identifying self-evident problems. Problems can emerge as significant because they reinforce already-existing assumptions about what is important or not. Policy decisions are implicated in the reproduction of areas that are deemed unworthy of attention or concern.

Drawing on the notion of frames, Colin McInnes and Kelley Lee (2012, p. 34) have argued that narratives about global health reflect 'a particular dominant narrative or set of narratives emphasising certain types of risks, the interests of certain population groups, the way in which the global nature of the problem is defined, and the need for certain high-level political responses'. The idea of framing has also been used to study issue-prioritisation in global health. Jeremy Shiffman (2009, p. 610) argues that the ascendance of an issue in the scale of priorities depends, first and foremost, on 'ideational portrayal', that is, on the effective communication of the importance of a certain issue 'in ways that appeal to political leaders' social values and concepts of reality'. In a second moment, institutions are required that can promote and sustain such portrayals. In a previous work, Shiffman and Smith (2007) identified a number of factors shaping prioritisation, organising them along four categories: the power of the actors putting forward a particular issue as a health priority; the strength and internal coherence of their reasoning; the political context in which these ideas are presented, which impacts upon their chances of resonating; and, finally, the characteristics of the issue, which determine the possibility that a credible case for its severity and potential resolution can be made.

This literature tells us that health agendas are not simply the result of predefined interests, but rather political sites of contestation where interests are being constituted and performed on the basis of values and ideological assumptions. Agenda-setting and issue-prioritisation in global health are political questions not simply because they are subject to the vagaries of day-to-day decisions and negotiations, but also because they are at the heart of the processes through which identities, responsibilities, and ideas of commonality and solidarity are shaped in global health. In order to fully understand neglect, we need to dig deeper into its meaning and enquire into what it tells us about what we have become as a global polity.

## The meaning of neglect

Neglect pertains not simply to particular diseases, but also to determinants (i.e., economic, social, infrastructural) and to groups. A disease can be considered neglected when it is not studied well enough, for instance, or when decisive steps are not taken to address it (e.g., neglected tropical diseases). A determinant is neglected when its role in outbreaks, disease incidence, or people's ability to deal with the occurrence of disease is not recognised or addressed (e.g., the quality of health-systems). A group is neglected when it is systematically placed in a position of vulnerability to disease, or is excluded from high-quality and affordable health care (e.g., undocumented migrants). In sum, neglect can be defined as a sustained process of making invisible a problem or condition, and/or the denial of resources necessary to understand or address it – this being at odds with the burden that this problem or condition has on individuals and societies. Neglect can happen as a combined effect of the actions/inactions of different actors: policymakers, donors, the media, and the general public.

When analysing neglect in global health, one important thing to consider is that neglect means more than disregard. In fact, neglect is a layered concept, which includes the failure to act in an adequate way to tackle a particular issue – even if that issue is not disregarded. In turn, 'to care' may mean different things. On the one hand, it can denote a feeling of empathy: to see a certain problem as important, as something that matters not just for oneself but also for others. On the other hand, 'to care' can also mean to act in a way that effectively tackles the problem. This means that the term neglect can be used to refer to at least four different situations. First, it can refer to a situation of neglect by invisibility, when an issue is simply disregarded or has not yet become visible – either because of its novelty or because the victims are silent (or being silenced). Second, we can have a situation of neglect by apathy, in which the issue is visible but not considered important by those with the ability to shape outcomes. Third, an issue can be visible and considered important but actors are not willing to act in order to address it – in this case, there is a situation of neglect by inaction. Finally, actors may seek to address the issue but do so in an inadequate way – neglect by incompetence.

Neglect is therefore not just about invisibility, but also about a moral landscape in which an issue is deemed as something that does not matter, and about a political arena in which effective solutions are not designed and implemented. This approach places neglect within a moral and political context in which the suffering of some is deemed less important than the suffering of others. It also shows that neglect does not just happen – it is rather produced or made to happen. At the crux of the production of neglect it is always possible to locate human agency, choices, actions, and inactions. Issues are rendered invisible in certain ways, by certain actors and following certain agendas. Neglect by apathy is the result of processes that shape the sphere of moral obligation – apathy is in fact a denial of empathy and a failure to care about the plight of others. Neglect by inaction is not simply absence of action – rather, it can be more aptly described as denial of response. Finally, neglect by incompetence also forces us to consider how resources are allocated and to question why adequate responses are not devised or applied.

This discussion points to the importance of seeing neglected health as intertwined with broader dynamics in world politics. On the one hand, neglect connects with the ways in which harm is reproduced at the global level (on harm, see Linklater, 2011, pp. 49–61). At the most basic level, neglect is complicit in the reproduction of the physical and/or psychological injuries that are attached to diseases. These include the stigmatisation and disrespect for the dignity of those suffering from neglected health problems. Neglect can also function as a multiplier of harm, when it enables damage to be done to the very mechanisms and institutions that are responsible for preventing or tackling health problems. Finally, we can talk of structural harm in relation to neglect: this pertains to situations when groups are neglected not exactly by the absence of rules and institutions, but by the fact that existing ones are skewed and place groups in positions of disadvantage.

On the other hand, neglect is connected with vulnerability: a group's or individual's susceptibility to harm, but also the inability to 'bounce back' and deal with harm (on vulnerability, see Goodin, 1985; Mackenzie, et al., 2014). Neglect is an important factor in the reproduction of vulnerabilities because it entails differentiated exposure to disease and an unequal distribution of capabilities to deal with it. The neglect of a certain disease may lead to less resources being available for prevention and cure, and therefore to immediate vulnerabilities, that is, to more people being exposed. Vulnerability may also be potential, when individuals or groups are socially and economically positioned in such a way that their health is prone to being inordinately affected by the slightest changes in circumstances and by decisions they cannot control or predict. These potential vulnerabilities go a long way in determining the incidence of a disease and its ability to decisively impact – or even cut short – the lives of those affected.

In sum, neglect is politically produced through the actions and inactions of those who would otherwise have the power to make a change. Importantly it involves the existence of groups that are systematically privileged in relation to others; and the presence of unequal relationships. Neglect simultaneously feeds from, and helps to reproduce, these inequalities.

## Emotions and the production of neglect

This chapter has argued that when analysing agenda-setting in global health we need to pay attention to the political processes through which problems are framed. Understanding the production of neglect thus calls for an engagement with the political imaginary in which certain policy options emerge as possible, necessary, or desirable solutions. Common accounts of neglect tend to ground their explanations on rational actors pursuing their predefined material interests (such as economic gain or strategic advantage). These accounts often overlook how interests themselves are being shaped by ideas. The literature mentioned earlier in this chapter, which emphasises the importance of frames in the social construction of our perceptions of what global health means and what its priorities should be, is a very important contribution to understanding how certain issues are left out. The framing literature allows us to see, for example, how the presence of a security-based rationality in global health decision-making has led to short-termist responses based on containment and crisis management, to the detriment of engaging with the underlying causes that allow problems to occur in the first place. In other words, a security framing of health problems can be complicit with the neglect of their deeper political, social, and economic determinants.

Whilst this literature has made an important contribution in emphasising the role of ideas, so far it has not engaged in sufficient depth with the affective dimension of framing. Neta C. Crawford (2000) has argued that the political role of emotions can be witnessed at different levels. On the one hand, emotions impact upon actors' perceptions of others' motives, thus shaping the content of relations. On the other hand, emotions also have effects at the level of cognition, that is, on actors' definitions of their interests and courses of action. This is because emotions influence the processes through which actors gather and process information about their environment; their calculation of risks, costs, and benefits; and their ability and receptivity to dialogue with other actors.

Emotions have been used to make sense of different modalities of engagement in world politics, helping to explain how actors establish various kinds of relations within an affective – and not simply rational – context (Mercer, 2006; Bleiker and Hutchison, 2008). But emotions can also be used to make sense of non-engagement or disengagement – in the case of neglect, the processes by which actors become disconnected or fail to connect with the suffering and ill health of others. Crucial for an affective analysis of neglect is abjection, defined as the act of casting away something or someone, but also to the process of debasing or rendering despicable. Abjection is intrinsically connected with the emotional dynamics through which certain groups are framed or emerge as alien (that is, outside the sphere of moral obligation); disgusting (triggering an unpleasant emotional reaction); and beyond any possibility of improvement. Abjection is an unavoidable feature of the cultural context in which certain groups are made invisible and some actors become emotionally desensitised to the needs and suffering of less privileged others.

Julia Kristeva (1982) engaged with the concept of abjection whilst discussing subject-formation. She defined abjection as an ambiguous relationship between self and other, characterised by a mixture of attraction and repulsion. The abject is something that simultaneously beckons and repels. Even though it lies at the margins of the self, the abject is not completely separable because it permanently unsettles and threatens to disrupt the integrity of the self. As Iris Marion Young (2011 [1990], p. 144) put it, the abject 'provokes fear and loathing because it exposes the border between self and other as constituted and fragile, and threatens to dissolve the subject by dissolving the border'. In other words, the abject emerges as dangerous by revealing the fault lines and limits in the self's constitution.

Abjection is important for an analysis of neglect because it is intrinsically tied to mechanisms of oppression. Young argues that instances of oppression like racism and sexism persist despite the adoption of anti-discrimination laws by becoming embodied and unconscious. Oppression happens not simply through official mechanisms but also in 'informal, often unnoticed and unreflective speech, bodily reactions to others, conventional practices of everyday interaction and evaluation, aesthetic judgments, and the jokes, images, and stereotypes pervading the mass media' (Young, 2011 [1990], p. 148). For Young, interactions between groups are thus underpinned by emotional dynamics of attraction and aversion. Specifically, oppression is supported by a process through which certain groups are rendered abject – that is, different, alien, and loathsome. Abject groups are defined by dominant discourses 'in terms of bodily characteristics, and constructs those bodies as ugly, dirty, defiled, impure, contaminated, or sick' (Young, 2011 [1990], p. 123).

Young's analysis of the complex mechanisms of oppression is highly relevant when thinking about neglect in global health. Drawing from this discussion, it becomes possible to conceive emotions as playing an important part in the international dynamics through which harm and vulnerability are reproduced. As was mentioned earlier, these dynamics are themselves implicated with the neglect of certain diseases, determinants, and groups – or, more precisely, on the neglect of certain health problems as they are experienced by groups that are placed in a position of subordination. When making sense of neglect in global health we must engage with the cultural and emotional processes through which interests are defined in tandem with an anxiety over certain groups and bodies. These groups and bodies are not simply marginalised or excluded. They are portrayed as morally tainted and a source of moral pollution. They are also deemed irredeemable, beyond possibilities of improvement. Taken together, these features mean that abject groups are placed outside the sphere of moral concern.

## Neglect in practice

The preceding discussion reveals neglect as a multifaceted phenomenon, which may occur at different levels and under many guises. In order to illustrate this, the chapter considers two cases that exemplify the ways in which neglect is produced in global health. The first case is water and sanitation. According to the World Health Organization (WHO) and the United Nations Children's Fund, in 2015 around 2.4 billion people did not have access to an improved sanitation facility, that is, one that hygienically separates human excreta from human contact (UNICEF and World Health Organization, 2015). Inadequate sanitation is directly related to poor water quality: also in 2015, and according to the same study, 663 million people did not use an improved source for drinking water – one that is protected from outside contamination, in particular by faecal matter. Poor sanitation and insufficient access to safe water are the direct causes or underlying conditions of several diseases (Mara and Feachem, 1999). According to World Health Organization (2013) figures, diarrhoea, which is directly related to the consumption of unsafe water, is the second leading cause of death in children under five years old (around 760 thousand child deaths annually). Several neglected tropical diseases are also connected to water and sanitation: examples include trachoma (the world's leading cause of preventable blindness) and soil-transmitted helminth infections like hookworm infection, ascariasis, and trichuriasis (Mara, et al., 2010). In addition, unavailability of safe water has been tied to school absenteeism and to the exacerbation of gender inequalities in education: women and children are often enrolled in the task of procuring water, and lack of water for hygiene in schools has more profound impacts on female attendance (Bartram and Cairncross, 2010; Hunter, et al., 2010). It has been estimated that improving sanitation and access to safe water – when combined with improvements in hygiene habits – could potentially prevent around 9.1% of the world's disease burden and 6.3% of deaths (Prüss-Üstün, et al., 2008).

The production of neglect in this case is partly due to invisibility, in the context of an agenda that is traditionally skewed towards high-profile communicable diseases. In line with international health efforts from the nineteenth century, global health is still predominantly geared towards containing the cross-border spread of diseases (so that they do not reach Western developed nations). This has resulted in the privileging of 'vertical' programmes of disease eradication (mostly those diseases that pose a threat to richer countries), in detriment of 'horizontal' interventions on infrastructure, primary health care and the strengthening of health systems that would directly impact upon safe water and adequate sanitation. However, as was mentioned, neglect should be approached as something more than an epiphenomenon of the (predetermined) interests of powerful nations and donors. It sits at the intersection of processes of meaning-construction and existing political, economic, and institutional structures. Those processes – and particularly the affective elements therein – mean that in the case of water and sanitation neglect is characterised by a mixture of invisibility and apathy. Indeed, it is now impossible to ignore the burden of issues related to water and sanitation upon global health. Making sense of the perpetuation of neglect needs to take into account an underlying logic of abjection. This pertains, on the one hand, to the nature of these issues, which are often deemed 'disgusting'. Issues related to excreta trigger an emotional reaction of unpleasantness and rejection, which makes wilful ignorance easier (on disgust, see Miller, 1997; Menninghaus, 2003). Politicians, opinion-makers, media, and celebrities thus tend to focus on issues (or 'causes') without such an affective baggage. On the other hand, the constitution of these issues as disgusting is boosted by the fact that problems related to inadequate water and sanitation are, to a great extent, issues of poverty. They arise from the unequal access to material resources, such as adequate housing and sewage infrastructure; they reveal discrepancies in access to education, namely education in hygiene. They are therefore issues that predominantly affect poor groups, which themselves have been perceived via discourses that frame them as fundamentally different, unable to help themselves but complicit in their own destitution, and mired in reprehensible habits. The 'disgusting' nature of water and sanitation issues, when conjoined with the anxiety over the poor, helps to explain the abjection that is at the heart of neglect.

The second case of neglect is Ebola. This may seem an unlikely case given the attention that Ebola received on the part of policymakers, the media, and the general public in the wake of the 2014 outbreak in West Africa. However, it can be argued that despite the great deal of attention received by Ebola, important dimensions of the problem remained invisible throughout the recent outbreak. The outbreak began in December 2013 in Guinea, with the Guinean Ministry of Health making an official declaration on 21 March 2014. A few days later, cases were confirmed in Liberia; in May, the first case in Sierra Leone was confirmed. By the end of June, Ebola was 'actively transmitting in more than 60 locations in Guinea, Liberia and Sierra Leone' (Médecins Sans Frontières, 2015). In August – after Western nationals had become infected – the WHO declared Ebola a 'public health emergency of international concern' (World Health Organization, 2014).

The framing of Ebola as a security issue and an emerging crisis needing to be contained happened to the detriment of seeing the outbreak from a broader perspective, that is, as the result of a series of events and conditions that stretch out into past choices and inactions. Seeing Ebola as an emerging crisis hindered a comprehensive engagement with the conditions that gave rise to the problem in the first place. What of the social and economic conditions that have turned Ebola into an endemic feature of this region? And the weak and inefficient health systems that have rendered some West-African countries unable to cope (Kruk, et al., 2015)? And the low levels of trust between politicians and the public, which, at least in the case of Liberia, seem to have considerably weakened the ability of health authorities to alter the trajectory of the epidemic (Epstein, 2014)? Finally, what about the global context in which the outbreak emerged, and the structural inequalities therein (Benatar, 2015)? These questions were not given sufficient attention.

The framing of the Ebola outbreak thus contributed to rendering the phenomenon visible in certain – and very limited – ways. In narratives about Ebola, the primary concern was the protection of the West vis à vis threatening infections coming from the outside. In spite of the visibility of the Ebola outbreak, the groups mostly affected by the disease, as well as of the social and economic conditions that made the outbreak possible, remained largely invisible. In addition, there was a process of abjection in place, as certain groups and practices were represented as alien, exotic, and disgusting – and directly linked to the spread of Ebola. In August 2014, American weekly news magazine *Newsweek* ran as its cover story an alarmist account of the dangers of the 'secret' trade of monkey meat into the US and Europe, which could become Ebola's 'backdoor' into the West. Indeed, the framing of Ebola in Western media cannot be separated from a persistent anxiety over certain kinds of groups, their habits and the threat they present to the integrity of the political community. This story was supported by an underlying narrative of the African continent as a place of despair and helplessness, about which little can be done except preventing problems from spilling over to other regions of the world. The *Newsweek* story can be understood in the context of the racialisation of Ebola, which in turn cannot be separated from the ensuing stigmatisation of West Africans living in the West (Dionne and Seay, 2015). Neglect was produced by the framing of Ebola as a racialised African problem deriving from backward practices and requiring a mixture of surveillance and containment. This happened to the detriment of seeing the outbreak as a problem of global health governance – of inequality, injustice, and the systematic reproduction of the vulnerability of certain groups. In the case of Ebola, then, neglect manifested itself not simply in the invisibility of certain groups and underlying conditions, but also in the re-inscription of the conditions for apathy and inaction.

## Conclusion

Neglect in global health is a complex phenomenon. It is deeply political not simply because it results from the day-to-day bargaining between competing interests, but also because it reveals how political communities shape their interests – and hence their identities – through cultural and affective processes. Neglect is not simply a status of invisibility. It is a process of making issues and groups simultaneously visible in certain ways and invisible in others. As a result of this, it is also a process by which moral horizons are defined and negotiated. At the heart of neglect there is a fundamental question about what we owe to others, and of our collective responsibility towards the health of others when we are not affected (at least directly). Neglect also raises the question of the extent to which we are able to recognise the fate of others as interlinked with our own.

Neglect reveals the paradoxes and limits of many narratives of global health – namely assumptions that we are somehow 'united'. Instead, neglect is connected with deep-seated divisions and inequalities – the mechanisms of reproduction of immediate and structural forms of harm and vulnerability in world politics. This means that overcoming neglect necessarily encompasses more than short-termist measures aimed at containing specific diseases or managing crises. Such superficial attention can only be expected to alleviate immediate forms of harm and vulnerability, whilst leaving deeper problems intact.

## References

Bartram, J. and Cairncross, S. (2010) 'Hygiene, sanitation, and water: forgotten foundations of health', *PLoS Medicine*, 7: e1000367.

Benatar, S. (2015) 'Explaining and responding to the Ebola epidemic', *Philosophy, Ethics, and Humanities in Medicine*, 10: 5.

Bleiker, R. and Hutchison, E. (2008) 'Fear no more: emotions and world politics', *Review of International Studies*, 34: 115–35.

Crawford, N.C. (2000) 'The passion of world politics: propositions on emotion and emotional relationships', *International Security*, 24: 116–56.

Dionne, K.Y. and Seay, L. (2015) 'Perceptions about Ebola in America: othering and the role of knowledge about Africa', *Political Science & Politics*, 48: 6–7.

Epstein, H. (2014) 'Ebola in Liberia: an epidemic of rumors', *New York Review of Books*, 61: 91–4.

Farmer, P. (1999) *Infections and Inequalities: The modern plagues*, Berkeley: University of California Press.

Fenwick, A. (2012) 'The global burden of neglected tropical diseases', *Public Health*, 126: 233–6.

Fidler, D.P. (2001) 'The globalization of public health: the first 100 years of international health diplomacy', *Bulletin of the World Health Organization*, 79: 842–9.

Goodin, R.E. (1985) *Protecting the Vulnerable: A reanalysis of our social responsibilities*, Chicago and London: University of Chicago Press.

Hotez, P.J. (2013) *Forgotten People, Forgotten Diseases: The neglected tropical diseases and their impact on global health and development*, Washington, DC: ASM Press.

Howard-Jones, N. (1950) 'Origins of international health work', *British Medical Journal*, 1: 1032–7.

Huber, V. (2006) 'The unification of the globe by disease? The international sanitary conferences on cholera, 1851–1894', *The Historical Journal*, 49: 453–76.

Hunter, P.R., MacDonald, A.M., and Carter, R.C. (2010) 'Water supply and health', *PLoS Medicine*, 7: e1000361.

Kristeva, J. (1982) *Powers of Horror: An essay on abjection*, New York: Columbia University Press.

Kruk, M.E., Myers, M., Varpilah, S.T., et al. (2015) 'What is a resilient health system? lessons from Ebola', *The Lancet*, 385: 1910–12.

Linklater, A. (2011) *The Problem of Harm in World Politics: Theoretical investigations*, Cambridge: Cambridge University Press.

Mackenzie, C., Rogers, W., and Dodds, S. (2014) 'What is vulnerability, and why does it matter for moral theory?' In: Mackenzie C., Rogers W., and Dodds S. (Eds.) *Vulnerability: New essays in ethics and feminist philosophy*, Oxford: Oxford University Press, pp. 1–29.

Mara, D., Lane, J., Scott, B., et al. (2010) 'Sanitation and health', *PLoS Medicine*, 7: e1000363.

Mara, D.D. and Feachem, R.G.A. (1999) 'Water- and excreta-related diseases: unitary environmental classification', *Journal of Environmental Engineering*, 125: 334–9.

Marmot, M. (2015) *The Health Gap: The challenge of an unequal world*, London: Bloomsbury.

McInnes, C. and Lee, K. (2012) *Global Health and International Relations*, Cambridge: Polity Press.

Médecins Sans Frontières. (2015) 'Pushed to the limit and beyond: a year into the largest ever Ebola outbreak', available at www.doctorswithoutborders.org/sites/usa/files/msf143061.pdf (accessed on 25 September 2017).

Menninghaus, W. (2003) *Disgust: Theory and history of a strong sensation*, Albany: State University of New York Press.

Mercer, J. (2006) 'Human nature and the first image: emotion in international politics', *Journal of International Relations and Development*, 9: 288–303.

Miller, W.I. (1997) *The Anatomy of Disgust*, Cambridge, MA: Harvard University Press.

Price-Smith, A.T. and Huang, Y. (2009) 'Epidemic of fear: SARS and the political economy of contagion', In: A.F. Cooper and J.J. Kirton (Eds.) *Innovation in Global Health Governance: Critical cases*, Farnham: Ashgate, pp. 23–48.

Prüss-Üstün, A., Bos, R., Gore, F., et al. (2008) *Safer Water, Better Health: Costs, benefits and sustainability of interventions to protect and promote health*, Geneva: World Health Organization.

Rushton, S. and Williams, O.D. (2012) 'Frames, paradigms and power: global health policy-making under neoliberalism', *Global Society*, 26: 147–67.

Schön, D.A. and Rein, M. (1994) *Frame Reflection: Toward the resolution of intractable policy controversies*, New York: Basic Books.

Shiffman, J. (2009) 'A social explanation for the rise and fall of global health issues', *Bulletin of the World Health Organization*, 87: 608–13.

Shiffman, J. and Smith, S. (2007) 'Generation of political priority for global health initiatives: a framework and case study of maternal mortality', *The Lancet*, 370: 1370–9.

UNICEF and World Health Organization. (2015) *Progress on Drinking Water and Sanitation – 2015 update and MDG assessment*, Geneva: World Health Organization.

World Health Organization. (2013) 'Diarrhoeal disease', available at www.who.int/mediacentre/factsheets/fs330/en/index.html (accessed on 25 September 2017).

World Health Organization. (2014) 'Statement on the 1st meeting of the IHR emergency committee on the 2014 Ebola outbreak in West Africa', available at www.who.int/mediacentre/news/statements/2014/ebola-20140808/en/ (accessed on 25 September 2017).

Young, I.M. (2011 [1990]) *Justice and the Politics of Difference*, Princeton and Oxford: Princeton University Press.

Zacher, M.W. and Keefe, T.J. (2008) *The Politics of Global Health Governance: United by contagion*, Houndmills: Palgrave Macmillan.

# 5

# The politics of funding research in global health partnerships

*Johanna T. Crane, Irene Andia Biraro, Tamer M. Fouad,*
*Yap Boum II, and David R. Bangsberg*

## Introduction: partnership and capacity building in global health science

Over the past 15 years, interest in 'global health' science has surged within North American research universities, resulting in a steep rise in academic departments, programmes, and institutes dedicated to global health research and education (Matheson, et al., 2014). Such programmes require international partners to enable global work and, more often than not, these partner institutions are in African countries. Although the term 'global health' is of relatively recent coinage, international health research has a long history. 'Tropical medicine' – a field born out of European colonialism – investigated infectious diseases like yellow fever, malaria, and yaws; and in the 1960s and 1970s the field of 'international health' worked hand-in-hand with international development in Africa to address questions of nutrition and maternal and child health (Giles-Vernick and Webb, 2013; Vaughan, 1991). Though the extent to which global health continues or is distinct from these older forms is a matter of some debate (Birn, 2009, 2014; Packard, 2016), there are some clear ways in which the field differs from its antecedents. First, the shift to global health has undoubtedly come with an unprecedented level of reliance upon, and faith in, quantitative metrics of impact and efficacy (Adams, 2016). Second, the field of global health itself claims a fundamental difference from older, paternalistic models of transnational medicine in that it aspires to equitable partnership between institutions and professionals in wealthy and poor nations. This was evident in a widely cited 2009 article in *The Lancet* in which a group of international authors representing the Consortium of Universities for Global Health argued for 'a common definition of global health' that emphasised 'the mutuality of real partnership, a pooling of experience and knowledge, and a two-way flow between developed and developing countries' (Koplan, et al., 2009, pp. 1994–5). 'The developed world', the authors noted, 'does not have a monopoly on good ideas' (Koplan, et al., 2009, p. 1994).

In this way, 'partnership' is central to the way in which global health science has been imagined by its leading practitioners. Many African researchers share a vision of 'good' partnerships or collaborations as rooted, if not necessarily in resource equity, in an equity of ideas and scientific contribution (Okwaro and Geissler, 2015; Okeke, 2018). This imagery of partnership serves as both a means of distinguishing global health from its antecedents and as a way to stake an ethical claim. By embracing 'partnership' as an ideal, global health programmes and professionals frame their relationship to the inequality that is part and parcel of scientific collaborations between high-income and low-income nations: the intent is not to exploit poverty for scientific or educational gain, but rather to work collaboratively with their host-country colleagues to improve health and reduce human suffering. In this vision, global health is imagined as a collaborative scientific endeavour in which 'real partnership' bridges international resource inequalities.

Relatedly, the notion of 'capacity building' has become central to the objectives of global health. Research partnerships and the funding that comes with them are not only used to 'co-produce' scientific knowledge, but also to build research and public health implementation capacity at under-resourced host institutions (Consortium of Universities for Global Health, n.d.; NIH, 2013). In other words, capacity building is seen as a mechanism for bridging inequalities and an indicator of a fair, non-exploitative partnership. Much like 'global health', the notion of 'capacity building' emerged as a way to signal a break with older, more paternalistic modes of engagement between wealthy former colonising powers and poorer formerly colonised nations (Geissler and Tousignant, 2016). In this vision, global health partnership is seen as enhancing research capacity by providing education, training, skills, and – less often – material and infrastructural support to the lower-income (often African) partners (Wendland, 2016). Nonetheless, despite these aspirations, evidence suggests that global health collaborations face considerable obstacles in achieving the goals of equitable partnership and lasting capacity building, and critics have noted that 'partnership' language may in fact mask inequalities and disagreements (Crane, 2010; Geissler, 2013).

In this chapter, we focus on the funding mechanisms and administrative practices commonly used in US global health research partnerships, and the barriers that these mechanisms and practices pose for equitable partnership. We do so in order to emphasise the importance of building African institutional capacity in the arena of fiscal administration, and to illustrate ways in which the fiscal and administrative structure of partnerships can undermine goals of equity and capacity building. Our analysis speaks specifically to US-funded global health research partnerships with institutions in Africa, as this is the dominant form taken by American academic global health partnerships.[1] Specifically, we first explain how US funding agencies' policies contribute to chronic underfunding of research overhead ('indirect') costs at foreign partner institutions; and, second, we describe how US universities rely upon administrative 'enabling systems' that avoid direct institutional partnership and externalise fiscal and legal risk to partners. Using the experiences of three of the authors with a US–Ugandan HIV research project, we then illustrate how these practices played out 'on the ground' using our project as a case study. We conclude by arguing that resource-rich institutions must acknowledge and take responsibility for their roles in undermining administrative capacity at underfunded partner institutions.

## Underfunding of foreign institutions

Research capacity at US universities expanded greatly during World War II and afterwards, when the federal government funneled increasingly generous grant monies into academic science. One practice that supported this expansion was the recognition and funding of both 'direct' and 'indirect' research costs by federal granting agencies such as the National Institutes of Health (NIH). 'Direct' costs are those attributable to a specific research project, such as researcher salaries or study-specific equipment and supplies. 'Indirect' costs (often referred to as 'overhead' or 'facilities and administration' costs) are those borne by the institution, and may include the provision of research space, electricity, human resources, accounting, and office supplies (NIH, 2011). Reimbursement for 'indirect' facilities and administrative costs helped US universities develop and maintain the infrastructure (such as buildings, laboratories, technologies, and administrative staff) needed to support robust research programmes. Today, agencies continue to pay for indirect research costs – most often as a percentage of direct costs – and as a result, universities continue to benefit from the ongoing investment in infrastructure that this funding structure allows. Within the US, where universities negotiate indirect cost rates directly with federal funding agencies, institutions are commonly reimbursed at rates of 50 per cent or more, meaning that for every dollar received for direct research costs, the principal investigator's home institution receives 50 (or more) cents to cover indirect, overhead expenses (Brainard, 2005).

Yet, this same funding structure that has helped build and maintain research capacity at US institutions may be undermining capacity at 'partner' institutions in low-income countries. Under US Department of Health and Human Services rules, indirect cost reimbursements for foreign institutions receiving NIH grant money are capped at a maximum of only 8 per cent. This figure represents an increase from the 0 per cent rate of the 1980s, a product of Reagan-era sentiments towards what was considered foreign 'aid'. The rule changed in the 1990s, when fears of 'emerging diseases' made the climate for international health funding more favourable. During this time, leaders at the National Institutes for Allergy and Infectious Diseases (NIAID) succeeded in lobbying for an increase to 8 per cent (the same amount offered to recipients of NIH training grants) but found that any amount greater than this was politically untenable (Crane, 2013). As our case study will illustrate, this funding structure may further exacerbate inequalities between well-funded and underfunded partners. The negative impact on foreign host institutions may then serve to justify US universities' preference for parallel administrative 'enabling systems' that externalise risk, maintain US control over accounting, and bypass direct partnership with host institutions, described later.

## Global health 'enabling systems' and institutional capacity building

Due in part to their inherently transnational nature, global health research partnerships can require a tremendous amount of administrative labour in order to ensure that fiscal, hiring, and accounting practices are in compliance with laws, regulations, and institutional policies in two or more different countries. This reality, and the challenges it brings, has given birth to global health 'enabling systems'. These are administrative structures and practices that facilitate, or enable, academic institutional partnerships between wealthy and poor nations. Designed by Northern universities, these modular systems are intended to smooth and monitor the flow of money and other resources to collaborators in poor countries, as well as to insulate Northern universities from legal and financial risk (Appel, 2012; Consortium of Universities for Global Health, n.d.). Overseen by offices with names like 'Global Operations Support' (University of Washington) and 'Global Support Services' (Harvard), enabling systems guide faculty through the legal and administrative steps involved in setting up an international research site.

The 'enabling system' approach is promoted by the Consortium of Universities for Global Health (CUGH), a US-based organisation with international membership that was founded in San Francisco in 2008, where it grew out of an administrative initiative at CUGH founding member University of Washington (UW). UW's Global Support Project was launched in 2006 by the university's Finance Office in response to increasing requests for cash abroad, primarily from faculty working in parts of Africa, and later became institutionalised as the university's office of Global Operations Support. Until 2018, UW faculty and staff led the CUGH committee on enabling systems (recently renamed the Global Health Operations Committee), and UW's global operations support system has been used as a model by other universities, including Duke and Harvard.[2] For these reasons, much of our description of enabling systems emphasises UW's approach, as the processes and procedures pioneered by UW serve as a template for the CUGH's work and for many universities seeking to develop global health enabling systems.

Many African nations hosting US global health partnerships do not have a mechanism for foreign universities (especially public universities run by US state governments) to register as legal entities and open bank accounts. This creates cash flow problems for US principal investigators, who have had to develop creative ways to get grant money to their field sites. At UW, as global health activities ramped up in the late 1990s and 2000s, faculty with international projects in Africa and elsewhere were routinely traveling to their field sites with large amounts of cash and depositing the grant money into personal bank accounts where it could then be used to pay for research space, supplies, and employees. Uncomfortable with the informality and lack of university oversight of this practice, in 2008 the UW's fledgling global support initiative recommended that the university establish a proxy non-profit corporation, dubbed 'UWorld', that could legally register (and thus open bank accounts) in host countries. This approach was quickly embraced by the CUGH and promoted at its inaugural meeting in 2008, where a UW administrator presented it as a way to be 'creative and compliant at the same time' (author fieldnotes). Although the US university administrators who organise these non-profit corporations see them as practical rather than political entities, such bodies do have an impact on global health governance. Their existence and practices raise important political questions about the ability and responsibility of funders, partner institutions, and African states to organise and deliver the resources that partnerships bring – what Hannah Brown calls a 'politics of sovereign responsibility' (Brown, 2015).

Since the founding of the CUGH, African global health leaders have raised concerns about proxy 'enabling systems' and their impact on African universities. At the organisation's first meeting in 2008, Nelson Sewankambo – Principal of the Makerere University School of Health Sciences in Uganda, CUGH board member, and one of the most senior and respected African researchers working in global health – argued that NGOs established by Northern universities were 'undermining local capacity' by setting up separate administrative bodies. He specifically named the UW's non-profit in Addis Ababa, Ethiopia, and urged the UW to instead help the University of Addis Ababa develop the capacity to manage the collaboration's finances. Tom Quinn of Johns Hopkins University, one of Sewankambo's long-time collaborators, echoed this statement, adding that international programmes tended to build independent structures because local ones were perceived as 'too difficult' (Crane, 2013).

Quinn's comment suggests that there is an additional factor driving the use of enabling systems: Western fears of mismanagement or corruption. These fears are stereotypes, but they are also not unwarranted in some cases. In many African countries – and certainly in Uganda – scientists and staff often share this mistrust of their own national government and public institutions.[3] African researchers, as well as their foreign colleagues, may understandably prefer to avoid entrenched bureaucracies and work through more nimble structures such as NGOs and proxy non-profits. Such experiences and perceptions then serve to justify the use of enabling systems which, like the case study of Uganda Research Institute (URI) illustrates below, detour around direct partnership with African institutions and instead establish a parallel administrative system that is more directly answerable to the US partner. The difficulties of working through entrenched and sometimes corrupt African bureaucracies are real (Smith, 2007). However, what gets lost in this picture – but what the case of URI clearly shows – is the fact that many of the administrative difficulties associated with global health are not specifically *African* but are rather *transnational* problems (McKay, 2012; Conteh and Kingori, 2010). URI's struggle to reconcile currencies, the lack of hiring documentation, and the organisation's fiscal precarity – all of these emerged from the transnational challenge of aligning systems and rules across countries and continents. They were American problems as much as Ugandan ones, though the burden was not equally shared.

The CUGH rightly describes proxy non-profits as 'enabling systems', as they are what *enable* partnerships such as the one in our case study to exist and persist. However, they may enable certain inequalities as well. On the ground, such systems may understandably raise sentiments of 'managerial disenfranchisement' from African partners (Brown, 2015). The dual capacity-building and capacity-eroding possibilities of enabling systems are reflected in the multiple dictionary definitions of the verb 'enable', which can mean 'to provide with the means or opportunity'; 'to make possible, practical, or easy'; or 'to give legal power, capacity, or sanction to' (Merriam-Webster, n.d.). Enabling systems are one way to provide the means or opportunity for partnership – they are intended to make partnership possible and practical. However, they do so by allocating legal power and capacity to non-profit corporations that act primarily on behalf of the US partner institution, rather than African public sector institutions. We should be cautious of the possibility that these administrative enabling systems may facilitate arrangements that are harmful to African institution-building, even as they make the logistics of partnership easier (Okeke, 2018). If so, such systems may reflect an alternate definition common in certain subfields of psychology, where 'enabling' refers to the facilitation of self-destructive behaviour by another (Merriam-Webster, n.d.).

Our case study, chronicled in the following, demonstrates how the use of a proxy non-profit administrative enabling system – coupled with low indirect cost reimbursements – failed to strengthen institutional capacity at a Ugandan university hosting a US-funded global health research programme.

## Case study: the partnership with Mbarara University of Science & Technology (MUST)

One of the authors [Bangsberg] was until 2016 the US director of an ongoing research partnership between Mbarara University of Science and Technology (MUST) in Mbarara, Uganda, and originally the University of California San Francisco (UCSF), but now Massachusetts General Hospital (MGH). Two of the other authors have been involved in this partnership as a research collaborator [Andia] and an anthropological observer [Crane]. The case study we outline here is based on these three authors' first-hand experiences working with this partnership from its inception in 2003 up to 2015.

The partnership began in 2003 when the US team initiated a study of access and adherence to antiretroviral medication at the HIV clinic affiliated with the MUST medical school. During the pilot phase, the Mbarara-based project manager was able to fund the study's then-small operating expenses (including staff salaries) using a petty cash account at a local bank. However, the limited banking infrastructure in Mbarara at the time meant this method required weekly trips to the capital city four hours away to withdraw money, and was thus not sustainable. As the study grew and gained more staff, the collaboration shifted to paying employees as independent contractors of UCSF. This too proved unsustainable, as the timing of invoice payments issued from a large state university accounting system were unpredictable and frequently delayed. Wiring transfers to Uganda incurred significant fees, and direct contracting to multiple employees made UCSF as well as the Ugandan employees legally vulnerable under Ugandan tax law. As a result, the collaboration used the now common 'enabling system' practice of establishing a proxy non-profit to act as the study's fiscal agent in Uganda. At the time, MUST did not have a grants management office, and from the UCSF perspective, setting up a small non-profit was considered a much more time efficient mechanism to meet US government accounting requirements than waiting for MUST to develop such an office *de novo*. From the MUST perspective, the need for a grants office was not evident. Like many African universities, its primary focus was on teaching and not research, and the research that did occur was typically conducted by students and self-funded, and thus did not require a grants office. MUST was also a very young university, only 25 years old, and did not have the funding or the administrative support to establish a new office at that time.

With legal assistance from both Ugandan and UCSF lawyers, a non-profit called the Uganda Research Institute (URI) was founded on behalf of the research collaboration. Due to conflict-of-interest regulations, no one directly employed by UCSF (such as the principal investigator (PI) or the project manager) was permitted to be a legal partner or member. As such, the UCSF team asked the Chief of Medicine at MUST [Andia] – also their principal collaborator – to head the organisation. URI was tasked with managing the study's finances and human resources in Uganda, services that were paid for by indirect cost reimbursements from the parent NIH grant.

Per the NIH policy described earlier, URI was limited to an indirect cost reimbursement rate of 8 per cent. By comparison, UCSF's reimbursement rate for on-campus research was 50.5 per cent that year; rates at private US universities are typically even higher (Committee on Finance, 2010). However, transnational research projects must negotiate multiple national and institutional bureaucracies and regulatory regimes, and thus entail administrative costs not typically required by domestic research collaborations. For example, fluctuating currency exchange rates posed significant challenges for URI. Because URI was funded by a US grant, the organisation's budget was drafted in dollars. However, many of its expenses – including payroll – had to be paid in Ugandan shillings, the value of which shifted on a daily basis. URI paid employees according to the current exchange rate, but was required to pay payroll taxes to the Uganda Revenue

Authority on the 15th of the following month, by which time exchange rates had changed. The result was that URI was responsible for paying and taxing employees at two different exchange rates.

As the number of studies within the collaboration grew, URI began to struggle to cover its operating expenses on 8 per cent indirect cost reimbursement provided by the NIH. By 2009, the collaboration had expanded to employ close to 60 local staff and oversaw not only the flagship adherence study, but many other smaller HIV-related projects including studies concerning alcohol use, food insecurity, prevention education, lipoatrophy, transportation, mortality, dermatology, and pediatric adherence. URI was responsible for hiring staff, overseeing payroll, withholding taxes, and providing accounting and facilities management for all of these studies, all at the fixed 8 per cent indirect rate. Because the grants funding most of these studies were quite small (some studies, in fact, had no funding at all), the indirect cost reimbursements yielded little additional resources and the organisation began running at a deficit.

In 2009, URI carried out an extensive financial audit in preparation for the five-year renewal of the organisation. The report highlighted some major audit queries, especially the use of cash flow and breaches of Ugandan labour laws. These problems stemmed from the collaboration's growth and structure. As the collaboration expanded, each new study joined URI with a different budget for similar cadres of staff. This, in combination with the exchange rate variability, meant that URI records showed several different salaries for each employee. Further still, many employees had been inherited from the collaboration's earlier days (when they were paid as independent contractors by UCSF), and there were no records (such as interview reports, job descriptions, or contracts) documenting that they were legally employed by URI and in accordance with Ugandan labour regulations.

Thus, in order to streamline its operations and prepare for renewal, URI's director and board of governors initiated a restructuring process. In order to ensure proper job documentation, URI asked all the staff to reapply for their positions. The organisation's corporate governance structures were also established, and mid-level managers were hired to oversee employees. The research staff were asked to follow new communication channels in which they would communicate with their PIs through their new line managers, and not directly as they had previously done. New financial regulations were also implemented in which all employees would be both paid and taxed at a single exchange rate, which was determined by averaging exchange rates for the previous year (2008). Unfortunately, the new averaged rate was lower than the current rate, meaning that staff would be getting less money. This was not favourable for the staff who then wanted to revert to the previous management systems. The staff requested audience with the US PI, who then made an emergency visit to Uganda to hold a resolution meeting.

The URI management upheld their position on the new reforms, and this gave the US PI a chance to approach the MUST administration about the more permanent solution of establishing an internal contracts and grants office. The subsequent founding of the MUST grants office in December 2009 was a collaborative effort involving significant technical assistance from the US team, the successful application of an International Extramural Associates Research Development Awards (IEARDA) NIH grant to build institutional capacity, and considerable research and advocacy within MUST by the collaboration's project manager and Associate Professor Nozmo Mukiibi F. B., who would become the new office's director and authorised signatory official. The office became the first central contracts and grants office at a Ugandan public university, and as such represents a significant advance to build local fiscal capacity. The research collaboration, which has since shifted its US home institution from UCSF to Massachusetts General Hospital (MGH), now works directly and exclusively through the MUST grants office. URI went ahead with their renewal independently, and continues to engage in public health work in Uganda.

The need for capacity building did not end with the establishment of the MUST grants office. Rather, the fledgling office presented several challenges that required ongoing support from the research collaboration. As a grants office within a public university, it was subject to Ugandan government procurement policies – which often delayed purchases of equipment by months and at times years – and the demands of international funding agencies. Much of the office's new accounting staff were relatively inexperienced recent university graduates who had learned accounting manually and had to be trained in using accounting software. In addition, the new office had little experience with US government accounting practices, and this led to compliance problems early on. At its inception, the grants office pooled the money from its different grants into a single bank account. (This was intended both to prevent corruption and to save money, as the office had to pay for each bank account it opened.) However, a 2012 audit report from Uganda's Office of the Auditor General found that this approach left the grants office unable to accurately assess the balance of funds for individual projects, making it out of compliance with US regulations regarding federal funding.

The MUST grants office shared the results of this audit with the MGH team, and requested help in meeting US federal guidelines. The MGH team, in turn, requested help from their Office of Research Management, which oversees research activities at MGH and other hospitals under the Partners HealthCare umbrella. With help from the Office of Research Management (including a week-long Ugandan site visit by the office's Vice President), MUST and MGH devised a multi-pronged solution that included installing QuickBooks accounting software and training staff in its use, creating an individual QuickBooks account for each grant, and linking each grant to a separate bank account. These changes required significant investments in travel and training by visiting MGH staff, which notably could not be charged to the parent NIH grants. Following these interventions, the MUST grants office passed an independent audit conducted according to US government 'Yellow Book' standards by PricewaterhouseCoopers at a cost of US$20,000. The cost of this audit, coupled with the significant investments in staff training, far exceeded the MUST grants' office budget, which is funded entirely through indirect cost reimbursements. In other words, *the grants could not pay for the capacity-building costs associated with their own administration.*

Like URI before it, the MUST grants office is limited to 8 per cent indirect cost reimbursements on NIH grants, which constitute the bulk of its funding. MUST policy encourages an indirect cost reimbursement rate of 15 per cent, which is sometimes met by private foundations or non-US government funders. But the university hesitates to demand more out of fear of discouraging collaborators. In addition (and somewhat ironically, given our argument), some outside partners use the jobs, infrastructure, and capacity building brought by their projects to argue against higher indirect cost reimbursements. In our case study, the bulk of the costs of staff training and the independent audit were absorbed by MGH. However, none of these expenses could be charged to the parent grants, and MGH was forced to find other means of paying for them.

## Conclusion

Foreign institutions in low-income countries such as Uganda are co-producing significant knowledge in the global health sciences. Much of this knowledge is produced in 'partnership' with US universities, yet US research funding and administrative structures can paradoxically undermine rather than build research and grants management capacities at African partner institutions. Thus 'partnerships' with American institutions may be forced into unequal and extractive relationships at a structural level, regardless of the good intentions of those involved.

The case study presented here reflects some important themes in the management of academic global health partnerships. Established just prior to the recent rise of 'global operations' and 'global support' offices at US universities, URI's difficulties demonstrate both the need for a more coordinated approach to transnational fiscal administration and the pitfalls of non-investment in administrative capacity building. In this respect, the promotion of global health 'enabling systems' by the CUGH is a double-edged sword. Some of the challenges experienced by URI – such as the coordination of multiple currencies and compliance with local labour law – are issues that better supported enabling systems are designed to handle smoothly. More established and better funded university-affiliated non-profits, such as UWorld (University of Washington) and Harvard Global (Harvard University) are able to leverage legal and administrative expertise and resources in ways that undoubtedly ease the administrative burden that transnational partnerships entail. Nonetheless, at the same time, the case of URI demonstrates that the use of such proxy non-profits can allow US universities to circumvent local bureaucracy while externalising the legal and financial risk associated with international work. For example, it was the Ugandan director of URI, not the American PI or his US institution, that risked liability for URI's non-compliance with Ugandan financial and labour laws. By avoiding direct partnership with host institutions and deflecting risk from US universities, such administrative enabling systems may undermine the ethic of partnership and the goal of local capacity building.

In addition, it is important not to romanticise 'partnership' and to acknowledge that genuine capacity building and real partnership involve considerable institutional costs and risks. In our case study, the establishment of a successful grants office at MUST required large, unbudgeted expenditures by the collaboration, and these expenditures were largely born by the US partner, MGH. In addition, in partnering directly with MUST rather than using a stand-in non-profit like URI, MGH opened itself up to significant financial and reputational risk regarding sub-recipient monitoring. Had the MUST grants office been found in violation of US federal accounting practices, MGH could have been charged with misappropriation of funds and been forced to repay all of the grants in question to the federal government. It was the MGH leadership's strong commitment to building capacity – and the recognition that this must include building grants administration capacity – that made MGH willing to accept this risk.

We recognise that there are legitimate reasons why both foreign and local researchers may wish to avoid working directly with African public institutions, many of which have entrenched bureaucracies and have suffered from decades of underfunding due to both international structural adjustment policies and poor national management (Mamdani, 2011; Pfeiffer and Chapman, 2010). Addressing these problems effectively will require investment and risk-taking not only by international partners like MGH, but also by African governments (Boum, 2018). Even questionable governments are capable of making productive investments in health care, as Mika's (2016) account of recent developments in Ugandan oncology shows.

At the same time, it is important to state that the use of 'enabling systems' to circumvent African institutions is not simply a novel way to mitigate (real or imagined) corruption. Rather, it is a new example of a longstanding problem. For the last generation, US policies and programmes have worked to de-capacitate the African public sector, first by supporting structural adjustment programmes that defunded public health and more recently by promoting NGOs and other para-statal bodies as the primary partners for US projects and grants (Pfeiffer and Chapman, 2010; Prince and Marsland, 2014; Geissler, 2015). Ironically, as Geissler and Tousignant point out, the rise of 'capacity building' as a concept and a goal of international aid coincided with the erosion of the public sector in recently independent African nations, often via economic programmes promoted by donor nations (2016; Barnhart and Diallo, 2016). As the 2014–2016 West African Ebola outbreak made abundantly clear, the need for health systems strengthening in Africa remains imperative for both African and global health (Packard, 2016; Pfeiffer and Chapman, 2015). Why, then, do global health 'partnerships' so often result in the opposite?

Part of the answer may have to do with how past efforts at partnership are and are not remembered (Graboyes and Carr, 2016). If the failure of a global health partnership is interpreted as resulting from 'African' problems, then future partnerships will likely act on this memory by avoiding direct engagement with African institutions and public systems perceived as unreliable and/or corrupt. This is the logic that sustains the notion and structure of enabling systems. But if the failure of a partnership is remembered as stemming from transnational problems, the role of both 'donor' and 'host' nations and their respective institutions are implicated. This, in turn, might allow us to imagine systems that foster engagement between institutions, rather than enable partnerships that maintain Northern control. Institutional memory about how and why some partnerships *succeed* is equally important. For example, international portrayals of Botswana's HIV treatment programme – a collaboration between the government of Botswana, the Merck Foundation, and the Gates Foundation – emphasised the role played by scientific and business expertise, and assumed that government bureaucracy was an impediment to innovation rather than a productive force helping the partnership succeed (Carpenter, 2010). Thus, the institutional memory of this project attributed its success to private philanthropy and industry involvement, and not to public sector facilitation, even though ethnographic research demonstrated that Botswana government bureaucrats played a crucial role in enabling the programme to succeed, both on an organisational and an interpersonal level. How partnerships are interpreted is not only about the past, but also about the future, as institutional memory shapes knowledge and practice about how to build a successful collaboration and what it means to engage in meaningful capacity building (Graboyes and Carr, 2016).

To conclude, building research capacity in low-income countries, and especially in Africa, is a widely accepted goal among global health stakeholders, including the NIH (Chu, et al., 2014; NIH, 2013). Yet, at the same time, funders and institutions in high-income countries systematically underfund partner institutions and advocate the establishment of parallel fiscal and administrative systems that may drain local research capacity. As Chu et al. (2014) have argued recently, global health partnerships may be made more equitable and less extractive by building African research capacity. This must include training in research and publication skills, improved technological infrastructure, greater local control over research agendas, and increased African authorship of scientific papers. In addition, it must include genuine fiscal and administrative capacity building with partner African institutions. Global health partnerships cannot continue to systematically underfund and undermine the very institutions and research capacities they purport to build.

## Notes

1   The specific funding mechanisms we describe here are likely different in other world regions. However, we expect that some of the challenges regarding control over funding and institutional capacity apply broadly.
2   On its website, the CUGH describes the Enabling Systems Committee's work as 'set[ting] up guiding principles to include university administrations' procedural and financial alignment with programmatic priorities in global health' and 'develop[ing] strategies to effectively respond to global opportunities and share best practices for accepting and managing international risk, financial services, academic human resources, legal frameworks, communication and outreach, information technologies, transparency in approach and efficiencies with international sites' (Consortium of Universities for Global Health, n.d.).
3   It is worth noting that there is also a common perception amongst many people in African countries that American and other foreign entities are corrupt in that they essentially enrich themselves with money intended to support African health and development. These suspicions, in part, reflect the vast differences in pay, housing, and benefits between foreign and African national staff, and the significant amount of 'global health' money that ultimately benefits American/foreign institutions and economies (Barnhart and Diallo, 2016).

## References

Adams, V. (2016) *Metrics: What counts in global health*, Durham and London: Duke University Press.
Appel, H. (2012) 'Offshore work: oil, modularity, and the how of capitalism in Equatorial New Guinea', *American Ethnologist*, 39(4): 692–709.
Barnhart, S. and Diallo, J. (2016) 'Is the global health industry too self-serving in the fight against AIDS?', available at www.humanosphere.org/opinion/2016/12/op-ed-is-global-health-industry-too-self-serving-in-the-fight-against-aids/ (accessed on 24 November 2017).
Birn, A.E. (2009) 'The stages of international (global) health: histories of success or successes of history?', *Global Public Health*, 4(1): 50–68.
Birn, A.E. (2014) 'Philanthrocapitalism, past and present: the Rockefeller Foundation, the Gates Foundation, and the setting(s) of the international/global health agenda', *Hypothesis*, 12(1): e8.
Brainard, J. (2005) 'The ghosts of Stanford', *Chronicle of Higher Education*, A16–A18.
Brown, H. (2015) 'Global health partnerships, governance, and sovereign responsibility in western Kenya', *American Ethnologist*, 42(2): 340–55.
Boum II, Y. (2018) 'Is Africa part of the partnership?', *Medicine Anthropology Theory*, 5(2): 25–34.

Carpenter, E.A. (2010) 'The invisible bureaucrat in Botswana's HIV drug therapy program', In: *Social Health in the New Millennium: A conference in honor of Steven Feierman*, University of Pennsylvania.

Chu, K.M., Jayaraman, S., Kyamanywa, P., and Ntakiyiruta, G. (2014) 'Building research capacity in Africa: equity and global health collaborations', *PLoS Medicine*, 11(3): e1001612.

Committee on Finance. (2010) 'Annual report on newly approved indirect costs and discussion of the recovery of indirect costs from research', available at http://regents.universityofcalifornia.edu/regmeet/nov10/f2.pdf (accessed on 20 November 2017).

Conteh, L. and Kingori, P. (2010) 'Per diems in Africa: a counter-argument', *Tropical Medicine and International Health*, 15(12): 1553–5.

Crane, J.T. (2010) 'Unequal "partners". AIDS, academia, and the rise of global health', BEHEMOTH-A Journal on Civilisation, 3(3): 78–97.

Crane, J.T. (2013) *Scrambling for Africa: AIDS, expertise, and the rise of American global health science*, Ithaca, NY: Cornell University Press.

Consortium of Universities for Global Health. (n.d.) 'Enabling systems', available at www.cugh.org/programs/enabling-systems (accessed on 16 June 2016).

Geissler, P.W. (2013) 'Public secrets in public health: knowing not to know while making scientific knowledge', *American Ethnologist*, 40:13–34.

Geissler, P.W. (Ed.) (2015) *Para-States and Medical Science: Making African global health*, Durham, NC: Duke University Press.

Geissler, P.W. and Tousignant, N. (2016) 'Capacity as history and horizon: infrastructure, autonomy and future in African health science and care', *Canadian Journal of African Studies / Revue Canadienne Des études Africaines*, 50(3): 349–59.

Giles-Vernick, T. and Webb, J. (2013) *Global Health in Africa: Historical perspectives on disease control*, Athens, OH: Ohio University Press.

Graboyes, M. and Carr, H. (2016) 'Institutional memory, institutional capacity: narratives of failed biomedical encounters in East Africa', *Canadian Journal of African Studies / Revue Canadienne Des études Africaines*, 50(3): 361–77.

Koplan, J.P., Bond, T.C., Merson, M.H., Reddy, K.S., Rodriguez, M.H., Sewankambo, N.K., and Wasserheit, J.N. for the Consortium of Universities for Global Health Executive Board. (2009) 'Towards a common definition of global health', *The Lancet*, 373: 1993–5.

Mamdani, M. (2011) 'The importance of research in a university', *Pambazuka News*, (526).

Matheson, A.I., Walson, J.L., Pfeiffer, J., and Holmes, K. (2014) 'Sustainability and growth of university global health programs', Center for Strategic and International Studies, available at www.csis.org/analysis/sustainability-and-growth-university-global-health-programs (accessed on 24 November 2017).

McKay, R. (2012) 'Documentary disorders: managing medical multiplicity in Maputo, Mozambique', *American Ethnologist*, 39(3): 545–61.

Merriam-Webster. (n.d.) 'Enable', available at www.merriam-webster.com/dictionary/enable (accessed on 1 June 2017).

Mika, M. (2016) 'Fifty years of creativity, crisis, and cancer in Uganda', *Canadian Journal of African Studies / Revue Canadienne Des études Africaines*, 50(3): 395–413.

NIH. (2011) 'Indirect costs', available at https://oalm.od.nih.gov/IndirectCostsFAQ#difference (accessed on 20 November 2017).

NIH. (2013) 'Building global health research capacity', available at https://report.nih.gov/NIHfactsheets/ViewFactSheet.aspx?csid=74&key=B#B (accessed on 20 November 2017).

Okeke, I. (2018) 'Partnerships for now?', *Medicine Anthropology Theory*, 5(2): 7–24.

Okwaro, F.M. and Geissler, P.W. (2015) 'In/dependent collaborations: perceptions and experiences of African scientists in transnational HIV research: transnational collaborations and HIV research', *Medical Anthropology Quarterly*, 29(4): 492–511.

Packard, R. (2016) *A History of Global Health: Interventions into the lives of other peoples*, Baltimore, MD: Johns Hopkins University Press.

Pfeiffer, J. and Chapman, R. (2010) 'Anthropological perspectives on structural adjustment and public health', *Annual Review of Anthropology*, 39: 149–65.

Pfeiffer, J. and Chapman, R. (2015) 'An anthropology of aid in Africa', *The Lancet*, 385(9983): 2144–5.

Prince, R. and Marsland, R. (2014) *Making and Unmaking Public Health in Africa: Ethnographic and historical perspectives*, Athens, OH: Ohio University Press.

Smith, D.J. (2007) *A Culture of Corruption*, Princeton, NJ: Princeton University Press.

Vaughan, M. (1991) *Curing Their Ills: Colonial power and African illness*, Stanford, CA: Stanford University Press.

Wendland, C. (2016) 'Opening up the black box: looking for a more capacious version of capacity in global health partnerships', *Canadian Journal of African Studies / Revue Canadienne Des études Africaines*, 50(3): 415–35.

# 6

# From global health to planetary and micro global health

## Theorising global health's present remodeling and scaling

*João Biehl and Yi-Ching Ong*

## Introduction – worlds on the edge

We live in interconnected, yet also radically unequal, insecure, and unhealthy worlds: worlds on the edge. The spread of infectious disease across borders, struggles over access to treatments, and the rise in chronic disease pose highly complex and often unpredictable challenges – realities that are, time and again, couched in the vocabulary of emergency, hinging on a temporality that insists on a break with the past, and a rhetoric of compassion, recovery, and progress even as conditions stagnate or worsen (Pinker, 2018; Easterbrook, 2018). Accelerating environmental change, the visible and invisible wounds of ongoing war and mass migration, and the tolls of poverty and discrimination within precarious health systems all create conditions of dire vulnerability. What algorithms generate insight about the medical and political dimensions of present and coming health challenges, or help navigate questions of accountability (especially those posed by local communities) and our ethical 'response-ability' (Haraway, 2007, p. 89), now and on the horizon?

Reflecting both on recent challenges – in particular, the West African Ebola outbreak (2014–2016) – and on emerging remodelings of the field, this chapter advocates for a critical and people-centred approach both to and within global health. We begin by scrutinising how global health acquired its contemporary configuration, followed by discussing prominent theoretical responses. With this understanding of global health as a plastic and expansive political, economic, and technological work-in-progress, we then consider how the field is being reconfigured through new movements (such as planetary health and humanitarian technology design). As we trace shifting relationships between theory, method, and praxis across scales and time, we examine how successes and failures are far from easy to predict or assess; rather, local worlds emerge as sites of continual experimentation. We therefore argue that an ethnographic focus on evidence and efficacy at the local level raises rather than lowers the bar for thoughtful inquiry and action.

The current moment calls less for the all-knowing hubris of totalising analytical schemes than for a human science (and politics) of the uncertain and unknown (Biehl and Locke, 2017; Petryna, 2015). Ethnography can serve as an 'empirical lantern' (Hirschman, 1998, p. 88) within and beyond theories of health in all their various forms, highlighting how the targets of interventions implode the units and models through which they are conceptualised, producing contrapuntal knowledge of how things are, what sustains their intractability, and how they might be otherwise (Biehl and Petryna, 2013a).

## Global health as 'open-source anarchy'

The West African Ebola outbreak was an 'acute-on-chronic' event, in the words of physician-anthropologist Paul Farmer (2011, p. 3): part and parcel of long-smoldering public health crises that humanitarian and global health interventions and politics as usual could not placate (or had even fueled), and with compounding deadly effects that people had to fight, at least initially, by themselves. As Jeremy Farrar, director of the Wellcome Trust, and Peter Piot, who helped to discover the Ebola virus, rightly pointed out, 'the particularly devastating course of this epidemic' could not be attributed to the 'biologic characteristics of the virus' alone (2014, p. 1545). It was, rather, the result of the combination of 'dysfunctional health systems, international indifference, high population mobility, local customs, densely populated capitals, and lack of trust in authorities after years of armed conflict' (Farrar and Piot, 2014, p. 1545; see also Piot, 2013). And, perhaps most importantly, it was 'a highly inadequate and late global response' (Farrar and Piot, 2014, p. 1545). The tragic limitations of this response were all too apparent as Ebola kept crossing borders – the grotesque disparities in risk and outcome between regions affected reflect both our technical prowess and the inequalities built into current world orders and value systems. In the aftermath of the epidemic, the limits of global health have again been exposed as funding and attention has been withdrawn, even as 'suffering certainly continues … in the form of clinical sequelae, lost livelihoods and loved ones, broken communities, food insecurity, and "stigma"' (Richardson, et al., 2017b, p. 80).

So, how did we get here?

Displacing earlier framings, such as colonial-era tropical medicine and postwar international health, the contemporary field of global health brings together a vastly diverse array of actors and interests in elastic relationships, and it has indeed become a big business (Brown, et al., 2006). Informed by various agendas, the World Health Organization, the World Bank, the Gates Foundation, pharmaceutical companies, governments, universities, and innumerable nongovernmental organisations are all working to address pressing health issues worldwide with unprecedented financial and technological resources (Biehl and Petryna, 2013a). Changes in the material and political capabilities of state and non-state actors, and changes in the world of ideas, now have more impact on each other than in the closed, state-centric system that prevailed during the Cold War. In this shifting matrix of actors and institutions, health variously emerges as an object of 'humanitarian reason' – as Didier Fassin (2011) would call it – and as an instrument of economic development, diplomacy, national security, or market expansion. Yet, even though these implicit agendas may collide or produce unintended consequences for communities and their health, global health players can become impervious to critique as they identify crises, cite dire statistics, and act upon these perceived needs. Likewise, declarations of crises' endings, and the attendant scaling back of efforts or shifting in priorities, are often presented as self-evident imperatives (Kenworthy, et al., 2018; Richardson, et al., 2017b).

Although activity in global health has increased markedly as new influxes of funding have entered the field, a concern for limited resources is still widely shared among scholars and practitioners – that is, 'socialization for scarcity' remains widespread, in Paul Farmer's words (Farmer, 2011, p. 254). This concern has partly manifested as an interest in finding cost-effective solutions that can be easily replicated and scaled up across a range of widely divergent contexts. In this vein, much of global health scholarship aims to develop models – more or less hypothetical – of such optimal interventions, and to identify and evaluate programmes that supposedly 'work' and that might lend themselves to replication and scaling.

Accordingly, evidence-based medicine and evidence-based policy have become the default languages for both public- and private-sector actors concerned with identifying problems and measuring outcomes (Adams, 2013a; Storeng and Béhague, 2014). This new landscape of evaluation is displacing the previous goals of interventions, making the provision of actual health services secondary to the development of reliable methodologies and the generation of comparable data. Metrics are presented as objective, value free, and abstracted from social and political contexts. Yet, in reality, as Vincanne Adams and colleagues (Adams,

2016) have noted, they operate as administrative apparatuses that shape health futures by reducing the noise of context and enabling business management rationalisations and decision-making.

The complex juxtaposition of agendas within the field of global health can be vividly seen in the case of treatment access, which has been one of the central tenets of global health activism and a professed goal of interventions since the mid-1990s (Nguyen, 2010). Public–private partnerships are booming and pharmaceutical companies have rebranded themselves as 'global health companies', making older treatments available and expediting access to newer ones (Biehl and Petryna, 2013b). We now see a multiplicity of actors, all vying for resources and influence while setting new norms for institutional response, sometimes providing the public health resources that states and markets have failed to furnish. In practice, the concerns of donors, not recipients, tend to predominate. Often, donors insist on funding disease-specific and technologically oriented vertical programmes at the expense of the public sector. Thus, in settings ranging from neoliberal Mozambique to urban North America, state-of-the-art facilities for HIV/AIDS coexist with dilapidated public hospitals (Pfeiffer, 2013).

Such narrowly targeted interventions may represent more than lost opportunities for investment in broader health systems – they also divert much-needed attention from addressing the complex patterns in which diseases manifest in individuals and populations, or what medical anthropologist Merrill Singer has termed 'syndemics' (Singer, et al., 2017). Co-infections, for example, are highly common, and notably so for the so-called 'Big 3' infectious diseases in global health (HIV/AIDS, tuberculosis, and malaria). And yet, while no one contracts or recovers from such diseases in a vacuum, much remains to be elucidated as to the biological pathways through which these diseases interact within individuals and populations, and how these interactions may complicate attempts at prevention and treatment (Griffiths, et al., 2011; Singer, et al., 2017). Beyond these biological interactions, much also remains to be understood as to how clusters of disease can emerge from sociopolitical environments of particular vulnerability. The vital importance of taking these interactions into account is evident from our recent experience with Ebola, where diminished access to health care during the epidemic led to increased mortality from malaria, HIV/AIDS, and tuberculosis (Parpia, et al., 2016). Similarly, population biologists warned that a 'second public health crisis' might follow Ebola, if concerted efforts to restore vital health services, such as childhood vaccinations for measles, were not made (Takahashi, et al., 2015).

Amid these calls for integration, however, multiple and fragmentary global health interventions remain more the rule than the exception, consolidating what anthropologist Susan Reynolds Whyte and her colleagues (2014) working in Uganda call 'projectified' landscapes of care. While enabling much-needed access to AIDS treatment, for example, the amalgamation of public–private interventions can endow states with new (sometimes abusive) powers while also diversifying claims to citizenship. We are left with what legal scholar David Fidler (2008, p. 260), would call an 'open-source anarchy' around global health problems – a policy space in which new medical technologies, ideas, strategies, rules, distributive schemes, and the practical ethics of health care are being assembled, experimented with, and improvised by a wide array of deeply unequal stakeholders within and across countries (Biehl, 2007).

Within this increasingly crowded landscape, the supposed beneficiaries of interventions are too often hidden from view, and appear either as having nothing to contribute or as unabashedly, uncritically receptive. While there have been some efforts to engage civil society and activists, a strong biomedical orientation remains pervasive, casting community engagement as politically necessary but 'scientifically' irrelevant (Biehl, 2007). As hopes for a magic bullet reign and the power of 'data' is ever more leveraged and fetishised, the visions of technocrats tend to outweigh other forms of practical and meaningful evidence. For example, 'technocratic ways of thinking' (Richardson, et al., 2017a, p. e255) in epidemiology may constrain the collection, use, and interpretation of data, yielding models that reinforce a biomedical paradigm in which individuals and their 'choices' are key drivers of disease spread, and obscuring the role of other crucial social and institutional drivers. Relatedly, as technocrats seek 'gold standard' practices that can be universally applied, emphasis has grown on interventions that can be readily packaged for many settings and assessed according to easily measured outcomes; such outcomes offer an illusion of precision, but may not predict the interventions' potential elsewhere, or reflect their true impact on communities (Adams, 2016). As even Angus Deaton, the recent Nobel laureate economist, has emphasised: 'Randomized control trials have been given a free pass in the name of rigor. But there are no magic bullets and there are no gold standards' (Deaton, 2012; see also Deaton 2013).

The human populations that constitute the subjects of health and development plans, however, are not flat and homogeneous – nor are they the source of problems or so-called cultural obstacles. Epistemological breakthroughs do not belong to experts and analysts alone; people's practical knowledge can help break open and transform paradigms (Biehl and Petryna, 2014). The Ebola crisis illustrates how core determinants of health resist technical and theoretical quick fixes, as it was ultimately sociocultural knowledge that proved crucial to enacting effective control efforts (Amon, 2014). Intended to minimise disease transmission, for example, curfews and quarantines failed to take into account historical and contemporary tensions between peoples and governments in Guinea, Sierra Leone, and Liberia, backfiring so spectacularly that in August 2015, Liberian troops ended up shooting at people protesting such draconian and ill-conceived measures. Social scientists on the ground have shown why curfews and quarantines were received so poorly, even violently; why rumors about Ebola needed to be taken seriously rather than dismissed as illogical or paranoid; and why bereaved families hid bodies, rather than surrendering them for sanctioned burial (Frankfurter, 2014). The recognition of history, politics, and culture productively liberate people from the decontextualised, faceless, and pliable role of 'victim' (Edelstein, et al., 2015; Global Citizen, 2015). As Amon describes in his analysis of the global health response to HIV/AIDS, behaviours that are officially denigrated as 'noncompliance' or 'ignorance' are often the result of 'structural and human rights barriers that … affect attempts to act on the information gained' (Amon, 2013, p. 102). If policy is to seriously engage with human rights – especially as 'the most fundamental principle of rights [is] that all individuals should be treated equally and with dignity' (Amon, 2013, p. 107) – 'people-centred' evidence for policy is vital (Biehl and Petryna, 2013a).

Moreover, a focus on the institutional cultures of various organisations themselves highlights how much of the responsibility for the epidemic lay not with culture itself – as if culture were something bounded, inherently irrational, or dangerous – but with particular decisions and disagreements within and among a global class of supposed saviors and scientific forecasters. Indeed, to this latter point, Eugene Richardson and colleagues argue that we should not only indict missing health care and governance infrastructures, but also an 'impoverished discursive infrastructure of contemporary public health … [that] implicate[d] marginalized individuals as sources of outbreaks' (Richardson, et al., 2017a, p. e255) and thus lent support to the rigid enforcement of containment strategies.

At stake, then, is not just technopolitical preparedness but also critical social scientific preparedness. As Andrew Lakoff notes, retrospective assessment of failures in global health is often followed by official vows to be better prepared for the next emergency (Lakoff, et al., 2015; Lakoff, 2017). So, what should such scientific preparedness look like? If we take seriously the role of science and the conceptual categories it produces in guiding the course of global health assessments and interventions, we must then also consider global health theories and their relationships to praxis with greater scrutiny. Richard Horton, editor-in-chief of *The Lancet*, has called for 'radical changes in behavior' in governance at the global scale (Horton, 2014b, p. 2186) – and this call could be extended to knowledge-making as well. To unpack nonmedical determinants – a lack of emergency preparedness, the capacity of frail or nonexistent health systems, myopic funding mechanisms, and slow-coming political action – we need to move out of our comfortable disciplinary silos and produce empirically rich, comprehensive, 'historically deep and geographically broad' (Farmer, et al., 2013, p. 2) analyses of the power constellations, institutions, processes, and ideologies that impact the form and scope of disease and health processes. This work can aid us in imagining how to develop human and institutional capacities that go beyond the repetition of history and that can help to defend, in a spirit of radical political openness, what Albert Hirschman (1971, p. 37) calls 'the right to a non-projected future as one of the truly inalienable rights of every person and nation'.

## Theorising global health

If global health has emerged as a prominent sphere of action and intervention, its consolidation as a field has called for new kinds of scrutiny (Janes and Corbett, 2009). A number of important critiques have emerged, destabilising assumed global health architectures and imperatives, and challenging our sense of what counts as 'global'. While unearthing the dominant epistemic and political modes that enable global health operations, social theorists have also thought critically about what kinds of interventions are actually workable, desirable, or ethical in the face of widespread disease, new vectors and disasters, toxic environments, and deadly health disparities (Biehl and Petryna, 2014; Das, 2015). Attending to these inquiries helps us to better grasp what is at work and at stake in contemporary global health, and to push our methods and analytics to better account for messy entanglements on the ground.

A first body of critique understands global health as a neocolonial or post-colonial imperial project. Historian of science Warwick Anderson, for example, not only argues that biomedicine is 'constitutively colonial' (2014, p. 381), but questions how too-easy binaries of domination and submission miss the complex post-colonial 'contact zones' in which relations of power unfold in multiple, shifting, and contested ways. Against the linear march of a triumphant narrative of globalisation, he attends to how global health both perpetuates and obscures colonial dynamics and to how global 'flows' rarely circulate smoothly. Such critiques resonate with the recent Ebola epidemic. Long before the outbreak erupted, the colonial legacy of the 'rubber plantation model of international health' shaped dramatic inequality in access to knowledge as well as resources (Dahn, et al., 2015). As early as 1982, scientific research warned of Ebola risk in the region, yet these findings – based on research carried out on the bodies of Liberian rubber workers by German scientists and published in a European journal – were never brought back to Liberia. The 'flows' of research were less 'flows' than lopsided allocations.

Where Anderson productively argues for a more multifaceted view of colonialism and post-colonialism, Jean and John Comaroff (2012), too, work to decentre global sovereignty, rejecting the conflation of 'the global' with the 'Euro-American'. 'Theory from the South', in the Comaroffs' telling, not only flips the West/non-West binary but destabilises it, casting the global South as 'a harbinger of history-in-the-making' (2012, p. 13). And indeed, countries in the global South are actively altering global health agendas for their own ends, through South–South partnerships, the circulation of generic pharmaceuticals, the contestation of trade and patent agreements, and the opening up of new markets (Cassier and Correa, 2008; Rajan, 2017). As in the case of Brazil (Biehl, 2007, 2013; Biehl and Petryna, 2013b), these countries are at once implicated in the broader landscapes of global health, and are forging novel dynamics for health care between markets, states, and citizens.

A second line of critique explores how global health reflects and shores up a capitalist neoliberal world order. Anne-Emanuelle Birn, for example, highlights how global health concerns merge with geoeconomic interests, increasingly under the purview of private-sector actors (Birn, 2014; Birn and Dmitrienko, 2005). The capacities and interests of public multilateral health agencies give way to an 'asymmetry of power' between private-sector actors and public interests, and philanthropic efforts to improve health and quality of life may in fact reinforce the very inequities they seek to overcome (Birn, 2014). Such arguments also dovetail with what Naomi Klein (2007) has called 'disaster capitalism', when, in moments of health emergency, the chaos of crisis is harnessed to implement controversial neoliberal policies while 'shock' prevents citizens from mobilising resistance. As both Klein and anthropologists Anne Lovell (2011) and Vincanne Adams (2013b) observed in the aftermath of Hurricane Katrina, the less obvious effects of disaster capitalism include the creation (and destruction) of infrastructures and mechanisms of social displacement and eviction, which get prolonged as a way of life while bureaucratic processes reproduce (rather than dismantle) conditions of vulnerability.

Physician-anthropologist Paul Farmer is one of the most vocal critics of the structural violence wrought by neoliberalism, taking on poverty and disease through a community-based approach that blends technological intervention with a focus on making health systems work. Farmer and Partners In Health (PIH), the organisation he cofounded, understand diseases as loci where biology, environment, and medicine have gone awry, and their notion of intervention accordingly tackles the structural conditions that perpetuate disease (Keshavjee, 2014). During the recent Ebola outbreak in Liberia and Sierra Leone, PIH-affiliated scholars argued forcefully that 'policies that pit[ted] prevention against care' (Cancedda, et al., 2016, p. S156) were counterproductive – while they aimed to prioritise prevention, they actually served to deter sick individuals from seeking health care and undermine community trust, thereby hampering efforts to identify, isolate, and treat Ebola-infected patients. PIH practitioners thus attempted to balance their approach to reflect emphasis on both prevention of new infections and caring for infected patients to improve their outcomes (Cancedda, et al., 2016). Furthermore, they challenged foreign interventionist approaches to the epidemic, hiring approximately two thousand local community members, including Ebola survivors, as community health care workers and contact tracers to work alongside two hundred foreign medics (Partners in Health, n.d.). Such hiring practices facilitated local trust and helped build up a more accessible community health care network that has persisted after Ebola subsided and foreign/silo interventions ended (Cancedda, et al., 2016; Richardson, et al., 2017a). Farmer's and PIH's work serves as a kind of critique in action, rejecting economic orthodoxies and taking a social justice approach to patient care.

A third critique of global health takes a more Foucauldian approach, focusing on the new regimes of governmentality and biosecurity reconfiguring discourse and practice around health and risk. As scholars like Andrew Lakoff and Stephen Collier (2008, p. 16) have argued, biosecurity in the realm of global health troubles traditional regulatory boundaries, as biological threats move without regard to borders, and globalisation becomes 'a key source of pathogenicity'. In this 'emergency modality of intervention', approaches shift from prevention to preparedness, creating new modes of surveillance and intervention, and encouraging technical responses without much concern for ongoing living conditions (Lakoff, et al., 2015; Lakoff, 2017). While these are compelling and important arguments on the level of institutional biosecuritisation, this critical body of work largely tends to overlook local perspectives, leaving little space for asking how people exist amidst, and lodge their own lived critiques of, such regimes of biosecuritisation. Furthermore, the trope of security functions through a largely Westernised notion of governmental operants and biopower. What other forms of securitisation exist elsewhere, and what clashes occur when they come into contact via global health interventions?

An emerging body of scholarship based on research undertaken in the global South offers an important swerve here, hinting at how critiques of governmentality might more fully account for the social and political. Katherine Mason's ethnographic work on SARS control efforts in Shenzhen, China, illustrates some of the 'microprocesses by which biosecurity discourses become intertwined with existing local discourses about who carries disease, who is dangerous, who belongs, and who does not' (Mason, 2012, p. 114). She evinces how an increasingly biosecuritised discourse around infectious disease outbreaks in China mutually legitimates and reinforces existing discrimination against migrant workers. In a similar vein, Brazilian public health and legal scholar Deisy Ventura explores how, in Brazil, 'the securitisation of the response to Zika turned the *Aedes aegypti* mosquito into public enemy number one' (Ventura, 2016, p. 3). She argues that the depiction of disease as a 'security threat' can also have other effects, including panic, haste, suspicion, and discrimination, as certain populations are labeled as vectors or 'at risk'. Such securitisation, Ventura argues, fosters a proliferation of surveillance techniques to prevent the spread of disease, exerting control not only over the microbial pathogens themselves but also over the myriad vectors that carry them (in other words, persons and goods). Moreover, the 'risk' Ventura foresees in her analysis dooms global health to ongoing periods of 'war' and 'truce' as opposed to a systematic practice addressing the infrastructural roots of socially determined health outcomes (Diniz, 2017).

A final sphere of critique has approached global health as a form of transnational humanitarianism. Perhaps best exemplified by the work of Fassin (2011), these critiques see global health as an extension of a broader form of humanitarian reason, which has become a dominant form of moral thinking in the West. Fassin (2012) cautions against taking the 'idea' of global health for granted, interrogating the assumptions of both 'global' – ultimately neither universal nor ever truly worldwide – and 'health' – where the politics of life are never a given. Attentive to how compassion in the face of suffering can be depoliticising, and to the ways humanitarian intervention has become an increasingly important form of global governance, Fassin and others rightly trouble our complacency about acting 'in the name of humanity', and highlight the inequality and violence that accompanies care (Redfield, 2013; Ticktin and Feldman, 2010; Han, 2012; Stevenson, 2014).

Yet, while critiques of global health as humanitarianism can nuance our thinking about rationality, interventionism, and morality, in certain forms their uptake can also elide the very possibility of engagement itself. Grossly oversimplifying the anthropological engagements with suffering, poverty, violence, and affliction as akin to critical and heroic impulses towards universal humanity and salvation (Robbins, 2013; Ticktin, 2014), such approaches can themselves produce a kind of myopia, missing ethnographic ambiguities and the complexities of how projects are actually conceptualised, implemented, and worked out, or desired by people themselves. Scholars like Farmer, engaged in the practical work of delivering care on the ground, highlight the deep ambiguities that coexist with new potentials and impasses, while also refusing to disengage from action in the face of radical injustice, despite inevitable double binds and ethical gray zones. Analytical distance too easily becomes a sanctioned form of moral detachment that dooms people differently than humanitarian reason – but dooms them nonetheless. The challenge here is to restore to the social sciences a sense of moral purpose and practical solidarity that might animate both critical thought and social action (Wilkinson and Kleinman, 2015; Briggs and Mantini-Briggs, 2016; Biehl and Locke, 2017).

## The plasticity of global health

Given the historical landscape of global health and the tensions raised by the critiques outlined previously, what should we make of ongoing attempts to remodel the field?

In what follows, we examine two distinct ways in which modes of conceptualising and acting in global health are shifting, as actors and institutions in the field search for alternatives. These two emerging frameworks – planetary health and humanitarian design – emphasise dramatically different scales of study and intervention, from the massive scope of geophysical and ecological change represented by planetary health (Horton, et al., 2014a), to the micro-worlds of humanitarian design (Redfield, 2016; Collier, et al., 2017). These differing scalar narratives function, as Nicholas King has argued, to 'invoke places and spaces at different geographic scales to explain events, enlist allies, and attract attention' (King, 2004, p. 63); and indeed, these narratives have been powerful in mobilising interest and material support. Following Bruno Latour's critical analysis of how the scale of health problems is reformulated to advance certain modes of science and health interventions (1983), we might therefore ask: what are the scientific premises at work here, and how might this shift approaches to intervention? Much remains to be seen as these initiatives continue to unfold, but we trace here how these frameworks aspire to and conceptualise change in global health, and how they represent both continuity and disjuncture with their preceding paradigms.

### Planetary health

Planetary health has emerged recently and with great fanfare as an extension of, or successor to, the field of global health. Judith Rodin (2015), President of the Rockefeller Foundation, idealistically termed it a vision of 'public health 2.0 – one that goes beyond the boundaries of our existing global health framework to take into consideration the natural systems upon which human health depends.' The manifesto outlining the goals of planetary health states that what is at stake is nothing less than the creation of 'a social movement to support collective public health action at all levels of society – personal, community, national, regional, global, and planetary … our vision is for a planet that nourishes and sustains the diversity of life with which we coexist' (Horton, et al., 2014a, p. 847). This new field sets out to provide a unifying framework for research and action that broadens the scope beyond the traditional ambit of human health and health care to include all the political, economic, social, environmental, and technological systems that impact human interactions with (and impact upon) Earth's geophysical and ecological systems. As signaled by its name, which invokes the grandeur of the cosmos, planetary health sets out to 'work at large scales, both spatially (from regional to global) and temporally (anticipating the effects of current trends across generations)' (Frumkin and Myers, 2017).

This turn to integrating environmental concerns with more conventional approaches to global health has been slowly gaining influence over time. Since the 1990s, the importance of interconnections between human health and the social, physical, and biological environments was advanced in academic circles through various eco-health and ecosystem approaches to public health (Wolf, 2015). In the 2000s, this movement gained further traction in international policy circles, as the One Health framework (which advocates for approaches that acknowledge interconnections between human, animal, and environmental health) was officially recognised by large organisations such as the United States' Center for Disease Control, the World Health Organization, the World Bank, and the United Nations. Growing concern for environmental sustainability among the broader international development community is also reflected in the transition from the Millennium Development Goals development era of 2000–2015 to the present era, guided by the Sustainable Development Goals and their concern for the 'triple bottom line … a combination of economic development, environmental sustainability, and social inclusion' (Sachs, 2012, p. 2206). Alongside this, concern over the implications and extent of human influence upon the environment has become increasingly widespread in the academic and popular discourse, as reflected by the rapid rise of the term 'Anthropocene' in recent years (Steffen, et al., 2011). Planetary health draws upon these coalitions of interest, but has benefited from a particularly concerted push to establish it as a distinctive field and framework for action. With funding from the Rockefeller Foundation and the Wellcome Trust, the field of planetary health has rapidly expanded – new academic journals dedicated to the field have been launched (including a subsidiary of *The Lancet*), and almost 20 universities have introduced programmes or classes in planetary health (Frumkin and Myers, 2017).

While it remains to be seen how exactly this surge of interest in planetary health research will manifest itself in new knowledge and on-the-ground interventions, we may nonetheless examine how planetary health intersects with some of the main critiques of global health. In its emphasis on envisioning and implementing more sustainable modes of living and organising, planetary health explicitly sets out to provide a counter-vision to a capitalist neoliberal world order and call into question patterns of overconsumption and unrestrained extraction (Horton, et al., 2014a). Other shifts in discourse, however, are less inherent to the planetary health framework and may represent potential areas for concern. Although planetary health sets out to advance principles of equity and inclusion, James Fairhead and colleagues (2012) point out that environmental issues have sometimes been conduits for colonial or neocolonial expressions of unequal power dynamics. They argue that 'notions of "green" (and what, and who, is green or not) come to be defined and mobilized in particular ways' (Fairhead, et al., 2012, p. 239), leading to contested policies such as 'green grabbing', or appropriation of resources for environmental ends that may involve significant alienation of afflicted communities. Such policies, they suggest, reflect an 'economy of repair' where powerful actors and states presume 'that unsustainable use "here" can be repaired by sustainable practices "there", with one nature subordinated to the other' (Fairhead, et al., 2012, p. 242). Careful attention will thus be required to guard against such potential exacerbation of existing global inequities as policies are pursued under the planetary health rubric.

Moreover, although framers of planetary health have called for transformation of the closed and hierarchical nature of knowledge production (Horton, 2013), robust institutional backing for this agenda has not been forthcoming. Decrying the production of knowledge from within disciplinary silos in academia, Richard Horton argues that,

> Planetary health demands more open knowledge systems – where valid knowledge comes from many societal sources, where universities are organized according to the problems society faces ... and where the products of research are available to all and in forms that meet the needs of diverse public communities.
>
> *Horton, 2013, p. 1012*

However, although similar calls for more interdisciplinary and democratic processes of science making have been made before, they have often met with both epistemological and institutional obstacles (Brondizio, et al., 2016).

A retrospective analysis of the One Health framework that prefigured planetary health may offer some insight. Meike Wolf argues that although the One Health framework aspired towards integrated and inter-disciplinary knowledge, in practice it was limited by a 'traditional biomedical model' of disease emergence and transmission that focused primarily on 'improved medical education and care as a solution to the problem of emerging zoonotic diseases' and neglected to situate human-animal encounters in a broader sociopolitical and cultural context (Wolf, 2015, p. 6). Studies that have attempted such contextualisation are relatively rare – a useful exemplar of possibilities in this line is Hannah Brown and Ann Kelly's work on viral hemorrhagic fever transmission, which elaborates the interactions between viral pathogen, animal reservoir, and human hosts and situates these biologically embodied encounters within a social context of care-giving and a historical context of post-colonial economies (Brown and Kelly, 2014). In doing so, Brown and Kelly point out the limitations of 'conceptualizing expertise as falling into discrete domains' and argue that 'a robust multi-dimensional approach to public health interventions rests on drawing together distinct ways of knowing rather than integrating different objects of knowledge' (Brown and Kelly, 2014, p. 294). Careful attention to, and integration of, insights from across the natural and social sciences will be crucial to ensuring that planetary health lives up to its aspirations to 'emphasize people, not diseases, and equity, not the creation of unjust societies' (Horton, et al., 2014a, p. 847; Brondizio, et al., 2016).

One of the key challenges for a more integrated science of planetary health is the current emphasis on 'large scales'. While this is necessary to call attention to the grand scope of the geophysical processes at work, and may even evoke a beneficial sense of shared purpose for some, care must be taken to attend to scales at which health is far from a shared experience. The threats of anthropogenic environmental change are sometimes presented as collective afflictions that can therefore spark collective action – as sociologist Ulrich Beck famously argued, 'poverty is hierarchic, [but] smog is democratic' (Beck, 1992, p. 36). As many subsequent critics of Beck have argued, however, this narrative of universalised environmental risk deflects attention from what we know about environmental hazards, which are often unequally distributed and dis-proportionately affect vulnerable communities with low socio-economic status (Brulle and Pellow, 2006). Reflecting on climate change in particular, historian Dipesh Chakrabarty suggests that 'the crisis ... will be routed through all our "anthropological differences" ... [thus] there is no corresponding "humanity" that in its oneness can act as a political agent' (2012, p.14). And indeed, current emergencies in health – from the Zika virus in northeastern Brazil to the water contamination in Flint, Michigan – speak to how bodies, infrastructures, technologies, and evidence are unequally shared and lived.

No longer a mere backdrop, environmental materials and infrastructures (from water management, sewage, and road systems, to birth control methods and pesticides) actually assume a central, often agentive role, interacting with communities in ways unaccounted for, and many times harmful (Barreto, et al., 2016; Bellinger, 2016). Even as we debate the necessity of transitioning to new modes of production and consumption, we still inhabit a 'chemical infrastructure' that forms the embodied 'legacy of a passing industrial capitalist age' (Nading, 2017, p. 145). Characterising these environmental effects on human bodies, however, poses notable challenges to toxicological research and epidemiological studies of causality. Confounding previous scientific intuitions, nonlinear relationships between exposure dose and effects, as well as significant health effects at very low doses, have been observed for many common environmental chemicals (Vandenberg, et al., 2012). Attention to temporality matters, as certain early periods in life may form 'critical windows' for development and thus influence health trajectories in later life; cumulative exposures over time also matter (Ben-Shlomo and Kuh, 2002). Work in this realm thus calls for greater scrutiny of both the distribution and accumulation of these exposures as well as what Margaret Lock has termed 'local biologies', (1993; 2017), or how bodies and suffering can vary according to historical and social conditions.

These epidemiological uncertainties and uneven exposures call for forms of evidence-making that are able to marry scientific rigor and political legitimacy, towards the goal of 'actionable knowledge' (Graeter, 2017, p. 141). Such practices are difficult to formulate, as afflicted individuals and communities are often either unable to marshal resources for systematic and sustained scientific inquiry, or find that the evidence they collect is officially disregarded, leaving them in a state of precarity (Shapiro, 2015). An indication of how evidence-making in planetary health might move forward, however, comes from Stefanie Graeter's work on industrial heavy metal pollution in the Mantaro Valley of Peru (2017). Graeter ethnographically traces a multi-year collaboration between the Catholic church and scientists working to document heavy metal contamination, arguing that this process of institutional 'accompaniment' was vital not only in its material support for research on these afflicted communities, but in its imbuing of 'scientific practices with moral credibility and trust' (Graeter, 2017, p. 121), thus yielding evidence that was suitable for leveraging political action. Graeter thus calls our attention to how new spaces for knowledge-making and action can emerge where precarity is actually a mobilising force and where 'those of no account are counted' (Rancière, 2001); only by insisting upon such spaces may we restore the place of the poor in the political and scientific community.

## Humanitarian design and micro-worlds in global health

While planetary health draws attention to supra-state phenomena and how the technological triumphalism of the industrial era has led us to the brink of disaster, the second framework emerging in global health – that of humanitarian design – brings attention to where states are absent or weak, and suggests that technological tinkering might provide some temporary relief. Design thinking began as a bundle of strategies and methods for engineers, architects, and urban planners looking to 'incorporate constituent or consumer insights' (Brown and Wyatt, 2010, p. 29) into products or solutions; but in the 1990s it began to burgeon into broader usage, as a framework for promoting creative innovation in business as well as academic sectors. In recent years, design thinking has crossed over into the sphere of social innovation, with influential design training institutions such as IDEO.org (the non-profit subsidiary of a large Silicon Valley-based international design consultancy) and the Hasso Plattner Institute for Design at Stanford (usually known as the d.school) launching initiatives that tout the transformative potential of design thinking for development and social innovation. This approach, which has also been termed 'human-centred design' by IDEO.org, places significant emphasis on the importance of user perspectives and feedback to the design process, and is therefore often presented as an antidote or alternative to technocratic top-down approaches to development interventions. This movement has gained the support and attention of prominent actors and institutions in the global health field; in 2013, Melinda Gates and Paul Farmer both cited 'human-centred design' as the innovation that was changing the most lives in the global South (Schwittay and Braund, 2017).

Recently, new global health initiatives have been launched that draw on the popular momentum of human-centred design to spur innovation. In 2014, the UK Department for International Development and IDEO.org co-launched Amplify, a challenge fund for design projects addressing eight development challenges, including women's safety, enhancing early childhood development, and reducing stigma around disabilities. Around the same time, the international non-profit PATH (together with the United States Agency for International Development, the Gates Foundation, and the Norwegian Agency for Development Cooperation) launched the Innovation Countdown 2030 initiative to 'identify, evaluate, and showcase high-impact technologies and interventions that can transform global health by 2030' (PATH, n.d.). Both of these initiatives reflect a contemporary belief in the power of innovation to increase impact – as economist Larry Summers and epidemiologist Gavin Yamey put it, 'today's health tools alone won't get us there … we'll need tomorrow's tools as well, including new medicines, vaccines, diagnostics, and other innovations' (PATH, 2015, p. 5). They also represent, however, a challenge to the structures and premises of mainstream innovation, which is depicted as a 'model running out of steam because it is too costly, elitist, and rigid and fails to address even basic socioeconomic needs' (PATH, 2015, p. 4). Amie Batson, PATH's Chief Strategy Officer, proclaimed that 'innovators are everywhere, not just in well-funded labs and technology companies in wealthy nations … today's innovation ecosystem is diffuse, with smart ideas coming from every corner of the globe and across every sector and discipline' (PATH, 2015, p. 8).

The forms of 'inclusive innovation' championed by Amplify and IC2030 aim to include marginalised communities in the innovation process, either through specifically developing products and services for their use, or through support for more local, grassroots innovation efforts (Schwittay and Braund, 2017; PATH, 2015). Both initiatives deliberately sought to solicit and seriously consider submissions from the global South, as a way of affirming a commitment to decentralising knowledge production – and in so doing they also seem to engage the critique of global health as a neo-imperial enterprise. This departure from traditional models is for the moment certainly incomplete. Schwittay and Braund (2017) point out that Amplify still maintained a somewhat conventional development structure wherein key positions of gatekeeping influence were located in the global North, with projects subject to vetting and selection by a committee comprised of IDEO.org designers in North America, DFID managers in London, and unnamed subject experts.

The perpetuation of hierarchies of expertise in humanitarian design initiatives has led some to dismiss these initiatives as a new form of 'soft cultural imperialism' (Johnson, 2011, p. 463). Nevertheless, Schwittay and Braund argue that the apparent reflexivity of Amplify and similar initiatives with regard to diverse sites of knowledge production may represent a genuine and potentially significant turn towards a more humble approach towards development and global health, suggesting that '[Amplify] can be seen as an approach to international development whose practitioners wonder whether they are asking the right questions where others have ready-made answers, [and] who examine the assumptions that most development interventions take for granted' (Schwittay and Braund, 2017).

The direct outcomes of this turn to humanitarian design – the products and services developed through these processes of 'inclusive innovation' – have likewise been subject to both critique and cautious defense. In particular, the proliferation of small-scale devices aimed for use in situations of disaster or extreme poverty – such as point-of-use water purifiers, rapid diagnostic kits, and other highly portable medical monitors – have provoked intense debate among social scientists (Moran-Thomas, 2013). Some scholars argue that these 'micro' devices create and function within 'microworlds'; that is, they operate on needs at both an individualised and individualising level (Redfield, 2016). This is inherent to their purpose and function; they are created for easy use and distribution so that they may provide some degree of relief in the face of defunct or absent state infrastructures and larger systems of care. But in so doing, do they end up drawing too much attention to individual or micro-level frames for causality and interventions in global health, and thereby undermine attention to larger questions of structural violence and state responsibility? And what should we make of the 'ever-closer entanglement of markets and morals' (Schwittay and Braund, 2017) that accompanies many of these devices, produced as they are under the umbrella of social entrepreneurship? Does this represent a covert triumph of neoliberal and technocratic logics under humanitarian guise?

Anthropologist Peter Redfield offers a measured analysis that seeks to temper a quick rush to dismissal even as it also offers cautionary guidance. Tracing the use of Band-Aids – a micro-device that has become synonymous with the idea of a temporary and ultimately inadequate solution – Redfield argues that the 'problem with Band-Aids is primarily one of scale and application … it follows that a critical response should not simply expose such deficiencies, but also explore them in relation to any desired alternative' (Redfield, 2017). A hasty critique that condemns 'micro' devices merely because of their small scale and temporary nature, he argues, 'run[s] the risk of trading one fetish for another: assuming that the real path to the future always lies in familiar "macro" technologies and planning' (Redfield, 2017). Similar to Schwittay and Braund, Redfield suggests that the turn towards 'micro' devices or to a 'micro global health', as we call it, might, in some instances, reflect a potentially productive disenchantment with larger projects; perhaps, even, a heightened willingness among some practitioners to 'hold in view the messiness and complexity of any project of change, ultimately recommending to proceed with caution' (Schwittay and Braund, 2017).

## Conclusion: peopling global health and multiplying theory

As we chart a path forward, seeking to avoid analytic myopia, moral detachment, and ready prescription, what might guide us in proceeding with due caution in global health's remodeling field? While all the spheres of critique mentioned previously point to the uneasy stakes of global health and its agendas, forms of research and practice, and consequences, none can fully account for the highly complex and uneven ways they unfold on the ground, nor the difficulties of engaging at all. A critical attitude and an empirical lantern is in order. That is, we advocate for charting the lives of individuals and institutions over time, chronicling people's varied interpretations of their conditions, all the while denaturalising operational categories. Doing this will require illuminating the concrete ways meso- and macro-level actors (and, increasingly, micro ones) impinge on local environments and lifeworlds and scrutinising how they become part of both new global regimes and people's struggles for survival and normativity in health (What is health?, 2009; Canguilhem, 1978). Close attention to the particular realities and to the various technologies and metrics in which they are cast highlights the productive and fraught coexistence between global health systems design and the alternative models people craft for 'engaging the real … [and for] worlding the world', as Clifford Geertz put it (2007, p. 222). They attune us to the places where global inequities and ideologies – neocolonialism, neoliberalism, governmentality, humanitarian reason and design – are reified, and also to the limits of those categories and the initiatives and items they are enveloped in.

Ethnography can thus capture the active embroilment of reason, life, and ethics, offering entry points into the plasticity of systems, theorisers, and norm-makers themselves and leaving space for pursuing new forms of critical and socially meaningful work in global health. Instead of withdrawing to a dispassionate 'armchair' position and easy cynical dismissal, this kind of work inhabits the tension between a critique *of* and a critique *in* global health, sustaining a space for inquiry and action, understanding *and* doing.

People and the worlds they navigate and the outlooks they articulate are more confounding, incomplete, and multiple than dominant analytical schemes tend to account for. The 'peoples' of global health tinker with alternative spaces of the 'global' in the pursuit of '*a* health' – troubling the inequalities of geopolitics and the hollow conceptions of truth and justice in preposterous social orders. Drawn to the unsettling of rationalities and ingrained commonsense, the critical global health we advocate for eschews a sense of theory as a totalising enterprise or as the privileged domain of elite knowledge-makers self-appointed to speak on behalf of benighted populations. Rejecting the division between those who know the world and those who must simply struggle to survive it, and upholding an equality of intelligences, our ethnographic forays can chronicle lived tensions between theory and practice and invoke both alternative conceptual frameworks and new kinds of imagination.

Ethnographic theory emerges from and in conversation with people and world-making practices, with various ways of knowing and relating. It is a way of staying connected to open-ended social processes and unknowns – a way of counter-balancing the generation of certainties and foreclosures by other disciplines. Keeping interrelatedness, precariousness, uncertainty, and curiosity in focus, our theorising is never detached from praxis, but directly shapes and channels anthropology's entanglements in processes of transformation. In this way, theory is multiple and multiplies, a 'tool box' that can be actionable, in the world and in our writing: 'it has to be used, it has to work' (Deleuze, 2004, p. 210; Biehl and Locke, 2017, p. 32). It is these immanent negotiations (of peoples, institutions, technologies, evidence, social forms, ecosystems, health, efficacy, and ethics) – in their temporary stabilisation, production, excess, and creation – that animate the unfinishedness of ethnography and critical global health.

## References

Adams, V. (2013a) 'Evidence based global public health: subjects, profits, erasures', In: J. Biehl and A. Petryna (Eds.) *When People Come First: Critical studies in global health*, Princeton: Princeton University Press, pp. 54–90.

Adams, V. (2013b) *Markets of Sorrow, Labors of Faith: New Orleans in the wake of Katrina*, Durham, NC: Duke University Press.

Adams, V. (2016) *Metrics: What counts in global health*, Durham, NC: Duke University Press.

Amon, J. (2013) 'The "right to know" or "know your rights"?: human rights and a people-centered approach to health policy', In: J. Biehl and A. Petryna (Eds.) *When People Come First: Critical studies in global health*, Princeton: Princeton University Press, pp. 91–108.

Amon, J. (2014) 'How not to handle Ebola', available at www.cnn.com/2014/09/12/opinion/amon-ebola-outbreak/ (accessed on 6 March 2018).

Anderson, W. (2014) 'Making global health history: the postcolonial worldliness of biomedicine', *Social History of Medicine*, 27(2): 372–84.

Barreto, M.L., Barral-Netto, M., Stabeli, R., Almeida-Filho, N., Vasconcelos, P.F.C., Teixeira, M., Buss, P., and Gadelha, P.E. (2016) 'Zika virus and microcephaly in Brazil: a scientific agenda', *The Lancet*, 387(10022): 919–21.

Beck, U. (1992) *Risk Society: Towards a new modernity*, translated by M. Ritter, London: Sage.

Bellinger, D. (2016) 'Lead contamination in Flint: an abject failure to protect public health', *New England Journal of Medicine*, 374: 1101–3.

Ben-Shlomo, Y. and Kuh, D. (2002) 'A life course approach to chronic disease epidemiology: conceptual models, empirical challenges and interdisciplinary perspectives', *International Journal of Epidemiology*, 31(2): 285–93.

Biehl, J. (2007) *Will to Live: AIDS therapies and the politics of survival*, Princeton, NJ: Princeton University Press.

Biehl, J. (2013) 'The judicialization of biopolitics: claiming the right to pharmaceuticals in Brazilian courts', *American Ethnologist*, 40(3): 419–36.

Biehl, J. and Petryna, A. (2013a) 'Critical global health', In: J. Biehl and A. Petryna (Eds.) *When People Come First: Critical studies in global health*, Princeton: Princeton University Press, pp. 1–22.

Biehl, J. and Petryna, A. (2013b) 'Legal remedies: therapeutic markets and the judicialization of the right to health', In: J. Biehl and A. Petryna (Eds.) *When People Come First: Critical studies in global health*, Princeton: Princeton University Press, pp. 325–46.

Biehl, J. and Petryna, A. (2014) 'Peopling global health', *Saúde e Sociedade*, 23(2): 376–89.

Biehl, J. and Locke, P. (2017) 'Introduction: ethnographic sensorium', In: J. Biehl and P. Locke (Eds.) *Unfinished: The anthropology of becoming*, Durham, NC: Duke University Press, pp. 1–40.

Birn, A.-E. and Dmitrienko, K. (2005) 'The World Bank: global health or global harm?', *American Journal of Public Health*, 95(7): 1091–2.

Birn, A.-E. (2014) 'Philanthrocapitalism, past and present: the Rockefeller Foundation, the Gates Foundation, and the setting(s) of the international/global health agenda', *Hypothesis*, 12(1): e8.

Briggs, C.L. and Mantini-Briggs, C. (2016) *Tell Me Why My Children Died: Rabies, indigenous knowledge, and communicative justice*, Durham, NC: Duke University Press.

Brondizio, E.S., O'brien, K., Bai, X., Biermann, F., Steffen, W., Berkhout, F., Cudennec, C., Lemos, M.C., Wolfe, A., Palma-Oliveira, J., and Chen, C.T.A. (2016) 'Re-conceptualizing the anthropocene: a call for collaboration', *Global Environmental Change*, 39: 318–27.

Brown, H. and Kelly, A.H. (2014) 'Material proximities and hotspots: toward an anthropology of viral hemorrhagic fevers', *Medical Anthropology Quarterly*, 28(2): 280–303.

Brown, T. and Wyatt, J. (2010) 'Design thinking for social innovation', *Development Outreach*, 12(1): 29–43.

Brown, T.M., Cueto, M., and Fee, E. (2006) 'The World Health Organization and the transition from "international" to "global" public health', *American Journal of Public Health*, 96(1): 62–72.

Brulle, R.J. and Pellow, D.N. (2006) 'Environmental justice: human health and environmental inequalities', *Annual Review of Public Health*, 27: 103–24.

Cancedda, C., Davis, S.M., Dierberg, K.L., Lascher, J., Kelly, J.D., Barrie, M.B., Koroma, A.P., George, P., Kamara, A.A., Marsh, R., and Sumbuya, M.S. (2016) 'Strengthening health systems while responding to a health crisis: lessons learned by a nongovernmental organization during the Ebola virus disease epidemic in Sierra Leone', *The Journal of Infectious Diseases*, 214(S3): S153–63.

Canguilhem, G. (1978) *On the Normal and the Pathological,* translated by C. Fawcett, R.S. Cohen (Ed.), Boston: D. Reidel.

Cassier, M. and Correa, M. (2008) 'Scaling up and reverse engineering: acquisition of industrial knowledge by copying drugs in Brazil', In: B. Coriat (Ed.) *The Political Economy of HIV/AIDS in Developing Countries: TRIPS, public health systems, and free access*, Cheltenham, UK: Edward Elgar, pp. 130–49.

Chakrabarty, D. (2012) 'Postcolonial studies and the challenge of climate change', *New Literary History*, 43(1): 1–18.

Collier, S.J., Cross, J., Redfield, P., and Street, A. (Eds.) (2017) 'Little development devices/humanitarian goods'. *Limn*: 9.

Comaroff, J. and Comaroff, J. (2012) *Theory From the South: Or, how Euro-America is evolving toward Africa*, Boulder, CO: Paradigm Publishers.

Dahn, B., Mussa, V., and Nutt, C. (2015) 'Yes, we were warned about Ebola', available at www.nytimes.com/2015/04/08/opinion/yes-we-were-warned-about-ebola.html (accessed on 6 March 2018).

Das, V. (2015) *Affliction: Health, disease, poverty*, New York: Fordham University Press.

Deaton, A. (2012) Lecture: 'How can we learn what works in health and development?', Global Health Colloquium, Princeton University, 5 October.

Deaton, A. (2013) *The Great Escape: Health, wealth, and the origins of inequality*, Princeton: Princeton University Press.

Deleuze, G. (2004) 'Intellectuals and power', In: D. Lapoujade (Ed.) translated by M. Taormina *Desert Islands and Other Texts, 1953–1974*, Los Angeles: Semiotext(e), pp. 206–13.

Diniz, D. (2017) *Zika: From the Brazilian backlands to global threat*, London: Zed Books.

Easterbrook, G. (2018) *It's Better Than It Looks: Reasons for optimism in an Age of Fear*, New York: Public Affairs.

Edelstein, M., Angelides, P., and Heymann, D. (2015) 'Ebola: the challenging road to recovery', *The Lancet*, 385: 2234–5.

Fairhead, J., Leach, M., and Scoones, I. (2012) 'Green grabbing: a new appropriation of nature?', *Journal of Peasant Studies*, 39(2): 237–61.

Farmer, P. (2011) *Haiti After the Earthquake*, New York: Public Affairs.

Farmer, P., Kim, J.Y., Kleinman, A., and Basilico, M. (2013) 'Introduction: a biosocial approach', In P. Farmer, et al. (Eds.) *Reimagining Global Health: An introduction*, Berkeley: University of California Press, pp. 1–14.

Farrar, J. and Piot, P. (2014) 'The Ebola emergency: immediate action, ongoing strategy', *The New England Journal of Medicine*, 371: 1545–6.

Fassin, D. (2011) *Humanitarian Reason: A moral history of the present*, Berkeley, CA: University of California Press.

Fassin, D. (2012) 'That obscure object of global health', In: M. Inhorn and E. Wentzell (Eds.) *Medical Anthropology at the Intersections: Histories, activisms, and futures*, Durham, NC: Duke University Press, pp. 95–115.

Fidler, D.P. (2008) 'A theory of open-source anarchy', *Indiana Journal of Global Legal Studies*, 15(1): 259–84.

Frankfurter, R. (2014) 'The danger in losing sight of Ebola victims' humanity', available at www.theatlantic.com/health/archive/2014/08/the-danger-in-losing-sight-of-ebola-victims-humanity/378945/ (accessed on 6 March 2018).

Frumkin, H. and Myers, S. (2017) 'Health at a planetary scale', available at www.politico.com/agenda/story/2017/09/13/planetary-health-challenges-000514 (accessed on 12 February 2018).

Geertz, C. (2007) 'To exist is to have confidence in one's way of being: rituals as model systems', In: A. Creager, E. Lunbeck, and M. Norton Wise (Eds.) *Science Without Laws: Model systems, cases, exemplary narratives*, Durham, NC: Duke University Press, pp. 212–24.

Global Citizen. (2015) 'Introducing "I survived Ebola"', available at www.globalcitizen.org/en/content/introducing-i-survived-ebola/ (accessed on 6 March 2018).

Graeter, S. (2017) 'To revive an abundant life: Catholic science and neoextractivist politics in Peru's Mantaro Valley', *Cultural Anthropology*, 32(1): 117–48.

Griffiths, E.C., Pedersen, A.B., Fenton, A., and Petchey, O.L. (2011) 'The nature and consequences of coinfection in humans', *Journal of Infection*, 63(3): 200–6.

Han, C. (2012) *Life in Debt: Times of care and violence in neoliberal Chile*, Berkeley, CA: University of California Press.

Haraway, D. (2007) *When Species Meet*, Minneapolis: University of Minnesota Press.

Hirschman, A.O. (1971) *Bias for Hope: Essays on development and Latin America*, New Haven, CT: Yale University Press.

Hirschman, A.O. (1998) *Crossing Boundaries: Selected writings*. New York: Zone Books.

Horton, R. (2013) 'Offline: planetary health – a new vision for the post-2015 era', *The Lancet*, 382(9897): 1012.

Horton, R., et al. (2014a) 'From public to planetary health: a manifesto', *The Lancet*, 383(9920): 847.

Horton, R. (2014b) 'Offline: can Ebola be a route to nation-building?', *The Lancet*, 384(9961): 2186.

Janes, C. and Corbett, K. (2009) 'Anthropology and global health', *Annual Review of Anthropology*, 38: 167–83.

Johnson, C. (2011) 'The urban precariat, neoliberalization, and the soft power of humanitarian design', *Journal of Developing Societies*, 27(3–4): 445–75.

Kenworthy, N., Thomann, M., and Parker, R. (2018) 'From a global crisis to the "End of AIDS": new epidemics of signification', *Global Public Health*, 8: 960–71.

Keshavjee, S. (2014) *Blind Spot: How neoliberalism infiltrated global health*. Berkeley, CA: University of California Press.

King, N.B. (2004) 'The scale politics of emerging diseases', *Osiris*, 19: 62–76.

Klein, N. (2007) *The Shock Doctrine: The rise of disaster capitalism*, New York: Picador.

Lakoff, A. and Collier, S. (2008) *Biosecurity Interventions: Global health and security in question*, New York: Columbia University Press.

Lakoff, A., Stehen Collier, S., and Kelty, C. (Eds.) (2015) *Ebola's Ecologies. Limn*: 5.

Lakoff, A. (2017) *Unprepared: Global health in a time of emergency*, Oakland, CA: University of California Press.

Latour, B. (1983) 'Give me a laboratory and I will raise the world', In: K. Knorr-Cetina and M. Mulkay (Eds.) *Science Observed: Perspectives on the social study of science*, London: Sage, pp. 141–170.

Lock, M. (1993) *Encounters with Aging: Mythologies of menopause in Japan and North America*, Berkeley, CA: University of California Press.

Lock, M. (2017) 'Recovering the body', *Annual Review of Anthropology*, 46: 1–14.

Lovell, A. (2011) 'Debating life after disaster: charity hospital babies and bioscientific futures in post-Katrina New Orleans', *Medical Anthropology Quarterly*, 25(2): 254–77.

Mason, K.A. (2012) 'Mobile migrants, mobile germs: migration, contagion, and boundary-building in Shenzhen, China after SARS', *Medical Anthropology*, 31(2): 113–31.

Moran-Thomas, A. (2013) 'A salvage ethnography of the Guinea worm: witchcraft, oracles and magic in a disease eradication program', In: J. Biehl and A. Petryna (Eds.) *When People Come First: Critical studies in global health*, Princeton, NJ: Princeton University Press, pp. 207–242.

Nading, A. (2017) 'Local biologies, leaky things, and the chemical infrastructure of global health', *Medical Anthropology*, 36(2): 141–56.

Nguyen, V.-K. (2010) *Republic of Therapy: Triage and sovereignty in West Africa's time of AIDS*, Durham, NC: Duke University Press.

Parpia, A.S., Ndeffo-Mbah, M.L., Wenzel, N.S., and Galvani, A.P. (2016) 'Effects of response to 2014–2015 Ebola outbreak on deaths from malaria, HIV/AIDS, and tuberculosis, West Africa', *Emerging Infectious Diseases*, 22(3): 433–41.

Partners in Health. (n.d.) 'Ebola', available at www.pih.org/programs/ebola (accessed on 16 April 2018).

PATH. (n.d.) 'Innovation Countdown 2030', available at http://ic2030.org/about/ (accessed on 16 April 2018).

PATH. (2015) 'IC2030 report: reimagining global health', available at http://ic2030.org/wp-content/uploads/2015/07/ic2030-report-2015.pdf (accessed on 16 April 2018).

Petryna, A. (2015) 'What is a horizon? Navigating thresholds in climate change uncertainty', In: P. Rabinow and L. Samimian-Darash (Eds.) *Modes of Uncertainty: Anthropological*, Chicago, IL: University of Chicago Press, pp. 147–64.

Pfeiffer, J. (2013) 'The struggle for a public sector: PEPFAR in Mozambique', In: J. Biehl and A. Petryna (Eds.) *When People Come First: Critical studies in global health*, Princeton, NJ: Princeton University Press, pp. 166–81.

Pinker, S. (2018) *Enlightenment Now: The case for reason, science, humanism, and progress*, New York: Viking Press.

Piot, P. (2013) *No Time to Lose: A life in pursuit of deadly viruses*, New York: W.W. Norton & Co.

Rajan, K.S. (2017) *Pharmocracy: Value, politics, and knowledge in global biomedicine*, Durham, NC: Duke University Press.

Rancière, J. (2001) 'Ten theses on politics', *Theory & Event*, 5(3).

Redfield, P. (2013) *Life in Crisis: The ethical journey of Doctors Without Borders*, Berkeley, CA: University of California Press.

Redfield, P. (2016) 'Fluid technologies: the bush pump, the LifeStraw® and microworlds of humanitarian design', *Social Studies of Science*, 46(2): 159–83.

Redfield, P. (2017) 'On Band-Aids and magic bullets', *Limn*: 9.

Richardson, E.T., Barrie, M.B., Nutt, C.T., Kelly, J.D., Frankfurter, R., Fallah, M.P., and Farmer, P.E. (2017a) 'The Ebola suspect's dilemma', *The Lancet Global Health*, 5(3): e254–6.

Richardson, E. T., et al. (2017b) 'The symbolic violence of "outbreak": a mixed-methods, quasi-experimental impact evaluation of social protection on Ebola survivor wellbeing', *Social Science & Medicine*, 195: 77–82.

Robbins, J. (2013) 'Beyond the suffering subject: toward an anthropology of the good', *Journal of the Royal Anthropological Institute*, 19(3): 447–62.

Rodin, J. (2015) 'Planetary health: a new discipline in global health', available at www.rockefellerfoundation.org/blog/planetary-health-a-new-discipline-in-global-health/ (accessed on 12 February 2018).

Sachs, J. D. (2012) 'From Millennium Development Goals to Sustainable Development Goals', *The Lancet*, 379(9832): 2206–11.

Schwittay, A. and Braund, P. (2017) 'Iterate, experiment, prototype', *Limn*: 9.

Shapiro, N. (2015) 'Attuning to the chemosphere: domestic formaldehyde, bodily reasoning, and the chemical sublime', *Cultural Anthropology*, 30(3): 368–93.

Singer, M., Bulled, N., Ostrach, B., and Mendenhall, E. (2017) 'Syndemics and the biosocial conception of health', *The Lancet*, 389(10072): 941–50.

Steffen, W., Grinevald, J., Crutzen, P., and McNeill, J. (2011) 'The anthropocene: conceptual and historical perspectives', *Philosophical Transactions of the Royal Society of London A: Mathematical, physical and engineering sciences*, 369(1938): 842–67.

Stevenson, L. (2014) *Life Beside Itself: Imagining care in the Canadian Arctic*, Berkeley, CA: University of California Press.

Storeng, K. and Béhague, D. (2014) '"Playing the numbers game": evidence-based advocacy and the technocratic narrowing of the safe motherhood initiative', *Medical Anthropology Quarterly*, 28(2): 260–79.

Takahashi, S., et al. (2015) 'Reduced vaccination and the risk of measles and other childhood infections post-Ebola', *Science*, 347(6227): 1240–2.

Ticktin, M. (2014) 'Transnational humanitarianism', *Annual Review of Anthropology*, 43: 283–9.

Ticktin, M. and Feldman, I. (Eds.) (2010) *In the Name of Humanity: The government of threat and care*, Durham, NC: Duke University Press.

Vandenberg, L.N., Colborn, T., Hayes, T.B., Heindel, J.J., Jacobs Jr., D.R., Lee, D.-H., Tshi Shioda, T., et al. (2012) 'Hormones and endocrine-disrupting chemicals: low-dose effects and nonmonotonic dose responses', *Endocrine Reviews*, 33(3): 378–455.

Ventura, D. (2016) 'From Ebola to Zika: international emergencies and the securitization of global health', *Cadernos de Saúde Pública*, 32(4).

'What is health? The ability to adapt [editorial]', (2009) *The Lancet*, 373(9666): 781.

Whyte, S.R. (Ed.) (2014) *Second Chances: Surviving AIDS in Uganda*, Durham, NC: Duke University Press.

Wilkinson, I. and Kleinman, A. (2015) *A Passion for Society: How we think about human suffering*, Berkeley, CA: University of California Press.

Wolf, M. (2015) 'Is there really such a thing as "One Health"? Thinking about a more than human world from the perspective of cultural anthropology', *Social Science & Medicine*, 129: 5–11.

# Part II
# Globalisation, neoliberalism, and health systems

# 7

# Boundaries of global health politics in the 'fourth world'

## Determinants of political will for hepatitis C treatment

*Jonathan García, Devynne Nelons, Tayler Tobey, and Katherine Marsi*

### Fourth world theory

Widespread mistrust of institutions, politically wielded stigma and discrimination, and deepening structural inequities – layered with climate change and political wars that displace waves of people from their homes – have contributed to greater exposure to disease among already vulnerable groups, and to the widening gap in access to health care and life-saving treatments. These are not 'third world' problems; nor are they problems of the 'first world'. The striking health disparities that require global health solutions exist within pockets of deep social and economic exclusion that exist in every society – what Manuel Castells termed the 'fourth world' (Castells, 2000, p. 348). This assumption, that all people in so-called developed or 'first world' countries have equitable access to health care and other social services, presents a critical political dilemma in addressing problems of the 'fourth world'. This chapter advances the concept of the fourth world as a useful framework for identifying and addressing health disparities that affect the most marginalised populations across societies. We discuss the rise in chronic hepatitis C virus (HCV) infection among people who inject drugs (PWID) in settings such as the United States, Canada, Australia, and the United Kingdom as a product of political, economic, social, and cultural marginalisation. The cost of treating HCV in these countries (i.e., due to their overall economic standing) doubly excludes the most vulnerable PWID from access to highly effective, life-saving treatment. We highlight the importance of social mobilisation to generate political will to address HCV treatment access.

The idea of the third world was analogous to the third estate of French commoners, which were exploited and neglected populations living in geopolitical non-alignment with neither the capitalist nor communist bloc (Wolf-Phillips, 1987). The phrase evolved to include issues regarding industrialisation and development and is most presently a term denoting an economic context rather than a geopolitical category. The first world or democratic-industrialised nations are terms often used to describe high-income or developed countries, whereas the term third world describes the category of lower-income countries, often used interchangeably with developing countries (Wolf-Phillips, 1987). This Three World Model does not capture the expansion in intra-country inequality. The increasing disparity in income *within* so-called developed or first world countries such as the United States, Canada, and Australia has prompted the adaptation of a Fourth World Theory (Castells, 2010).

In 1999, Manuel Castells presented this theory at the United Nations Research Institute for Social Development conference,

> This world is composed of people, and territories, that have lost value for the dominant interests in informational capitalism. Some of them because they offer little contribution as either producers or consumers. Others because they are uneducated or functionally illiterate. Others because they become sick or mentally unfit. Others because they could not afford the rent, became homeless, and were devoured by life in the streets. Others who, unable to cope with life, became drug addicts or drunks. Others because, in order to survive, they sold their bodies and their souls, and went on to be prostitutes of every possible desire.
>
> *Castells, 1999, p. 10*

The fourth world is brought on by poverty and inequality resulting in extreme polarisation (Castells, 2010). Its boundaries are drawn around pockets of social exclusion, often where groups in high-income countries encounter the challenges and conditions experienced by marginalised groups in low- and middle-income countries – or worse. These challenges are further exacerbated by the economic and social isolation of their relative social status in the high-income countries. Castells (2010) describes four processes that drive relative social differentiation: *inequality*, *polarisation*, *poverty*, and *misery*. *Polarisation* is a process of expanding inequality that occurs explicitly when the growth of the lower and upper ends of wealth distribution outpace the middle and thereby increase the disparity between the two extremes of social class while diminishing the middle. Extreme poverty is the bottommost distribution of wealth, which is referred to by Castells as *misery* and includes a number of additional social and economic disadvantages. Castells notes that in the US, 'extreme poverty refers to those households whose income falls below 50 per cent of the income that defines the poverty line' (Castells, 2000, p. 349). In addition, Castells argues that these excluded groups become 'perversely integrated' into society through informal and illegal economies that support globalisation. Due to these processes brought on by globalisation, the fourth world exists inside most countries – across the categories of low-, middle-, and high-income. The health problems that 'global health' needs to address are as present in the South Bronx as they are in Soweto. The problem is that 'global health' did not really change the paradigm to capture extreme marginalisation and neglect that are globally pervasive. Rather than simply rebranding international health and tropical medicine as global health, the notion of the fourth world advances a concept of health in a truly global system.

## Case of HCV treatment access in the fourth world

In this case study, we focus on the fourth world inhabited by people who inject drugs (PWID) living with HCV in so-called developed countries. Across societies, PWID with HCV share experiences of exclusion during globalisation that result in misery, homelessness, and discrimination. One way in which globalisation alters the health outcomes of low-income individuals and families is by re-shaping housing affordability and housing markets (Labonté, et al., 2015). The housing instability that results has been repeatedly linked to poor health outcomes and limited access to health services (Kim, et al., 2009; Fullilove, 2010). Studies show a significant association between homelessness and HCV infection, noting that PWID in unstable housing are considerably more likely to contract HCV (Topp, et al., 2013). In some populations, as many as 90 per cent of PWID have contracted the virus, a number that continues to expand in areas of unequal economic development (Kim, et al., 2009). Collectively, the combination of unstable housing, high rates of unemployment, prolonged injection drug use, as well as stigma and discrimination associated with drug use contribute to the ongoing social exclusion for individuals living with HCV in the fourth world (Van Boekel, et al., 2013; Neale, 2008). Substance use is reported as a major contributing factor to homelessness in urban communities, emphasising the comorbidity of substance use and other mental disorders (O'Toole, et al., 2004).

For PWID with chronic HCV in the fourth world, accessing treatment is uniquely difficult. This presents a clear example of fourth world exclusion as the rapid technological developments in HCV treatment function to further marginalise PWID. The cost to treat HCV infection with direct-acting antivirals (DAA) in high-income countries including Canada, the United Kingdom, and the United States are US$53,123; US$43,226; and US$84,000, respectively, for a 12-week treatment with sofosbuvir (Iyengar, et al., 2016). In contrast, countries such as Egypt, Brazil, and India are able to deliver the same treatment regimen for US$3,117; US$9,708; and US$1,861 respectively (Iyengar, et al., 2016). These values are adjusted using the purchasing power parities for GDP (national currency per US dollar). The dramatic contrast in pricing between low-, middle-, and high-income countries is largely due to legal and political considerations, and not always associated with average ability to pay or health system capacity. Swathi Iyengar, et al. (2016) argue that,

> Paying for sofosbuvir and ledipasvir/sofosbuvir in national health systems would consume large proportions of their total pharmaceutical budget. The potential total cost of treatment presents a financial and ethical dilemma for payers and physicians. Some national health systems have therefore restricted access to these medicines to small groups of patients, despite the fact that almost all patients with chronic hepatitis C infection are likely to benefit from treatment with these medicines.
>
> *Iyengar, et al., 2016, p. 3*

The pharmaceutical companies that develop treatments such as sofosbuvir can extend permission for production to external manufacturing companies via voluntary licensing, which dramatically lowers prices. This allows outside companies in certain countries to produce a generic version of the medication. Tiered pricing models, cost sharing, and subsidy programmes allow low-income countries and middle-income countries (LMIC) to offer treatment options at a lower cost (Iyengar, et al., 2016; Andrieux-Meyer, et al., 2015; MSF, 2015). Political will and civil society advocacy were crucial for increasing access to HCV treatment worldwide, providing examples from successful countries such as Brazil and Thailand (WHO, 2016), where threatening to file for compulsory licensing allowed for the production of generic medications. As described in detail in other chapters in this book (Vieira and Di Giano, Chapter 31; and Cueto, Chapter 24), Brazil has led the global resistance to restrictive intellectual property laws. In Thailand, civil society groups have effectively mobilised to file a patent opposition to allow access to direct-acting antivirals for HCV treatment (WHO, 2016). Additionally, countries that employ single payer health care systems are usually more equipped to control cost and better negotiate affordable rates with pharmaceutical companies. For this reason, countries such as the US with highly privatised insurance models pay a disproportionate amount for drug treatments (Rosenthal and Graham, 2016). The national cost of HCV-related health care in the US was roughly US$6.5 billion in the year 2011 and nearly double that amount in 2014 (Trooskin, et al., 2015). Although the costs to research and develop sofosbuvir were estimated at US$100 million (and no greater than US$11 billion), Gilead Science, Inc., the creator and manufacturer of sofosbuvir, is predicted to gross nearly US$200 billion in profit for a 20-to-1 return on their investment (Trooskin, et al., 2015). Despite discounted pricing, market competition, and exclusivity arrangements, the persistent restriction of HCV treatment coverage by insurers has sharpened the disparities in access to treatment (Trooskin, et al., 2015).

These costs combine with absence of political will to generate greater geographic disparities within the US. A 2017 report, produced by the Center for Health Law and Policy Innovation at Harvard about Medicaid access for people living with chronic HCV, revealed the vast variation in access to life-saving medications across different states (NVHR and CHLPI, 2017). This variation was determined by restrictions to direct-acting antivirals according to 1) liver damage restrictions, which limit access to those with most damage, 2) prescriber restrictions, which require specialised providers to prescribe medications, and 3) sobriety restrictions, which in some states require up to 12 months proof of sobriety before receiving treatment (NVHR and CHLPI, 2017). These analyses found that treatment was most restricted in Arkansas, Louisiana, Montana, Oregon, and South Dakota; and most accessible in Alaska, Connecticut, Massachusetts, Nevada, and Washington (NVHR and CHLPI, 2017). With growing concern for the 'nation's opioid crisis' (Pearson and Soh, 2018) and the prevalence of injected methamphetamine and heroin use (Lansky, et al., 2014), these restrictions limit what essentially constitutes a cure for HCV in increasingly vulnerable populations. The boundaries of the fourth world are drawn around pockets of social exclusion and poverty in these states, and the high-income status of the US only serves to further exclude these populations. Political unwillingness to expand Medicaid and local-level priority-setting driven by structural stigma further exacerbate these geographic disparities.

In fact, stigma and discrimination augment marginalisation among PWID living in the fourth world. Health policy and messaging emphasise risk behaviours like injection drug use that stigmatise vulnerable groups (Butt, 2008). Stigma against PWID can vastly limit their access to treatment, especially when they need to navigate prescriptions through specialty providers. For people living with HCV, the health care system is the place they are most likely to experience stigma (Treloar, et al., 2013). When patients hear that HCV treatment is rationed based on arbitrary and unfounded guidelines regarding degree of liver damage and risk of re-infection, seeking care becomes linked in patients' minds with submitting to or enduring stigma. Access to treatment is thus limited by structural stigma against PWID in which 'gate keepers' frequently employ subversive means of denying care to HCV patients (Treloar, et al., 2013). PWID often delay or avoid diagnosis and treatment, leading to continued risk of disease transmission, or remove themselves from the pool of treatment applicants entirely when they believe they will be passed over for treatment regardless of their need.

In response to these dimensions of social and economic marginalisation, there has been budding social mobilisation for HCV treatment activism across different cities and states in the US. In New York, organisations such as VOCAL-NY, which mobilise around homelessness and healthy equity (e.g., access to overdose prevention and HIV prevention) for PWID, have also taken up HCV treatment access as a key item in their political agenda. Organisations like VOCAL-NY have created a positive community identity among drug users to fight stigma. They have effectively pressured the city and state health departments through community organising, town hall meetings, founding the NYS Hepatitis C Coalition, conducting budgeting advocacy to 'drop harmful restrictions for coverage for HCV treatment, granting access to thousands' and passing the 'Hep C Screening Law to expand standing order HCV testing, the first of its kind in the country' (Vocal-NY.org, 2018, n.p.). In response to disparities in access in Louisiana, community mobilisation efforts, including allied health officials, have started to consider pursuing acting under US Code Section 1498 to lower the prices of HCV treatment, arguing that it is a public good (Tribble, 2017). These instances of mobilisation are reminiscent of, and sometimes borrow from, methods for social mobilisation used in the global South, in countries such as Brazil (ABIA, 2014, 2017) and social movement organisations such as the International Treatment Preparedness Coalition (ITPC, 2017). One lesson learned from the global South, and from the US in the case of Cipro for Anthrax in 2001, is to threaten the use of 'compulsory licensing':

> When HIV programmes for antiretroviral treatment began in 2003, a number of countries relied on compulsory licensing to import or manufacture affordable generic versions of first-line HIV medicines. Compulsory license issuance remains a backbone flexibility enshrined under international law that can be used to promote public health and increase access to essential HCV medicines.
>
> *MSF, 2015, p. 4*

For social mobilisation to become effective, however, it will be important for local organisations to form broader networks that pressure the US government to ally with communities of people living with HCV.

## Concluding remarks

Barriers to accessing HCV treatment created by intellectual property policies, structural stigma, and rationing of treatment disproportionately impact PWID living in the fourth world. Born of urbanisation, globalisation, and neoliberalism, deficits in employment and housing create risk environments that cultivate inequality, polarisation, poverty, and misery. For an already highly stigmatised population, the effects of living in the fourth world create a lasting sense of socio-economic, cultural, and political disenfranchisement.

The fourth world framework proposed by Castells is useful for understanding the politics of global health on several levels. First, by highlighting that global health disparities, inequalities, and social exclusion occur in pockets of highly vulnerable populations (in both high-income and LMIC countries), we are able to notice the shared experience of marginalisation across societies and work towards developing social solidarity. Second, this concept counterbalances decisions made to scale-down programmes in national settings where on-average health capacity has improved or infection rates have stabilised. Instead, it emphasises the complex disparities that occur within countries that affect the most vulnerable groups. Third, by identifying large-scale economic processes and policies (e.g., intellectual property laws, treatises) and political will as determinants of extreme marginalisation, we are able to mobilise to change these structures that perpetuate suffering.

## References

ABIA (2014) 'Brasil é excluído de licença que autoriza produção de genéricos para remédio contra hepatite C', available at http://abiaids.org.br/brasil-e-excluido-de-licenca-que-autoriza-producao-de-genericos-para-remedio-contra-hepatite-c/27134 (accessed on 28 March 2018).

ABIA (2017) 'GTPI participa de protesto global contra Gilead', available at http://abiaids.org.br/gtpi-participa-de-protesto-global-contra-gilead/30841 (accessed on 28 March 2018).

Andrieux-Meyer, I., Cohn, J., de Araújo, E.S.A., and Hamid, S.S. (2015) 'Disparity in market prices for hepatitis C virus direct-acting drugs', *The Lancet Global health*, 3(11): e676–77.

Butt, G. (2008) 'Stigma in the context of hepatitis C: concept analysis', *Journal of Advanced Nursing*, 62(6): 712–24.

Castells, M. (1999) 'Information technology, globalization, and social development', UNRISD discussion paper 114, September, available at http://citeseerx.ist.psu.edu/viewdoc/download?doi=10.1.1.130.5730&rep=rep1&type=pdf (accessed on 20 March 2018).

Castells, M. (2000) 'The rise of the fourth world', In: D. Held and A. McGrew (Eds.), *The Global Transformations Reader: An introduction to the globalization debate*, Cambridge: Polity Press, pp. 348–54.

Castells, M. (2010) 'The rise of the fourth world: informational capitalism, poverty, and social exclusion', In: Castells, M., *End of Millennium*, Oxford, UK: Wiley-Blackwell.

Dunn, J.R. and Hayes, M.V. (2000) 'Social inequality, population health, and housing: a study of two Vancouver neighborhoods', *Social Science & Medicine*, 51(4): 563–87

Fullilove, M.T. (2010) 'Housing is health care', *American Journal of Preventive Medicine*, 39(6): 607–8.

ITPC (2017) 'High-, middle-, or low-income: pharma greed is not justified in any country!', available at http://itpcglobal.org/high-middle-low-income-pharma-greed-not-justified-country/ (accessed on 18 March 2018).

Iyengar, S., Tay-Teo, K., Vogler, S., Beyer, P., Wiktor, S., de Joncheere, K., and Hill, S. (2016) 'Prices, costs, and affordability of new medicines for hepatitis C in 30 countries: an economic analysis', *PLOS Medicine*, 13(5): e1002032.

Kim, C., Kerr, T., Li, K., Zhang, R., Tyndall, M.W., Montaner, J.S., and Wood, E., (2009) 'Unstable housing and hepatitis C incidence among injection drug users in a Canadian setting', *BMC Public Health*, 9(1): 270.

Labonté, R., Cobbett, E., Orsini, M., Spitzer, D., Schrecker, T., and Ruckert, A. (2015). 'Globalization and the health of Canadians: "Having a job is the most important thing"', *Globalization and Health*, 11: 19.

Lansky, A., Finlayson, T., Johnson, C., Holtzman, D., Wejnert, C., Mitsch, A., Gust, D., Chen, R., Mizuno, Y., and Crepaz, N. (2014) 'Estimating the number of persons who inject drugs in the United States by meta-analysis to calculate national rates of HIV and hepatitis C virus infections', *PLOS ONE*, 9(5): e97596.

Medecins Sans Frontiere (MSF). (2015) 'Strategies to secure access to generic hepatitis C medicines', available at www.msfaccess.org/sites/default/files/MSF_assets/HepC/Docs/HepC_brief_OvercomingbarriersToAccess_ENG_2015.pdf (accessed on 21 March 2018).

National Viral Hepatitis Roundtable (NVHR) and Center for Health Law and Policy Innovation (CHLPI). (2017) 'Hepatitis C state of Medicaid access report', available at https://stateofhepc.org/resources/ (accessed on 21 March 2018).

Neale, J., (2008) 'Homelessness, drug use and hepatitis C: a complex problem explored within the context of social exclusion', *International Journal of Drug Policy*, 19(6): 429–35.

O'Toole, T.P., Gibbon, J.L., Hanusa, B.H., Freyder, P.J., Conde, A.M., and Fine, M.J. (2004) 'Self-reported changes in drug and alcohol use after becoming homeless', *American Journal of Public Health*, 94(5): 830–35.

Pearson, C. and Soh, C. (2018) 'Midwest and mid-Atlantic state face provider shortage to address opioid epidemic' available at http://avalere.com/expertise/life-sciences/insights/midwest-and-mid-atlantic-states-face-provider-shortage-to-address-opioid-ep (accessed on 21 March 2018).

Rosenthal, E.S. and Graham, C.S. (2016) 'Price and affordability of direct-acting antiviral regimens for hepatitis C virus in the United States', *Infectious Agents and Cancer*, 11: 24.

Topp, L., Iversen, J., Baldry, E., Maher, L., and Collaboration of Australian NSPs (2013). 'Housing instability among people who inject drugs: results from the Australian needle and syringe program survey', *Journal of Urban Health*, 90(4): 699–716.

Treloar, C., Rance, J., and Backmund, M. (2013) 'Understanding barriers to hepatitis C virus care and stigmatization from a social perspective', *Clinical Infectious Diseases*, 57(suppl 2): S51–S55.

Tribble, S.J. (2017) 'Louisiana proposes tapping a century-old patent law to cut hepatitis C drug prices', available at www.washingtonpost.com/national/health-science/louisiana-proposes-tapping-a-century-old-patent-law-to-cut-hepatitis-c-drug-prices/2017/05/02/fc611990-2f76-11e7-9534-00e4656c22aa_story.html?utm_term=.713d9181a82d (accessed on 21 March 2018).

Trooskin, S.B., Reynolds, H., and Kostman, J.R. (2015) 'Access to costly new hepatitis C drugs: medicine, money, and advocacy', *Clinical Infectious Diseases*, 61(12): 1825–30.

Van Boekel, L.C., Brouwers, E.P., Van Weeghel, J., and Garretsen, H.F. (2013) 'Stigma among health professionals towards patients with substance use disorders and its consequences for healthcare delivery: systematic review', *Drug & Alcohol Dependence*, 131(1): 23–35.

Vocal-Ny.org. (2018) 'Hepatitis C', available at www.vocal-ny.org/?p=275 (accessed on 21 March 2018).

WHO. (2016) 'Global report on access to hepatitis C treatment', available at http://apps.who.int/iris/bitstream/handle/10665/250625/WHO-HIV-2016.20-eng.pdf;jsessionid=FEF58B63303FE5E700418910439006CA?sequence=1 (accessed on 21 March 2018).

Wolf-Phillips, L. (1987) 'Why "third world"?: origin, definition and usage', *Third World Quarterly*, 9(4): 1311–27.

# 8

# Sabotaged bodies, sacrifice, and lost youth under punitive neoliberalism

*Luis L. M. Aguiar*

Our social world is rife with neoliberal thought, and is organised to promote the virtues and values of profit, entrepreneurship, and sacrifice (Judt, 2010). In the following I tell a story on how this unfolds in Canada focusing on young men labouring in the physically and emotionally demanding camps of extractive industries in the northern interior of the country. To secure workers, industry entices them with high wages and free airfare whilst beating them with hard labour, long hours, and isolation. And, to escape an economy failing them 'at home', young (mostly) men fall under the influence of slick peddlers of new economic goldrushes and migrate to camps readying themselves to slash and turn terrains into 'rewarding' landscapes to new investors in capitalism. In this scenario, high wages and looong shifts, combined with managerial control, fuel rugged masculinity masking the abuses and health consequences to young men's bodies bull's eyed for profit-making. Here, '[h]ealthy bodies [are] needed but deformities, pathologies, sickness are often produced' (Harvey, 2000, p. 103). While health issues can be separated from workers' labour experiences, they are best understood when tied to the totality of the capitalist labour process since what is most important is that '[c]apital continuously strives to shape bodies to its own requirements' (Harvey, 2000, p. 115). Today, this is facilitated by weakened trade unions, individualising social movements, austerity, and a neoliberal state. This reality transcends borders and is manifest in both the global North and South (Moody, 1997; Herod, 2018). The discussion that follows highlights some of the issues raised here.

## Etching finance capital into our bones

The fordist regime of capital accumulation (the post war social compromise between labour, capital, and the State for the benefit of all three) had to go since it no longer served capital's needs, nor the working class' need (Herod, 2018). It was argued that without an increase in profitability there would be no growth in employment, jobs, wage levels, and indeed the standard of living (Harvey, 2005). Neoliberal intellectuals cemented this thinking in society through their work in academic publishing, and growing visibility in pop culture and media circles (Beder, 2000). They argued that the working class now had a free path to success because unions and their contract language no longer stood in their way as unions' power declined and their legitimacy questioned (Harvey, 2005). Society was more 'open' than ever before, since achievement could only be hindered by one's psychological and emotional character flaws since barriers and obstacles to achievement had been removed (Sennett, 1998; Hoffman and Casnocha, 2012). The male white working class was too politically and organisationally weak to effectively resist this ideology, which also entailed economic restructuring leading to wholesale devastation of their communities and sense of self-worth. Jobs were eliminated, unions hemorrhaged members and had few clues how to respond to this assault on the working class and its organisations (Cowie, 2010). De-industrialisation created desperate people[1] with few options because of the decimation of industrial jobs and the rollback of the welfare state. Economic restructuring fragmented the spaces of production, disrupting communities as identities fragmented, making solidarity and political organising difficult (Clement and Vosko, 2003).

The stage was set for the introduction and implementation of neoliberalism. Bourdieu (1998) says neoliberalism undertook an unprecedented assault on the welfare state, which he considered one of the greatest human inventions. It is in this instance that we get the rise of finance capital through the deregu-lation of financial markets, which amongst other things allowed banks to collude with capital's wishes to both introduce and implement mechanisms for the production of precarity and the liquidity of money wholesale (the circulation of money made easier and quicker) (Albo, et al., 2010). The result was the massification of credit cards and the introduction of debit cards, lines of credit, overdraft 'protection', etc., and 'putting' money in consumers' pockets to prop up demand for capital goods while wages stagnated or declined (Kaletsky, 2010). In other words, the attack on working class jobs, wage stagnation, and re-defined employment relationships could not stand in the way of putting money in workers' pockets to consume and prevent capitalism from experiencing overproduction and underconsumption (Harvey, 2010). Finance capital corralled and trapped the working class into the spaces of banks and other financial institutions. The goal was to access working people's money more rapidly and circulate it quickly in the seamless management of money, at the same time as banks shedded workers by replacing them with machines and new technologies versed in the 'invisible' movement of money. Banks' real coup was to convince working people that the banks could manage and grow workers' money better than they could themselves. And to do so, banks needed access to clients' money. It is in this instance that we get lines of credit (readilines), repeated mortgage restructuring, and 'easier' means of borrowing money. Given these changes, it is no surprise Canadians' debt continues to rise even with the exclusion of calculations of mortgage payments (Walks, 2013). The 'financialisation of daily life' is entrapment (Martin, 2002).

This finance-led regime of accumulation is propped up by a neoliberalism of individualism feeding into, and fed by, finance and monetary 'rewards' (Mirowski, 2013). But this process does not simply lead to economic and political development. It is also one that socialised the population into accepting that it is in this way that debt chasers can self-actualise, and fulfil their life ambitions (Martin, 2002). The current young generation has grown up with nothing else but finance-led capitalism where money is easily available and debt a matter of life (Cairns, 2017). Canadian youth are 'financialised' having internalised 'entrepreneurial attitudes to personal success' and accepted the centrality of the finance industry in organising their lives through their interactions with financial institutions like banks (Mulcahy, 2017, p. 222). This experience is not an individual act or case-by-case adoption. Rather, it is so much more widespread and pernicious as 'the working class responds by reorganizing and adapting their lifestyles' (Mulcahy, 2017, p. 230). Canadian youth are 'reorganizing and adapting their lifestyles' to the omnipresence of fictitious money and credit cards, lines of credit, 'easy' borrowing, mortgages, personal investment portfolios, etc., and remaking them-selves into the 'entrepreneurial subjectivity' (Scharff, 2016) of the self in contemporary 'finance-led regime of accumulation' (Mulcahy, 2017, p. 230). Housing, for example, is scarce and exorbitantly priced, and rental options limited in a tight housing market often laced with landlords' racist practices (Demographia, 2012; Lewis and Berg, forthcoming). Working class youth are told that future prosperity lies in the North where money is large and sacrifice larger. The option to go North is no option at all for young men at a time when personal debt is no longer a temporary strategy towards deferred gratification but indeed a fact of life most people (young and not so young) are burdened with (Horton, 2017, pp. 284–5). And at a time when one's worth is assessed by the toys one owns, debt 'weighs' heavy in the lives of Kelowna, British Columbia residents. In mapping urban debtscapes by city and neighbourhood in Canada, Walks (2013) found Kelowna ranks second in the country in indebtedness, measuring household debt as a percent of disposable income. Kelownians' indebtedness is rivalled only by Vancouverites who rank first in the country (Walks, 2013). This debt load is exacerbated by statistics showing that Canadian youth who are 23 years old or younger face a rate of labour market instability of 35 per cent. That is, finding permanent full time employment is a difficult proposition for Canadian young people (Galarneau, et al., 2013). In this climate choice is a symptom of people's ongoing vulnerability, insecurity, and precarity, and not a reach-and-grab at various viable opportunities. Today, Canadians 'expect that living standards will decline in a stagnant economy and fewer young people will achieve the middle class lifestyles of their parents' generations' (Lowe and Graves, 2016, p. 3). Future prospects look grim since 'if current trends continue unchecked [there is no evidence that checks are in place] in 10 years Canadian society will have more insecurity, less opportunity, and a reduced quality of life' (Lowe and Graves, 2016, p. 3). Issues of inequality are even more pressing and visibly striking in small cities like Kelowna, where the disparity between the rich and the poor has grown by an alarming rate since the new millennium (Van Emmerik, 2017).

What follows next in this chapter is a Millsian (1967) account of history and biography of an intimate experience of the working life of a person close to my heart. It is a tragic course indicative of experience of the contemporary working class and the assault on their bodies in the age of finance capital, precarity, and austerity (Lorey, 2015; Mulcahy, 2017; Stanley, 2014). Neoliberalism does not speak of assault or torture but of persistent reinvention of self in a climate of opportunity and entrepreneurialism (as if this isn't oppressive too!). Yet the entrepreneurialism of some is at the expense of the disciplining and advantaging of the many. The abuses of labour is pervasive today especially with the austerity programme demanding further commitment to the desires of capital and the need for profit (Bramall, 2016). The 'neutral' language of business and the labour market silences these abuses. Individual responsibility and responsibilisation are evoked as features of the new citizen-worker no longer in need of the nanny state since he/she now relies on his/her own initiative and personal motivation to succeed (Pimlott-Wilson, 2015). Structural barriers and built-in inequalities in capitalism are relegated to the dustbin of history as neoliberalism promotes its ideology and influence. Since we live at the time of the 'end of history' (the end of alternatives to socio-economic re-organising), only personal motivation and aspiration matters in aiming higher towards achievement (Pimlott-Wilson, 2015, p. 289). This is a disservice to human beings increasingly tied to the swing of the labour market, the neoliberal model, and the latter's insistence on making a distinction between 'winners' and 'losers'. Winners and losers according to whom, for whom, and by whose standards and evaluation?

Neoliberalism remains pervasive but in the hinterlands of the nation, economic change is accentuated differently and workers indentify in ways that correspond to the specificities of place (Aguiar, et al., 2005). In this case study, a changing economy expels young working class male workers while a corresponding industry in the North absorbs them into its ranks to transform ruggedscapes on the interior into oil and gas industrial investment. The expulsion in one place and the absorption of working class youth in the labour market in another is not unconnected or conincidental (Sassen, 2014). I see this as the process of primitive accumulation exacerbated by austerity in the interior of the country and workers as victims to capital's seduction. This seduction means bodily sacrifice and torture justified by a lack of options in the centre and the finance-led industry's creation of debt chasers. The following is how I experience this through the lens of watching my son resist and accommodate to a new reality of work and economic anxiety in austere Canada (Evans and McBride, 2017).

## Young men and 'camping' in the North

3:00pm. 3:00pm every third Tuesday of the month, I drive my son to the Kelowna airport to board a plane taking him to northern Alberta and the open fields of the interior of the province where the controversial resource economy of heavy industry and manual labour is found (Dorow and O'Shaughnessy, 2013; Shrivastava and Stefanick, 2015). A pre-paid company airfare ticket awaits him at the check-in counter, as does a regularly scheduled direct flight to Fort McMurray (Fort Mac). It is a short flight into the interior, but it might as well be to the other side of the country given the social distance between him and me, and between him, his co-workers, and the outside world. The exchange of snapchats, mobile phone texts, and even the occasional Skype conversation only confirm the distance between us rather than annihilate it.

Once in Fort Mac, a chartered bus picks him up and others with coordinated flight patterns descending on the airport originating from Kelowna and elsewhere (Barnetson and Foster, 2016; Dorow, et al., 2015).[2] The bus takes the workers on another 90-minute ride into the camp where they will remain for stints of three weeks at a time. The camp is isolated, self-contained, and 'self-sufficient'. In and out access is restricted to company personnel and vehicles, as well as registered delivery trucks and employed cleaners and kitchen staff. Rides are between the camp and the workplace (and of course the airport) since supervisors provide all necessities for the 'campers': accommodations, food, cleaning/cleaners, and even a gym and pool. It is an oasis resort in the hinterlands of Canada. What else could it be? What more could they want? Well, in some instances workers respond by changing the name of their camp to represent more accurately their experience. For instance, Wapasu camp is re-baptised 'Wapatraz'.[3] The employer organises the social reproduction of labour to minimise labour turnover and desertion. Labour retention is an industry onto itself (Government of Alberta, 2013). It is key in assembling workers and keeping them ready for the hard labour of resource industry. It is also a means of 24-hour surveillance and disciplining of labour power. Residents of Fort Mac protest company practices of fly in and fly out (FIFO) mobile workers who come and go 'just in time' while living temporarily in isolated and isolating work sites far from the city (Dorow and O'Shaughnessy, 2013, p. 131). Locals argue the restricting of workers to the camps and work sites prohibits their mobility thereby preventing them from visiting the city and contributing to the local economy (King, 2014). To add insult to injury, multinationals hire FIFO workers even when the local labour market has available skilled workers for hire (CBC News, 2015). But restricting workers' mobility (geographically and in the labour market) is an aggressive labour control ploy to retain workers and tie them to specific employers (Aguiar, et al., 2011).

The isolation of the camp, and more importantly that of the workers, succeeds in keeping workers undistracted from outside sources so they can be easily and readily available to mount corporate-rented buses to attack the hard soil awaiting digging and churning it over in the early stage of transforming the vast landscape. The natural Gaia of the land is neutered and new artifices constructed as 'man' only now breathes life where organic matter existed, shifted, and moved since time immemorial (Lovelock, 1995). First Nations' communities, animals, trees, foliage, streams, rivers, ecologies, and patterns of slow moving earth – culture and nature – are forever gone, displaced, or threatened to make room for the more important activity of bulldozing land to lay pipelines while smirking at environmentalists (Slowey and Stefanick, 2015; Keeling and Sandlos, 2015). Young male bodies too willing or naïve to comprehend that capital takes from them more than their time (oh, it takes so much more!), provide the labour power from which surplus value is extracted to make landscapes yield their 'buried' treasures (Barnetson, 2015; Lowe, 1995; Stuckler and Basu, 2013). It is said (shouted, even in the Kelowna media) that the wages are good, and these 'boys' have 'earned' this hard labour as sentence for past mistakes, poor life choices, and misguided life trajectories (Patterson, 2014). They have turned their backs on neoliberalism's generosities of opportunities by deregulating legislation and undoing institutional rigidities, promoting creative industries and cities, emboldened entrepreneurialism, and reinvigorating individualism (Keyes, forthcoming). These boys are lucky to have jobs given their uninspired aspirational goals or poor university programme choices (Roberts and Evans, 2012; Currid-Halkett, 2017). Besides, is there anything better than hard labour to re-think one's career choices? But, a more accurate assessment might be that neoliberalism dismissed and discarded them at one end (the inflexibility of the model to accommodate different interests and aptitudes at different stages in one's intellectual development) to then re-capture them at another end (as young adults without 'options' in a labour market in constant flux) (Giroux, 2016). The conditions for primitive accumulation must be activated, prioritised, and praised.

In the Okanagan, the restructuring of industry moves rapidly away from manufacturing to the 'soft' industries of wellness, play, and luxury (Aguiar and Marten, 2011). Workers' vulnerability is advantageous to the buyers of labour power. Hardened neoliberals say this labour experience is penance for their undisciplined ways, and dutiful submission is the least they can do for business leaders so kind to absorb them despite their 'mistakes' and 'deficiencies'. Are they not lucky to have a job? Did they not fail to heed the call to improve themselves for new times, new realities, new skills, and new attitudes (Bröckling, 2016)? Shouldn't they be grateful to business elites' benevolence in offering them jobs? They 'chose' to seek no alternatives. As if! Are alternatives theirs to find in a society interwoven with neoliberal values, scrutinised, and policed for their adherence and practise? For real? And yet Marx reminds us, '[t]o be a productive workers is therefore not a piece of luck but a misfortune' (cited in Harvey 2000, p. 106). Is it they who failed the gurus and lackeys of neoliberalism or the other way around? Have they not been restructured out of the post-industrial economy of the Okanagan Valley (Aguiar and Marten, 2011)? What better way to address youth unemployment in an uncertain economic future than by encouraging them to go North (Galarneau, et al., 2013; Capital News, 2014)? A local employment policy of precarity and youth displacement, I fear. Or, one side of the primitive accumulation processes (i.e., generating a workforce) in the resource industry of a finance-led regime of accumulation. The other side is legislative; laws are enacted to facilitate the enclosure of land and land grabs (Sassen, 2014). Critics argue this is the case with Bill 24 in the province of British Columbia. This bill deregulates legislation protecting agricultural land in the province and seeks to re-designate large tracts of this land as non-agricultural for the purpose of non-farming activities in the name of economic sustainability and investment. Some add that the introduction of this bill is to 'offer' land to the oil and gas industries (Aguiar and Marten, 2019).

Left unarticulated are Kelowna elites' failure to accommodate different aptitudes in a working population maladjusted to an economy structured on the low wages of the industries of 'wellness', 'play', retail, and serving (Aguiar, et al., 2005). 'Greens and Grapes', 'Silicon Vineyard', 'Work Hard, Play Hard' are all marketing slogans confirming the Okanagan Valley as 'cradle of free enterprise' (Seymour, 2017, p. A1; Keyes, forthcoming) where the bourgeoisie organises the economy to grow wealth and exacerbate inequality by increasing profit through the exploitation of low-wage workers. As a result, low wages persist for the servant and invisible working class for whom a campaign for increasing the minimum wage is a political goal and not a move towards a living wage for workers living in the fifth most expensive city in Canada (Auyero, 2015; Bush, 2017). An Okanagan Valley regional luxury economy is afoot, and if you are not rich or willing to succumb to low-wage service work or perform luxury work in high end hotels, golf courses and resorts, wineries, and car dealerships in the region, then you are screwed! But this reality is unexamined since statements and assumptions about opportunity, entrepreneurialism, and smugness of place form the common sense neoliberal belief system in the interior of British Columbia (Keyes, forthcoming; Keyes and Aguiar, forthcoming).

'We Love It Here!' This is another local slogan, but what precisely is it that we love about the valley? The hours of sunshine? The low wages? The low population density? The high cost of real estate? We know slogans are not innocent and neither is branding of cities (Aguiar, et al., 2005). Complicity affirms consent, and progressive resistance is largely absent in 'the Bible belt of Canada' where entrenched structures of political conservatism and leadership persist stretching back to the early twentieth century but most powerfully and thoroughly consolidated in the post war period under the 'leadership' of the Bennett family. The Bennetts 'provided' the province with two Premiers, and an 'inside man' to the province's most recent leader's inner circle (Palmer, 1987; Shaw, 2017). Here the state governs on the behalf and behest of the bourgeoisie! (Miliband, 1977). Furthermore, the most recent Premier was elected to the legislature by running for a seat in West Kelowna after failing to win a seat in her own riding in Vancouver (Shaw, 2013). She established her constituent office and residence in West Kelowna during her second term as Premier. On 9 August 2017, she lost the election and subsequently quit politics altogether (Ghoussoub, 2017).

I won't see my son for almost three weeks. When he returns, he packs into one week all those activities he thought about while digging holes and moving soil in the dead of night in a field he holds no affection for. And, he begins to despise it with each passing 'tour of duty'. If he did see the fields in the long days and bright sun of the northern sky, would he think differently of the abuse he metes out on a patch of land instructed by supervisors indifferent to lands existing for millennia? Would he identify the traces and implications for climate change of the resource industry? It's hard to say. He sees so little of what he does. The landscape of labour is not visible beyond one work assignment at a time, one shift at a time. The forest is indeed invisible for the trees. Today, as in the past, the 'regeneration' of nature is purported to be the way towards economic growth, prosperity, and community health (Walsh-Dilley, 2017). This is in spite of the perilousness of communities standing in the way of fast encroaching forces of climate change abetted by the ongoing colonialism of First Nations' Peoples (Marino, 2015).

At home, my son does not speak about work; he is uninterested in re-telling (re-living) the brutality of his manual labour for my benefit. What happens in the North stays in the North. I hardly see him as he moves about consuming activities, friends, and spaces at a pace an addict would admire. This 'addiction' is fed by local businesses claiming their economic survival is contingent on young men abusing their bodies in the North in exchange for wages. Who cares for their lost youth and tormented and tortured bodies so long as their wages keep the local economy humming? Besides, are they not free to choose such an experience? Are they not free to choose this class relationship? Tch! A local conspiracy for the ongoing abuse of young men persists, is normalised, even 'healthy' to their development as responsible adults and community members in doing their share to prosper the Okanagan economy. I watch and think; how can this persist? How did my son not resist the hypnotic spell of money and the 'easy' access to it in the hinterlands of the country? How can I help him see through this smokescreen of ideological bliss?

Today the flat landscapes of the hinterlands are reinvented and re-affirmed as 'Gold Mountain' to a hyper masculinised Canadian youth driven by consumerism (Yee, 2014). My son's friends have been 'going North' for half a dozen years. A rite of passage for working class boys? Screw you! One must resist capital's interests in defining our personal, experiential, and intellectual growth and development discourses. Yet, a passage it is nonetheless, and one through which young and vibrant bodies endure, to be shortly tamed and disciplined to the interests of profit-seeking *nouveau riche*. Toughness, brutishness, restlessness, eagerness, independence, sense of adventure, malleability – features of Canadian youth – roll into a carrot and stick mantra of 'fair day's wages for a fair day's work'. Unless visibly scarred on the body, corporeal suffering is denied and dismissed.

It was a matter of time before my son too followed his friends into the 'untamed wilderness' of the northern Alberta 'frontier' to offer his services to the corporate gods in Calgary engorging themselves by robbing Canadian boys of their time, innocence, and bodies – of their youth. Here age discrimination is endorsed as youth continue to spoil their bodies for someone else's cash pleasures. To blame his friends for pressuring him to join them would be to give them too much credit, and to assume my son's easy complicity with their pressure tactics. To blame a lack of career aspirations is to blame the victim and to ignore, dismiss, and devalue structures of discrimination and exploitation in the formative years of young men and women, my son included (Roberts and Evans, 2012). Marx in the *Communist Manifesto* reminds us, '[the bourgeoisie] has converted the physician, the lawyer, the priest, the poet, the man [sic] of science, into its paid wage laborers' (Marx and Engels, 1998). The lure of easy money is a ruse for the ongoing proletarianisation of Canadian youth. God damn it! The latter works in the service of the former. *All that is solid melts into air* (Marx and Engels, 1998).

Our ride to the airport is usually quiet and sombre. There is a hug, a wave, and then I stand by the car as my son turns and heads into that moving corridor of people contraption we call airport. There, he is temporarily held hostage until taken from me and delivered to awaiting bosses at another port for disembarking human cargo. If someone were watching us dis-embrace and then followed him with their eyes, they would be unable to tell he is on his way to the land of body torturing for enhancing the lifestyles of elites in some fancy high-rise floor in a downtown building in Calgary. He dresses smartly – usually in shorts with a tight fitting t-shirt outlining his sculpted body. A small and stylish backpack drapes across his back with room barely for his ID essentials. If the sun is shining, and in the summer it usually is in Kelowna, he dons a pair of sunglasses. He bears a new haircut; he looks good. The dark glasses reflect, or do they repel the surroundings thereby creating a cocooning personal space necessary to undertake the plight ahead to isolation and social deprivation? I suspect the glasses hide gentle tears welling in his eyes as pain and suffering soon replace love and joy. (They do in mine.) In his bodily set-up, he seems more like someone going to some athletic competition or onto an excursion at some university campus, than someone boarding a plane to the land of exploited youth, sabotaged bodies, and suffering.

My son has always been a sharp dresser, but attire seems to take an enhanced meaning in his journey to the interior of the country. Dressing stylish and sharp is a way to fend off the advances of capital and its attempt to stamp ownership on his body regardless of where he may be. In fact, his toned body is hard unlike any other time since he was born, even when he played elite soccer. It is a way for him to impress control on his body, and in doing so, preempt capital from reaching into him from the inside. It is a way to assert control over his body; a conscious effort to do so before capital makes advances on it. Working on the body in the camp gym during long periods of isolation in unknowable lands with little to do except eat, sleep, and work is a necessary life diversion, a life-saving activity. It is a lifeline where he and his co-workers make friends and establish acquaintances. Exercise is a way to cope, a means to stay sane. The gymscape interrupts the control exercised by supervisors and 'caretakers' in the camp and work site. It is my son's space of resistance. In this activity, he expresses class-consciousness in refusing to allow the capitalist labour process to capture his body and use it and abuse it until he is no longer wanted or useful for capital accumulation (Lowe, 1995). How long can he keep resisting? Or, might I fear it to be an ongoing training exercise in readying the body for the hard labour of capitalist exploitation (Kelley, 1997)? Is the gymscape a serendipitous locale where the corporation encourages bodies to ready themselves to the rhythms of work and the physical fitness necessary to endure hard labour in the landscape of suffering? The fetishising of the hard body in the gymscape parallels closely, I'm afraid, the intensity of the labour process of laying pipes and burrowing holes. Will capital eventually 'break' him? How sad and devastating that will be. Capital inculcates its values in various ways. God damn it! *All that is solid melts into air* (Marx and Engels, 1998).

## Institutionalising practices

What of the institutionalising practices in place for new and older recruits in the camps? For capital, exploiting workers' labour power isn't the only activity in the labour process; workers must also be taught how to labour. Here strict rules of social behaviour apply – from what to wear, and how to, and what and when to eat and sleep. They are imposed and policed by company thugs threatening expulsion if violation of 'agreed-upon' conduct occurs. Institutionalisation *a la* Goffman seems to work in tandem with a Foucauldian diagnosis of caring practices of the self in the name of employability and pursuit of a paycheque. 'Iron Pete' describes it like this,

> I mentioned that there are [three] wings in the camp. They are laid out in a horse shoe shape and each has a 'brass alley' leading to the buses that stage in the middle. The buses come and go in coordinated waves. All bus activity is regulated by the red 'x' or the green check mark over the alley doors that tell you whether you can go through or not. If one is watching from a distance they would see the lines slowly forming on one side of the alley as the workers queue together followed by a tsunami-like out-pouring as the sign turns green and everyone rushes to get a good seat on their respective buses. If you are at the end of your line your bus may be full and then you have to catch the overflow bus which leaves 10 minutes later and may get you to work after the start time. If you are past the prescribed time and the light clicks red you are in some trouble. You then have [three] options: 1) call in sick; 2) call

work and they may send someone to pick you up; 3) wait for the later bus and arrive just before lunch. All of these options suck so one wants to be at the bus line early if possible.

*Anonymous, 2012*

Few camp returnees speak openly about their work and experiences as to do so will release emotions and open wounds buried deep in their psyche. It is also difficult to know their thoughts since neoliberalism is chameleon-like, adapting to the circumstances as necessary, even legitimising individuality so long as it dovetails with supporting 'winners'. What we can say is that these are not boys working at 'accumulation of experiences' to enhance their resumes to extend social advantages of the already advantaged (Holdsworth, 2017, pp. 296–7). Instead, they are examples of people who have 'internaliz[ed] uncertainty' (Pimlott-Wilson, 2015, p. 289) thereby making their way the best they can in these times of precarity and uncertainty (Standing, 2014). Their *economic refugee* migrant status produced and expulsed from the post-industrial economy of the Okanagan Valley means this internalisation might be financially beneficial, but also socially taxing, body torturing, and anxiety inducing. Tony MacKenzie explains the consequences of 'doing time' in Fort Mac: 'When I'm at work, I'm constantly thinking about home. It's challenging to go away and leave your family … you miss the little things, like a hockey game or a dance recital. So you're making those sacrifices' (Capital News, 2014, p. A3).

Further, '[p]recarization is not an exception, it is rather the rule' (Lorey, 2015, p. 1). Having created uncertainty and insecurity via neoliberalist policies, capital banks on young people (but not only) to replenish labour ranks in industries with difficulties in recruiting and retaining workers (Harvey, 2005). No wonder money is such an appeal. It is the only thing that brings workers back. Abra (a fly in/fly out worker) explains:

> I know that sounds bad, that it was all about the money, but that's really what draws most people up there to Fort Mac. You stay in for about 21 days in a row, you're working 12-hour days, then you usually get a week off. So it's hard … but when you come out your bank account is full.

*Capital News, 2014, p. A6*

Perhaps the bank account grows. What also grows is debt as FIFO workers chase debt to keep up with the Joneses in a community heavily indebted and largely defined by a luxury economy of boats, expensive cars, golf club memberships, lavish monster homes, and ski hill weekend trysts. One might say people suffer from 'financial melancholia' as a 'psychological syndrome of being trapped by past debt obligations' (Davies, et al., 2015, p. 12). For debt chasers (FIFO), 'debt panic' invokes feelings of shame and guilt and often sensing that one is trapped in a 'prison' (Davies, et al., 2015, p. 11). There is an economic price too in that '[d]ebt creates a future where one is always paying for the past' (Davies, et al., 2015, p. 32). Under these circumstances, it becomes difficult to contribute to the local economy when one is constantly trying to catch-up on one's debt payment instead of consuming new items in the economy (Davies, et al., 2015, p. 37). The irony would be too rich, if the experience wasn't so sad! FIFO workers also experience the distancing of social and familial relationships. That is, the re-integrating to home life isn't smooth nor without the ominous presence of the institutionalised camp self. The latter makes for awkward social interactions even with loved ones:

> My husband does three weeks on and one week off. Of course, this includes travel home and to camp (now he already lost two of his seven days off), leaving him with five days at home. It takes us two days to get used to each other and then he is already in transition mode again … i.e. thinking and preparing himself for the return trip. We have a two year old baby boy. He doesn't understand that it is his dad at home. My baby is more freaked out by 'the stranger' in our midst than happy. I am ashamed to confess that having my husband come home is disruptive to the baby's routine. We try and do fun things when

my husband is home. I don't want to burden him then with menial tasks and give him a honey-do list. So I have to do it all by myself; including maintenance and repairs, or hire someone to do the work. So, our overall lifestyle changed and a large chunk of the 'extra' money he earns is consumed by our fun week and work done around the house.

*Capital News, 2014, p. A3*

Going North to earn wages to ease living in the Okanagan, ironically, has instead created strife in the home and intensified the domestic labour of women. Alas, the more things change, the more they stay the same.

## Notes

1  Think of songs like 'Fast Car' by Tracy Chapman and 'Atlantic City' by Bruce Springsteen.
2  http://globalnews.ca/news/1104019/flying-between-kelowna-and-fort-mcmurray-just-got-easier/, accessed 21 August 2017.
3  See the commentary section in the following: http://adventuresofironpete.blogspot.ca/2012/03/wapasu-lodge-aka-camp-kearl.html?m=1, accessed 1 September 2017. This is not my son's camp.

## References

Aguiar, L. and Marten, T. (2011) 'Shimmering white Kelowna and the examination of painless white privilege in the Hinterland of British Columbia', In: A. Baldwin, L. Cameron, and A. Kobayashi (Eds.) *Rethinking the Great White North: Race, nature, and the historical geographies of whiteness in Canada*, Vancouver, BC: UBC Press, pp. 127–44.

Aguiar, L. and Marten, T. (2019) 'Bill 24, climate change and cerebral farmers in the British Columbia interior', *BC Studies*, forthcoming.

Aguiar, L.L.M., Tomic, P., and Trumper, R. (2005) 'Work hard, play hard: Selling Kelowna, BC, as year-round playground', *Canadian Geographer*, 49(2): 123–39.

Aguiar, L., Tomic. P., and Trumper, R. (2011) 'Mexican migrant agricultural workers and accomodations in the Okanagan Valley, British Columbia'. Metropolis British Columbia, Working paper series, no.11–04, Vancouver, British Columbia: Metropolis British Columbia.

Albo, G., Gindin, S., and Panitch, L. (2010) *In and Out of Crisis: The global financial meltdown and left alternatives*, Oakland, CA: PM Press.

Anonymous. (2012) 'Wapasu Lodge aka Camp Kearl', available at http://adventuresofironpete.blogspot.ca/2012/03/wapasu-lodge-aka-camp-kearl.html?m=1 (accessed on 1 September 2017).

Auyero, J. (2015) *Invisible in Austin: Life and labor in an American city*, Austin, TX: University of Texas.

Barneston, B. (2015) '"Politically, how do you make it relevant?...kill more young people." The prospects for greater enforcement of teen employment laws in Alberta, Canada', Relations Industrielles/Industrial Relations, 70(3): 558–83.

Barnetson, B. and Foster, J. (2016) 'Dead quiet in the hinterlands: The construction of workplace injuries in western Canada newspapers, 2009–2014', *Labour & Industry*, 26(2): 75–89.

Beder, S. (2000) *Selling the Work Ethic: From puritan pulpit to corporate PR*, New York, NY: ZED.

Bourdieu, P. (1998) *Acts of Resistance: Against the new myths of our time*, Cambridge, UK: Polity Press.

Bramall, R. (2016) 'Introduction: the future of austerity', *New Formations*, 87: 1–10.

Bröckling, U. (2016) *The Entrepreneurial Self: Fabricating a new type of subject*, London and Thousand Oaks, CA: Sage.

Bush, D. (2017) 'British Columbia's NDP government decision to "slowly raise" the minimum wage to $15', available at www.kelownacapnews.com/news/the-1300-km-commute-part-2-the-community/ (accessed on 3 September 2017).

Cairns, J. (2017) *The Myth of the Age of Entitlement: Millennials, austerity, and hope*. Toronto, ON: University of Toronto Press.

Capital News. (2014) 'The 1,300km commute: the people, the community, getting there', available at www.kelownacapnews.com/news/the-1300-km-commute-part-3-getting-there/ (accessed on 4 October 2017).

CBC News. (2015) 'Suncor making amends after Fort Hills hiring policy excluded Fort McMurray workers', available at www.cbc.ca/news/canada/edmonton/suncor-making-amends-after-fort-hills-hiring-policy-excluded-fort-mcmurray-workers-1.3315618 (accessed on 1 September 2017).

Clement, W. and Vosko, L. (Eds.). (2003) *Changing Canada: Political economy as transformation*, Montreal/Kingston: McGill/Queen's University Press.

Cowie, J. (2010) *Stayin' Alive: The 1970s and the last days of the working class*, New York, NY: The New Press.

Currid-Halkett, E. (2017) *The Sum of Small Things: A theory of the aspirational class*, Princeton, NJ: Princeton University Press.

Davies, W., Montgomerie, J., and Wallin, S. (2015) *Financial Melancholia: Mental health and indebtedness*, Political Economy Research Centre, Goldsmiths: University of London.

Demographia. (2012) *8th Annual Demographia International Housing Affordability Survey: 2012 ratings for metropolitan markets*, Bellevile, Illinois: Performance Urban Planning.

Dorow, S. and O'Shaughnessy, S. (2013) 'Fort McMurray, wood buffalo, and the oil/tar sands: revisiting the sociology of "community"', *Canadian Journal of Sociology*, 38(2).

Dorow, S., Cassiano, M., and Doerksen, C. (2015) 'Live-in caregivers in Fort McMurray: a socioeconomic footprint', available at www.onthemovepartnership.ca/wp-content/uploads/2015/01/Live-in-Caregivers-in-Fort-McMurray-Report-Overview-Dorow-et-al-Jan-2015.pdf (accessed on 5 October 2017).

Evans, B.M. and McBride, S. (2017). *Austerity: The lived experience*, Toronto, Canada: University of Toronto Press.

Galarneau, D., Morissette, R., and Usalcas, J. (2013) What has Changed for Young People in Canada? Catalogue no. 75-006-x. Ottawa, ON: Statistics Canada, Government of Canada.

Ghoussoub, M. (2017) 'Christy Clark resigns as leader of B.C. Liberal Party', available at www.cbc.ca/news/canada/british-columbia/christy-clark-resigns-as-leader-of-b-c-liberal-party-1.4226286 (accessed on 5 October 2017).

Giroux, H. (2016) *The Terror of Neoliberalism: Authoritarianism and the eclipse of democracy*, Boulder, CO: Paradigm Publishers.

Government of Alberta. (2013) 'Retaining your staff', available at www.albertacanada.com/files/albertacanada/retainingyourstaff.pdf (accessed on 31 August 2017).

Harvey, D. (2000) *Spaces of Hope*, Berkeley, CA: University of California Press.

Harvey, D. (2005) *A Brief History of Neoliberalism*, New York, NY: Oxford University Press.

Harvey, D. (2010) *The Enigma of Capital and the Crises of Capitalism*, New York, NY: Oxford University Press.

Herod, A. (2018) *Labor*, Medfor, MA: Polity.

Hoffman, R. and Casnocha, B. (2012) *The Start-Up of You*, New York, NY: Crown Business.

Holdsworth, C. (2017) 'The cult of experience: Standing out from the crowd in an era of austerity', *Area*, 49(3): 296–302.

Horton, J. (2017) 'Young people and debt: Getting on with austerities', *Area*, 49(3): 280–7.

Judt, T. (2010) *Ill Fares the Land*, New York, NY: Penguin.

Kaletsky, A. (2010) *Capitalism 4.0: The birth of a new economy in the aftermath of crisis*, New York, NY: Public Affairs.

Keeling, A. and Sandlos, J. (2015) *Mining and Communities in Northern Canada: History, politics, and memory*, Calgary, AB: University of Calgary Press.

Kelley, R.D.G. (1997) Yo' mama's disfunktional! Fighting the cultural wars in urban America, Boston, MA: Beacon Press.

Keyes, D. (forthcoming) 'Okanagan in print: typographical Heimlich fantasies of the entrepreneurial whiteness', In: D. Keyes and L. Aguiar (Eds.) *Hinterland of Whiteness: White fantasies in the Okanagan Valley, British Columbia*, Vancouver, BC: UBC Press, pp. 255–90.

Keyes, D. and Aguiar, L. (Eds.) (forthcoming) *Hinterland of Whiteness: White fantasies in the Okanagan Valley, British Columbia*, Vancouver, BC: UBC Press.

King, T. (2014) 'Fly-in, fly-out is our biggest threat', available at www.fortmcmurraytoday.com/2014/11/06/fly-in-fly-out-is-our-biggest-threat (accessed on 1 September 2017).

Lewis, S. and Berg, L. (forthcoming) 'White supremacy, surveillance, and urban Aboriginal women in the Kelowna, BC, housing market', In: D. Keyes and L. Aguiar (Eds.) *Hinterland of Whiteness: White Fantasies in the Okanagan Valley, British Columbia*, Vancouver, BC: UBC Press, pp. 187–217.

Lorey, I. (2015) *State of Insecurity: Government of the precarious*, New York, NY: Verso.

Lovelock, J. (1995) *Gaia: A new look at life on Earth*, New York, NY: Oxford University Press.

Lowe, D. (1995) *The Body in Late-Capitalist USA*, Durham, NC: Duke University Press.

Lowe, G. and Graves, F. (2016) *Redesigning Work: A blueprint for Canada's future well-being and prosperity*, Toronto, ON: University of Toronto Press.

Marino, E. (2015) *Fierce Climate, Sacred Ground: An ethnography of climate change in Shishmareff, Alaska*, Fairbanks, Alaska: University of Alaska Press.

Martin, R. (2002) *Financialization of Daily Life*, Philadelphia, PA: Temple University Press.

Marx, K. and Engels, F. (1998) *The Communist Manifesto: A modern edition*, New York, NY: Verso.

Miliband, R. (1977) *Marxism and Politics*, New York, NY: Oxford University Press.

Mills, C.W. (1967) *The Sociological Imagination*, New York, NY: Oxford University Press.

Mirowski, P. (2013) *Never Let a Serious Crisis Go To Waste*, New York, NY: Verso.

Moody, K. (1997) *Workers in a Lean World: Unions in the International Economy*, New York, NY: Verso.

Mulcahy, N. (2017) 'Entrepreneurial subjectivity and the political economy of daily life in the time of finance', *European Journal of Social Theory*, 20(2): 216–35.

Palmer, B.D. (1987) *Solidarity: The rise & fall of an opposition in British Columbia*, Vancouver, BC: New Star Books.

Patterson, W. (2014) 'The 1,300 km commute (Part 2: the community)', available at www.kelownacapnews.com/news/the-1300-km-commute-part-2-the-community/ (accessed on 1 September 2017).

Pimlott-Wilson, H. (2015) 'Individualising the future: the emotional geographies of neoliberal governance in young people's aspirations', *Area*, 49(3): 288–95.

Roberts, S. and Evans, S. (2012) '"Aspirations" and imagined futures: the im/possibilities for Britain's young working class', In: W. Atkinson, S. Roberts, and M. Savage (Eds.) *Class Inequality in Austerity Britain: Power, difference and suffering*, Malden, MA: Palgrave/Macmillan, pp. 70–89.

Sassen, S. (2014) *Expulsions: Brutality and complexity in the global economy*, Cambridge, MA: The Belknap Press of Harvard University.

Scharff, C. (2016) 'The psychic life of neoliberalism: mapping the contours of entrepreneurial subjectivity', *Theory, Culture & Society*, 33(6): 107–22.

Sennett, R. (1998) *The Corrosion of Character: The personal consequences of work in the new capitalism*, New York, NY: W.W. Norton & Company.

Seymour, R. (2017) '"Team Okanagan" liberals cruise to victory as fortunes of party less certain', *The Daily Courier*, A1–2.

Shaw, R. (2013) 'Christy Clark to seek Kelowna seat in byelection; Ben Stewart resigning', available at www.timescolonist.com/news/local/christy-clark-to-seek-kelowna-seat-in-byelection-ben-stewart-resigning-1.313362 (accessed on 5 October 2017).

Shaw, R. (2017) 'Christy Clark: B.C.'s modern-day W.A.C. Bennett?', available at http://vancouversun.com/news/politics/christy-clark-b-c-s-modern-day-w-a-c-bennett (accessed on 5 October 2017).

Shrivastava, M. and Stefanick, L. (Eds.) (2015) *Alberta Oil and the Decline of Democracy in Canada*, Athabasca, Alberta: Athabasca University Press.

Slowey, G. and Stefanick, L. (2015) 'Development at what cost? First Nations, ecological integrity, and democracy', In: M. Shrivastava and L. Stefanick (Eds.) *Alberta Oil and the Decline of Democracy in Canada*, Athabasca, Alberta: Athabasca University Press, pp. 195–224.

Standing, G. (2014) The Precariat: The new dangerous class, New York, NY: Bloomsbury Academic.

Stanley, L. (2014) '"We're reaping what we sowed": everyday crisis narratives and acquiescence to the age of austerity', *New Political Economy*, 19(6): 895–917.

Stuckler, D. and Basu, S. (2013) *The Body Economic: Why austerity kills*, New York, NY: HarperCollins.

Van Emmerik, K. (2017) 'Kelowna is one of Canada's fasting-growing cities', available at https://globalnews.ca/news/3237406/kclowna-is-one-of-canadas-fasting-growing-cities/ (accessed on 5 October 2017).

Walks, A. (2013) 'Mapping the urban debtscape: the geography of household debt in Canadian cities', *Urban Geography*, 34(2): 153–87.

Walsh-Dilley, M. (2017) 'Book review: the mushroom at the end of the world: on the possibility of life in capitalist ruins', available at http://journals.sagepub.com/doi/10.1177/0309132517698562 (accessed on 5 October 2017).

Yee, P. (2014) *Tales from Gold Mountain*, Toronto, ON: Groundwood.

# 9

# 'Willingness to pay'

## How health care user fees spread around the world, 1965–2015

*Aaron Shakow and Salmaan Keshavjee*

### User fees and global health

Worldwide, one of the hottest topics in public life today is health care and who should pay for it. Since at least the 1970s, it has been recognised that one way to ration access to this often-expensive social service is to charge patients at the point of service delivery. When payment is demanded up front, many people avoid the doctor's office, even if they are sick, and the poorer they are, the more pronounced this effect. Yet for years, development specialists urged poor countries to recoup the costs of health care directly from individuals rather than relying on public financing.

Ultimately the viability of user fees as an exercise in health policy rested on two empirical questions: (a) could the health system raise enough money at the point of service delivery to improve care even when the central state expenditure was minimal?; and (b) could a process be developed for assessing people's ability to pay which ensured that the poor majority would not be priced out of the market?

By the late 2000s, a global consensus had emerged: the answer to both questions was 'no'. Among the poor, the evidence shows, user charges at the point of service delivery have a consistently detrimental impact on health (Keshavjee, 2014). Meanwhile, removing user fees leads to improvements in health system usage without significantly affecting quality (James, et al., 2005; Ansah, et al., 2009; UNICEF, 2009b; Yates, 2009). In its 2008 World Health Report, the World Health Organization (WHO) advised countries to 'resist the temptation to rely on user fees' (WHO, 2008, p. 26). The United States had already forbidden multilateral lenders from making the institution of user fee policies a condition of loan funding (United States Congress, 2000). Between 2000 and 2010, numerous African countries, where user fees had become widespread over the previous two decades, abolished them (Riddé and Morestin, 2011).

Even the U.N. Children's Fund (UNICEF), which was a leading advocate for 'community financing' through user fees after launching its Bamako Initiative in 1988, eventually repudiated the policy (UNICEF, 2009a). It was, however, a battlefield conversion. In 2007, UNICEF grudgingly admitted for the first time that health programmes on the Bamako Initiative model were rarely brought to scale, and that 'even in those countries where Bamako has been deemed a success, poor people viewed price as a barrier … a large share did not use essential health services despite exemptions and subsidies' (UNICEF, 2007, p. 36). In the same report, though, it still claimed that 'calls for the immediate and universal elimination of user fees for health care services may prove overly simplistic or unrealistic' (UNICEF, 2007, pp. 57, 85).

A background paper for the World Development Report of 2004 gives insight into the intractability of received wisdom with regard to user fees, despite ample peer-reviewed evidence that they are harmful and administratively unsound. Written by key architects of the Bamako Initiative at UNICEF and the World Bank, it argued that forcing poor people to pay for their own medicines transforms them: 'From mere recipients of health care, *consumers* became active partners whose voice counted' (Knippenberg, et al., 2003, p. 4). This was not an empirical, knowledge-based position. It was an ideology.

## Health care fees and neoliberalism

The belief that consumer choice should outweigh impact on household finances and access to essential health care in evaluating a policy reflects a deep commitment to the principle that private administration is not just more efficient than its public analogue, but also morally superior. This principle is a core tenet of neoliberalism, a movement that arose among academic economists during the 1940s in opposition to the state-centred Keynesian approach that informed the design of international development institutions after World War II (Steil, 2013). Disciples of Keynes such as James Meade and Joan Robinson explicitly called for redistribution to serve the principle of social justice (Robinson, 2017). Neoliberals, by contrast, were anti-egalitarian, advocating an approach that saw 'the market' as the optimal distributor of social goods. Citizens became 'consumers', and 'choice' in a market setting became the moral basis of society (Nozick, 1974). This ideological frame is firmly embedded in today's health-sector user-fee policies (Clarke, et al., 1994).

Underlying neoliberal ideology in health care were two doctrines: 'rational choice', which proposed that consumers in a free market always make decisions in their own interest; and 'human capital', which defined support to citizens (vis-à-vis health, education, and other public goods) as an investment in the instruments of capitalist production (Foucault, et al., 2008; Mirowski, 2013). Because such investments were held to be 'the most distinctive feature of our economic system', US neoliberals paid careful attention to health care (Schultz, 1961, p. 17). In order to capture the bureaucratic state, their premises were expressed in a technical idiom of planning and administration. An intimate relationship thus developed between the scholarly apparatus of neoliberalism and management approaches that used systems theory as a guide to the organisation of industrial and scientific production ('managerialism') (Mirowski, 2002; Lewis, 2007).

Both disciplines attempted to restrict choices about public allocation to purely economic parameters, using procedures like cost-benefit analysis – deliberately in some cases – to place important political-philosophical debates in public health such as equality or equity versus autonomy outside the scope of debate. In other words, the so-called 'separation thesis' (that business decisions transcend ethical reasoning) was being applied, with little self-reflection or transparency, to the public sector (Durkheim, 1992; Wicks, 1996; Werhane, 1999).

Recognisably neoliberal policy ideas and planning tools were already percolating through the health sector as early as the 1960s. In many cases this trend was inspired by a desire to defend the expansion of state social services from its institutional critics (who were often, paradoxically, self-conscious neoliberals). Long before neoliberal principles like privatisation and 'choice' received explicit institutional support from the governments of Margaret Thatcher in the United Kingdom and Ronald Reagan in the United States they were endorsed by prominent advocates of statist liberalism.

Similarly, although the international financial crisis that began in 1982 with Mexico's default on sovereign debt was a key milestone in the neoliberal colonisation of global health, the process was by then already well advanced. Indeed, one can go so far as to say that global health as we know it was *created* through the transmission of neoliberal ideas to countries around the world. As far back as the 1960s, the WHO was in close consultation with neoliberal economists who were calling into question the universal access to care offered by the British National Health Service and the Medicare programme in the United States. A decade later, the neoliberal preference for privatisation and central state retrenchment was imbedded in WHO and UNICEF's 'Health For All' campaign, which, though bold in its call for increased access to basic health care for the world's poor, explicitly endorsed fiscal decentralisation and a preference for village health care institutions over secondary and tertiary-care facilities as part of its 'Health For All' campaign.

Global health and neoliberalism were linked by a network of bureaucracies, procedures, and documentary forms which asserted a global model of liberal governmentality. Neoliberalism took the shape of policies which travelled along that network, and also a vocabulary of terms and metaphors applied to an 'elaborate [transnational] social system, affected by attitudes, values and ideologies as much as by profiles of illness, economics and technology' (Mechanic, 1979; Lee and Goodman, 2002, p. 109).

These policies were promoted by numerous international development agencies. Yet, they contradicted the principle of health as a human right espoused by many of the same agencies (Hayek, 2013). Instead, they substituted a vision of autonomous 'choice' – for individuals, village communities, and states. Even key actors who identified publicly with the social-welfare state and associated ideas of social and economic rights came to support approaches that embraced the neoliberal principle of autonomy (Nicholson, et al., 2016). These tensions in the nascent institutions of global health can be seen as a refraction of fissures in the domestic politics of health care in wealthy industrialised countries, particularly the United States of America.

## American health care: state funding and cost control

US health care costs were rising sharply in the postwar period. Between 1950 and 1965, prices for hospital-based care in the United States grew at 7 per cent annually, 5 percentage points above the general rate of price inflation (Hanft, 1967). The percentage of these costs underwritten by the state, however, was relatively low (Abel-Smith, 1963). In 1962, US national health expenditure was US$31.75 billion, 5.4 per cent of GDP, but the government share was only 25 per cent (Reed and Rice, 1964). This pattern shifted, however, with the passage of Medicare and Medicaid legislation in 1965 under President Lyndon B. Johnson (Starr, 1982).

Given bitter opposition to Medicare legislation by the American Medical Association (AMA) and other trade groups, congressional leaders did not have the appetite for a second battle over cost controls, which were described by the AMA and its Republican allies in Cold War terms as 'socialised medicine'. The law gave hospitals and practitioners substantial autonomy to set prices – and predictably, after the passage of Medicare the price of hospital-based services rose every year at 14 per cent (Patterson, 1997). As the government contribution grew, reducing costs and promoting efficiency became a sovereign priority (Richmond and Fein, 2005). The sharply increased recurrent costs for health care also became a target for critics like management guru Peter Drucker, who declared in 1968 that 'modern government has become ungovernable' under the new bureaucracy, and that its functions should be transferred en masse to NGOs or private corporations (Drucker, 1992, p. 220; Bel, 2006).

To fend off this reaction, Johnson and his successors fell back on 'operational research', an approach to policy analysis that had gestated in England and the United States during World War II, and was then adopted by neoliberal economists of the Chicago School (Mirowski, 2002). Operational research in health care began to flower in the late 1950s as an outgrowth to the neoliberal interest in 'human capital' (Kiker, 1966; Blaug, 1976). However, it also served the practical needs of hospitals in the United States and the United Kingdom, where many officials were keen to fend off criticism about public health expenditures (Flagle, 1961; Flagle, 1962; Porter, 1995). It overlapped with the 'systems analysis' approach developed by the RAND Corporation for the US military. When Ford C.E.O. Robert McNamara was appointed to head the US Defense Department in 1961, systems analysis – whose emblem was the 'cost-benefit ratio' – became a prerequisite for all budget submissions (Fisher, 1971; Halberstam, 1993). The month after Lyndon Johnson signed Medicare into law in 1965, he announced that McNamara's 'programme budgeting' methods would be adopted by all Federal agencies, especially the Department of Health, Education and Welfare (Novick, 1965).

As some saw early on, key conceptual features of cost-benefit analysis were neoliberal in essence. By implying that only economic rationality was relevant to budget allocations, it effectively negated consideration of political commitments such as equity in health care access – while simultaneously presenting itself as a procedure that 'has no politics' (Wildavsky, 1966). As the World Bank's 1981 *World Development Report* observed, 'The value of services is hard to measure … if they are supplied free by the public sector' – evading the possibility that universal access to services might be the point of departure, in which case it was the *fulfillment* of that (non-scalar) value which a policy analysis ought to assess (World Bank, 1981c, p. 17).

To be sure, much depended on the way in which cost-benefit studies were embraced by decision makers. Yet, when budgets were justified mainly in terms of cost, the combination of implicit bias and political pressure almost invariably produced cheaper policies – a dynamic became clearer when cost-benefit analysis was officially re-imposed on all federal agencies by Ronald Reagan in 1981 (Shabecoff, 1981).

## Neoliberalism, 'community financing', and global health

The bureaucratic instinct for self-preservation that drove the adoption of systems analysis in the United States during the 1960s also affected international development agencies, which were under pressure to finance similar expansions of social services in post-colonial countries. At the World Bank, for example, lending to governments before the 1970s had focused exclusively on import substitution and investment in so-called 'productive sectors', meaning industry and agriculture (World Bank, 1964). The basic mathematical tool for modeling the development process was the capital/productivity ratio, which has no room for 'soft' indicators like health (Myrdal, 1971). As the agency's Vice President Robert Garner had put it in 1949: 'We can't go messing around with education and health. We're a bank!' (Kapur, et al., 1997, p. 111).

It was primarily neoliberal economists who focused on health care during this period: because it was central to the enlightenment model of governmentality, because it swelled public budgets that they were keen to redirect towards private-sector institutions, and because it was key to re-imagining the value framework for individual human life (Fisher, 1897; Becker, 1962; Mushkin, 1962; Schultz, 1962). Thus, where mainstream development economics provided no rationale to expand social services in poor countries, neoliberals seemed to offer a lifeline. In the early days of 'global health', egalitarian internationalists were already showing a distinct affection for analytical frameworks developed to promote autonomous and hierarchical social relations.

As a technocratic agency par excellence, the WHO was an early convert to the concept of operational research (WHO, 1950). It was imbedded most self-consciously in the work of its tuberculosis office, which focused at first on the logistics of BCG vaccine delivery.

By 1964, the quantitative programme budgeting framework developed by RAND and implemented at the McNamara Defense Department was percolating into WHO's operational planning – first in tuberculosis interventions, and then throughout the organisation as a whole (WHO, 1964; Candau, 1966; Brogger, 1967). Such exercises troubled many officials – both because they uncritically applied economic models across very different national settings, and because they masked an unacknowledged moral choice. As one critic argued: 'To convert the goal of health into simple economic expression … could never satisfy the multiple ideals or moral, humanitarian, and social principles of the [public-health] profession' (Macchiavello, 1961, p. 16).

Nonetheless, WHO plunged forward. In 1967, it recruited a prominent neoliberal critic of national health services to evaluate the national tuberculosis control programme in India (Feldstein, et al., 1973). An unsigned analysis in WHO's annual budget justification for fiscal 1968 urged universal application of cost-benefit analysis and other programme budgeting approaches (WHO, 1967).

Meanwhile, Robert McNamara had moved on from the US Defense Department to the World Bank. Four years into his tenure, as he reorganised the Bank around 'programme budgeting' and decentralisation to regional offices in consultation with McKinsey & Co., McNamara moved decisively into the field of health care (Galambos and Milobsky, 1995). In 1972, with technical experts gathering at the World Health Assembly to discuss the link between health and economic development, the World Bank extended a substantial loan to Indonesia for health care infrastructure in collaboration with WHO and UNICEF (WHO, 1972). McNamara began to echo WHO rhetoric with calls for 'establishing growth targets in terms of essential human needs' (McNamara, 1981, p. 212).

His next step was to formalise a World Bank health policy. Published in 1975, it endorsed cost-benefit analysis in health planning, but warned against uncritical use of such tools and discouraged exclusive reliance on the private sector. Health care, the document argued, echoing Kenneth Arrow's well-known analysis (Arrow, 1963), was subject to certain fundamental 'market failures': poorly informed consumers, a lack of competition amongst providers, externalities associated with infectious diseases, and the unaffordability of services by the poor, all of which justified a primary role for the public sector in financing and providing health services (World Bank, 1975).

As the WHO and UNICEF embarked on planning for the 1978 Conference on Primary Health Care in Alma Ata, Kazakhstan, McNamara stressed World Bank's support for examining 'inexpensive health delivery systems ... designed around community-based health workers who can provide the poor with a broad spectrum of simple and effective services' (McNamara, 1981, pp. 326–7). He directed the Bank's policy research department to investigate resource requirements for a 'Basic Human Needs' approach to international development that would include a commitment to building decentralised health and education infrastructure (Burki and Voorhoeve, 1977; Streeten and Burki, 1978). The *World Development Report* for 1980 explicitly appealed to the guarantee of health and education in the Universal Declaration of Human Rights, and it promoted the argument that 'human development' in these areas is critical 'not only in alleviating poverty directly, but also in increasing the incomes of the poor, and GNP growth as well', meaning that 'some steps we all have long known to be morally right ... make good economic sense as well' (McNamara, 1980, p. iii). A staff-written background paper for the 1980 report argued that 'the use of prices and markets to allocate health care is generally not desirable' (Golladay and Liese, 1980, p. 28).

## Community financing and 'Health For All'

Meanwhile, the thrust of global health was in the opposite direction. What is striking in retrospect about the Alma Ata Declaration is the extent to which it embedded neoliberal prescriptions from the start. In country after country, WHO and UNICEF advisers urged some combination of aid and loan funding, training for theoretically unpaid community members, and up-front user fees.

In Sierra Leone, for example, the primary health care pilot project aimed to 'shif[t] a substantial degree of authority and responsibility to local health development committees at both the chiefdom and district levels.' The 'community orientation' of the project 'could reduce dependence on the central government's revenues. This would be particularly important in the area of pharmaceuticals for Sierra Leone' (World Bank, 1981b, p. 112). In the mid-1980s Bank staff reported approvingly that the primary health care projects in Sierra Leone were recouping between 40 and 78 per cent of the cost of drugs from patients through user fees (World Bank, 1986).

These reports highlight an unresolved tension in the primary health care movement, and in the liberal model of development more generally. The Alma Ata Declaration urged that primary health care be made 'universally accessible to individuals and families in the community ... at a cost that the community and country can afford' (Art. 6). However, despite a clear statement in the official meeting report that 'individual payment on a fee-for-service basis is certainly not a solution that can be widely applied', references in the declaration to 'the community' as a key source of financing left the possibility of such payments wide open. 'Members of the community can contribute ... financial and other resources to primary health care', the report suggested in a passage on local participation. It stressed the importance of policies 'to ensure that the community controls ... the funds it invests in primary health care' (WHO and UNICEF, 1978, pp. 51,71).

While it was the government's responsibility to 'ensure that essential drugs are available at the various levels of primary health care at the lowest feasible cost', the emphasis at Alma Ata on decentralisation meant that financing, too, was being mandated as a local responsibility (WHO and UNICEF, 1978, p. 52). Community members were asked to contribute 'their own resources, in cash and kind, in order to develop primary health care in accordance with the programme they have worked out' (WHO and UNICEF, 1978, p. 68).

In WHO's 1978 elaboration of the financing issues associated with primary health care, it encouraged clinics at the village level to charge 'small fees' for drugs and governments 'to find new types of local institutions through which health care can be cooperatively developed with financing partly by the local people themselves', giving them 'both the right and the incentive to participate in the running of the program' (WHO, 1978, p. 28). Members of the study group did caution that 'care should be taken, in the worldwide enthusiasm for maximum local participation or self-reliance in health program development, that this movement is not exploited to relieve national governments of their responsibility' (WHO, 1978, p. 29). But clearly if 'international organizations, multilateral and bilateral agencies, nongovernmental organizations, funding agencies, and other partners in international health' ignored the recommendation at Alma Ata to 'channel increased technical and financial support into' primary care, then these 'small fees' would become more and more central to the success of the larger enterprise (WHO and UNICEF, 1978, pp. 31–2).

In the period after the Alma Ata conference, experiments in 'community financing' proliferated. The mandate claimed by WHO and UNICEF for primary health care as a centrepiece of liberal development led aid agencies and governments to try and recover some of its costs from patients through local health financing strategies. They were by no means unprecedented. Shortly after Cameroon's decolonisation in 1960, for example, the Directorate of Private Sector Support (DASP) began retaining the services of village-level health workers by allowing them to keep the markups from pharmaceuticals sales (USAID, 1980; Molem, 2008). This practice of funding recurrent salary costs of key public-sector health personnel at the village and district level through user fees was one precedent of decentralised financing strategies for primary health care that some observers call 'neoliberal'.

Another popular model, introduced via USAID and other bilateral development agencies, was the revolving drug fund. In revolving credit arrangements, an initial capital investment is replenished by beneficiaries, often with the proceeds from sale of a commodity. A common feature of many agricultural development projects in the 1960s and 70s, revolving funds were envisioned by bilateral donors as a way to help small farmers pay for key inputs like seed and fertiliser without locking donors into permanent support (Lieberson, 1985). By the mid-1970s, the model had begun to find its way into social-sector development projects as well, and the 'Health For All' declaration made it attractive to governments seeking to offload recurrent costs – particularly in the financial turmoil that followed the Mexican default on its sovereign debt in the summer of 1982 (Stinson, 1982; Cross, et al., 1986).

Left unstated was the fact that revolving funds in poor farming communities had been widely unsuccessful, with the start-up capital soon dissipating in the face of poverty and high administrative costs (Lieberson, 1985). Moreover, the migration of the model from so-called productive economic sectors to health care rested on a striking unspoken premise: that user fees for health services and user fees for farm commodities are analytically equivalent (Abel-Smith, 1980).

In this sense, revolving drug funds were neoliberal per se. They were inspired by a concept of 'human capital' that had, in the early 1960s, become a special project of the University of Chicago economist Gary Becker, a leading figure in the Mont Pelerin Society (Allende, 1939). Becker proposed that the benefits of social services to the individual could be monetised just like any other commodity by assessing their additional contribution to a worker's economic productivity (Becker, 1975).

Becker illustrated his broader theory of human capital with an analysis of education, but it was soon taken up by health economists. They contributed another characteristically neoliberal argument that would become prominent in certain rationalisations of cost recovery during the 1980s: the claim that markets assert a self-organising rationality on consumption. Because the consumer is rational, 'the demand for medical care must be derived from the more fundamental demand for "good health"' (Grossman, 1972, p. 248). Because that fundamental demand drives people's attempts to access health services, 'the importance of the cash price and the time cost of care as barriers to medical consumption would be very small', even in poor communities (Heller, 1976, p. 2). If so, then the high recurrent costs of drugs and personnel can be recovered from patients without depressing their willingness to use the formal health system, allowing for cost-savings by governments (or bilateral funders) (Heller, 1979).

The question of whether user fees depressed utilisation of health services in very poor communities was never examined in particularly good faith. Already by 1979 it was widely understood by health economists that direct costs to consumers had a rationing effect and that the imposition of copayments for curative care would decrease its utilisation (Abel-Smith, 1980). Rationing by price was a core hypothesis of the RAND Corporation's Health Insurance Experiment, whose final results were published in 1988, but circulated much earlier (Aron-Dine, et al., 2013). In USAID publications from just before Reagan took office, the imposition of charges was described as a way to 'discourage the use of in-patient curative care' (PADCO, 1980, p. 51).

The effect was familiar to WHO experts as well. 'If it becomes known that a clinic gives treatment to every patient free of charge', wrote the tuberculosis researcher Wallace Fox three years after Sierra Leone's independence from Great Britain, 'this can be depended upon to result in patients presenting … earlier … and hence to improved prospects of cure' (Fox, 1964, p. 137). In developing countries where infectious diseases accounted for most encounters with public health services, the preventive effect of curative care raised serious questions about the World Bank dichotomy of 'preventive' versus 'curative' health services (Russell, 1986).

In retrospect, the 'community financing' approach seems to have had little to do with programme effectiveness or patterns of consumer behaviour, and everything to do with a ferocious debate about the costs of government in the developing world. After the first oil crisis in 1974, recurrent expenditures became a heavy burden for poor countries on top of debt payments that often included interest on loans taken out by colonial rulers for the infrastructure of colonial rule. Because official donors and development banks typically reserved their support at the time for capital expenditures, and with 'petrodollars' readily available elsewhere, current accounts shortfalls were often financed in the mid-1970s by commercial debt – a 'solution' encouraged by development agencies, including WHO (Wood, 1986; Kapur, et al., 1997).

After two further global economic shocks in 1979 and 1982, the strategy became self-defeating, as creditors pursued outstanding debt with the assistance of the very same agencies. By early 1979 (at the outset of the second oil shock) the 'recurrent cost problem' came to be seen as a rationale to 'favor programs and investments with lower recurrent expenditure implications' and to encourage governments to impose 'fees for the use of project services … in such social sectors as health and education' (Heller, 1979, p. 41).

Two meditations on the 'recurrent cost problem' were published in December 1981. Side by side, they illustrate the stark choice that confronted advocates of international development at the time. The first was in a book intended by World Bank Vice President Mahbub ul Haq as a blueprint for the World Bank's shift to the 'Basic Human Needs' agenda:

> The question of finance is peculiarly difficult. For many basic needs projects recurrent costs are quite heavy in relation to capital costs. This means that any system must allow for continuing financial support, rather than a once-for-all commitment to capital costs. The obvious solution – levying [user] charges to cover recurrent costs – may be both difficult to administer and undesirable because the social benefits of the projects very often far exceed the private benefits to the individual consumer.

This is clearly true … [of] health, education, or sanitation projects, where the community at large benefits as well as the participating individuals … Since a major objective of basic needs programs is to provide universal access – especially for the very poor – any system of charges is likely to debar the very people for whom the programs are essential.

*Streeten, et al., 1981, p. 149*

After Ronald Reagan's election to the US presidency, however, Haq resigned and the 'human needs' agenda was abandoned. Other opinions began to take priority, such as those contained in a regional review prepared by USAID's Africa Bureau:

Major elements of the above program do not generate revenues to pay for their operating expenses … Policy measures to reduce the recurrent cost problem include reconsideration of certain policies, such as free education, free primary health care, free potable water; and the principle of the state as the primary employer and producer … The real tax base should be increased through macro-policy reform that accelerate private sector production, and introduce user charges for public services.

*USAID, 1981, p. 6*

The primary health care movement had been closely aligned with Haq's push for 'basic human needs' (Kapur, et al., 1997). Yet, by the early 1980s it was the second approach that came to permeate WHO and UNICEF through well-funded collaborations like the Strengthening Health Systems Delivery (SHDS) project, a joint initiative of USAID and WHO's Africa office that provided more than US$28 million between 1975 and 1986 'to develop the capability to plan, implement, and manage effective and economically feasible' delivery of primary health care in 20 Central and West African countries (WHO, 1977, p. 13; Robinson, 1983). The revolving drug-fund experiments of the 1970s proved to be the point of entry for a campaign by development agencies in the following decade to privatise health care in developing countries using their sovereign debt as a lever.

Meanwhile, the vision of primary health care was itself being downsized. Many people dismissed the Alma Ata Declaration's sweeping goal of 'Health for All by the Year 2000' as overblown and unrealistic, and poor countries struggled to move forward with weak guidance and financial support from bilateral donors and multilateral agencies (Cueto, 2004). Into this breach came a counterattack which drew selectively from particular topics of discussion at Alma Ata like maternal health and substituted them for the broader agenda (Newell, 1988). At a World Bank-funded conference in 1979, Rockefeller Foundation staff proposed that the 'primary health care' brand be applied to just four health services: immunisation, oral rehydration (to fight pediatric diarrhea), breastfeeding, and the use of antimalarial drugs. The response to this suggestion by aid agencies was enthusiastic (Chorev, 2012). The World Bank, USAID, and many other funders of international health began to limit their direct funding to these four specific interventions under the 'Selective Primary Health Care' banner, meaning by default that other health services in the developing world had to be sustained by a different stream of financing.

Soon the Bank's policy apparatus took steps to make this trend explicit. One of the last documents to reach McNamara's desk before his resignation in June 1981 was the so-called 'Berg Report', which definitively situated Africa as a primary focus of the Bank's emerging emphasis on reorienting government health policy (Stein, 2008). Lead author Elliot Berg urged development institutions to 'play a basic role in designing projects so as to emphasize user charges and cost recovery', and 'to develop approaches that conserve fiscal resources while expanding the provision of basic services.' The Berg Report's goal of promoting 'decentralized, self-financing approaches' to health in developing countries was to be achieved by a dramatic shift in fiscal responsibility from national capitals to villages, principally 'provision of primary rural health care through … paramedics funded by village revolving funds' (World Bank, 1981a, p. 44).

Berg's call for 'paramedicals funded by village revolving funds' represented another conscious effort to colonise the Health For All agenda – with its focus on 'barefoot doctors' and other lay providers – in order to shrink the scope of central government activities rather than to increase the agency of village communities or to expand health services.

Soon after the Berg Report came out, the World Bank moved to create an empirical justification for its two principal recommendations for the health sector: administrative decentralisation from national authorities to the village level, and 'cost recovery' or user fees for the population at large. An economist in the Country Policy Department, Nancy Birdsall, began poring over household survey data from rural Mali, trying to calculate the price elasticity of demand for health services – that is, whether raising the price made people use it less. The explicit premise of the exercise was that 'services as they are now constituted and financed would be impossibly expensive to extend to the whole population', so that governments had to explore 'other options' like charging cash fees (World Bank, 1982, pp. 251–2). Indeed, under heavy pressure from the Bank, Mali passed legislation in 1983 and 1984 mandating 'various forms of community participation' in health care financing, including user fees (Brunet-Jailly, 1991, p. 10; Koita and Brunet-Jailly, 1989). The idea that demand for health care was price-inelastic drew from a decade of neoliberal health economics focused on 'cost-sharing' in industrialised countries, but budget administrators at development agencies required no footnotes to see its appeal (Abel-Smith, 1980).

Birdsall's work was circulated internally in 1983 (Birdsall and Chuhan, 1987). The following year a second, much larger, research project was launched in Peru. Supervised by David de Ferranti, a longtime RAND Corporation staffer, it represented a collaboration with the Peruvian government, USAID, PAHO, the West German development agency GTZ, and the U.N. statistical agency, based on a massive survey of over 12,000 households sampled with strict attention to statistical methodology to ensure that they were representative of the country as a whole (World Bank, 1984).

Meanwhile, the American government was moving decisively to reshape public health care institutions in the developing world. 'Recent changes in policy and economic environments have increased the prominence of issues of local financing and non-governmental support of the health system', reported one USAID consultant in 1984 as he explored how to shift the burden of recurrent health sector costs in Sierra Leone from public agencies to patients. 'A political philosophy eschewing the public sector's role in remedying social problems has caused donor countries to reevaluate their roles in foreign assistance programs.' Thus: 'The principal motivation for this study is the policy decision, US Government-wide, that government is to be the provider of services of last resort. That is, alternatives to publicly financed services must be sought and exploited...' (Meyer, 1984).

By the end of 1986 USAID had officially determined that the 'inability to cover recurrent costs of preventive health care' was likely an outcome of 'excessive government spending on personal, curative care and excessive utilization of secondary and tertiary care facilities.' American aid should therefore support 'development of private services, fees-for-service, [and] efficient resource allocation and utilization' (USAID, 1986, p. 7). A few months later, the American aid agency published the results of a five-year, 16-country survey of health care community financing projects that had received US funding between 1981 and 1986. It offered not only an analysis of relevant considerations, but perhaps more importantly, a palette of possible project designs for subsequent support (Stinson, et al., 1987).

The World Bank's Peru study was completed around the same time. It showed unequivocally that 'user fees can generate substantial revenues, but are accompanied by substantial reductions in aggregate consumer welfare, with the burden of the loss on the poor', so that 'undiscriminating user fees would be regressive both in terms of access and welfare' (Gertler, et al., 1987; Manning, et al., 1988, p. 19). However, David de Ferranti did not appear as an author, and the report was not published initially by the World Bank (Gertler, et al., 1988). In the period between planning and execution, de Ferranti had become one of the Bank's most prominent advocates of 'cost recovery' in poor countries, and this apparently led him to distance himself after the findings contradicted his chosen approach – even though it was a study for which he had formal responsibility.

'The conventional and still growing faith that health care should be totally paid for and administered by government needs to be vigorously challenged', de Ferranti insisted in an influential 1985 policy paper, one of ten he wrote or coauthored on the subject after 1981. 'There appears to be considerable scope for having users bear a larger share of health care costs, preferably through a combination of fees for services and fees for coverage' (de Ferranti, 1985, n.p.). He subsequently contributed to an official statement of World Bank policy on user fees along with Birdsall and Elliot Berg's former student John Akin, who had been one of the most consistent and effective advocates of the argument that out-of-pocket payments would not decrease utilisation of health services in poor countries (Akin, et al., 1981; Keshavjee, 2014). It outlined an 'approach [that] would reduce government responsibility for paying for the kinds of health services that provide few benefits to society as a whole', which is to say that 'most curative care, whether provided by the government or non-government sector, should be paid for by those who receive the care' (World Bank, 1987, pp. 1–2).

Two months later, the Peru data, showing the damaging effects of user fees on the poor, was published by the National Bureau for Economic Research. The paper drew little attention.

## The Bamako Initiative

The slogan of 'community financing' had captured the imaginations of development agencies. At the annual meeting of WHO's Africa office in 1987 Jim Grant, the executive director of UNICEF, proposed a scheme that was necessary, in his view, to save primary health care from drowning in a sea of red ink (Grant, 1987). Given the state of the global economy, Grant argued, the best that African governments could hope for was to avoid 'disproportionate cut-backs'. Thus 'the social sectors themselves must produce internal restructuring to put higher priorities on those programs which result in the most benefit to the vulnerable' (Grant, 1987, p. 82). These structural adjustments were to be guided by a sharp distinction between curative care – whose recurrent costs should be recovered from poor patients – and preventive care – which were less suitable targets for user fees (Grant, 1987). Grant's formulation seemed clearly to draw upon the World Bank policy paper published that spring by de Ferranti, Birdsall, and Akin (World Bank, 1987).

Grant proposed to fund the expansion of primary health care to developing countries by asking patients to pay for their own drugs through revolving drug funds. 'The local costs of the PHC [primary health care] system', he argued, should be 'financed in good part though essential drugs purchase' by patients. Since medicines are the focal point of modern curative care it was reasonable to think that they could pay for other recurrent expenditures. In any case it was better for people to buy medicines in public facilities with regulated mark-ups than in an unregulated private sector. 'Even if people pay two or three times what UNICEF pays for the drugs', these prices 'are very affordable for most' (Grant, 1987, p. 87). Grant offered the audience an enthusiastic vision of 'an expanded PHC system throughout Africa within five years, which would meet the essential drug needs of the great majority … and which would be largely locally financed and managed' (Grant, 1987, p. 86).

In the first Bamako Initiative annual report, UNICEF described no fewer than 24 action plans, with four countries already in the implementation stage, all within a few hundred miles of Bamako – Benin, Guinea, Nigeria, and Sierra Leone (UNICEF, 1989). In September 1989, they met in Sierra Leone to plan the next steps. The delegations described a situation far less promising than the one Grant had imagined. 'People are asked to pay many taxes and contributions', they reported, 'as well as to construct health facilities.' However, 'there is a limit to the amount that people can contribute.' They reported significant difficulty determining who should be exempted from payment and who should bear the burden for out-of-pocket costs of 'the poorer people'.

Theoretically this evaluation was to be a community responsibility but 'community participation is complex … Health committees which are supposed to represent the people should be composed in such a way that they are representative and competent.' In many instances, it appears, there was significant pressure on these bodies from the paramount chiefs and other local vested interests (Marquez and Seims, 1987, p. 61). Worst of all, they noted, was an apparent bootstrap problem: the failure to provide quality services before the implementation of 'community financing' was causing people to opt out of the public system altogether, shrinking the funding base for fee-based service expansion (UNICEF, 1990). Evaluations of the Bamako Initiative from all over the world in the mid-1990s suggested that the revolving drug funds had failed to have a significant impact on the availability of medicines and other important supplies and did not raise significant amounts of money. Fee exemptions seemed to be ineffective at ensuring access in settings with a high proportion of very poor patients (Keshavjee, 2014).

It was just over half a century since the Labour government had announced to every British household that the National Health Service 'will provide you with all medical, dental, and nursing care. Everyone – rich or poor, man, woman or child – can use it or any part of it. There are no charges, except for a few special items' (Webster, 2002, p. 24). That famous pamphlet also inspired the government health services established in a number of post-colonial states, and its continued grassroots appeal inspired them to cling tenaciously to the principle of free care, long after their ability to deliver had vanished in a sea of debt. Decolonisation officially presumed that independent states would confer on their citizens the same rights as industrialised countries, a central feature of the American rhetoric of development after World War II. It became, among other things, important to people's national allegiance. It could not be casually abandoned.

## Conclusion

The global inflationary crises of the 1970s and their aftermath turned the aspirations of post-colonial states for a National Health Service equivalent to the system in the United Kingdom into a bureaucratic fiction. Many citizens were already operating informally on a fee-for-services basis. But instead of approaching this situation as a public-health and a moral problem, committing their authority and resources to closing the gap between wealthy and poor nation-states in a postwar international system that treated them formally as equivalent and interchangeable, development institutions elected simply to draw lines of quarantine that allowed clear distinctions to be imposed between them – equal, but separate.

As we've shown, many features of this approach can be seen in the structure and premises of WHO's 'Health For All' campaign. How could an egalitarian movement be transformed so quickly into a mechanism for stratification of rich countries from poor ones? The answer is that neoliberalism in global health during its formative period in the 1980s reflected a permanent tension within the liberal state system itself rather than an ideology of the moment. It grew out of a tendency to address failures of egalitarian ideals within a given group not by trying to widen the institutional criteria for inclusion ('social justice'), or by working to alter the relevant traits of group members who are disfavored ('social change'), but rather, by arbitrarily re-classifying those members outside the boundaries of the group itself – a 'liberal strategy of exclusion' (Mehta, 1999, p. 46). It is not simply that the 'neoliberal' strategy was thoroughly steeped in the terminology of egalitarianism, but also that it was in many cases free-riding on existing institutions, cashing out strategies (like cost-effectiveness analysis or fiscal decentralisation) designed to mitigate the high costs of statism, but for the purposes of public savings and private enrichment rather than social inclusiveness.

During the past decade the policy discussion over user fees has shifted decisively back towards the prevalent view among health economists in the 1970s – before development agencies became mesmerised by the so-called 'recurrent cost problem' – that charging patients at the point of service delivery is likely to impede access to care in very poor communities (Robert and Riddé, 2013). Many countries in Africa started to remove user fees in the 2000s and reported significant increases in health services utilisation (Riddé and Morestin, 2011). David de Ferranti himself seems to have quietly thought the better of his position on community financing as early as 1995, telling an interviewer that 'the Bank' (as he put it) had been wrong to encourage ministries of health to introduce user fees when there may have been 'better ways to get to better places' (Lee and Goodman, 2002, p. 110).

By then de Ferranti was director of the Bank's Human Development Department, and even after this admission of error he did not change his public stance. Indeed in 1996 he wrote in the foreword to a case study of Sierra Leone that the country's approach (based on 'community financing' and user fees) allowed it to 'use available resources more productively, and ... increas[e] accountability to households' (Siegel, et al., 1996).

In the absence of any public accountability for their errors of analysis, both UNICEF and the World Bank continued to promote the Bamako Initiative as a success in West Africa well into the 2000s, and resource-poor countries like Sierra Leone continued to engineer 'cost recovery' into their public health systems, even though the Bank had formally acknowledged the risks of imposing fee-for-service care in poor communities (Johnson and Stout, 1999).

Plainly, the durability of UNICEF's commitment to 'cost recovery' speaks to an intense ideological commitment. Today, by contrast, the received wisdom within development agencies favors public provision of universal health coverage (UHC) financed with tax revenues, and opposes direct payment at the point of service delivery, a position that has received public support from the U.N. General Assembly and numerous mainstream development economists, including David de Ferranti (Savedoff, et al. 2012; Boseley, 2016).

This movement towards more equitable distribution of health care resources is welcome. But absent hoped-for public funding, UHC could easily become a vessel for imposition of very different policies, for example expansion of unregulated private insurance markets. The precedent of WHO's primary health care campaign should make us wary about the ease with which the resource needs of egalitarian liberalism can give its neoliberal counterpart a lever with which to undermine it. There is little doubt that delivering the fruits of modern medicine to the world's more than seven billion inhabitants cannot be achieved by governments alone and will require input from the private sector. The challenge lies in ensuring that this egalitarian endeavor benefits from existing resources, including capital, without allowing 'the market' and its hierarchical relationships to arbitrate the distribution of essential social goods or to frame the moral basis of society.

# References

Abel-Smith, B. (1963) *Paying for Health Services: A Study of the Costs and Sources of Finance in Six Countries*, Geneva: World Health Organization, pp. 45–6.

Abel-Smith, B. (1980) 'Report on the seminar', In: *Sharing Health Care Costs: Proceedings of an international seminar held at Wolfsberg, Switzerland, 20–23 March 1979*, Washington, DC: NCHSR.

Akin, J., Guilkey, D., and Popkin, B. (1981) 'The demand for child health services in the Philippines', *Social Science and Medicine*, 15(4): 249–57.

Allende, S. (1939) '*La Realidad Médico-social Chilena (síntesis)*, Santiago: n.p., 195–8.

Ansah, E.K., et al. (2009) 'Effect of removing direct payment for health care on utilization and health outcomes in Ghanaian children: a randomised controlled trial', *PLoS Med*, 6(2): e1000033.

Aron-Dine, A., Einav, L., and Finkelstein, A. (2013) 'The RAND health insurance experiment, three decades later', *Journal of Economic Perspectives*, 27(1): 197–222.

Arrow, K. (1963) 'Uncertainty and the welfare economics of medical care', *American Economic Review*, 53: 941–73.

Becker, G. (1962) 'Investment in human capital: theoretical analysis', *Journal of Political Economy,* 70(5, Part 2, Suppl.): 9–49.

Becker, G. (1975) *Human Capital: A theoretical and empirical analysis, with special reference to education*, 2nd ed., New York: National Bureau of Economic Research.

Bel, G. (2006) 'The coining of "privatization" and Germany's National Socialist Party', *Journal of Economic Perspectives*, 20(3): 187–94.

Birdsall, N. and Chuhan, P. (1987) 'Willingness to pay for health and water in rural Mali: do WTP questions work?', Washington, DC: World Bank.

Blaug, M. (1976) 'The empirical status of human capital theory: a slightly jaundiced survey', *Journal of Economic Literature*, 14(3): 827–55.

Boseley, S. (2016) 'From user fees to universal healthcare: a 30-year journey', *The Guardian*, available at www.theguardian.com/society/sarah-boseley-global-health/2012/oct/01/worldbank-healthinsurance (accessed 5 November 2016).

Brogger, S. (1967) 'Systems analysis in tuberculosis control: a model', *American Review of Respiratory Disease*, 95(3): 419–34.

Brunet-Jailly, J. (1991) 'Health financing in the poor countries: cost recovery or cost reduction?', Washington, DC: World Bank.

Burki, S. and Voorhoeve, J. (1977) 'Global estimates for meeting basic need: background paper', unpublished discussion paper.

Candau, M.G. (1966) *The Work of WHO 1965: Annual report of the Director-General to the World Health Assembly and to the United Nations*, Geneva: World Health Organization.

Chorev, N. (2012) *The World Health Organization between North and South*, Ithaca: Cornell University Press.

Clarke, J., Cochrane, A., and McLaughlin, E. (1994) 'Mission accomplished or unfinished business? The impact of managerialization', In: C. Cochrane and E. McLaughlin (Eds.) *Managing Social Policy*, London: Sage, pp. 226–42.

Cross, P., et al. (1986) 'Revolving drug funds: conducting business in the public sector', *Social Science and Medicine*, 22(3): 335–43.

Cueto, M. (2004) 'The origins of primary health care and selective primary health care', *American Journal of Public Health*, 94: 1864–74.

de Ferranti, D. (1985) 'Paying for health services in developing countries: an overview', Washington, DC: World Bank.

Drucker, P. (1992) *The Age of Discontinuity: Guidelines to our changing society*, London and New Brunswick, NJ: Transaction Publishers.

Durkheim, E. (1992) *Professional Ethics and Civic Morals*, London: Routledge.

Flagle, C. (1961) 'Conference on operational research in the health services of Great Britain', *Operations Research*, 9(3): 417–8.

Flagle, C. (1962) 'Operations research in the [U.S.] health services', *Operations Research*, 10(5): 591–603.

Feldstein, M., et al. (1973) *Resource Allocation Model for Public Health Planning: A case study of tuberculosis control*, Geneva: World Health Organization.

Fisher, G. (1971) *Cost Considerations in Systems Analysis: A Report prepared for the Office of the Assistant Secretary of Defense (systems analysis)*, New York: American Elsevier Publishing Co.

Fisher, I. (1897) 'Senses of "capital"', *The Economic Journal*, 7(26): 199–213.

Foucault, M., Burchell, G., and Davidson, A. (2008) *The Birth of Biopolitics: Lectures at the Collège de France, 1978–79*, New York and Basingstoke, UK: Palgrave Macmillan.

Fox, W. (1964) 'Realistic chemotherapeutic policies for tuberculosis in the developing countries', *British Medical Journal*, 1(5376): 135–42.

Galambos, L. and Milobsky, D. (1995) 'Organizing and reorganizing the World Bank, 1946–1972: a comparative perspective', *Business History Review*, 69: 156–90.

Gertler, P., Locay, L., and Sanderson, W. (1987) 'Are user fees regressive? The welfare implications of health care financing proposals in Peru', Washington, DC: National Bureau of Economic Research.

Gertler, P., Locay, L., Sanderson, W., Dor, A., and van der Gaag, J. (1988) 'Health care financing and the demand for medical care', Washington, DC: World Bank.

Golladay, F. and Liese, B. (1980) *Health Issues and Policies in the Developing Countries: A background study for the World Development Report*, Washington, DC: World Bank.

Grant, J. (1987) 'Toward maternal and child health for all: a Bamako Initiative', In: World Health Organization, Regional Committee for Africa, *Report of the Regional Committee: Thirty-seventh session, Bamako (Mali), 9–16 September 1987*, Brazzaville: WHO.

Grossman, M. (1972) 'On the concept of health capital and the demand for health', *The Journal of Political Economy*, 80(2): 223–55.

Halberstam, D. (1993) *The Best and the Brightest*, New York: Ballantine Books.

Hanft, R. (1967) 'National Health Expenditures, 1950–65', *Bulletin of the United States Social Security Administration*, 30(2): 3–13.

Hayek, F. (2013) *Law, Legislation and Liberty: A new statement of the liberal principles of justice and political economy*, London and New York: Routledge.

Heller, P. (1976) 'A model of the demand for medical and health services in west Malaysia', USAID.

Heller, P. (1979) 'The underfinancing of recurrent development costs', *Finance & Development*, 16(1): 38–41.

James, C., et al. (2005) 'Impact on child mortality of removing user fees: simulation model', *British Medical Journal*, 331 (7519): 747–9.

Johnson, T. and Stout, S. (1999) *Investing in Health: Development effectiveness in the health, nutrition, and population sector*, Washington, DC: World Bank.

Kapur, D., Lewis, J., and Webb, R. (1997) *The World Bank: Its first half-century*, Vol. 1: History, Washington, DC: Brookings Institution Press.

Keshavjee, S. (2014) *Blind Spot: How neoliberalism infiltrated global health*, Berkeley and Los Angeles: University of California Press.

Kiker, B.F. (1966) 'The historical roots of the concept of human capital', *Journal of Political Economy*, 74(5): 481–99.

Knippenberg, R., et al. (2003) 'Increasing clients' power to scale up health services for the poor: the Bamako Initiative in West Africa', Washington, DC: World Bank.

Koita, A. and Brunet-Jailly, J. (1989) 'Mali', In: B. Abel-Smith and A. Creese (Eds.) *Recurrent Costs in the Health Sector: Problems and Policy Options in Three Countries*, Washington, DC and Geneva: USAID and WHO.

Lee, K. and Goodman, H. (2002) 'Global policy networks: the propagation of health care financing reform since the 1980s', In: K. Lee, K. Buse, and S. Fustukian (Eds.) *Health Policy in a Globalising World*, Cambridge and New York: Cambridge University Press, pp. 97–119.

Lewis, D. (2007) *The Management of Non-Governmental Development Organizations*, London: Routledge.

Lieberson, J. (1985) 'A synthesis of A.I.D. experience: small-farmer credit, 1973–1985', Washington, DC: USAID.

Macchiavello, A. (1961) *Methods of Evaluation of the Contribution of Health Programs to Economic Development*, Washington, DC: Pan-American Health Organization.

Manning, W., Newhouse, J., Duan, N., et al. (1988) *Health Insurance and the Demand for Medical Care: Evidence from a randomized experiment*, Santa Monica, CA: RAND Corp.

Marquez, L. and Seims, L.R. (1987) 'Community health worker incentives', In: L.R. Marquez, A. Brownlee, J. Molzan, et al. (Eds.) *Community Health Workers: A comparative analysis of PRICOR-funded studies*, Chevy Chase, Md.: Center for Human Services, pp. 53–63.

McNamara, R. (1980) 'Foreword', In: *World Development Report 1980*, Washington, DC: World Bank.

McNamara, R. (1981) *The McNamara Years at the World Bank: Major policy addresses of Robert S. McNamara, 1968–1981*, Baltimore and London: Johns Hopkins University Press.

Mechanic, D. (1979) *Future Issues in Health Care: Social policy and the rationing of medical services*, London and New York: The Free Press.

Mehta, U.S. (1999) *Liberalism and Empire: A study in nineteenth-century British thought*, Chicago and London: University of Chicago Press.

Meyer, J. (1984) 'Private sector research retrieval and analysis project: Sierra Leone', USAID Report No. JDMCG/TR-84/6, 2 June, Doc. No. PN-AAQ-965, pp. 1–2.

Mirowski, P. (2002) *Machine Dreams: Economics becomes a cyborg science*, Cambridge and New York: Cambridge University Press.

Mirowski, P. (2013). *Never Let a Serious Crisis Go to Waste: How neoliberalism survived the financial meltdown*, London: Verso.

Molem, C.S. (2008) 'Decentralisation of health care spending and HIV/AIDS in Cameroon', In: M. Sama and VK. Nguyen (Eds.) *Governing Health Systems in Africa*, Dakar: Council for the Development of Social Science Research in Africa, pp. 60–81.

Mushkin, S. (1962) 'Health as an investment', *Journal of Political Economy*, 70(5, Part 2, Suppl.): 136–57.

Myrdal, G. (1971) *Asian Drama: An inquiry into the poverty of nations*, U.K. and New York: Penguin.

Newell, K. (1988) 'Selective primary health care: the counter revolution', *Social Science and Medicine*, 26(9): 903–6.

Nicholson, T., et al. (2016) 'Double standards in global health: medicine, human rights law and multidrug-resistant tuberculosis treatment policy', *Health and Human Rights Journal*, 18(1): 85–101.

Novick, D. (1965) *Program Budgeting*, Cambridge, MA: Harvard University Press.

Nozick, R. (1974) *Anarchy, State and Utopia*, Oxford and Cambridge, MA: Blackwell.

Patterson, J. (1997) *Grand Expectations: The United States, 1945–1974*, Oxford and New York: Oxford University Press.

Planning and Development Collaborative (PADCO). (1980) Integrated Improvement Program for the Urban Poor: An orientation for project design and implementation, n.p.

Porter, T. (1995) *Trust In Numbers: The pursuit of objectivity in science and public life*, Princeton, NJ: Princeton University Press.

Reed, L.S. and Rice, D.P. (1964) 'National health expenditures: object of and source of funds, 1962', *Bulletin of the United States Social Security Administration*, 27(8): 11–21.

Richmond, J. and Fein, R. (2005) *The Health Care Mess: How we got into it and what it will take to get out*, Cambridge, MA and London: Harvard University Press.

Riddé, V. and Morestin, F. (2011) 'A scoping review of the literature on the abolition of user fees in health care services in Africa', *Health Policy and Planning*, 26: 1–11.

Robert, E. and Riddé, V. (2013) 'Global health actors no longer in favor of user fees: a documentary study', *Globalization and Health*, 9: 29.

Robinson, I. (1983) *An Inventory of A.I.D.-assisted projects with pharmaceutical components*, Washington, DC: United States Public Health Service.

Robinson, J. (2017) *Economics: An awkward corner*, Abingdon, U.K. and New York: Routledge.

Russell, L. (1986) *Is Prevention Better Than Cure?*, Washington, DC: Brookings Institute.

Savedoff, W.D., et al. (2012) 'Political and economic aspects of the transition to universal health coverage', *Lancet*, 380: 924–32.

Schultz, T. (1961) 'Investment in human capital', *The American Economic Review*, 51(1): 1–17.

Schultz, T. (1962) 'Reflexions on investment in man', *Journal of Political Economy*, 70(5, Part 2, Suppl.): 1–8.

Shabecoff, P. (1981) 'Reagan order on cost-benefit analysis stirs economic and political debate', The New York Times, 28.

Siegel, B., et al. (1996) 'Health reform in Africa: lessons from Sierra Leone', World Bank Discussion Paper No. 347, Health Sector Reform Series, Washington, DC: World Bank.

Starr, P. (1982) *The Social Transformation of American Medicine: The rise of a sovereign profession and the making of a vast industry*, New York: Basic Books.

Steil, B. (2013) *The Battle of Bretton Woods: John Maynard Keynes, Harry Dexter White, and the making of a new world order*, Princeton and Oxford: Princeton University Press.

Stein, C. (2008) *Beyond the World Bank Agenda*, Chicago and London: University of Chicago Press.

Stinson, W. (1982) *Community Financing of Primary Health Care*, Washington, DC: American Public Health Association.

Stinson, W., et al. (1987) *Community Financing of Primary Health Care: The PRICOR experience; a comparative analysis*, Washington, DC: USAID.

Streeten, P. and Burki, S. (1978) 'Basic needs: some issues', *World Development*, 6(3): 411–21.

Streeten, P., et al. (1981) *First Things First: Meeting basic human needs in developing countries*, Washington, DC: World Bank.

UNICEF. (1989) *Revitalizing Primary Health Care: The bamako initiative; progress report*, New York: United Nations.

UNICEF. (1990) *Report on the International Study Conference on Community Financing in Primary Health Care: Held at the Cape Sierra Hotel, Freetown, Sierra Leone, 23–30 September 1989*, New York: UNICEF.

UNICEF. (2007) *State of the World's Children 2008: Child survival*, New York: UNICEF.

UNICEF. (2009a) *Maternal and Child Health: The social protection dividend*, New York: UNICEF.

UNICEF. (2009b) *Removing User Fees in the Health Sector in Low-Income Countries: A multi-country review*, New York: UNICEF.

United States Congress. (2000) 'Foreign operations, export financing, and related programs appropriations, 2001', 106th Congress, Public Law 106–429, 6 November 2000, §1900A-61.

USAID. (1980) *Second Health Officers Conference Report, Abidjan, Ivory Coast, 8–13 December 1980*, Washington, DC: USAID.

USAID. (1981) *An Assessment of West African Agricultural Development*, Washington, DC: USAID.

USAID. (1986) '*Policy paper: health assistance (revised)*', Washington, DC: USAID.

Webster, C. (2002) *The National Health Service: A political history*, 2nd ed., Oxford and New York: Oxford University Press.

Werhane, P. (1999) *Moral Imagination and Management Decision Making*, New York: Oxford University Press.

WHO. (1950) 'Division of co-ordination of planning and liaison', In: *Report of the Standing Committee on Administration and Finance to the Fifth Session of the Executive Board*, Annex XI: 2,13.

WHO. (1964) 'Expert committee on tuberculosis', Eighth Report, Geneva: World Health Organization.

WHO. (1967) 'Proposed regular programme and budget estimates for the financial year 1 January – 31 December 1968 with proposed programmes and estimated obligations under other available sources of funds', *Official Records of the WHO No. 154*, Geneva: World Health Organization, App. 6, p. XLIX.

WHO. (1972) 'The contribution of health programmes to socio- economic development', Report on the technical discussions, Geneva: World Health Organization.

WHO. (1977) 'Phase II SHDS project, World Health Organization comments', unpublished.

WHO. (1978) *Financing of Health Services: Report of a WHO study group*, Geneva: WHO.

WHO. (2008) 'World Health Report 2008: Primary Health Care (Now More Than Ever)', available at www.who.int/whr/2008/en/ (accessed on 14 December 2015).

WHO and UNICEF. (1978) *Alma-Ata 1978: Primary health care*, Geneva: WHO.

Wicks, A. (1996) 'Overcoming the separation thesis: the need for a reconsideration of business and society research', *Business and Society*, 35(1): 89–118.

Wildavsky, A. (1966) 'The political economy of efficiency: cost-benefit analysis, systems analysis, and program budgeting', *Public Administration Review*, 26(4): 292–310.

Wood, R. (1986) *From Marshall Plan to Debt Crisis: Foreign aid and development choices in the world economy*, Berkeley and Los Angeles: University of California Press.

World Bank. (1964) 'The economy of Sierra Leone', Washington, DC: World Bank.

World Bank. (1975) 'Health Sector Policy Paper', Washington, DC: World Bank.

World Bank. (1981a) *Accelerated Development in Sub-Saharan Africa – An agenda for action*, Washington, DC: World Bank.

World Bank. (1981b) 'Sierra Leone: prospects for growth and equity', unpublished.

World Bank. (1981c) *World Development Report 1981*, Washington, DC: World Bank.

World Bank. (1982) 'Demand for and willingness to pay for services in rural Mali', In: *The World Bank Research Program: Abstracts of current studies 1982*, Washington, DC: World Bank.

World Bank. (1984) 'Health care demand and resource mobilization: the case of Peru', In: *The World Bank Research Program: Abstracts of current studies 1984*, Washington, DC: World Bank.

World Bank. (1986) 'Sierra Leone: health and population sector support project; staff appraisal report', unpublished.

World Bank. (1987) *Financing Health Services in Developing Countries: An agenda for reform*, Washington, DC: World Bank.

Yates, R. (2009) 'Universal health care and the removal of user fees', *Lancet*, 373: 2078–81.

# 10

# The politics of health systems strengthening

*Katerini T. Storeng, Ruth J. Prince, and Arima Mishra*

## Introduction

The 2014–2015 Ebola epidemic in Guinea, Liberia, and Sierra Leone brutally exposed the consequence of the neglect of national health systems. Historian of science Guillaume Lachenal describes the epidemic as the logical consequence of two decades of political choices and actions, starting with the systematic undermining of African health care systems by neoliberal reforms and perpetuated by the political and institutional landscape of global health (Lachenal, 2014). In the affected countries, and across many other poor countries, health care delivery has been left largely to a patchwork of nongovernmental organisations (NGOs), public–private partnerships (PPPs), and medical humanitarian organisations that sidestep the state (Prince and Marsland, 2013). In Liberia, for instance, the Ebola epidemic unfolded in a context where three quarters of government-owned health facilities were managed by NGOs (Moran, 2015).

The Ebola epidemic has hardened political consensus that strengthening health systems is essential for future epidemic preparedness. Recent health systems initiatives by former sceptics like the Bill & Melinda Gates Foundation continue a decade-long trend towards greater attention and resources to this issue. This trend has been driven not only by concerns about containing epidemics like Ebola, but also by global health actors' greater appreciation that weak health systems present 'bottlenecks' to the achievement of their organisational objectives and threaten broader development agendas (Hafner and Shiffman, 2012). However, as the recent debates about the Ebola epidemic illuminate, despite greater political priority, both the concept of health systems strengthening and the agenda to achieve this objective remain vague.

A decade ago, the WHO defined health systems holistically as 'all organisations, people and actions whose primary intent is to promote, restore or maintain health' (WHO, 2007, p. 2). In practice, however, global health actors imbue the notion with vastly different meanings and propose a range of potentially contradictory approaches. This reflects not just technical disagreement about policies and programmes, but also deep fault lines in public health ideologies. One major fault line concerns the relative power that states and private-sector actors should have over the stewardship of health systems. Another concerns the tension between a focus on technology-based medical care and a conceptualisation of health as a social phenomenon requiring more complex forms of intersectoral policy action (WHO, 2010a, p. 2). While some conceive of a health system as a 'core social institution' (Freedman, 2005), others approach it as a technical apparatus and focus on improving implementation and management structures, with relatively little attention to the politics and power governing social relations (Storeng and Mishra, 2014). Many discussions about health systems focus exclusively on the public sector, with too little emphasis on how rampant privatisation and decimated public health systems reproduce 'structural violence' and inequality (Foley, 2010; Biehl and Petryna, 2013). As we discuss in this chapter, debates about health systems and how to strengthen them thus cut to the core of the politics of global health.

## The recent history of national health systems

Expanding access to health care through building health care facilities, training, and employing health care workers and providing equipment and medicines was a key commitment of many post-colonial governments. Latin American countries such as Chile and Argentina implemented comprehensive health care systems in the 1950s (Birn, et al., 2016). On the eve of independence from Great Britain, India issued the progressive Bhore Committee Report (GoI, 1946), committing the government to building a robust health system with universal access to health care services. While newly independent African countries followed more piecemeal approaches, building up a national health care system remained a central development goal (Turshen, 1999).

Nationalist, anti-imperialist, and mission movements in many recently decolonised nations played key roles in developing and diffusing core concepts like 'health for all', which became central in the WHO's work in the 1970s (Fee, et al., 2008). The Alma-Ata Declaration on primary health care, which WHO member states signed in 1978, emphasised strong, publicly funded health systems as core to the achievement of 'health for all', based on the understanding that improved health systems could potentially help alleviate social inequality as part of overall social and economic development (Cueto, 2004).

Development policies in the 1980s and early 1990s, however, undermined years of progress in building up countries' health systems. In the early 1980s, international agencies and donors largely replaced the comprehensive Alma-Ata Declaration with 'selective' primary health care that addressed the main causes of mortality through targeted 'cost-effective' interventions. UNICEF's GOBI strategy for child survival (growth monitoring, oral rehydration, breast-feeding, and immunisation) became the flagship of this approach (Cueto, 2004). Meanwhile, African governments facing fiscal crises implemented structural adjustment programmes as conditions for loans from the World Bank and the International Monetary Fund (IMF), which included economic reforms to reduce state spending and encourage the private sector. In African countries, health sector reforms introduced as part of these programmes removed state responsibility for health care provision and protection at a time when citizens were most in need of them (Standing, 2002; Pfeiffer and Chapman, 2010).

Coinciding with the height of the AIDS epidemic, the lack of medicines, equipment, and funds to pay salaries or repair buildings forced demoralised health professionals to leave the public system. Abandoned by their governments, patients without the means to pay for private health care were left to rely on the goodwill of foreign donors and NGOs, while those who could afford it sought privatised health care (Prince, 2013). NGOs, supposed to fill the gaps left by incapacitated public health systems, could not compensate for a systemic approach, and often instead became the 'velvet glove' of further privatisation (Pfeiffer and Chapman, 2010; Pfeiffer, 2003). By the late 1990s, many African countries saw increased mortality and morbidity rates and drastically lowered life expectancies, especially among the poor who could least afford to pay the 'cost-sharing' user fees imposed by structural adjustment programmes.

In India, meanwhile, the government's neoliberal reforms encouraged the growth of a large heterogeneous unregulated private sector catering to more than 80 per cent of outpatient and 60 per cent of in-patient care, including a recent surge in corporate private hospitals providing secondary and tertiary care. India's weak and fragmented public health system continues to focus on select preventive and disease specific programmes, contributing to large-scale health disparities along the lines of caste, class, gender, and region (Baru, et al., 2010, Duggal, et al., 2005). The Government's current National Health Policy (2002) candidly acknowledged that liberalisation and privatisation have compromised most of the public health goals envisioned in earlier national health policies (1983), which conformed to the spirit of the WHO's Health for All vision (Sen, 2012).

## Health systems strengthening in the era of global health

The transition from 'international' to 'global' health during the past two decades has ushered in another stage in the fragmentation of national health systems (Brown, et al., 2006). The system of intergovernmental collaboration established after the Second World War and overseen by the WHO has given way to an 'unruly melange' (Buse and Walt, 1997) of overlapping global health initiatives dominated by powerful players operating within a neoliberal framework, notably the World Bank and private foundations (Rushton and Williams, 2011; Hanrieder, 2015; Clinton and Sridhar, 2017). The most important of these is the Bill & Melinda Gates Foundation, which shortly after its establishment in 1999 oversaw the formation of two major global public–private partnerships (PPPs) for health: Gavi, the Vaccine Alliance and the Global Fund to Fight AIDS, Tuberculosis and Malaria. These partnerships pioneered joint decision-making among the Gates Foundation, multilateral agencies, donor bodies, the pharmaceutical industry, and civil society organisations (Buse and Harmer, 2007), and often rely on NGOs as implementing partners, with the state playing a coordinating role. Within a decade, more than 100 different PPPs for global health formed. Meanwhile, the Gates Foundation has acquired immense power over the global health agenda. One illustration of this is that the Foundation is in official relations with the WHO and is its second largest donor, with a global health budget that has surpassed the WHO's regular budget (McGoey, 2016).

In donor-dependent countries, the power to set agendas, priorities, and approaches lies largely in the hands of such external donors and initiatives (Prince, 2016). Most often, these actors follow a model of health care delivery based on vertical disease interventions (targeting a single disease such as malaria or tuberculosis) or selected interventions (such as providing rotavirus vaccinations to children under 5). In this model, health problems are approached as technical challenges requiring market-based solutions like improved diffusion of technological or medical innovations – what historian Anne-Emmanuelle Birn (2005, p. 514) has labelled 'technology as public health ideology'.

Donor-funded global PPPs for health have widely been praised for their innovation and ability to save lives. At the same time, they have introduced new forms of administrative oversight, audit, and accountability, injecting corporate practice and culture into the field (Merry and Conley, 2011). Their business-oriented approach has amplified competition between initiatives, increased bureaucratisation, and undermined coordinated and sustainable health action on the ground (e.g., McCoy, 2009; Storeng, 2014). High-volume global funds from such partnerships have been shown to disrupt the policy and planning processes of recipient countries, for instance by distracting governments from coordinated efforts to strengthen health systems and by introducing 're-verticalisation' of planning, management, and monitoring and evaluation systems (Biesma, et al., 2009). While the World Bank and the IMF now acknowledge that structural adjustment policies had a negative impact on health in many African countries, today's global health initiatives have done little to reinvest in public health care systems or in the professionals running them, leaving them, in the words of historian Steve Feierman, in a 'situation of normal emergency' (Feierman, 2011, p. 185).

For example, in Kenya, the national health care system struggles to provide care in conditions of chronic underinvestment, and the delivery of health care services continues to rely heavily on the private sector and on NGOs. Weak, with inadequate infrastructure, it struggles to operate in the 'shadowlands' of well-resourced, global health programmes, with negative effects on the motivation and commitments of public sector workers (Prince and Otieno, 2014). Although the Kenya government signed the 2001 Abuja Declaration pledging to allocate 15 per cent of the government budget to health, the health budget has declined, to 5.3 per cent of the total government budget in 2013. Low public investment ensures that the burden of paying for health care falls largely on individual patients, whether they can afford it or not. Since 2013, the government has provided antenatal care, and services for children under 5 have free of charge in public facilities, but the policy of 'cost sharing' remains, requiring patients to pay for everything else, from bandages to medicines and IV fluid. In this system, doctors have to tailor their prescriptions to the size of the patient's pocket, with the consequence that many patients receive sub-optimal treatment.

With growing evidence of their unintended effects, global public-private partnerships for health have come under growing pressure to be more mindful of how they affect national health systems. From around 2005, such pressure galvanised some of the most prominent partnerships – including Gavi and the Global Fund – to expand their disease-specific remit to direct portions of their funding to general health system strengthening, so-called 'HSS support' (Storeng, 2014). However, these schemes focus primarily on strengthening delivery systems for targeted interventions in line with the public health vision of their major donor, prompting critics to refer to it as the 'Gates approach' to public health. Indeed, HSS investments often operate more at the level of rhetoric than reality, given the fundamental distrust in the state that is characteristic of the powerful organisations that fund these initiatives.

Although they claim to support national health systems, the reality is that in many countries, service delivery depends on the continued goodwill of donors and NGOs, raising doubts about sustainability and about countries' ability to development and implement coherent national health plans (McCoy, 2009). More generally, donors' predilection for investing in combating single, infectious diseases where potential exists to save lives through medical commodities has contributed to neglect of non-communicable but fatal diseases such as diabetes and cancer, for which specialist diagnostic and treatment equipment barely exists in many poor countries (Livingstone, 2012).

Health workers' frustrations at these conditions recently erupted in national medical workers' strikes in Kenya and Zimbabwe. In Kenya's strike, which lasted 100 days between December 2016 and March 2017, doctors and nurses demanded not only better pay but also improved working conditions and a reform of public hospitals; they wanted the government to employ more doctors and provide more medicines and better medical equipment. The doctors' union presented the strike as a struggle to protect and save the public health care system in the face of massive privatisation and allegations of corruption at government ministries. On blogs and social media, doctors and their supporters argued that public hospitals were becoming hospitals 'for the poor' while middle classes with private health insurance could choose private facilities. The strike was hugely controversial – during lively debates on social media, some Kenyans accused the doctors of breaking their Hippocratic Oath, of personally benefitting from the strike (as some government doctors own private health care facilities) and of using arguments about the public good to cover their desire to protect their middle-class lifestyles and identities. Whatever the truth claims, the strike demonstrated that the issue of a functioning public health care system is deeply emotional and linked to contested visions regarding citizenship, development, and progress. It also drew attention to the huge inequalities in access to health care and to the political and corporate interests driving the expanding private health care sector.

In India, the Government's commitment to achieve the UN's Millennium Development Goals (MDGs) and mounting civil society pressure to address health inequity led to an ambitious health system strengthening effort in the early 2000s, known as the National Rural Health Mission (NRHM). The NRHM, formalised in 2005, revived the spirit of the WHO's primary health care approach and sought to undertake 'architectural correction' of the public health system. Specifically, the NRHM outlined a series of measures to improve health outcomes and restore rural people's trust in the health system. These included strengthening decentralised health planning and inter-sectoral collaboration; integrating vertical health programmes; introducing more flexible health financing; integrating alternative systems of medicine; and improving community ownership of health. However, its implementation unfortunately followed more of a programme than a 'mission' mode. In practice, its comprehensive vision was on many levels reduced to a targeted drive to improve vaccination and institutional delivery rates as part of the government's broader effort to meet the MDG targets for child survival and maternal health (MDGs 4 and 5) (Rao, 2017; Mishra, 2014).

## 'Universal health coverage' and health systems strengthening

Since the quelling of the Ebola crisis, concerns about 'fragile' national health care systems have been pushed up the policy agenda. Calls for a more progressive, comprehensive approach – to invest in public health systems and ensure that the costs of health care do not exclude the poor – are gaining currency.

Much current debate is articulated under the banner of Universal Health Coverage (UHC), which former WHO Director General Margaret Chan has described as 'the single most powerful concept public health has to offer' (Chan, 2012, n.p.). The WHO defines UHC as ensuring that all people can use the health services they need, without financial hardship (WHO, 2010b). The WHO's call to achieve UHC worldwide by 2030 is being hailed as the most progressive policy objective since WHO's 1978 call for 'Health for All in the Year 2000' through investment in primary health care systems (Rodin and de Ferranti, 2012). A number of countries (e.g., Brazil, Ghana, Mexico, Rwanda, Turkey, Thailand, China, and India) are implementing reforms to expand the availability of health care, and, at the time of writing (May 2017), more than 80 countries had asked the WHO for UHC implementation assistance (Lagomarsino, et al., 2012; WHO, 2014; Mishra and Seshdari, 2016).

While UHC measures include a focus on the health workforce, medicines, and information systems, questions of health financing and social protection through tax-based or insurance systems form their cornerstone (Savedoff, et al., 2012). In most low- and middle-income countries, health insurance cover has been limited to groups such as civil servants or those in formal employment. UHC reforms propose to extend health insurance coverage by including people in the informal economy (the majority of the population in many countries), the unemployed, and the poor. However, the ways UHC addresses such issues remains unclear. There are different models of moving towards UHC (Lagomarsino, et al. 2012). UHC can be employed within different political ideologies (Funahashi, 2016; Reich, et al. 2016) and interest groups have different stakes in it (Mills, et al., 2012). Furthermore, the question of what is *universal* in UHC is a matter of negotiation. In 'resource-poor' countries, UHC means an extremely circumscribed range of services (Schmidt, et al., 2015).

UHC is, therefore, not a universal model but a forum for experimentation and contestation (Schmidt, et al., 2015). In India, for example, a key tension in debates about UHC is between the language of comprehensive primary health care necessary for addressing the social determinants of health (espoused in the National Rural Health Mission) and universal access to health services (e.g., through empanelled hospitals, package of services). While one is inter-sectoral and comprehensive in outlook, the other is about numbers of services and coverage, with considerably more space for the private sector (Sengupta and Prasad, 2011; Mishra and Seshdari, 2016). The UHC debate not merely lays bare the tensions in public health ideologies but also deep asymmetries of power. For example, the High Level Expert Committee Report on UHC commissioned by the Government of India was almost silent on the growing role of the private sector in the various subsystems of health service provision (Baru, 2012). Srivatsan and Shatrugna (2012) rightly remind us to the need for 'progressive hegemony' around the concept of UHC to make it feasible and meaningful. This would require, they argue, the Government to engage in negotiations with different groups of people ranging from political parties (national and regional), local government representatives, professional associations, academic bodies, civil society, and private sector so that their 'ideas, needs and constraints are woven into the broader picture' (Srivatsan and Shatrugna, 2012, p. 63).

## Conclusion

Today's most powerful global health actors have belatedly come to espouse commitment to health systems as part of a broader commitment to UHC. The Rockefeller Foundation, which began to focus on health systems a decade ago through country-level work in Bangladesh, Ghana, Rwanda and Vietnam, has recently refined its 'Transforming Health Systems' initiative, with a focus on UHC (Rockefeller Foundation, 2017). USAID recently published its first dedicated HSS 'vision' (USAID, 2015) and even the Gates Foundation, known for its embrace of technological approaches to health and its vehement opposition to 'HSS support' (Storeng, 2014), has publicly committed to health system strengthening through its 'Integrated Delivery' strategy (Bill & Melinda Gates Foundation, 2017).

Within the new UHC rhetoric, however, the polysemic nature of the concept of health systems strengthening becomes evident yet again. Progressive rationales for health systems strengthening that focus on ensuring health equity co-exist with a discourse of global health security that conceives of health systems strengthening in instrumental terms. For instance, a major report on Ebola published in *The Lancet* talks not of fragile public health systems, but of 'inadequate national investment and donor support for building national health systems *capable of detecting and responding to disease outbreaks*' (Moon, et al., 2015, p. 2208, emphasis added). The authors draw (disputable) links with general health system strengthening, arguing that,

> strategic investments for International Health Regulation core capacities can and should also strengthen broader health systems. For example, health information systems can support surveillance and monitoring of outbreaks and routine health services; training and payment of community health works and civil society service providers can help achieve universal health coverage, while providing an essential trained workforce during emergencies.
>
> *Moon, et al., 2015, p. 2209*

Such win-win rhetoric is strongly reminiscent of earlier, but unsubstantiated, arguments that investments in disease-specific PPPs will confer system-wide benefits (Storeng, 2014).

What seems clear is that high-level commitments to health system strengthening do not foment commitment to publicly funded health systems with a strong focus on equity and sustainability (Birn, et al., 2016). Instead, critics are concerned that unquestioned preference for the PPP model of health care 'provision' and global push for private-sector financing models 'collectively undermine the human right to universal health care and the achievement of the SDGs' (Lethbridge, 2017).

Historian Anne-Emmanuelle Birn and colleagues even suggest that recent 'health systems' initiatives including UHC signal the continuation of a decades-long co-optation of progressive social justice aims by neoliberal global health actors (Birn, et al., 2016).

Historically, national forces relating to class, economic interests and political power have shaped both progressive and regressive approaches to public health (Birn, et al., 2016). As global institutions' influence over countries' approaches to public health continue to grow unabatedly, political challenges over health have increasingly been reframed as technical issues. Unfortunately, this seems to be happening regarding UHC and its formulation of a health system. Growing dissatisfaction with current approaches has led to greater recognition of health systems as social institutions in which politics and power are central (Storeng and Mishra, 2014). It also lays behind calls from anthropologists to public health specialists for greater focus on the 'software' of health systems, including quality, responsiveness, and resilience (Kieny and Dovlo, 2015) and the need to revive a people-centred approach (Biehl and Petryna, 2013). Such a focus must come to terms with the enduring tension between political and technical approaches that is at the heart of contemporary debates about health systems and universal health coverage.

## References

Baru, R. (2012) 'A limiting perspective on universal coverage', *Economic and Political Weekly*, XLVII(8): 64–6.

Baru, R., Acharya, A., Acharya, S., Kumar, A.S., and Nagaraj, K. (2010) 'Inequities in access to health services in India: caste, class and region', *Economic and Political Weekly*, XLV(38): 49–58.

Biehl, J. and Petryna, A. (Eds.) (2013) *When People Come First: Critical studies in global health*, Princeton, NJ: Princeton University Press.

Biesma, R.G., Brugha, R., Harmer, A., Walsh, A., Spicer, N., and Walt, G. (2009) 'The effects of global health initiatives on country health systems: a review of the evidence from HIV/AIDS control', *Health Policy and Planning*, 24(4): 239–52.

Bill & Melinda Gates Foundation. (2017) 'Integrated delivery – strategic overview', available at www.gatesfoundation.org/What-We-Do/Global-Development/Integrated-Delivery (accessed on 29 May 2017).

Birn, A. E. (2005) 'Gates's grandest challenge: transcending technology as public health ideology', *Lancet*, 366(9484): 514–19.

Birn, A.-E., Nervi, L., and Siqueira, E. (2016) 'Neoliberalism redux: the global health policy agenda and the politics of cooptation in Latin America and beyond', *Development and Change*, 47(4): 734–59.

Brown, T. M., Cueto, M., and Fee, E. (2006) 'The World Health Organization and the transition from "international" to "global" public health', *American Journal of Public Health*, 96(1): 62–72.

Buse, K. and Harmer, A.M. (2007) 'Seven habits of highly effective global public-private health partnerships: practice and potential', *Social Science & Medicine*, 64(2): 259–71.

Buse, K. and Walt, G. (1997) 'An unruly mélange? Coordinating external resources to the health sector: a review', *Social Science & Medicine*, 45(3): 449–63.

Chan, M., (2012). 'Address to the sixty-fifth World Health Assembly', available at www.who.int/dg/speeches/2012/wha_20120521/en/ (accessed on 29 May 2017).

Clinton, C. and Sridhar, D. (2017) *Governing Global Health: Who runs the world and why?*, Oxford University Press.

Cueto, M. (2004) 'The origins of primary health care and selective primary health care', *American Journal of Public Health*, 94(11): 1864–74.

Duggal, R., Gangolli, L.V., and Phadke, A. (2005) *Review of Health Care in India*, Mumbai: CEHAT.

Fee, E., Cueto, M., and Brown, T.M. (2008) 'WHO at 60: snapshots from its first six decades', *American Journal of Public Health*, 98(4): 630–33.

Feierman, S., (2011) 'When physicians meet: local medical knowledge and global public goods', In: W. Geissler and C. Molyneux (Eds.) *Evidence, Ethos and Experiment: The anthropology and history of medical research in Africa*, London: Berghahn Books, p. 171.

Foley, E.E. (2010) *Your Pocket is What Cures You: The politics of health in Senegal*, New Brunswick, New Jersey and London: Rutgers University Press.

Freedman, L. (2005) 'Achieving the MDGs: Health systems as core social institutions', *Development*, 48: 19–24.

Funahashi, D.A. (2016) 'Rule by good people: health governance and the violence of moral authority in Thailand', *Cultural Anthropology*, 31(1): 107–30.

GoI. (1946) *Report of the Health Survey and Development Committee (Bhore Committee Report)* Volume 1, Delhi: Government of India.

Hafner, T. and Shiffman, J. (2012) 'The emergence of global attention to health systems strengthening', *Health Policy and Planning*, 28(1): 41–50.

Hanrieder, T., (2015) *International Organization in Time: Fragmentation and reform,* Oxford: Oxford University Press.

Kieny, M.P. and Dovlo, D. (2015) 'Beyond Ebola: a new agenda for resilient health systems', The *Lancet*, 385(9963): 91–2.

Lachenal, G. (2014) 'Ebola 2014. Chronicle of a well-prepared disaster', available at http://somatosphere.net/2014/10/chronicle-of-a-well-prepared-disaster.html (accessed on 29 May 2017).

Lagomarsino, G., Garabrant, A., Adyas, A., Muga, R., and Otoo, N. (2012) 'Moving towards universal health coverage: health insurance reforms in nine developing countries in Africa and Asia', *The Lancet*, 380(9845): 933–43.

Lethbridge, J. (2017) 'World Bank undermindes right to universal healthcare', available at www.brettonwoodsproject.org/2017/04/world-bank-undermines-right-universal-healthcare/?utm_source=IHP+Newsletter&utm_campaign=05c7d031e4-EMAIL_CAMPAIGN_2017_04_14&utm_medium=email&utm_term=0_14504ce43d-05c7d031e4-298051801 (accessed on 20 May 2017).

Livingstone, J. (2012) *Improvising Medicine: An African oncology ward in an emerging cancer epidemic*, Durham, NC: Duke University Press.

McCoy, D. (2009) 'Global health initiatives and country health systems', *The Lancet*, 374(9697): 1237.

McGoey, L. (2016) *No Such Thing as a Free Gift: The Gates Foundation and the price of philanthropy*, London: Verso Books.

Merry, S.E. and Conley, J.M. (2011) 'Measuring the world: Indicators, human rights, and global governance', Current Anthropology, 52(S3): S83–95.

Mills, A., Ally, M., Goudge, J., Gyapong, J., and Mtei, G. (2012) 'Progress towards universal coverage: the health systems of Ghana, South Africa and Tanzania', *Health Policy and Planning*, 27 (Suppl 1): i4–12.

Mishra, A. (2014) '"Trust and teamwork matter": Community health workers' experiences in integrated service delivery in India', *Global Public Health*, 9(8): 960–74.

Mishra, A. and Seshdari, S. R. (2016) 'Unpacking the dicourse on universal health coverage in India: Implications for health', *Social Medicine*, 9(2): 86–92.

Moon, S., Sridhar, D., Pate, M.A., Jha, A.K., Clinton, C., Delaunay, S., … Piot, P. (2015) 'Will Ebola change the game? Ten essential reforms before the next pandemic. The report of the Harvard–LSHTM Independent Panel on the Global Response to Ebola', *The Lancet*, 386(10009): 2204–21.

Moran, M. (2015) 'Surviving ebola. The epidemic and political legitimacy in Liberia', *Current History*, 114(772): 177–82.

Pfeiffer, J. (2003) 'International NGOs and primary health care in Mozambique: the need for a new model of collaboration' *Social Science & Medicine*, 56(4): 725–38.

Pfeiffer, J. and Chapman, R. (2010) 'Anthropological perspectives on structural adjustment and public health', *Annual Review of Anthropology*, 39(1): 149–65.

Prince, R.J. (2013) 'Situating health and the public in Africa', In: R.J. Prince and R. Marsland (Eds.) *Making and Unmaking Public Health in Africa: Ethnographic and historical perspectives*, Athens, Ohio: Ohio University Press, pp. 1–53.

Prince, R.J. (2016) 'Public health and global interventions in Africa', *Current History*, May: 163–8.

Prince, R.J. and Marsland, R. (2013) (Eds.) *Making and Unmaking Public Health in Africa: Ethnographic and historical perspectives*, Ohio: Ohio University Press.

Prince, R.J. and Otieno, P. (2014) 'In the shadowlands of global health: observations from health workers in Kenya', *Global Public Health*, 9(8): 927–45.

Rao, S. (2017) *Do we care? India's health system*, Delhi: Oxford University Press.

Reich, M.R., Harris, J., Ikegami, N., Maeda, A., Cashin, C., Araujo, E.C., … Evans, T.G. (2016) 'Moving towards universal health coverage: lessons from 11 country studies', *The Lancet*, 387(10020): 811–16.

Rodin, J. and de Ferranti, D. (2012) 'Universal health coverage: the third global health transition?', *The Lancet*, 380(9845): 861–62.

Rockefeller Foundation. (2017) 'Transforming health systems: Building strong health systems and advancing universal health coverage', available at www.rockefellerfoundation.org/our-work/initiatives/transforming-health-systems/ (accessed on 29 May 2017).

Rushton, S. and Williams, O.D. (Eds.) (2011) *Partnerships and Foundations in Global Health Governance*, London: Palgrave Macmillan.

Savedoff, W.D., de Ferranti, D., Smith, A.L., and Fan, V. (2012) 'Political and economic aspects of the transition to universal health coverage', *The Lancet*, 380(9845): 924–32.

Schmidt, H., Gostin, L.O., and Emanuel, E.J. (2015) 'Public health, universal health coverage, and Sustainable Development Goals: can they coexist?' *The Lancet*, 386(9996): 928–30.

Sen, G. (2012) 'Universal health coverage in India: a long and winding road', *Economics and Politics Weekly*, XLVIL(8): 45–52.

Sengupta, A. and Prasad, V. (2011) 'Developing a truly universal Indian health system: the problem of replacing "Health for All" to "Universal access to health care"', *Social Medicine*, 6(2): 69–72.

Srivatsan, R. and Shatrugna, V. (2012) 'Political challenges to universal access to health care', *Economic and Political Weekly*, XLVII(8): 61–63.

Standing, H. (2002) 'An overview of changing agendas in health sector reforms', *Reproductive Health Matters*, 10(20): 19–28.

Storeng, K.T. (2014) 'The GAVI Alliance and the "Gates approach" to health system strengthening', *Global Public Health*, 9(8): 865–79.

Storeng, K.T. and Mishra, A. (2014) 'Politics and practices of global health: critical ethnographies of health systems in context', *Global Public Health,* 9(8): 858–64.

Turshen, M. (1999) *Privatizing Health Services in Africa*, New Brunswick: Rutgers University Press.

USAID. (2015) 'USAID's vision for health systems strengthening', Washington, DC: U.S. Agency for International Development.

WHO. (2007) 'Everybody business: strengthening health systems to improve health outcomes: WHO's framework for action', Geneva: World Health Organization.

WHO. (2010a) 'A conceptual framework for action on the social determinants of health', Geneva: World Health Organization.

WHO. (2010b) 'The World Health Report. Health systems financing: the path to universal coverage', Geneva: World Health Organization.

WHO. (2014) '500+ Organizations Launch Global Coalition to Accelerate Access to Universal Health Coverage (press release)', available at www.who.int/universal_health_coverage/universal-health-coverage-access-pr-20141212.pdf?ua=1 (accessed on 29 May 2017).

WHO. (2015) 'Tracking universal health coverage: first global monitoring report. Joint WHO/World Bank Group report', Geneva: World Health Organization.

# 11

# National and subnational politics of health systems' origins and change

*Radhika Gore*

## Introduction

In analyses of the global community's response to health threats, researchers rightly cast the state as one of a range of actors, where others include intergovernmental organisations, civil society groups, and private actors (Storeng, et al., Chapter 10, in this volume). However, while transnational and non-state actors play expanding roles in global health governance, states do not merely submit to external power but continue to be sovereign entities in the international system and are central actors in the provision of health services (Ricci, 2009). Each state confronts and addresses health threats based in part on its institutional capacity, history, political priorities, and relations within society.

The global response to HIV, for instance, suggests how state policies and progress in addressing this epidemic have varied based on the nature of national ethnic conflict (Lieberman, 2009), political salience of cultural norms (Altman, 2006), integration of state agencies with societal groups and organisations (Swidler, 2006), intensity of civic activism (Nunn, 2009), and bureaucratic organisation and capacity (Parkhurst and Lush, 2004), among other factors.

The variance in states' responses to health issues thus derives in part from the distinctiveness of their health systems and health politics. The state may be conceptualised as a unitary actor on the global health stage, but it is simultaneously a manifold, multilevel entity within its borders (Sharma and Gupta, 2006). Understanding the politics of global health therefore requires understanding how public health challenges and debates are refracted not only through the governing structures and machinations of the *global* health community, but also through health system institutions and actors *within states*. Key to this understanding is a foundational grasp of the national and subnational politics of health systems' origins and evolution.

This chapter discusses an example of how to chart such an inquiry, specifically, how to examine the historical and institutional processes that shape a health system and affect state response to a health-related issue. The issue considered here is urbanisation – a trend evident across low- and middle-income countries (Montgomery and Ezeh, 2005) – with an aim to explain the state's inattention to primary care in urban India. Urbanisation, like other sociopolitical processes such as decentralisation and privatisation, has a particular social-scientific definition but is diverse in its manifest features and health impacts across countries. Urbanisation refers to 'a demographic and land change process' wherein the setting for human habitation is increasingly the city (Seto, et al., 2010, p. 170). Forms of the urban and processes of urbanisation, however, vary widely across the globe (Brenner, 2013). States differ in how they promote and respond to urban change, with critical effects on health care services for urban populations.

A focus on urbanisation helps expand the purview of issues typically explored in political analysis of health systems. Health systems researchers have tended to concentrate on disease- and programme-specific issues, issues 'often driven by global actors and agendas', thereby neglecting to study national and subnational sociopolitical developments, institutions, and associated 'political cultures and practices' that influence how health systems are organised and function (Sheikh, et al., 2011, p. 4). Urban health research is a case in point – much of it concerns the study of how urban living and working conditions affect health (Friel, et al., 2011). It offers evidence of how cities expose the poor to unhealthy physical and social environments in conditions of concentrated poverty. But it yields scant insight into the national and subnational politics that define the organisation and workings of urban health care services (Friel, et al., 2011; Stren, et al., 2003). We know that public health care facilities offer low-quality, difficult-to-access services in cities (Das and Hammer, 2014; Seeberg, et al., 2014), but we know less about why this low quality persists (Mills, 2014).

In India, urban health care has received marginal attention in both health policy and urban development programmes. Public provision of primary care in cities, a responsibility that falls to municipal governments, has been incommensurate with urban population growth and is widely unpopular relative to an avid, largely unregulated private health care sector that accounts for over 70 per cent of all outpatient visits (NSSO, 2015). In this chapter, I explain reasons for deficiencies in state-provided urban primary care by (a) conceptualising the link between urban space and population health, (b) based on this conception, analysing the policy debates and conflicts that mark the origins of the national health service apparatus and its scope in cities, and (c) estimating the possibility for local collective action to forge its change.

## Linking urban and health politics

Conceptualising the link between health and urban politics is a critical starting point in this inquiry, since it brings into view how a health system develops concurrently with state institutions across the state's manifold agencies and locations. An essential move here is to view cities not just as physical sites where people are exposed to risk of disease but as spaces produced by multiple processes such as 'capital investment, state regulation, collective consumption, [and] social struggle' (Brenner, 2013, p. 95). Because of their complexity and dynamism, urban sites are usefully defined not solely in terms of empirical *facts*, such as land area, population size, and demographics, but with reference to constitutive historical *processes* that engender urban space and associated health services.

These processes are inherently political in that they involve potential conflicts of visions and goals among actors. Political leaders, administrators, business groups, and community organisations may diverge in their imaginary or ideas and expectations about the urban, espousing contradictory frames and holding different meanings about common issues and how they should be resolved (Brenner, 2013). Issues of economic growth and development are a key theme in such conflicts, as urbanisation processes are centrally implicated in flows of capital, labour, and culture (Harvey, 1985).

In India, for instance, in recent decades the state has aimed to develop cities' potential for growth and connections to the global economy (Goldman, 2011) and invested marginally in basic public services in cities (Coelho and Maringanti, 2012). Liberalisation reforms have encouraged a growing private sector in health care provision and medical education that is especially dense in urban areas (Baru, 2003; Rao, et al., 2011). Local social mobilisation, which can theoretically contribute to improving public health care services (Evans, 2009), has in practice been uncommon and challenging to sustain in urban India (Agarwal, et al., 2008; More, et al., 2012). Both urban space and urban health care are thus implicated in common, multilevel processes, which shape the organisation and evolution of state-provided urban primary care.

Studying the politics of state-provided urban primary care therefore entails examining imaginaries of the urban as reflected in the state's mandate for health and urban development and in local social contestations. I review selected health and urban policy documents, administrative data, and related social-science literature to examine how the state has conceived and responded to urban populations and health needs, particularly for providing urban primary care. The reviewed policy texts and data cover two key periods: years just following India's independence in 1947, marking policy debates over seminal blueprints for India's health system; and from the 1980s to the present, marking the beginning and deepening of liberalisation reforms in India.

To study social mobilisation, I review health and social science literature analysing current health-related collective action in cities. My analysis is informed by fieldwork in three Indian cities, where I conducted 24 in-depth interviews with staff from 17 non-governmental organisations (NGOs) in Mumbai, Pune, and New Delhi. Although I do not present data from the interviews in this chapter, my discussions with and observation of NGO activities help guide my analysis of the literature.

## The origins and evolution of state-provided urban primary care

### *The demographic and political salience of India's majority rural population*

The village in rural India has, in colonial and post-colonial nationalist thought and policy, been the emblematic site of social and economic 'backwardness', in need of social ascencion, disease eradication, population control, and poverty reduction (Thakur, 2014). India's population was over 80 per cent rural as of 1951 (around independence) and remains high at about 70 per cent rural (Ministry of Home Affairs, 2011). This demographic reality partly explains the rural orientation of India's health system. However, the persistent marginalisation of urban areas in health policy despite a steadily growing urban population – decadal population growth rates have been over 30 per cent in urban areas compared to under 22 per cent for rural areas since the 1960s (YASHADA, 2014, p. 46) – suggests the political rather than purely demographic salience of urban and rural populations in India.

Rural populations presented an urgent political question in newly independent India, where the challenge that confronted the state was to reconcile twin imperatives: to achieve economic growth based on modern industry and to establish legitimacy over a vast, heterogeneous, and mainly agricultural nation (Chatterjee, 1997), characterised by 'regional patriotisms' and numerous monolingual and religious communities (Kaviraj, 2000, p. 151). It was through state-led planning and administration of development – rational, apolitical, and universal – that the state would 'claim its legitimacy as … the will of the nation' and set into motion national economic and social development (Chatterjee, 1997, p. 279).

The health of the public was a central concern in development plans, though national policy debates evince multiple, competing ideas about health: health was 'at once, a basic human right, a tool for the improvement of the "Indian race", making it more efficient and more governable, and health was an instrument for economic development' (Amrith, 2007, p. 117). The National Planning Committee (NPC) of the Indian National Congress party, which formed the first government in independent India, described poverty as a root cause of disease. It also underscored that, along with destitution, the 'appalling ignorance of the masses and their religious and social prejudices', weakened and debilitated the Indian masses, resulting in a population chronically ill and susceptible to epidemics (NPC, 1947, p. 21). Ultimately, in the ascendant view within policy debates, improving the public's health was less a goal in itself and more a means to achieve economic productivity and progress.

In arguing for 'the economic value of public health', national leaders upheld and reinforced the Bhore Committee report, a major and influential colonial government-commissioned survey of health and health infrastructure in India conducted in the years just preceding independence (Amrith, 2006, p. 63). The Bhore Committee's findings and proposals inspired and set standards for subsequent development of India's health system (Amrith, 2007). In its recommendations, the Committee proposed the state, as opposed to social reformers or volunteers, as the essential driver of health programmes with rural populations as their main focus.

Urban populations were not wholly ignored in health plans but were not their primary target. The Bhore Committee acknowledged that urbanisation posed health risks and it found major deficiencies in urban health care services: hospitals in urban areas were more plentiful than in rural areas but their physical infrastructure was 'hopelessly out of date' (GoI, 1946, p. 39). Thus, at the moment of independence, the state had evidence of both rural and urban health risks and health care deficiencies. But the emphasis of seminal national health plans and subsequent programmes converged on the rural.

Despite noting gaping inadequacies across the health system, national leaders ultimately did not direct policy and budgetary attention to undertake systemic health reform. Rather than comprehensive reforms, national health initiatives in the 1950s and 1960s focused on eradicating specific communicable diseases (tuberculosis and malaria chief among them) and instituting population control measures through top-down, technocratic, biomedical interventions, guided and funded by international agencies (Amrith, 2007; Rao, 2004). The health system lumbered ahead with a meagre bureaucratic and service delivery infrastructure, having 'retained the decentralized, fractured structure of the public health services' of the colonial state (Amrith, 2006, p. 81). Retaining the colonial administrative apparatus also meant inheriting weak structures of municipal governance (Weinstein, et al., 2014), a point I return to later in this chapter.

Policy debates in areas other than health, notably in industrial policy, further undermined the possibility of reforming urban health care. Business leaders framed influential proposals that aligned industrial policy with state imperatives of nation-building and economic growth, but their commitments to social justice and redistribution were largely rhetorical (Chibber, 2003). They argued for centralised coordination of economic policy rather than dispersed policy-making power across subnational governments, thereby augmenting the centre's control over cities (Chibber, 2003). They emphasised public investment in infrastructure rather than basic services in cities, and in hospitals and medical education rather than primary care services (Priya, 2005).

Central government attention to urban primary care emerged in 1982 in the form of a commissioned report that delineated norms for urban health care infrastructure (Kapadia-Kundu and Kanitkar, 2002). In the following year the centre introduced 'urban health posts' – community-level primary care facilities – in ten states (MOHFW, 2013). Yet the centre neither implemented the recommended norms nor sustained the health posts, leaving municipal governments devoid of guidelines and funds to upgrade urban primary care (Kapadia-Kundu and Kanitkar, 2002). Municipal health services, where they exist, are focused on child survival and reproductive health across India's health system, reflecting the selective view of primary care that international agencies promoted globally in the 1980s (see Storeng, et al., Chapter 10, in this volume).

Recent health reforms reaffirm the dominance of the rural in national policy and planning. The National Rural Health Mission, launched in 2005, aimed to 'provide accessible, affordable and quality health care to the rural population' (MOHFW, 2005, p. 5). A similar scheme – the National Urban Health Mission – was proposed in 2006 and drafted in 2008 to address health care needs of urban populations, but was launched only in 2013, eight years after the launch of the rural programme (MOHFW, 2013). Thus, throughout the decades following independence, improvements to state-provided urban health care lagged rural health care reforms. As a central government planning document observed,

> Unlike the rural health services there have been no efforts to provide well-planned and organized primary, secondary and tertiary care services in geographically delineated urban areas. As a result, in many areas primary health facilities are not available; some of the existing institutions are underutilized while there is over-crowding in most of the secondary and tertiary centers.
>
> *Planning Commission, 2002, p. 89*

As I next discuss, like central government health schemes, municipal governments, too, have failed to address urban health care.

## Weak municipal governance capacity and the economic salience of cities

In India's federal system, at state level, the responsibility for rural primary care falls to the department of health. The responsibility for urban primary care falls to municipal governments, who in turn report to the department of urban development, whose focus is not on health care but on transportation, energy, roads, water supply, and sanitation in cities (see Figure 11.1 for the example of Maharashtra state). Municipal governments have long held limited autonomy. Their continuing weak power *vis-à-vis* state governments is not solely a function of path dependence but reflects the salience of cities in national economic plans, initially as physical sites of modern industry and later as motors of economic growth under liberalisation reforms.

In the first decades of independence, 'the center remained largely silent on urban policy questions' (Weinstein, et al., 2014, p. 45), adopting no definitive policies to address urban growth, land use, land prices, and housing, among other urban issues (Shaw, 1996). This left urban poverty as well as the capacities, responsibilities, and powers of municipal governments largely unaddressed. In the 1960s, the centre made funds available for state governments to draft master plans and decide urban land use. But these stand-alone plans hewed to modernist ideals of planned urbanisation (Shaw, 1996) and neglected the unsettled predicament of migrants – rising cadres of informal, self-employed, and casual labour in cities (Bhowmik, 2009). In the late 1960s, when support for modernist ideals retreated, policymakers backed populist proposals to support small–medium towns in an attempt to deconcentrate major cities, but these initiatives did little to strengthen municipal governance or improve basic services (Weinstein, et al., 2014).

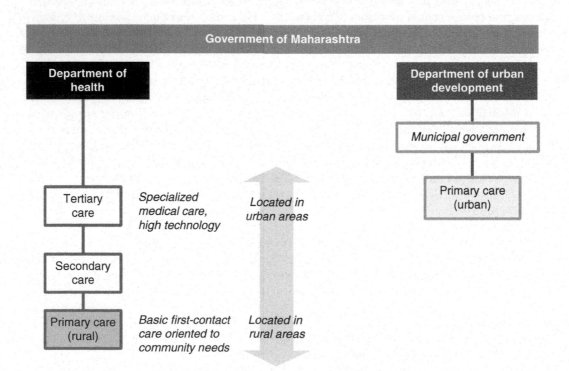

*Figure 11.1*  Organisation of health care services in Maharashtra state

Beginning in the 1980s, the state's view of urban spaces and populations shifted in ways that again undermined reform of urban public services. Under liberalisation, national urban development programmes emphasised cities not just as emblems of modernity and sites of industry but as drivers of growth through their connections with global markets (Fernandes, 2004). Ideas about modernity and technology had shaped national development plans in newly independent India, and they continued to do so under liberalisation. But the position of the urban poor in those plans changed. Whereas early state programmes 'tended to depict [urban] workers or rural villagers as the archetypical citizens and objects of development, ... mainstream national political discourses increasingly depict the middle classes as the representative citizens of liberalising India' (Fernandes, 2004, p. 2416).

The fate of decentralisation laws enacted in 1992 further illustrates liberalisation's inimical effects on state-provided urban health care. Constitutional Amendment Acts (CAAs) in 1992 sought to achieve decentralised, participatory local self-government in rural and urban jurisdictions. However, implementation of the acts has proceeded more effectively in rural than urban areas, one reason being that they do not mandate that state governments devolve powers to municipal governments but only give them the discretion to do so (Murthy and Mahin, 2016). States have been reluctant to devolve powers, fearing a loss of control over the direction and spoils of urban economic growth and arguing circularly that municipal governments have low administrative capacity to actually take on the task of delivering public services (Murthy and Mahin, 2016). As a result, most municipal governments 'still face resource constraints to even carry out their routine functions' (Kundu, 2014, p. 616). In rural areas, under the CAAs, states created administrative and political procedures and institutions for local decision-making, enabling a measure of participatory health planning and monitoring down to the village level (Shukla, et al., 2014). Such correspondence between local government and community-level health planning eludes urban areas (MOHFW, 2014).

Urban renewal initiatives in the 2000s aimed to address municipal governments' insufficient fiscal powers, outdated administrative processes, and absence of channels for citizen participation (JNNURM, 2011). But in practice they have emphasised upgrades to infrastructure such as roads and transportation – investments to boost cities' economic viability, not basic public services or municipal governance (Coelho and Maringanti, 2012). The state's approach, moreover, reinforces cultural shifts under liberalisation that render the poor invisible (Mander, 2017). National discourses of development now reference 'a new set of elite "citizens"' who are 'undeniably urban', and whose concerns lie afield from those of the vulnerable, impoverished populations who were previously prioritised in the 'narrative of national development' (Bhan, 2014, p. 556). State-provided primary care is peripheral to the concerns of this new urban elite, who widely use private providers as surveys of health care-seeking in cities suggest (Gupta, et al., 2009).

Municipal governments' weak capacity, coupled with the state's economic policies in recent decades, has implied low priority for reform of urban health care. The state's policy neglect of urban primary care has consequences that lie beyond the health disparities it creates, such as intra-city inequalities in health status (Agarwal, 2011; Subbaraman, et al., 2012). As I next discuss, by giving a fillip to private health care, liberalisation policies may have diminished prospects for local collective action to improve urban health care.

## Prospects for collective action to improve urban health care

The state's early emphasis on a technocratic approach to health set the conditions for muted collective action for health care in India. In late-colonial society, self-help groups, voluntary and charitable organisations, and neighbourhood associations had played a role in publishing and circulating 'ideas about health and healthiness' (Amrith, 2009, p. 13). But in independent India, national leaders substituted an institutionalised, rational, planning-based approach for the individual charity and sympathy-based, unorganised efforts of elite interventions in health (Amrith, 2009). The state effectively negated civic engagement in health when it failed to communicate to citizens the idea of 'health as a right and an entitlement of citizenship' (Amrith, 2009, p. 13).

Yet the current scene of community activism for public services in urban India suggests that factors other than a historically low civic awareness about health may be simultaneously at work. Evidence suggests that local mobilisation for other urban public services (water, sanitation) is more robust than for health care. One reason for weaker collective action for health, I argue, is the ready availability of *private* alternatives. The health system's organisation – a dominant, largely unregulated private sector and chronically under-resourced public sector – reinforces a muted popular understanding of health as a right. The ready accessibility of private services counteracts people's grievances – their sense of a deficiency or injustice in need of redress – about state-provided health care.

Public expenditure on health care in India is 1.2 per cent of GDP, low relative to 4.1 per cent in Brazil and South Africa (Marten, et al., 2014). By contrast, private sector involvement in health care is notable for its history, magnitude, fervency, and diversity (Baru and Nundy, 2008; Bhat, 1993). Private providers have accounted for over 70 per cent of all outpatient transactions in urban India since at least the late 1980s (NSSO, 1998; 2015). State monitoring of health care providers and facilities, such as through licensing, registration, and accreditation to assure quality standards, has been weak (Sheikh, et al., 2015) and actively contested by private stakeholders (Srinivasan, 2013). As a result, people can purchase health care and related services (diagnostics, drugs, insurance) as commodities in a sizeable and largely unregulated market.

Public investment in water and sanitation in cities is also inadequate, but the private provision of these services is far less extensive. The state remains a significant, if deficient, supplier of these public goods. For instance, informal and formal private suppliers of water have been slow to gain a foothold in water supply markets in urban India (Water and Sanitation Program, 2011). One-third of urban households depend on shared, community, and public toilets, and one-third of the lowest-income households lack any access to toilets (Wankhade, 2015). But private sector interventions to test new technologies and business models, including community-based and commercial approaches to operate and maintain public toilets, are yet to be scaled up (Dasra, 2012).

Parallel to the state's more significant role in water and sanitation, social mobilisation for these services appears more robust than for health care. For example, researchers have documented the politics of slum-dwellers' collectives in Mumbai (Roy, 2009); mobilisation among the urban poor to collectively press for sanitation services in informal settlements in Mumbai (McFarlane, et al., 2014); and dissident responses of lower-middle-class residents in Bangalore's periphery to market-oriented water reforms (Ranganathan, 2014).

In contrast, efforts by NGOs to mobilise urban communities for improved health care have been few and difficult to sustain (Agarwal, et al., 2008; More, et al., 2012). One challenge that distinguishes mobilisation for health care versus other public services is that 'access to health care is not limited by distance or scarcity' (More, et al., 2012, p. 2). The urban poor navigate a heterogeneous health sector, encompassing public and private clinics and hospitals, individual practitioners, alternative healers, and drug shops, and tend to use the less qualified, less expensive segment of a spectrum of private providers (Das and Das, 2006; Seeberg, et al., 2014). The large private sector enables the poor to avoid state facilities, thus deflecting their potential grievances against health care as an inadequacy in need of redress. In this way, the national political economy of urban development and health care combines with the local politics of access to public goods in cities to forestall improvements to state-provided urban primary care.

## Conclusion

This case study shows how national and subnational politics shape the organisation and development of India's health care services in urban settings. State health programmes have focused on rural rather than urban populations, while urban development initiatives have focused on infrastructure to ensure cities' economic viability rather than on basic services. Attempts to empower municipal governments have been few and ineffective, caught between the centre's interest in cities as drivers of economic growth and state governments' reluctance to devolve power to cities. As a result, urban primary care has received marginal attention across levels of the state (central, state-level, municipal); across state agencies (health, urban development); and across time (post-colonial to liberalisation). Concurrently, the private sector's expansion in health care presents urban residents a ready alternative to deficient state services, thereby potentially diminishing the likelihood of social mobilisation for urban health care.

Historical conditions and processes can produce alternate configurations of health systems in other states. In Brazil, for instance, political barriers to universal health care appeared high in 1988, in the midst of Brazil's transition to democracy after two decades of military rule (Falleti, 2010). The health system was highly centralised, municipalities had little role in managing and providing health care, and private entities absorbed national funding for health through contracts. Two decades later, municipalities were responsible for delivering basic health care, and the private sector, though still prevalent, became less significant as a contractor (Falleti, 2010). These health system changes were wrought gradually over time. As the military expanded its territorial reach and sought to legitimate its rule in rural areas, its penetration into society enabled reformist elements – 'leftist health care organizations' who championed public social medicine – to introduce and eventually institutionalise principles of universalism and decentralisation (Falleti, 2010, p. 40) and expand primary care access (Paim, et al., 2011).

The Brazil case highlights the distinct national and subnational politics that undergird its health system's evolution. It suggests that social movements have played a more significant role in shaping health system reform in Brazil than in India. In both cases, historical processes that constitute a health system are critical to explaining its development and anticipating state response to global health threats.

## References

Agarwal, S. (2011) 'The state of urban health in India: comparing the poorest quartile to the rest of the urban population in selected states and cities', *Environment and Urbanization*, 23: 13–28.

Agarwal, S., Satyavada, A., Patra, P., and Kumar, R. (2008) 'Strengthening functional community provider linkages: lessons from the Indore urban health programme', *Global Public Health*, 3(3): 308–25.

Altman, D. (2006) 'Taboos and denial in government responses', *International Affairs*, 82(2 HIV/AIDS-special issue), 257–68.

Amrith, S. (2006) *Decolonizing International Health: India and Southeast Asia, 1930–65*, Basingstoke and New York: Palgrave Macmillan.

Amrith, S. (2007) 'Political culture of health in India: a historical perspective', *Economic and Political Weekly*, 42(2): 114–21.

Amrith, S. (2009) 'Health in India since independence', working paper 79, Brooks World Poverty Institute, The University of Manchester.

Baru, R. (2003) 'Privatisation of health services: a South Asian perspective', *Economic and Political Weekly*, 38(42): 4433–7.

Baru, R. and Nundy, M. (2008) 'Blurring of boundaries: public-private partnerships in health services in India', *Economic and Political Weekly*, 43(4): 62–71.

Bhan, G. (2014) 'The impoverishment of poverty: reflections on urban citizenship and inequality in contemporary Delhi', *Environment and Urbanization*, 26(2): 547–60.

Bhat, R. (1993) 'The public/private mix in health care in India', *Health Policy and Planning*, 8(1): 43–56.

Bhowmik, S. (2009) 'Labor sociology searching for a direction', *Work and Occupations*, 36(2): 126–44.

Brenner, N. (2013) 'Theses on urbanization', *Public Culture*, 25(1): 85–114.

Chatterjee, P. (1997) 'Development planning and the Indian state', In: P. Chatterjee (Ed.) *State and Politics in India*, New Delhi: Oxford University Press, pp. 271–98.

Chibber, V. (2003) *Locked in Place: State-building and late industrialization in India*, Princeton: Princeton University Press.

Coelho, K. and Maringanti, A. (2012) 'Urban poverty in India: tools, treatment and politics at the neo-liberal turn', *Economic and Political Weekly*, 47(47 and 48): 39–43.

Das, J. and Hammer, J. (2014) 'Quality of primary care in low-income countries: facts and economics', *Annual Review of Economics*, 6: 525–53.

Das, V. and Das, R. (2006) 'Urban health and pharmaceutical consumption in Delhi, India', *Journal of Biosocial Science*, 38(1): 69–82.

Dasra. (2012) *Squatting Rights: Access to toilets in urban India*, Sulabh International, Dasra, Omidyar Network, and Forbes Marshall.

Evans, P. (2009) 'Population health and development: an institutional–cultural approach to capability expansion', In: P. Hall and M. Lamont (Eds.) *Successful Societies: How institutions and culture affect health*, Cambridge University Press, pp. 104–27.

Falleti, T. (2010) 'Infiltrating the state: the evolution of health care reforms in Brazil, 1964–1988', In: J. Mahoney and K. Thelen (Eds.) *Explaining Institutional Change: Ambiguity, agency, and power*, New York: Cambridge University Press, pp. 38–62.

Fernandes, L. (2004) 'The politics of forgetting: class politics, state power and the restructuring of urban space in India', *Urban Studies*, 41(12): 2415–30.

Friel, S., Akerman, M., Hancock, T., et al. (2011) 'Addressing the social and environmental determinants of urban health equity: evidence for action and a research agenda', *Journal of Urban Health*, 88: 860.

GoI. (1946) *Report of the Health Survey and Development Committee (Bhore Committee Report) Volume 1*, Delhi: Government of India.

Goldman, M. (2011) 'Speculative urbanism and the making of the next world city', *International Journal of Urban and Regional Research*, 35(3): 555–81.

Gupta, K., Arnold, F., and Lhungdim, H. (2009) *Health and Living Conditions in Eight Indian Cities, National Family Health Survey (NFHS-3), India, 2005–06*, Mumbai: International Institute for Population Sciences; Calverton: ICF Macro.

Harvey, D. (1985) *The Urbanization of Capital: Studies in the history and theory of capitalist urbanization*, Baltimore, MD: Johns Hopkins University Press.

JNNURM. (2011) *Implementation of the 74th Constitutional Amendment and Integration of City Planning and Delivery Functions*, New Delhi: Ministry of Urban Development, Government of India.

Kapadia-Kundu, N. and Kanitkar, T. (2002) 'Primary healthcare in urban slums', *Economic and Political Weekly*, 5086–9.

Kaviraj, S. (2000) 'Modernity and politics in India', *Daedalus*, 129(1): 137–62.

Kundu, D. (2014) 'Urban development programmes in India: a critique of JnNURM', *Social Change*, 44(4): 615–32.

Lieberman, E. (2009) *Boundaries of Contagion: How ethnic politics have shaped government responses to AIDS*, Princeton: Princeton University Press.

Mander, H. (2017) 'Public goods, exclusion and 25 years of economic reforms: a blotted balance sheet', In: *India Exclusion Report 2016*, New Delhi: Yoda Press, pp. 1–30.

Marten, R., et al. (2014) 'An assessment of progress towards universal health coverage in Brazil, Russia, India, China, and South Africa (BRICS)', *The Lancet*, 384(9960): 2164–71.

McFarlane, C., Desai, R., and Graham, S. (2014) 'Politics of sanitation: informality and the constitution of urban metabolic life in Mumbai', In: K. Shrestha, H. Ojha, H. McManus, P. Rubbo, and K. Dhote (Eds.) *Inclusive Urbanization: Rethinking policy and practice in an age of climate change*, New York and London: Routledge, pp. 67–86.

Mills, A. (2014) 'Health care systems in low- and middle- income countries', *The New England Journal of Medicine*, 370: 552–7.

Ministry of Home Affairs. (2011) *Census of India 2011: Rural urban distribution of population (provisional population totals)*, New Delhi: Registrar General and Census Commissioner, Ministry of Home Affairs, Government of India.

MOHFW. (2005) *Framework for Implementation: National rural health mission, 2005–2012*, New Delhi: Ministry of Health and Family Welfare, Government of India.

MOHFW. (2013) *National Urban Health Mission: Framework for implementation*, New Delhi: Ministry of Health and Family Welfare, Government of India.

MOHFW. (2014) *Making the Urban Health Mission Work for the Urban Poor: Report of the Technical Resource Group for the National Urban Health Mission*, New Delhi: Ministry of Health and Family Welfare, Government of India.

Montgomery, M. and Ezeh, A. (2005) 'The health of urban populations in developing countries: an overview', In: S. Galea and D. Vlahov (Eds.) *Handbook of Urban Health: Populations, methods, and practice*, New York: Kluwer, pp. 201–22.

More, N.S., et al. (2012) 'Community mobilization in Mumbai slums to improve perinatal care and outcomes: a cluster randomized controlled trial', *PLoS Medicine*, 9(7): e1001257.

Murthy, S. and Mahin, M. (2016) 'Constitutional impediments to decentralization in the world's largest federal country', *Duke Journal of Comparative and International Law*, 26: 79–139.

NPC. (1947) *National Planning Committee Series (report of the sub-committee): National health, Chair: S.S. Sokhey*, Bombay: Vora & Co.

NSSO. (1998) *Morbidity and Treatment of Ailments: NSS 52nd round*, National Sample Survey Organization, Ministry of Statistics and Programme Implementation, Government of India.

NSSO. (2015) *Key Indicators of Social Consumption in India – health: NSS 71st round*. National Sample Survey Organization, Ministry of Statistics and Programme Implementation, Government of India

Nunn, A. (2009) *The Politics and History of AIDS Treatment in Brazil*, New York: Springer-Verlag.

Paim, J., et al. (2011) 'The Brazilian health system: history, advances, and challenges', *The Lancet*, 377(9779): 1778–97.

Parkhurst, J. and Lush, L. (2004) 'The political environment of HIV: lessons from a comparison of Uganda and South Africa', *Social Science & Medicine*, 59(9): 1913–24.

Planning Commission. (2002) *Tenth Five Year Plan 2002–2007, Volume II: Sectoral policies and programmes*, Planning Commission, Government of India.

Priya, R. (2005) 'Public health services in India: a historical perspective', In: L. Gangolli, R. Duggal, and A. Shukla (Eds.) *Review of Healthcare in India*, Mumbai: Centre for Enquiry into Health and Allied Themes, pp. 41–73.

Ranganathan, M. (2014) 'Paying for pipes, claiming citizenship: political agency and water reforms at the urban periphery, *International Journal of Urban and Regional Research*, 38(2): 590–608.

Rao, M. (2004) *The Unheard Scream: Reproductive health and women's lives in India*, New Delhi: Zubaan and Panos Institute.

Rao, M., et al. (2011) 'Human resources for health in India', *The Lancet*, 377(9765): 587–98.

Ricci, J. (2009) 'Global health governance and the state: premature claims of a post-international framework', *Global Health Governance*, 3(1): 1–18.

Roy, A. (2009) 'Civic governmentality: the politics of inclusion in Beirut and Mumbai', *Antipode*, 41(1): 159–79.

Seeberg, J., et al. (2014) 'Treatment seeking and health financing in selected poor urban neighbourhoods in India, Indonesia and Thailand', *Social Science & Medicine*, 102: 49–57.

Seto, K., Sánchez-Rodríguez, R., and Fragkias, M. (2010) 'The new geography of contemporary urbanization and the environment', *Annual Review of Environment and Resources*, 35: 167–94.

Sharma, A. and Gupta, A. (2006) 'Introduction: rethinking theories of the state in an age of globalization', In: A. Sharma and A. Gupta (Eds.) *The Anthropology of the State: A reader*, Blackwell Publishing Ltd., pp. 1–41.

Shaw, A. (1996) 'Urban policy in post-independent India: an appraisal', *Economic & Political Weekly*, 31(4): 224–8.

Sheikh, K., et al. (2011) 'Building the field of health policy and systems research: framing the questions', *PLoS Medicine*, 8(8): e1001073.

Sheikh, K., Saligram, P., and Hort, K. (2015) 'What explains regulatory failure? Analysing the architecture of health care regulation in two Indian states', *Health Policy and Planning*, 30(1): 39–55.

Shukla, A., Khanna, R., and Jadhav, N. (2014) 'Using community-based evidence for decentralized health planning: insights from Maharashtra, India', *Health Policy and Planning*, 33(1): e34–45.

Srinivasan, S. (2013) 'Regulation and the medical profession: Clinical Establishments Act, 2010', *Economic and Political Weekly*, 48(3): 14–6.

Stren, R., McGee, T., Moser, C., and Yeung, Y. (2003) 'The challenge of urban governance', In: M. Montgomery, R. Stren, B. Cohen, and H. Reed (Eds.) *Cities Transformed: Demographic change and its implications in the developing world*, Washington, DC: The National Academies Press, pp. 355–409.

Subbaraman, R., et al. (2012) 'Off the map: the health and social implications of being a non-notified slum in India', *Environment and Urbanization*, 24(2): 643–63.

Swidler, A. (2006) 'Syncretism and subversion in AIDS governance: how locals cope with global demands', *International Affairs*, 82(2): 269–84.

Thakur, M. (2014) 'Understanding ruralities: contemporary debates', working paper, New Delhi: Centre for the Study of Social Systems, Jawaharlal Nehru University.

Wankhade, K. (2015) 'Urban sanitation in India: key shifts in the national policy frame', *Environment and Urbanization*, 27(2): 555–72.

Water and Sanitation Program. (2011) *Trends in Private Sector Participation in the Indian Water Sector: A critical review*, World Bank.

Weinstein, L., Sami, N., and Shatkin, G. (2014) 'Contested developments: enduring legacies and emergent political actors in contemporary urban India', In: G. Shatkin (Ed.) *Contesting the Indian City: Global visions and the politics of the local*, Chichester: John Wiley and Sons, pp. 39–64.

YASHADA (Yashwantrao Chavan Academy of Development Administration). (2014) *Maharashtra Human Development Report 2012: Towards inclusive human development*, New Delhi: Sage Publications India Pvt Ltd.

# Part III
# The changing shape of global health governance

# 12

# Reforming the World Health Organization

*Yanzhong Huang and Gabriella Meltzer*

The World Health Organization (WHO) was established in 1948 to ensure 'the attainment by all peoples of the highest possible level of health' (WHO, 2006, p. 2). Over the past seven decades, the organisation has made significant achievements towards fulfilling this lofty goal. Yet from the outset, the resources and capabilities at the organisation's disposal have been incommensurate with the scope and scale of the challenges it has sought to address. The discrepancy between the WHO's mandate and capacities has become even more glaring with the rise of additional global health challenges over the past three decades, including HIV and AIDS, pandemic influenza, and noncommunicable diseases (NCDs). WHO is striving to tackle these challenges, but its leading role in global health continues to be undermined by problems of prioritisation, underfunding, leadership, and internal and global governance issues, all of which set the context for reforming the organisation.

This chapter addresses the WHO's years-long reform process, analysing its successes and failures to adapt to the shifting global health landscape. It begins with an overview of the organisation's history since its establishment in 1948. Despite key achievements such as the eradication of smallpox, and response to the 2003 SARS outbreak, the organisation faces tremendous governance challenges in sustaining its leadership in global health in the twenty-first century. The chapter will then examine the reform process by discussing how the reform was conceived, what measures were pursued, and their effectiveness. Particular attention is paid to the role of the global South in pushing for these reforms. The 2014 Ebola outbreak in West Africa epitomised the aforementioned governance challenges and signalled the lack of progress in the WHO reform. Unfortunately, the Ebola crisis thus far has not spurred fundamental change in WHO management, governance, or financing structures.

## The establishment of WHO

By the close of the Second World War in 1945, significant portions of the world laid in shambles. The period during and immediately following the war witnessed the greatest population migration to date, creating ripe conditions for the spread of infectious diseases among millions of refugees lacking adequate shelter, nutrition, or primary health care. In addition, rates of sexually transmitted and tropical vector-borne diseases skyrocketed among troops who had been stationed far from their countries of origin. The severe damage inflicted upon countries' infrastructures and economic systems crippled their ability to respond to burgeoning epidemics.

This situation highlighted the need to create an international regime to collectively address crises that threatened geopolitical and social stability (Lee, 2008). In light of the absence of health as a major, stand-alone priority on the United Nations (UN) agenda, Brazil and China submitted a joint declaration calling for a specialised conference with the goal of establishing an international health agency specifically devoted to health. Their request culminated with the convening of the June 1946 International Health Conference, which laid the groundwork for the WHO's prototype (Lee, 2008). The WHO constitution officially came into force on 7 April 1948, and the agency was formally established as a UN entity in September 1948.

The newly created health organisation has a three-tiered institutional structure. Its headquarters is located in Geneva. The World Health Assembly (WHA) is the decision-making body. Held annually in Geneva and attended by delegations from all member states, the WHA determines WHO policies, appoints the WHO director-general, supervises financial policies, and reviews and approves programmatic budgets. The executive board, composed of 34 individuals technically qualified in the field of health, offers expert technical assistance and gives effect to the WHA's decisions and policies. Day-to-day operations of the WHA are conducted in Geneva through the secretariat, which is led by the director-general (DG). The next level of the organisational structure features six WHO regions, each with a regional office. Subject to the general authority of the DG, the regional office is the administrative organ of the regional committee and carries out the decisions of both the WHA and the executive board within the region. Below the regional level are 149 WHO field offices in countries, territories, or areas. It is worth noting that the WHO was created at a time when regional health entities had already been in place. Among them is the Pan American Health Organization (PAHO) in the Western Hemisphere, the oldest health organisation in the international community. It took a year for the two groups to agree that PAHO would become one of the regional arms of WHO, while remaining self-governing (McCarthy, 2002).

As a specialised agency for global health, the WHO is intended to 'act as the directing and coordinating authority on international health work' (WHO, 2006, n.p.). This involves coordinating global responses to international public health emergencies and developing health-related norms and standards. Unlike many other UN agencies, the WHO has constitutional authority to convene experts, governments, and other actors to negotiate and monitor normative instruments – both legally binding treaties and nonbinding rules or instruments that promise to create expectations about future conduct ('soft law') (Klock, 2012). Despite this powerful mechanism, the WHO does not have the authority to enforce compliance and must rely on national governments to implement the international law (Gostin and Sridhar, 2014). The organisation has a dual mandate to be both a political body where states debate and negotiate on sometimes divisive health issues, as well as a technical agency that uses its health expertise to provide technical assistance and guidance. As a technical agency, it serves as a 'knowledge broker' in global health – collecting, analysing, and disseminating information and evidence for policy making and capacity building.

## An assessment of historical WHO interventions

Since its founding, the WHO has made disease prevention and control one of its top priorities. In June 1948, the first WHA identified malaria, tuberculosis (TB), sexually transmitted diseases, maternal and child health, 'sanitary engineering', and nutrition as top priorities. WHO has since launched a series of global campaigns against tuberculosis (1947–51), malaria (1955–70), smallpox (1967–80), polio, diphtheria, whooping cough, tetanus, TB, and measles through the Expanded Programme on Immunization or EPI (1974–present), onchocerciasis (1974–present), HIV/AIDS (1987–96), and polio through the Global Polio Eradication Initiative or GPEI (1988–present). To the extent that these campaigns focused on infectious diseases, the twenty-first century saw a growing interest in the WHO to tackle NCDs. The WHO Global Action Plan for the Prevention and Control of NCDs 2013–20 signalled a potential paradigm shift by providing a road map and a menu of policy options for national and international actors to attain, among other global targets, a 25 per cent relative reduction in premature mortality from NCDs by 2025 (WHO, 2017a).

The campaign against smallpox was a huge success. The last endemic case of smallpox was recorded in Somalia on 26 October 1977 (Henderson, 1987). D.A. Henderson, the disease epidemiologist who led the eradication effort, attributed the success to the WHO, which 'alone among the international organizations, has the requisite scientific expertise and channels of communication with the national authorities for the monitoring and coordination of health programs' (Henderson, 1987, p. 537). The results were less rosy for the Global Malaria Eradication Program. While the global campaign led to the elimination of malaria in many regions in the world, it has not achieved major success in sub-Saharan Africa, which accounts for 80 per cent of today's burden of malaria. As a result, the aspiration of global eradication was abandoned in 1969 (Tanner and de Savigny, 2008). Experts pointed out that the malaria campaign placed too much emphasis on technical solutions (e.g., insecticides, vaccines, and drugs), while failing to integrate those tools into the pre-existing health and social systems prevailing in endemic areas (Lee, 2008). The need to focus beyond simply developing better tools led to the launch of the Roll Back Malaria initiative in 1998, which emphasises achieving targets for control through country level capacity building and health systems strengthening (WHO, 2000, p. 1).

WHO's experience in malaria eradication highlights the tension between a disease-specific 'vertical' approach and a systematic or 'diagonal' approach. As early as 1978, the Alma-Ata Declaration identified primary health care (PHC) as the key to attain the goal of Health For All. Focusing on community-based health workers, affordable technologies, integrated care, and the need to address underlying structural causes of poor health, the PHC campaign represented an antithesis to the top-down, high-tech based and disease focused western biomedical model. Later, it also took on large corporations and transnational industries to control the risk factors of poor health. The Framework Convention on Tobacco Control (FCTC) is the first international treaty negotiated under the auspices of WHO. Adopted by the WHA in 2003 and entered into force in 2005, FCTC has since become one of the most rapidly and widely embraced treaties in United Nations history (WHO, 2015b). In March 2005, the WHO launched the Commission on the Social Determinants of Health (CSDH), which brings together a global network of policymakers, researchers, and civil society organisations to support tackling the social causes of poor health and avoidable health inequalities.

Beginning in the 1980s, globalisation and the growing risk of human exposure to infectious diseases resulted in the increased interaction between health and security. This development parallels WHO efforts to tackle trans-border spread of acute infectious diseases from a security perspective. Securitisation efforts were not new, but apparently gained momentum when the WHO confronted severe acute respiratory syndrome (SARS), the 'first severe infectious disease to emerge in the globalized society of the twenty-first century' (Fidler, 2004, p. 801). During the outbreak, WHO issued travel alerts and advisories, and set up global virtual laboratory networks to identify the exact coronavirus that spawned SARS cases in patients. In addition, under the leadership of then Director-General Gro Harlem-Brundtland, the WHO successfully put mounting political pressure on the Chinese government to allow its experts into the country and reveal the true nature of the outbreak.

The growing threat of a public health emergency of international concern (PHEIC) and renewed WHO authority during SARS accelerated the negotiation process for the revision of the International Health Regulations (IHR), an international legal instrument that is binding for all the WHO member states (Fidler, 2004). Entered into force in June 2007, the IHR requires countries to build certain core surveillance and response capacities to uphold public health security. As shown in the 2009 H1N1 pandemic, despite its limitations, the revised IHR has provided a more robust framework for responding to public health emergencies of international concern (PHEIC) (Wilson, et al., 2010). In the wake of the pandemic, the WHO sponsored the landmark Pandemic Influenza Preparedness Framework for virus sharing and access to affordable vaccines for countries in the global South. Today, the WHO remains the chief reference body for support in handling global health threats.

## The challenges

Despite its achievements, the WHO has struggled to maintain its legitimacy and comparative advantage in a rapidly changing global health landscape. As far as challenges are concerned, five sets of issues remain at the forefront: institutional identity, funding, DG leadership, internal governance, and management.

### Institutional identity problem

One of the major issues the WHO faces is defining its role in global health governance. Throughout its 70-year history, the WHO has consistently been challenged by its member states to reduce the number of objectives laid out in its constitution, while simultaneously taking on greater responsibilities. While they advocate for a leaner and stronger WHO (WHO, 2017d), they disagree over the core missions and identity of the health agency. Should the WHO focus on the development of global norms and standards or expand its role as an operating agency? Should it be politically active (e.g., taking on powerful special interests) or play a more restricted, largely technocratic role? How should it balance the objectives of disease prevention, health promotion, and treatment? Lack of a clear idea of its core mission led to WHO efforts to compete for leadership as an operating agency, as shown in its launch of the 3 by 5 Initiative in 2003, which sought to provide three million people living with HIV/AIDS in low- and middle-income countries with life-prolonging antiretroviral treatment (ART) by the end of 2005. The failed initiative led one think tank scholar to ask the organisation to 'stop chasing numbers in order to achieve the desired bureaucratic outcome and instead focus on testing and evaluation, responsible treatment, and monitoring of AIDS patients' (Adelman, 2006).

The uncertainty is complicated by disagreement over the philosophical approach to global health. Should WHO emphasise sustained interventions into specific health concerns and diseases or tackle the broader determinants of health? While a growing consensus has emerged that an epidemic today is just too complex to be tackled by one single approach, WHO activities continue to be shaped by a strong focus on disease-specific problems (Lee, 2008). This tension can be traced back to the deep ideological differences between the East and West camps during the Cold War: while communist regimes envisioned an organisation that would embrace social medicine, democratic camps sought to confine its role to disease surveillance and control (Lee, 2008). With the end of the Cold War, the tension today is no longer a reflection of East–West political divide or North–South conflict but rather the indication of the competition of different approaches to global health challenges in the context of sustained funding and capacity problems. As WHO programmes have expanded beyond control of specific infectious diseases to tackling issues such as poverty and diseases, intellectual property rights and access to affordable drugs, and health inequities, donors began to question the organisation's performance and priorities, which contributed to the funding crisis since the 1990s (Bollyky, 2012).

### Funding crisis

Closely associated with the issue of institutional identity is a crisis in funding, which exacerbates the gap between the WHO's mandate and actual capabilities. Although rising global health challenges demand the investment of greater resources and capacity, funding for WHO has never matched the problems its member states task it to address. WHO has an operating annual budget of about US$2 billion, which is one-third that of the US Centers for Disease Control and Prevention (CDC). Worse, WHO's budget planning and prioritisation is heavily dependent upon voluntary donations allocated according to donor interests. Its budget consists of two separate sources of funding: assessed contributions (ACs) from WHO's 194 member states and voluntary contributions (VCs) from member states and non-government funders, including the United States, United Kingdom, Bill & Melinda Gates Foundation, and GAVI Alliance. ACs are wholly flexible and predictable (agreed upon in advance), but they are only a small portion of the WHO budget. VCs are larger in size, but are voluntary and guided by donor priorities, meaning they do not have the same predictability and flexibility as ACs.[1] For the two-year period 2010–11, 80 per cent of WHO money came from VC and only 20 per cent of its budget was completely under organisational control. This has severely constrained WHO's ability to plan a realistic budget.

The fragmented and franchised financing structure has also led to the use of the WHO's regular funding to subsidise outside funding for special projects like polio eradication (because much of the earmarked funds are not allowed to include overhead). In addition, there are sustainability issues. A stagnant budget comprised of member assessments and voluntary contributions is not able to keep up with increasing demands, inflation, and global economic sluggishness. In 2007, WHO's expenditures started to exceed its revenues, and by 2010, the organisation faced a significant deficit (Garrett, 2013). Also, VCs to WHO funding are heavily skewed towards the US government and Gates Foundation. In 2010, the US government was contributing 15.5 per cent of VCs. The second largest voluntary donor, the US-based Bill & Melinda Gates Foundation, contributed 15.2 per cent. The lack of predictable, flexible, and sustainable funding has seriously compromised its ability to fulfil its core functions. For example, only 3 per cent of its 2012–13 budget addressed NCDs.

## Problematic director-general (DG) leadership

The WHO's identity and funding issues are exacerbated by problematic DG leadership. According to the WHO constitution, the DG is the chief technical and administrative officer of the organisation. In light of growing global health challenges and the international health agency's sustaining budget woes, having a capable and visionary WHO DG is not only central to its day-to-day administration, but also crucial for maintaining its leadership in global health governance. Although each DG has achieved varying degrees of success in terms of reforming the organisation and fulfilling its mandate, not all demonstrated the leadership needed to effectively run the organisation. In April 2016, with support from the Rockefeller Foundation, Council on Foreign Relations's Global Health programme conducted a 'straw poll' asking respondents to choose their favourite DGs.[2] When asked to rank the top two DGs of the agency since 1973,[3] an overwhelming majority (67 per cent) ranked Dr. Gro Harlem Brundtland as their first choice. This is not surprising: during her tenure as WHO DG, Brundtland made sweeping changes throughout the organisation, used WHO's treaty-making power to negotiate the Framework Convention on Tobacco Control, and issued the first travel advisories in the organisation's 55-year history during the 2003 SARS epidemic.

In contrast, no respondent ranked Hiroshi Nakajima as his or her first choice. Although the respondents did not explain why they ranked Nakajima so poorly, Gostin and Sridhar have noted that the former WHO DG was accused of 'cronyism and corruption, an autocratic management style, and financial mismanagement' (Gostin and Sridhar, 2014, p. 133). Considered by American journalist Barton Gellman as a 'master of back-room manoeuvring', Nakajima as WHO DG had a famous conflict with then head of the WHO's AIDS programme, Jonathan Mann, which resulted in Mann's resignation (Gellman, 2000). Nakajima's unwillingness to cut budgets or use resources more efficiently to meet new challenges dampened donor countries' enthusiasm surrounding the WHO and its organisational capacities. In turn, the Clinton and Bush administrations in the United States, along with their European partners, channelled their loss of confidence in the WHO leadership towards creating alternative global health initiatives dedicated to those efforts Nakajima would not financially or politically support – specifically HIV/AIDS, tuberculosis, maternal and child health, and polio eradication, to name a few (Lee, 2008). As a result, the WHO ceded its leadership over HIV/AIDS prevention and control to organisations such as UNAIDS and the Global

Fund to Fight AIDS, Tuberculosis and Malaria. Dissatisfaction with the WHO leadership and the demand for greater control over spending by major donors also led to efforts to supplant the WHO core funding with extra-budgetary support. It was in the wake of this leadership crisis that Dr. Gro Brundtland took the helm and navigated the sinking WHO ship through treacherous waters.

## Internal governance and management issues

A fair performance assessment of the WHO leadership would have to take into account internal governance issues. The WHO constitution grants regional offices significant autonomy in the policy process. Their management, governance, and spending decisions are not closely monitored by any central authority (The Economist Group Limited, 2014). WHO regional directors are appointed by governments in the region, not by the WHO DG. Their allegiances are therefore to the region rather than to the headquarters in Geneva. Given the lack of close oversight and control over regional offices, such an institutional setup makes it difficult for Geneva to align regional and country offices closely with overall WHO strategies and priorities, although it may create certain protection against overly top-down decision-making.

Other organisational and institutional issues have widened the internal governance gap. To make the organisation more efficient and accountable, its management should be staffed by properly trained professionals for budgeting, financial, and administrative roles. The constitution places a premium on geographical basis and the internationally representative character of staff recruitment, which often leads to an opaque and inward-looking appointment process that de-emphasises competencies and qualifications related to WHO's core functions. Scholars have complained that WHO staff has become bloated, mediocre, and ineffective in translating scientific and technical knowledge into effective guidance for member states (Hoffman and Røttingen, 2014; Horton, 2015). On the one hand, the WHO is critically short on experts to cover new global health challenges, such as NCDs. On the other hand, there are few non-medical experts to cope with the issues of global health diplomacy and governance. According to a study published in *Public Health*, of the one-third of the WHO staff deemed professionals, nearly half are medical specialists, only 1.6 per cent are social scientists, and 1.4 per cent are lawyers. While doctors are crucial for the WHO to exercise its technical leadership, this staff composition means that the organisation does not have the capacity to understand local traditions and cultures, manage international relations, and perform some of its core functions such as creating rules and principles for global health (Hoffman and Røttingen, 2014).

Meanwhile, global health is not governed by a single regime centred on the WHO but rather a 'regime complex', or 'a collective of partially overlapping and non-hierarchical regimes' (Raustiala and Victor, 2004, p. 277). WHO must balance the member-state driven decision-making with the need to work within a broader governance context characterised by the involvement and influence of states, other intergovernmental institutions (e.g., World Bank), and non-state actors (e.g., Gates Foundation). The Gates Foundation's global health budget, for example, is about twice the size of WHO's core budget. Proliferation of additional global health entities not only threatens to marginalise WHO's global health leadership, but is also responsible for overlapping mandates, poor coordination, and wasted resources. Member states' priorities, for instance, are often in conflict with major donors that are in control of different resources, such as the US government and the Gates Foundation.

## The 2010 WHO reform process

In January 2010, Margaret Chan launched the WHO's years-long reform process with a convening of member state representatives to discuss the 'predictability and flexibility of WHO's financing'. This was in the aftermath of the global economic crisis, where the WHO was concerned about its financial sustainability with the weakening US dollar, alongside an overstretched agenda and a need to compete with countless other multilateral and non-state organisations for political and financial support. These preliminary discussions, along with external evaluations, prompted Chan and the WHO to undertake a far more wide-reaching reform effort to address fundamental questions about the WHO's mission and priorities, internal governance, interaction with other global health entities, and managerial operations to enhance account-ability and efficiency. Participants concluded that the main challenges facing the organisation included a 'lack of clear organizational priorities', 'lack of predictable and flexible financing', and 'highly decentralized organizational structure' (U.S. Government Accountability Office, 2012, p. 11).

The 128th meeting of the WHO Executive Board in January 2011 established a three-pronged approach towards reform that would ultimately guide the remainder of the process to this day: (1) 'greater focus to meet the expectations of member states in addressing health priorities'; (2) 'greater coherence in global health through better governance'; and (3) 'an organization that was fit for purpose through management reforms' (WHO, 2017d, p. 9). This approach was ratified by the 129th World Health Assembly, which met in the spring of that year (WHO, 2017c).

As mentioned previously, the WHO's agenda was merely growing and becoming quite overextended with each passing year and an increasingly complex global health landscape. Given the growing attention on the social determinants of health and health disparities, microbial dynamics of infectious diseases, glo-balisation, and an epidemiological transition accompanying modernisation, the organisation simply did not have the capacity to shoulder, or even define, the necessary components of its global health governance model. As Chan said in her address to the WHA,

> The level of WHO engagement should not be governed by the size of a health problem. Instead it should be governed by the extent to which WHO can have an impact on the problem. Others may be positioned to do a better job.
>
> *WHO, 2017b, n.p.*

With this in mind, Chan presented the following programmatic priorities to the member states, which were agreed upon in 2012 (WHO, 2012, p. 5):

---

**Communicable diseases:** reducing the burden of communicable diseases, including HIV/AIDS, tuberculosis, malaria, and neglected tropical diseases.

**Noncommunicable diseases:** reducing the burden of noncommunicable diseases, including heart disease, cancer, lung disease, diabetes, and mental disorders as well as disability, and injuries, through health promotion and risk reduction, prevention, treatment and monitoring of noncommunicable diseases and their risk factors.

**Promoting health through the life course:** reducing morbidity and mortality and improving health during pregnancy, childbirth, the neonatal period, childhood and adolescence; improving sexual and reproductive health; and promoting active and healthy ageing, taking into account the need to address determinants of health and internationally agreed development goals, in particular the health-related Millennium Development Goals.

**Health systems:** support the strengthening, organization with a focus on integrated service delivery and financing, of health systems with a particular focus on achieving universal coverage, strengthening human resources for health, health information systems, facilitating transfer of technologies, promoting access to affordable, quality, safe, and efficacious medical products, and promoting health services research.

**Preparedness, surveillance and response:** surveillance and effective response to disease outbreaks, acute public health emergencies and the effective management of health-related aspects of humanitarian disasters to contribute to health security.

---

In each of these programmatic areas, the WHO, based on its determined comparative advantages, would carry out the following core functions (Vijayan, 2007, p. 41):

1. **providing leadership** on matters critical to health and engaging in partnerships where joint action is needed;
2. shaping the **research agenda** and stimulating the generation, translation and dissemination of valuable knowledge;
3. setting **norms and standards** and promoting and monitoring their implementation;
4. articulating **ethical and evidence-based** policy options;
5. providing **technical support**, catalysing change, and building sustainable institutional capacity; and
6. **monitoring** the health situation and assessing health trends.

In addition to these efforts to better establish its organisational priorities, the WHO also developed strategies to tackle its managerial and governance woes. Governance highlights include greater alignment between the WHO Executive Board and regional committees for joint input; stricter guidelines for the nomination and election of regional directors and the DG; and better streamlining of strategic decision-making and handling of relationships with non-state actors. From a managerial standpoint, the WHO sought to overhaul its human resources operations with a staffing and financing structure reflective of the aforementioned priorities; more efficient technical and policy support to member countries' stated needs; and the creation of a 'culture of evaluation' based on accountability, risk management, and transparency (Clift, 2013). According to the WHO's budget documents submitted to the WHA in May 2013, about US$1 billion was cut from 2011–12 spending, and the agency laid off or left unfilled roughly 20 per cent of staff positions. In order to enhance WHO's credibility, Chan also promised accountability and outcomes measurement, as delineated in the Figure 12.1 (Garrett, 2013).

## Participation of the global South: the case of BRICS[4]

The global South has a long history of engaging in the WHO. Brazil and China, for example, were founding members of the organisation. In 2006, China received the support of many countries in the global South in leading a successful campaign to elect Dr. Margaret Chan as WHO DG (Huang, 2010). Five years later, she ran for the same office virtually unopposed – thanks to China's continued political

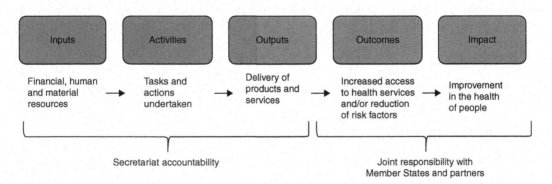

*Figure 12.1* Accountability and outcomes measurement flow chart

support. With strong support from China and the rest of the global South, Chan was initially in an ideal position to initiate the reform process.

Participation of the BRICS countries (excluding Russia) epitomises the involvement of the global South in WHO reform. While they did not publicly coordinate their reform efforts, BRICS representatives met privately to mobilise their diplomatic power to further their interests in the formulation of the WHO agenda. Following Margaret Chan's official launch of the WHO reform, BRICS's health ministers first met in 2011 in Beijing, where they issued the Beijing Declaration, committing them to active participation in WHO reform efforts. This support was reiterated at the BRICS's health ministers' meetings in New Delhi (2012) and Cape Town (2013). While none of the resulting documents led to any formal action, they symbolically established BRICS and other developing countries as a bloc of influence within the WHO whose priorities could no longer be ignored in favour of those of wealthier donor member states (Gautier, et al., 2014).

The BRICS nations collaborated at the highest political level, but they did not necessarily unite as an entire group around specific elements of reform. Rather, there were 'natural pairings' around certain key issue areas (Gautier, et al., 2014). For example, Brazil and India prioritised reforming intellectual property policies and expanding universal access to medicines; Brazil, China, and India pushed for reform in drug manufacturing and sharing of health technologies; China, India, and Brazil promoted the elevation of primary health care and community engagement; and China and India stressed the importance of health security and surveillance. Brazil successfully advocated for the addition of social determinants of health in the programmatic agenda, as well as for the establishment of an Ethics Committee to monitor conflicts of interest with regards to non-state actors. Universal access to health technologies was also incorporated into reforms, and Russia helped advance the WHO's recognition of noncommunicable diseases. Their level of involvement in WHO reform debate also varies, with Brazil the most active among BRICS, followed by India, South Africa, China, and Russia (the least active) (Gautier, et al., 2014). But these more fundamental, rather than operational, concerns highlight the ideological influence of BRICS on WHO reform (Gautier, et al., 2014).

Despite these issue-based pairings, BRICS converged philosophically in their vision of WHO's roles and functions. Unlike the European Union and United States that pushed for a more limited mandate focused only on standards and norms settings, BRICS advocated for a broader mandate that would include in-country assistance and technical guidance. Paradoxically, despite their call for a broader mandate for the WHO, countries in the global South were reluctant to provide the health agency with the necessary authority and resources to push meaningful reforms forward. In May 2001, when the United States reduced its budgetary contributions from 25 per cent to 22 per cent, other member states, notably China, Cuba, and Pakistan, protested, saying this would increase the financial burden on developing countries. The total share of contributions by the BRICS countries to the WHO for its 2012–13 regular budget was only 7.3 per cent (Huang, 2012). Also, BRICS favoured strengthening the power of member states rather than broadening membership to include non-state actors. Some BRICS countries (Brazil, India, and South Africa) might have been supportive of the involvement of non-state actors, but they were reluctant to involve the corporate sector and influential private foundations in WHO decision-making (Gautier, et al., 2014). This contrasted with the position of countries in Europe and America, which support multi-stakeholder participation in global health governance.

## Assessment of the 2010 reform process

The reforms enacted under Chan's leadership had a mixed reception among those in the global health community. In 2012, Charles Clift of Chatham House argued that while these reforms were admirable, a number of inherent structural and constitutional problems identified in previous evaluations were not directly addressed. The steps for reform at no point articulated WHO's place in the global health system;

rather, there were only vague guidelines as to how to interact with the overly general category of 'other stakeholders', which at this point had far outnumbered the WHO in number and financial resources (Gautier, et al., 2014). The five programme priorities (communicable diseases, noncommunicable diseases, promoting health through the life course, health systems, and corporate services/enabling functions) identified by the WHO replicated efforts of other international agencies or initiatives, such as the Global Fund to Fight AIDS, Tuberculosis and Malaria; UNICEF (children's health); the World Bank (health system strengthening); and the UNFPA (reproductive health). They also created a zero-sum game in budget-related decision-making, sustaining the boom and bust budgeting cycle for WHO emergency response (Hoffman and Røttingen, 2014). The WHO's 2014–15 biannual budget saw a 21 per cent increase in programme funding devoted to NCDs. However, only 5.7 per cent of the budget was devoted to outbreak and crisis response, representing a 51.4 per cent decrease from what had been provided in the previous two-year budget. Badly weakened by budget cuts, the WHO's outbreak and emergency response units were curtailed to such a level that the unit devoted to the science of pandemic and epidemic diseases had only one technical expert on Ebola and other haemorrhagic diseases.

Another glaring issue echoed in the reforms, as noted by many observers, was Chan's reluctance to incite opposition from member states. As a legacy of donor earmarking that began in the Nakajima years, countries continue to approach the WHO for technical and financial support to address their specific health needs. And while the list of programmatic and technical priorities is strong rhetorically, David Stuckler commented in 2014 that it would be difficult for the WHO to reject those funds demanding actions that do not fall under its newly stated jurisdiction. Additionally, the reforms did not address the autonomous nature of the WHO's six regional offices, where directors are still 'chosen by, and often beholden to, local ministers of health', creating a plethora of managerial problems in countries plagued by corruption (The Economist Group Limited, 2014, n.p.).

When accounting for the lack of significant progress of WHO reform, member states, which help shape the WHO's priorities and resources and the secretariat's mandate, are heavily to blame for not providing the secretariat with the necessary authority and resources to advance reforms. They turned down proposals to create the Committee C for all WHO stakeholders or host a multi-stakeholder World Health Forum. In May 2015, they also rejected Margaret Chan's proposal to increase assessed contributions by 5 per cent to ensure the full financing of the budget. As the leading donor in global health and the source of WHO's largest assessment contribution, the US government could be a lead catalyst in the WHO reform process. Yet, it is often hesitant to take on such a role.

However, the WHO Secretariat is equally to blame for its lack of transformational leadership. Unlike other international organisations such as the World Bank, the WHO often cedes its leadership in agenda setting to major funders, allowing the latter to cherry pick projects for implementation. Laurie Garrett also noted in an article in *Foreign Affairs* that Chan 'seemed to defer too much to national governments' wishes and agendas, even when they were in conflict with the organization's primary mission' (Garrett, 2015, p. 94). Prior to the Ebola crisis, the WHO leadership had failed to act on the proposal of an independent pandemic review committee to establish a rapid-response contingency fund. It was these and other problems that created the perfect storm for the failure in WHO's initial response to the 2014 Ebola outbreak.

## 2014 Ebola outbreak

The West African Ebola outbreak, which reached its peak in 2014, revealed the lack of progress of the WHO in actually implementing the reform measures articulated since 2010. In a report commissioned by the WHO to assess its response, a group of independent experts concluded that the 'WHO does not have the capacity or organizational culture to deliver a full emergency public health response' (WHO, 2015a, p. 15). As Laurie Garrett noted, the WHO's response to Ebola was 'limited, uncoordinated, and dysfunctional' (Garrett, 2015, p. 85).

That said, the WHO Secretariat did not completely neglect the initial outbreak. In April 2014, the WHO mobilised technical support and resources to aid the impacted countries, and had deployed 113 technical experts to assist local health authorities. Adam Kamradt-Scott has noted that this response was commensurate to past Ebola outbreaks, in which the WHO had sent very limited numbers of personnel to assist on the ground. That, according to him, '[was] understandable when recalling that the international organization was never intended to be a "first responder" agency, but rather the "directing and coordinating authority" in international health' (Kamradt-Scott, 2016, p. 405).

Nevertheless, the Ebola spread in West Africa did not follow the same pattern as past Ebola outbreaks. The first case of the Ebola outbreak in West Africa was reported in Guinea in March 2014, and from there, rapidly spread to neighbouring Liberia and Sierra Leone. Observing disaster on the horizon, Doctors Without Borders warned the international community that Ebola's spread was 'unprecedented'. In contrast, WHO authorities based in Geneva responded that the outbreak was 'relatively small still' (Kelland, 2016, n.p.).

On the surface, the false perception of the extent of the 2014 outbreak was a result of 'inadequate understanding of the nature of the outbreak, poor decision-making within the WHO, and over-deference to political considerations' (Schaefer, 2015, n.p.). A closer look, however, revealed fundamental institutional and constitutional arrangement problems within the WHO, which the 2010 reforms sought, but failed, to address. The member state-driven decision-making apparently led the WHO to defer to the optimism of Guinea, whose minister of health assured his international counterparts at the 67th WHA in May 2014 that the outbreak in his country was 'yielding very encouraging results' and was now 'essentially under control' (Kamradt-Scott, 2016, p. 405). The Africa regional office also failed to serve as an effective intermediary between Geneva and the country offices. During the Ebola outbreak, pressures from the government of Guinea, which feared the domestic consequences of prematurely declaring the outbreak a public health emergency of international concern (PHEIC), reportedly led the regional office to initially downplay the seriousness of the problem to Geneva and even withhold information about new infections (Boseley, 2014).

By mid-June 2014, it became apparent that the outbreak was displaying profoundly unique epidemiological characteristics. With a cumulative 440 cases (150 of which were new ones from 28 May through 10 June), WHO authorities in the West African region requested Margaret Chan to declare a PHEIC, invoking the 2005 international health regulations (IHR) (Briand, et al., 2014).[5] However, they were met with no response from Geneva. As cases and fatalities climbed, meetings were held throughout July 2014 at WHO headquarters with a variety of traditional, multilateral stakeholders that amounted to little more than rhetoric. It was not until 8 August 2014, with a total of 1,800 reported Ebola cases, that Director-General Chan finally declared a PHEIC (Kamradt-Scott, 2016). Misplaced confidence in rapid mobilisation of external funds in an international health crisis nevertheless only delayed the WHO's surge capacity in responding to the Ebola outbreak. Garrett writes that,

[A]s late as the end of February 2015, after the worst of the crisis had passed, less than half of the finances, personnel, and supplies promised by the global community had actually materialized on the ground. If the aid had arrived earlier, the epidemic would undoubtedly have been contained faster and with fewer fatalities.

*Garrett, 2015, p. 86*

Described by Sheri Fink as a 'technical agency that is heavy on technical know-how but light on logistical muscle' (Fink, 2014, n.p.), the WHO in the response to Ebola was largely side-lined by a separate UN response team and member states such as the United States. By the time the epidemic was declared over on 13 January 2016, this Ebola outbreak had killed five times more people than all other known outbreaks combined, totalling 28,637 reported cases and 11,315 deaths across West Africa (BBC News, 2016).

Critics linked the hobbled WHO response to shortcomings in the WHO reform process. The 2010 reform did not lead to profound changes in the WHO's funding or governance structure, which continued to be characterised by the prevailing tensions between the regional WHO and its headquarters; the central WHO's shrinking budget and overreliance on donor nations; and an overcrowded international health space in which the WHO is unable to assert its dominance and responsibilities as a coordinating and norms setting body. All of these trends, none of which were adequately addressed in Chan's 2010 reform efforts, came to a head during this mismanaged, and entirely preventable, loss of life. Worse yet, some of the reform measures were implemented in a way that was counterproductive for effective response to global health challenges. Hans Troedsson, WHO assistant director-general for general management, admitted that while the decision to lay off almost 1,000 staff members in the African region in 2011 was able to save cost in the immediate term, it led to the loss of potentially invaluable professional administrative officers (Ravelo, 2017). Keiji Fukuda, WHO assistant director-general in charge of outbreak response, indicated that the layoff negatively affected WHO's ability to respond to major outbreaks and pandemics (Fink, 2014).

## Post-Ebola WHO reform

Following the outbreak's conclusion, the WHO convened an independent commission led by David Nabarro, Special Envoy of the UN Secretary-General on Ebola, to assess its performance and make recommendations for improvement. Its conclusions fell under three major categories: the 2005 International Health Regulations, WHO's health emergency response capacity, and the organisation's role within the wider global health architecture:

1. **International health regulations**: The committee recommended that the WHO develop core capacities for all countries party to the IHR with the financial assistance of the World Bank; strengthen all levels of the organisation to identify health risks and declare emergencies; consider incentives and disincentives for individual country reporting or lack thereof; and establish an intermediate emergency alert level for earlier stages of health crises.
2. **Emergency response capacities**: The committee recommended growth of member countries' assessed contributions by 5, rather than 0, per cent; contribution to a $100 million emergency contingency fund; member state political will and an internal WHO organisational culture geared towards emergency response; the establishment of a Center for Emergency Preparedness and Response within WHO overseen by an independent board; more appropriate staffing procedures to fit the needs of vulnerable countries; reestablishment of the WHO as an authoritative convening body for international cooperation, as well as research and development; and the engagement of local communities and empowerment of regional officials.
3. **WHO engagement with other parties**: The committee recommended improved coordination of the PHEIC with emergency measures taken by other humanitarian organisations; a better internal understanding within WHO of the broader humanitarian system; a special recognition by the United Nations system as a whole of health as a top-priority global security risk; and the appointment of a special UN envoy in the case of health emergencies (WHO, 2015a).

In response to the policy recommendations, the WHO added emergency capacities as a new field of reform (WHO, 2016). Focusing on consolidating the resources and capabilities of WHO work in outbreaks and emergencies, the reform aims to build 'one single Programme, with one workforce, one budget, one set of rules and processes and above all one clear line of authority' (WHO, 2016, n.p.).

It is quite unfortunate that despite all the 'autopsies' and recommendations following the outbreak, the WHO appears to not have actually internalised or implemented these policy prescriptions. It is interesting that while the Ebola crisis led to the death of more than 11,000 people, none of the WHO staff thus far has borne personal responsibility for the crisis. As Yanzhong Huang noted in May 2016,

> the Ebola crisis has not spurred fundamental change in the WHO management, governance, or financing structures.... No far-reaching reform measures have been unveiled to tackle the root causes of the problem, namely, organizational ineffectiveness, a lack of clarity in priorities, and insufficient funding.
>
> *Huang, 2016, n.p.*

This view was shared by a piece in the January 2017 issue of *The Lancet*, where the Harvard-London School of Hygiene and Tropical Medicine commission retrospectively analysed the outcome of this institutional soul-searching. They concluded that there has yet to be a dedicated, concerted undertaking to address the typical, old problems of the WHO: its insecure financing, unclear organisational identity, limited transparency and accountability, and vulnerability to political pressure from its member states (Moon, et al., 2017).

To be fair, fixing these problems is not easy. They require changes in the WHO constitution. Yet article 60 of the constitution states that WHA decisions on important questions, including amendments to the constitution, must be made by a two-thirds majority of the members present and voting. With the surprising outcomes of the 2016 Brexit vote and the 2016 US presidential election, it is becoming ever clearer that political tides are shifting away from globalisation and a heralding of multilateralism towards nationalism and populism. In an already precarious financial situation, this politically and historically unprecedented situation will require the WHO to re-evaluate not only its primary sources of revenue, but also its programmatic subordination to the will of the United States and United Kingdom.

Still, the WHO DG can play a key role in taking the initiative of pushing the reform forward. As Gostin and Friedman of Georgetown University wrote in *The Lancet* in October 2014, 'Global health leadership can be built, but only if genuine leaders choose to build it' (Gostin and Friedman, 2014, p. 1324). Unfortunately, while Chan has admitted that the outbreak 'shook this organization to its core', she viewed the Secretariat as 'servants' to member states and preferred to wait for consensus from them before taking any further action. In the absence of reforming the underlying institutional and structural problems, however, it is unlikely the organisation can regain the world's confidence in its leadership over global health.

## Conclusion

The World Health Organization was created to serve as the lead international agency to tackle health issues worldwide. While some single-pronged initiatives proved successful, the shifting global health governance landscape over the past decades have only underscored the inadequacies of the health agency in addressing the new global health challenges. Plagued by a fundamental mismatch between its mandate and the resources and capabilities at its disposal, the organisation is increasingly unable to assert its global health leadership, which led to the 2010 reform process. The reform efforts nevertheless failed to adequately address WHO's inherent management, financing, and leadership flaws. These issues were brought to the forefront during the agency's initial mishandling of the 2014 West African Ebola outbreak. Post-Ebola emergency capacity building efforts have not spurred fundamental changes in the organisation.

In May 2017, the 69th WHA met and elected Dr. Tedros Adhanom Ghebreyesus – an Ethiopian politician, diplomat, and public health expert – to be its new director-general. In light of its sustained financing and governance challenges, the election of Tedros as the first WHO DG from Africa and the first non-physician to become WHO DG opened a new window for WHO reform. In doing so, he will have to demonstrate the needed experience, skills, and leadership in working with member states and other stakeholders to tackle the WHO's structural and governance challenges and steer the agency in a direction that can make it a true guardian of health around the world.

## Notes

1 More than 17 per cent of its 2014–15 programme budget, for example, was allocated for polio eradication, a top priority of the Gates Foundation, a chief donor.
2 See www.surveymonkey.com/r/5DL59LJ. The survey received a total of 56 responses. It is important to note that this pool of respondents is not representative of all those invested in the future of global health governance, but may prove indicative of general opinion on the subject.
3 Since 1973, six individuals have served as the WHO director-general: Halfdan Mahler (1973–88), Hiroshi Nakajima (1988–98), Gro Harlem Brundtland (1998–2003), Jong-wook 'J.W.' Lee (2003–6), Anders Nordstrom (2006–7, interim), and Margaret Chan (2007–present).
4 Since global South as a term is used to refer to what used to be called the third world, it strictly speaking does not include Russia. For analytical convenience, here we use BRICS to highlight the contribution from emerging economies that represent the global South.
5 A PHEIC has immediate ramifications for all 196 nations privy to its conditions under the 2005 IHR, and the four countries with reported cases (Guinea, Liberia, Sierra Leone, and Nigeria) were given specific instructions based on recommendations of the WHO Emergency Committee: declaration of a national emergency, activation of disaster-management mechanisms, establishment of emergency operations centres, and limitation of international or local travel based on the extent of infection.

## References

Adelman, C.C. (2006) 'Let's learn from global health failures', *The New York Times*, available at www.nytimes.com/2006/05/23/opinion/23iht-edadelman.html (accessed on 29 March 2018).

BBC News. (2016) 'Ebola; mapping the outbreak', available at www.bbc.com/news/world-africa-28755033 (accessed on 3 November 2017).

Bollyky, T. (2012). 'Reinventing the World Health Organization', available at www.cfr.org/expert-brief/reinventing-world-health-organization (accessed on 29 March 2018).

Boseley, S. (2014) 'World Health Organisation admits botching response to Ebola outbreak', *The Guardian*, available at www.theguardian.com/world/2014/oct/17/world-health-organisation-botched-ebola-outbreak (accessed on 3 November 2017).

Briand, S., Bertherat, E., Cox, P., et al. (2014) 'The international Ebola emergency', *New England Journal of Medicine*, 371(13): 1180–3.

Clift, C. (2013) 'The role of the World Health Organization in the international system', available at www.chathamhouse.org/publications/papers/view/189351 (accessed on 3 November 2017).

Fidler, D.P. (2004) 'Germs, governance, and global public health in the wake of SARS', *The Journal of Clinical Investigation*, 113(6): 799–804.

Fink, S. (2014) 'Cuts at WHO hurt response to Ebola crisis', *The New York Times*, available at www.nytimes.com/2014/09/04/world/africa/cuts-at-who-hurt-response-to-ebola-crisis.html (accessed on 29 March 29, 2018)

Garrett, L. (2013) 'The survival of "global health" – part 1: WHO's Margaret Chan sets the stage', available at http://lauriegarrett.com/blog/2013/5/21/the-survival-of-global-health-part-one-whos-margaret-chan-sets-the-stage (accessed on 3 November 2017).

Garrett, L. (2015) 'Ebola's lessons', Foreign Affairs, available at www.foreignaffairs.com/articles/west-africa/2015-08-18/ebolas-lessons (accessed on 7 November 2017).

Gautier, L, et al. (2014) 'Reforming the World Health Organization: what influence do the BRICS wield?', *Contemporary Politics*, 20(2): 163–81.

Gellman, B. (2000) 'Death watch: the global response to AIDS in Africa', available at www.washingtonpost.com/wp-dyn/content/article/2006/06/09/AR2006060901326.html?sid=ST2010111801753 (accessed on 3 November 2017).

Gostin, L.O. and Friedman, E.A. (2014) 'Ebola: a crisis in global health leadership', *The Lancet*, 384(9951): 1323–5.

Gostin, L.O. and Sridhar, D. (2014) 'Global health and the law', available at www.nejm.org/doi/full/10.1056/NEJMra1314094?af=R&rss=currentIssue&#t=article (accessed on 2 November 2017).

Henderson, D.A. (1987) 'Principles and lessons from the smallpox eradication programme', *Bulletin of the World Health Organization*, 65(4): 535–46.

Hoffman, S. and Røttingen, J.A. (2014) 'Split WHO in two: strengthening political decision-making and securing independent scientific advice', *Public Health*, 128(2): 188–94.

Horton, R. (2015) 'Offline: a pervasive failure to learn the lessons of Ebola', *The Lancet*, 386(9998): 1024.

Huang, Y. (2010) 'Pursuing health as foreign policy: the case of China', *Indian Journal of Global Legal Studies*, 17(1): 125–6.

Huang, Y. (2012) 'Health agency overshadowed but vital', available at http://nytweekly.com/columns/intelarchives/08-03-12/ (accessed on 3 November 2017).

Huang, Y. (2016) 'How to reform the ailing World Health Organization', available at www.cfr.org/expert-brief/how-reform-ailing-world-health-organization (accessed on 3 November 2017).

Kamradt-Scott, A. (2016) 'WHO's to blame? The World Health Organization and the 2014 Ebola outbreak in West Africa', *Third World Quarterly*, 37(3): 401–18.

Kelland, K (2016) 'Special Report – The World Health Organization's critical challenge: healing itself', available at https://af.reuters.com/article/worldNews/idAFKCN0VH0Z5.

Klock, K.A. (2012) 'The soft law alternative to the WHO's treaty powers', *Georgetown Journal of International Law*, Washington, DC: Georgetown University Law Center.

Lee, K. (2008) *The World Health Organization*, London; New York: Routledge.

McCarthy, M. (2002) 'A brief history of the World Health Organization', *The Lancet*, 360(9340): 1111–2.

Moon, S., Leigh, J., Woskie, L., et al. (2017) 'Post-Ebola reforms: ample analysis, inadequate action', *BMJ*, 356: j280.

Raustiala, K. and Victor D.G. (2004) 'The regime complex for plant genetic resources', *International Organization*, 58(2): 277–309.

Ravelo, J.L. (2017) 'WHO's budget and the tasks for the next director-general', available at www.devex.com/news/who-s-budget-and-the-tasks-for-the-next-director-general-90385 (accessed on 29 March 2018).

Schaefer, B. (2015) 'What World Health Organization did wrong on Ebola response', available at http://dailysignal.com/2015/08/15/what-world-health-organization-did-wrong-on-ebola-response/ (accessed on 3 November 2017).

Tanner, M. and de Savigny, D. (2008) 'Malaria eradication back on the table', *Bulletin of the World Health Organization*, 86(2): 82–3.

The Economist Group Limited (Ed.) (2014) 'Too big to ail', *The Economist*.

U.S. Government Accountability Office. (2012) 'World Health Organization: reform agenda developed, but U.S. actions to monitor progress could be enhanced', *GAO-12-722*.

Vijayan, S. (2007) 'A World Health Organization primer', *Medscape General Medicine*, 9(4): 41.

WHO. (2000) 'Roll back malaria: report by the secretariat', available at http://apps.who.int/gb/archive/pdf_files/EB106/ee4.pdf (accessed on 3 November 2017).

WHO. (2006) 'Constitution of the World Health Organization', available at www.who.int/governance/eb/who_constitution_en.pdf (accessed on 2 November 2017).

WHO. (2012) 'WHO reform: report by the director general', available at http://apps.who.int/iris/bitstream/10665/79742/1/A65_40-en.pdf (accessed on 3 November 2017).

WHO. (2015a) 'Report of the Ebola interim assessment panel', available at www.who.int/csr/resources/publications/ebola/report-by-panel.pdf (accessed on 3 November 2017).

WHO. (2015b) 'The WHO framework convention on tobacco control: an overview', available at www.who.int/fctc/about/en/ (accessed on 3 November 2017).

WHO. (2016) 'Global policy group statement on reforms of WHO work in outbreaks and emergencies', available at www.who.int/dg/speeches/2016/reform-statement/en/ (accessed on 3 November 2017).

WHO. (2017a) 'Global Action Plan for the Prevention and Control of NCDs 2013–2020', available at www.who.int/nmh/events/ncd_action_plan/en/ (accessed on 2 November 2017).

WHO. (2017b) 'WHO director-general calls for a change', available at www.who.int/dg/speeches/2011/eb_20110117/en/ (accessed on 3 November 2017).

WHO. (2017c) 'WHO reform process', available at www.who.int/about/who_reform/process/en/ (accessed on 3 November 2017).

WHO. (2017d) 'Ten years of transformation: making WHO fit for purpose in the 21st century', available at www.who.int/about/who_reform/report-2017.pdf (accessed on 3 November 2017).

Wilson, K., Brownstein, J., and Fidler D. (2010) 'Strengthening the international health regulations: lessons from the H1N1 pandemic', *Health Policy and Planning*, 25(6): 505–9.

# 13

# Health governance

## A neglected and an uncharted path of governance in Africa

*Oyewale Tomori*

## Governance

Governance is too complex for a simple definition. Broadly, governance encompasses 'the collective action and mechanism of a society to achieve common and agreed goals' (Dodgson, et al., 2002, p. 6). Governance therefore should, on a daily basis, embrace and have positive effect on every aspect of societal activities, from politics to economy and from health to social activities. There are two major players in the act of governance: the governor and the governed. The governor may include the government, the board/chief executive of a company, or the decision maker in a public or private setting, each holding the reins of power or controlling the instrument of power. The governed are the individuals who make up the society, a group or a company, who benefit or suffer the effect of governance. Ideally and in the strict sense of the word, governance should be of benefit to all involved; however, in reality and for many nations, especially in Africa, poor governance has been responsible for the undesirable state of social and economic development.

Good governance should be based on the following principles (Graham, et al., 2003):

- A mutually agreed development programme produced through participation and broad consensus;
- Maintenance of processes and mechanism for implementation of the programme while making the best use of available resources;
- Monitoring and evaluation of the programme to ensure effectiveness and efficiency;
- Regulating the behaviour of a wide range of actors to ensure adherence to the rule of law, fairness, and equity for all;
- Establishing and implementing transparent and effective accountability mechanisms.

## Health governance

Health governance is the component of governance focusing on the 'actions and measures adopted by a society for the promotion and protection of the health of its population' (Dodgson, et al., 2002, p. 6). The concept of health governance is broadened by the WHO to include a wide range of steering and rule-making related functions carried out by governments/decision makers, as they seek to achieve national health policy objectives that are conducive to universal health coverage (WHO, 2006). This fits appropriately into the original definition of health by the WHO, formulated in 1948, as 'a state of complete physical, mental and social well-being and not merely the absence of disease or infirmity' (WHO, 2006, p. 1).

Over the years, with the changes in age distribution of populations and pattern of diseases and illnesses, the classical WHO definition of health has come under some criticisms (*The Lancet*, 2009). One proposed definition of health is 'the ability to adapt and to self-manage' (Huber, et al., 2011, p. 1) but there is still no consensus on a replacement or modification for the classical WHO definition of health. There is a need for further debate on the definition of health as it may affect other health-related issues. In spite of the criticism of WHO definition of health, the current WHO concept of health governance remains valid, as a political process that involves balancing competing influences on and demands of health (WHO, 2011a).

A recent study on governance for health in the twenty-first century, commissioned by the WHO Regional Office for Europe, defines governance for health as 'the attempts of governments or other actors to steer communities, countries or groups of countries in the pursuit of health as integral to wellbeing through both a "whole-of-government" and a "whole-of-society" approach' (Kickbusch and Gleicher, 2012, p. 4). Furthermore, governance for health 'promotes joint action of health and non-health sectors, public and private partnerships, and citizens for common good' (Kickbusch and Gleicher, 2012, p. 4). The requirements of governance for health include 'a synergistic set of policies, many of which reside in sectors other than health and outside of government and which must be supported by structures and mechanisms that facilitate collaboration. The engagement of people is a defining factor' (Kickbusch and Gleicher, 2012, p. ix).

## Global health governance

Global health governance (GHG) is a term that has evolved over time and is still evolving. The numerous scholarly works on the subject were analysed by Lee and Kamradt-Scott (2014, p. 1) and they concluded that 'the rapid growth in scholarship has not only created considerable variation in the definition, but also confusion in the application of global health governance'. What is now generally accepted as GHG is a transition from international health governance (IHG) of the 1990s, when international health was governed by nation-states and multilateral organisations with state members (Ng and Ruger, 2011). During the IHG period, health funding was provided by donors to recipient national governments in bilateral agreements and the responsibility for health delivery service was carried out by the government. The WHO coordinated such global issues as the eradication of smallpox and international disease reporting and outbreak control through the International Health Regulations (IHR). New concern with GHG came in the wake of accelerated globalisation with increasing economic interdependence, and rapid and extensive international movements of people and products. However, this period was characterised by a lack of clear definition of roles and delineation of functions by the numerous GHG stakeholders, with stakeholders playing any or all of the roles 'as sources of funding, as originators of initiatives, and as implementers, monitors, and evaluators' of the project (Ng and Ruger, 2011, p. 2). From the plethora of definitions and meanings of GHG, three concepts and distinct uses of the term global health governance were identified (Lee and Kamradt-Scott, 2014). These are (a) globalisation and health governance; (b) global governance and health; and (c) governance for global health. Globalisation and health governance is primarily concerned with the health-related institutions that govern collective responses to such issues as global spread of infectious diseases, antibiotic resistance, or health outcomes of wars, famine, and climate change (Moon, 2008; Hein, et al., 2009). Global governance and health addresses the roles, influence, and impacts of institutions outside the health sector, such as the World Bank, International Monetary Fund (IMF), and World Trade Organisation (WTO). The impact, for example, of the World Bank Structural Adjustment policy on health of populations in low- and middle-income countries has become a global governance and health issue (Lee and Kamradt-Scott, 2014). The focus of governance for global health is on access to medicines, health equity, or primary health care (Dickerson and Grills, 2012), or principles such as human rights (Gable, 2007; Meier and Onzivu, 2014) and social justice (Brown, 2012). The good governance for global health must be accountable, transparent, responsive, equitable and inclusive, effective, efficient, and participatory and should be found at levels that extend from local communities to multinational organisations (Gostin, 2014).

## African perspective of governance and health governance

Regarding the definition and practice of governance and health governance, African countries have generally adopted, with minimal adaptation, the global definitions and dictates of bilateral partners and international agencies.

### Governance in Africa

A cursory history of governance in Africa can be divided into three periods: pre-colonial, colonial, and post-colonial. The pre-colonial period was marked by inter-regional wars among the different African groups, during which the powerful made slaves of the weak. The colonial period probably commenced in full force with the 1884 Scramble for Africa, when Europe imposed its will on Africa at the end-point of a gun barrel. The majority of African countries obtained independence in the 1960s. During the immediate post-independence and post-colonial period, political leaders in many African countries imposed their will on their citizens by force of arms and intimidation.

The Organization of African Union (OAU) preceded the African Union (AU) that came into force in 2001 and was formally inaugurated in 2002 (Elias, 1965; AU, 2002). The AU charter listed 14 objectives to be pursued in order to make Africa strong, united, and developed. Objective seven is focused on governance, the promotion of democratic principles and institutions, popular participation and good governance, while objective 14 is concerned with the eradication of preventable diseases and the promotion of good health. How well have African countries met these objectives? Between 2001 and 2012, African leaders, through the mechanism of the AU, set up four institutions on good governance (AU, 2007a). These are the New Partnership for Africa's Development (NEPAD) in 2001, the African Peer Review Mechanism (APRM) in 2002, and the African Charter on Democracy, Elections and Governance in 2007, the African Governance Architecture (AGA) in 2010.

The goals of NEPAD are in line with those of the United Nations Millennium Declaration, and good public governance is a central core for successful attainment of the socio-economic objectives of NEPAD (Mekolo and Resta, 2005).

The APRM was created,

> [T]o foster the adoption of policies, standards and practices leading to political stability, high economic growth, sustainable development and accelerated sub-regional and continental economic integration through sharing of experiences and reinforcement of successful and best practices, including identifying deficiencies and assessing the needs of capacity-building.

*APRM, 2003, p. 2*

The APRM has a country self-assessment mechanism with set objectives for monitoring and evaluating democracy and good political governance (nine objectives), economic governance and management (five objectives), corporate governance (five objectives), and socio-economic development (six objectives).

The African Charter on Democracy, Elections and Governance (ACDEG) has 13 objectives, including promotion and adherence to:

[T]he universal values and principles of democracy and respect for human rights; the principle of the rule of law premised upon the respect for, and the supremacy of, the Constitution and constitutional order in the political arrangements and the holding of regular free and fair elections to institutionalize legitimate authority of representative government as well as democratic change of governments.

*AU, 2007a, p. 3*

Although member states of the African Union adopted the charter in 2007, the charter did not come into force until 2012 (five years later), the time it took for a sufficient number of countries to sign and approve the charter. The last country to sign the charter did so in 2015 (AU, 2007b).

The African Governance Architecture (AGA) is a mechanism for dialogue between stakeholders mandated to promote good governance and bolster democracy in Africa, with the overall goal of strengthening good governance and consolidating democracy in Africa (AU, 2010).

The Mo Ibrahim Foundation is an African foundation, established in 2006 with one focus: 'the critical importance of governance and leadership in Africa. It is our belief that governance and leadership lie at the heart of any tangible and shared improvement in the quality of life of African citizens' (Mo Ibrahim Foundation, 2017, p. 1).

## Index of governance in Africa

The Mo Ibrahim Foundation (MIF) defines governance as the provision of the political, social, and economic goods that a citizen has the right to expect from his or her state, and that a state has the responsibility to deliver to its citizens (Ibrahim, 2006). The MIF publishes the Ibrahim Index of African Governance (IIAG), an annual assessment of the quality of governance in every African country, and uses four main conceptual categories: Safety & Rule of Law, Participation & Human Rights, Sustainable Economic Opportunity, and Human Development (Mo Ibrahim Foundation, 2016a). The IIAG analyses more than 90 indicators built up into 14 sub-categories, four categories, and one overall measurement of governance performance. These indicators include official data, expert assessments, and citizen surveys, provided by more than 30 independent global data institutions. The foundation also awards annually the Mo Ibrahim Prize, to recognise and celebrate African executive leaders who have developed their countries and strengthened democracy and human rights.

The 2016 IIAG report provides a summary of trends of governance performance in Africa over the period of 2006 to 2015. According to the report, there has been a very slight improvement in overall governance performance at the continental level. The African average score 'of 50.0 in 2015, is up only one point from the score registered a decade earlier and reflects the trend of improvement seen across the majority of countries over the past ten years' (Mo Ibrahim Foundation, 2016a, p. 1). Of the 53 countries participating in the assessment, 37 countries showed improvement in overall governance, representing 70 per cent of African citizens. Only 13 of the 37 countries recorded progress in each of the four dimensions of governance. There were '16 countries which registered a negative trend in Overall Governance since 2006' (Mo Ibrahim Foundation, 2016a, p. 18), all declining in Safety & Rule of Law. The report noted that 'war and civil unrest, leading to decline in Safety & Rule of Law are the common factors in the countries showing the worst degree of decline in overall governance' (Mo Ibrahim Foundation, 2016a, p. 18). The Ibrahim Prize was established in 2007, and the Prize Committee has only been able to award the prize to deserving African leaders in 2007, 2008, 2011, and 2014. It has not awarded the prize in 2009, 2010, 2012, 2013, 2015, and 2016, because the Prize Committee, 'after in-depth review, did not select an African leader worthy of the Prize' (Mo Ibrahim Foundation, 2016b, p. 1).

The poor state of governance in Africa has contributed significantly to the state of underdevelopment. The period of the first 10 to 20 years of independence in some African countries, especially where political leaders undemocratically remained in office, was characterised by human rights abuse, civil wars, and insurgencies. The confidence and impunity of some African leaders to remain in power through undemocratic means may have been encouraged by the strict adherence by OAU/AU member states to the clause stipulating 'non-interference in the internal affairs of States' found in article III of the original charter of the OAU (OAU, 1963, p. 4). African leaders who abhor good governance and the practice of democracy have been protected by this article. Today, Africa still has no less than ten leaders who have stayed in power uninterrupted, for between 25 and 39 years, often with constant shifts of the goal post of democracy. However, there appears to be a flickering light at the end of the dark and long tunnel of poor governance in Africa, with the decision of the AU in January 2017 to call on the outgoing President of the Islamic Republic of the Gambia, (Yahya Jammeh),

> to respect the Constitution of the Gambia, the ECOWAS and the AU Constitutive Act and the African Charter on Democracy, Elections and Governance, by handing over power, on 19 January 2017, as stated in the Constitution, to the newly-elected President of The Gambia, Adama Barrow, as decided by the people of the country.
>
> *AU, 2017a, p. 2*

Yahya Jammeh had attempted to reverse the outcome of the presidential election held in The Gambia on 1 December 2016, which he lost to the leader of opposition Adama Barrow.

## Health and health governance in Africa

African countries, individually and collectively through the AU, the WHO African Region (WHO-afro), and other international and regional groups, have through resolutions and agreements focused actions and adopted measures for the promotion and protection of the health of Africans. The enthusiasm of African leaders (including Ministers of Health) for adopting resolutions and making declarations on good governance was far less than for health and health matters. Over the past ten years, African leaders have, on the average, adopted four resolutions/declarations per year on health and less than one on good governance (AU, 2017b; WHO-afro, 2017). Despite the surfeit of health resolutions, Africa's health indices remain much below accepted and acceptable standards. The clear lesson is that the health of African citizens will continue to suffer in the absence of good governance.

In 2000, African leaders joined other heads of state in adopting the Millennium Declaration, which was designed to improve social and economic conditions in the world's poorest countries by 2015. A set of eight goals was devised to track progress. Three of these goals relate specifically to health; while two more have health components (UN, 2000). In 2001, heads of state of AU at a meeting in Abuja, Nigeria, signed the Abuja Declaration and Frameworks for Action on Roll Back Malaria. Member nations pledged to increase health budgets to at least 15 per cent of the state's annual budget and urged donor countries to 'fulfil the yet to be met target of 0.7 per cent of their GNP as Official Development Assistance (ODA) to developing countries' (OAU, 2001, pp. 5–6).

Ten years after the Abuja Declaration, the African Union Commission reported that six AU member states (Botswana, Burkina Faso, Malawi, Niger, Rwanda, and Zambia), met the 15 per cent benchmark (Olajide, 2010). The WHO, on the other hand, reported that in 2010, only one African country (Tanzania) had reached that target, while 26 had increased health expenditures and 11 had actually reduced health expenditures. Nine others had not had a noticeable negative or positive trend (WHO, 2011b). In another report, UNAIDS puts the number of AU countries meeting the target in 2011 at six (Liberia, Madagascar, Malawi, Rwanda, Togo, and Zambia) (UNAIDS, 2013). It is obvious the agencies are using different assessment criteria for measuring country performance.

An assessment conducted 15 years after Abuja Commitment provided a more comprehensive analysis of country performance. The report concluded that,

[M]ost African governments have increased the proportion of total public expenditure allocated to health in the early 2000s. The average level of per capita public spending on health rose from about US$70 in the early 2000s to more than US$160 in 2014. Domestic resources for health in Africa accounted for about 76 [per cent] in 2014, and external aid has increased from 13 [per cent] to 24 [per cent] of total health expenditure over the same period.

*WHO, 2016, p. 8*

However, the report cautioned on the many challenges to health financing which may prevent achievement of, or even the sustenance of, the current level of success. The report (WHO, 2016) highlighted the following challenges,

- Of every US$100 of state fund, it is estimated that an average US$16 is allocated to health, of which less than US$4 goes to the right health services.
- Despite rapid economic growth and availability of more resources to government, budgetary priorities changed with reduced proportionate allocation to health.
- Funding of the health sector has been inconsistent and unpredictable.
- Weak links between health and public financial management lead to budget under spending, with serious impediments hampering successful access of allocated funds.

These challenges, if not addressed, will compromise government capacity for sustaining long-term progress, hamper effective planning, and undermine implementation and efforts to achieve equity service coverage.

## From the Millennium Development Goals (MDGs) to the Sustainable Development Goals (SDGs)

Africa's Millennium Development Goal (MDG) progress was monitored by the Africa Union Commission (AUC), Economic Commission for Africa (ECA), Africa Development bank (AfDB), and United Nations Development Programme–Regional Bureau for Africa (UNDP-RBA). A recent UNDP report (2015) concluded that Africa was on track, attaining almost three out of the eight MDGs: MDG 2 (Achieve universal primary education), MDG 3 (Promote gender equality and empower women), and the targets related to MDG 6 (Combat HIV/AIDS, malaria and other diseases). The report, while adopting a positive slant on Africa MDG progress, cautions that more effort is needed if the gains of the MDGs are not to be reversed. Indeed, a closer look at individual country MDG performance gives only a faint hope of Africa's ability to successfully reach the Sustainable Development Goals (SDGs), given the challenges ahead. Some of the African countries with huge populations are not yet on track to achieve the MDG health goals; 'millions of children are out of primary schools, youth unemployment is rising, and current economic situation with exchange difficulties are creating the environment for a reversal of the gains of the MDGs' (UNDP, 2015, pp. XV, 47, and 52). It is essential for each country to assess its performance and identify her 'true' successes and glaring failures. Reports of such assessments should be widely disseminated and made subjects of national debates and discussion. They should be used as tools to stimulate governments to increase allocations and devote resources to programmes that will benefit and improve the socio-economic status and well-being of the society. Many African countries overly depend on external donors for their social and economic programmes. There is a low regard for, and scant interest in, sourcing local resources to contribute to development programmes and health-related issues, such as disease prevention and control. Where domestic resources are available, they are often diffuse, non-discrete, and difficult to quantify. African countries need to devise a mechanism and a framework for quantifying and acknowledging domestic input.

Sustaining progress in such activities as the MDGs is dependent on the level of preparedness of a nation to absorb shocks, be it economic or health related. The World Bank estimated that in 2015, the three countries of Guinea, Liberia, and Sierra Leone suffered a loss of US$2.2 billion in the gross domestic product (GDP) due to the Ebola virus disease outbreak (World Bank, 2016). This is an example of the adverse effect and reversal of years of sustained economic growth, by disease epidemics. We must move away from considering health as a non-revenue-yielding activity of the government and appreciate that the growth and sustenance of the economy depends on maintaining a healthy population, quite apart from the fact that disease is a revenue-destroying venture.

## Conclusion

On my way to a meeting organised by the AU, I watched the film *Queen of Katwe*. I cried for Africa and for her people, while watching the film. The film is based on the life of a 10-year-old girl living in one of the slums of Africa. The film traced the dramatic change in her life on meeting a soccer and chess coach at a missionary programme. Her life of constant struggle and suffering in the slums near the city centre was transformed when she learned the game of chess and became a national and international champion. As her life moved between the squalor and disease of the slum and the cities where she participated in and won national and international competitions, I reflected on the differences in the life of the millions of the poor people in Africa living below the poverty line, and of the very few rich people living, especially those living far above their legitimate means. The film made it easy to contrast the suffering and the poor state of health of the slum dwellers with the life of the leaders living in seeming states of complete physical, mental, and social well-being and absence of disease. I shed some tears for the pain and agony of the slum dwellers and also reflected on the inequity and injustice of poor governance that separated the citizens of a nation. I also cried for joy when the young chess prodigy and slum dweller proudly raised the flag of her country after winning a chess competition outside her country. With the young girl representing the ordinary citizen and the coach a leader of the society, the film showed that with natural talent, determination, and courage combined with purposeful and committed leadership and guidance of the coach, the great majority of citizens of African nations can rise above the slum and the poverty line, living in good health and enjoying social well-being.

It may be beneficial for good governance in Africa if at the next gathering of African heads of states, the film *Queen of Katwe* is screened during a plenary session at which all African heads of state are in attendance. African governments have for a long time paid lip service to and not seriously considered good governance as a framework for economic and social development. Without good governance, funds allocated for health, education, and other development activities are likely to be wasted, yielding poor outcomes. Civil societies, and other stakeholders, must be frontline advocates for the establishment and institutionalisation of good governance. During the first annual African governance forum, Kofi Anan, former UN Secretary General, said 'there is no single issue of greater importance to the economic and political future of Africa than good governance, and it must command the full and lasting attention of Africans' (ECA, 1997, p. 1). The comment was made 20 years ago, and it is even more relevant today for the development and health of the people of Africa.

## References

African Peer Review Mechanism (APRM). (2003) 'Africa's self-assessment for good governance', available at http://aprm-au.org/ (accessed on 19 September 2017).

African Union (AU). (2002) 'Consultative act of the African Union', available at www.au2002.gov.za/docs/key_oau/au_act.htm (accessed on 19 September 2017).

African Union (AU). (2007a) 'African Charter on Democracy, Elections and Governance', available at www.achpr.org/instruments/charter-democracy/ (accessed on 19 September 2017).

African Union (AU). (2007b) 'Communique', available at www.peaceau.org/uploads/647.psc.comm.gambia.13.01.2017-1.pdf (accessed on 7 October 2017).

African Union (AU). (2010) Available at http://aga-platform.org/244925257-The-African-Governance-Architecture-AGA-and-Platform-Notebook.pdf (accessed on 19 September 2017).

African Union (AU). (2011) 'Meeting the Abuja promise by African governments to commit 15% of total national budgets to health', available at www.ppdafrica.org/docs/policy/abuja-e.pdf (accessed on 19 September 2017).

African Union (AU). (2017a) 'Communique', available at www.peaceau.org/uploads/647.psc.comm.gambia.13.01.2017-1.pdf (accessed 7 October 2017).

African Union (AU). (2017b) 'OAU/AU treaties, conventions, protocols & charters', available at www.au.int/web/en/treaties (accessed on 19 September 2017).

Brown, G.W. (2012) 'Distributing who gets what and why: four normative approaches to global health', *Global Policy*, 3: 292–302.

Dickerson, C. and Grills, N. (2012) 'The world health organization engaging with civil society networks to promote primary health care', *Global Health Governance*, 6(1): 1–13.

Dodgson, R., Lee, K., and Drager, N. (2002) 'Global health governance: a conceptual review', available at http://apps.who.int/iris/bitstream/10665/68934/1/a85727_eng.pdf (accessed on 19 September 2017).

Economic Commission for Africa (ECA). (1997) 'ECA first African governance forum', available at www.africa.upenn.edu/Urgent_Action/apic_72097.html (accessed on 19 September 2017).

Elias, T.O. (1965) 'The Charter of the Organization of African Unity', *The American Journal of International Law*, 59(2): 243–67.

Gable, L. (2007) 'The proliferation of human rights in global health governance', *Journal of Law, Medicine and Ethics*, 35(4): 534.

Gostin, L.O. (2014) *Global Health Law*, Cambridge: Harvard University Press, pp. xvi and 541.

Graham, J., Amos, B., and Plumtre, T. (2003) 'Principles for good governance in the 21st century', Policy Brief No.15, Institute of Governance Ottawa, available at http://unpan1.un.org/intradoc/groups/public/documents/UNPAN/UNPAN011842.pdf (accessed on 19 September 2017).

Hein, W., Burris, S., and Shearing, C. (2009) 'Conceptual models for global health governance', In: K. Buse, W. Hein, and N. Drager (Eds.) *Making Sense of Global Health Governance*, Palgrave Macmillan, pp. 72–98.

Huber, M., Knottnerus, J.A., Lawrence, W., Green, L.W., et al. (2011) 'How should we define health?' *BMJ*: 343.

Ibrahim, M. (2006) 'The Mo Ibrahim Foundation invests in governance and leadership to catalyse Africa's transformation', available at https://web.archive.org/web/20121019024858/http://www.moibrahimfoundation.org/overview/ (accessed on 19 September 2017).

Kickbusch, I. and Gleicher, D. (2012) 'Governance for health in the 21st century', available at www.euro.who.int/__data/assets/pdf_file/0019/171334/RC62BD01-Governance-for-Health-Web.pdf?ua=1 (accessed on 19 September 2017).

Lee, K. and Kamradt-Scott, A. (2014) 'The multiple meanings of global health governance: a call for conceptual clarity', *Globalization and Health*, 10: 28.

Meier, B.M. and Onzivu, W. (2014) 'The evolution of human rights in WHO policy and the future of human rights through global health governance', *Public Health*, 128(2): 179–87.

Mekolo, A. and Resta, V. (2005) 'Governance progress in Africa: challenges and trends', available at http://unpan1.un.org/intradoc/groups/public/documents/un/unpan021509.pdf (accessed on 19 September 2017).

Mo Ibrahim Foundation. (2016a) 'A decade of African governance 2006–2015: 2016 index of African governance report', available at http://s.mo.ibrahim.foundation/u/2016/10/01184917/2016-Index-Report.pdf (accessed on 19 September 2017).

Mo Ibrahim Foundation. (2016b) 'Ibrahim prize for achievement in African leadership', available at http://mo.ibrahim.foundation/prize/ (accessed on 19 September 2017).

Mo Ibrahim Foundation. (2017) available at http://mo.ibrahim.foundation/about us (accessed on 19 September 2017)

Moon, S. (2008) 'Medicines as global public goods: the governance of technological innovation in the new era of global health', *Global Health Governance*, 2(2): 1–23.

Ng, N. and Ruger, J. (2011) 'Global health governance at the crossroads', *Global Health Governance*, 3(2): 1–37.

Olajide, A. (2010) 'Ten year review: Abuja Declaration on health financing in Africa', available at www.who.int/pmnch/media/membernews/2011/20110329_abujadeclaration.pdf (accessed on 19 September 2017).

OAU. (1963) 'OAU Charter', available at www.au.int/web/sites/default/files/treaties/7759-file-oau_charter_1963.pdf (accessed on 19 September 2017).

OAU. (2001) 'Abuja Declaration on HIV/AIDS, tuberculosis and other related infectious Diseases –OAU/SPS/ABUJA/3', available at www.un.org/ga/aids/pdf/abuja_declaration.pdf (accessed on 19 September 2017).

*The Lancet*. (2009) 'What is health? The ability to adapt', *The Lancet*, 373: 781.

UN. (2000) 'Goal 4: reduced child mortality', available at www.un.org/millenniumgoals/childhealth.shtml (accessed on 19 September 2017).

UNAIDS. (2013) 'Abuja +12 shaping the future of health financing in Africa', available at www.unaids.org/sites/default/files/media_asset/JC2524_Abuja_report_en_0.pdf (accessed on 19 September 2017).

UNDP. (2015) 'MDG report: lessons learned in implementing the MDGs', available at www.undp.org/content/undp/en/home/librarypage/mdg/mdg-reports/africa-collection.html (accessed on 19 September 2017).

WHO. (2006) 'Constitution of the World Health Organization', available at www.who.int/governance/eb/who_constitution_en.pdf (accessed on 19 September 2017).

WHO. (2011a) 'Governance', available at www.who.int/healthsystems/topics/stewardship/en/ (accessed on 19 September 2017).

WHO. (2011b). 'The Abuja Declaration ten years on', available at www.who.int/healthsystems/publications/abuja_report_aug_2011.pdf?ua=1) (accessed on 19 September 2017).

WHO. (2016) 'Public financing for health in Africa: from Abuja to the SDGs', *WHO*, xv: 47–52

WHO-afro. (2017) 'Regional committee sessions', available at www.afro.who.int/en/who-in-the-african-region/governance/regional-committee-for-africa.html (accessed on 19 September 2017).

World Bank. (2016) '2014–2015 West Africa ebola crisis: impact update', available at http://pubdocs.worldbank.org/en/297531463677588074/Ebola-Economic-Impact-and-Lessons-Paper-short-version.pdf (accessed on 19 September 2017).

# 14

# Learning from research on experiences of health diplomacy in Africa

*Rene Loewenson and Bente Molenaar-Neufeld*

## Background

From 2012 to 2014, the Regional Network for Equity in Health in East and Southern Africa (EQUINET) implemented a research programme in east and southern Africa (ESA) that examined the role of global and south–south health diplomacy in addressing selected key challenges to health and strengthening health systems in the region.

Global Health Diplomacy (GHD) refers to the processes through which states, non-state actors, and intergovernmental organisations negotiate responses to health challenges or use health in negotiations to achieve other political, economic, or social objectives. While health has been brought into foreign policy processes for several centuries, GHD is still an emergent concept, without a shared definition (Lee and Smith, 2011). While there is no articulated 'African approach' to GHD, a thematic analysis of published literature on African negotiations in global health found that these often invoked a liberation ethic, African unity, and developmental foreign policy (Loewenson, et al., 2014). Shared positions have been built by the Africa Group at the World Health Assembly (WHA) and in continental and regional bodies on intellectual property, medicines access, migration of health workers, control of breast milk substitutes, food security, debt cancellation, and fair trade (SADC, 2009; Loewenson, et al., 2014).

There have been debates about whether it is in the best interest of public health to raise health in foreign policy (Hoffman, 2010; Gagnon, 2012; Haynes, et al., 2013; Loewenson, et al., 2014). Fidler (2005) has suggested that health can be brought into foreign policy in various ways: (i) as regression, when health is purely addressed as a security issue, overriding public health norms and values; (ii) as remediation, when health is addressed through traditional foreign policy and has no special, transformative, or ethical role in international relations, or (iii) as revolution, as a right, goal and shared global responsibility that has a transformative role in foreign policy. The review of literature on African negotiations in global health found concerns over the loss of sovereignty, on the role of private actors, and over weak attention to underlying determinants of health (Loewenson, et al., 2014). At the same time globalisation, the level of external financing of African health systems, and rising international interest in African resources have intensified global and international negotiations (AU, UNECA, 2007; Amosu, 2007). Drawing on specific experiences of GHD within the ESA region, we explored whether health and health system goals have been advanced in GHD processes and what factors have affected this. We did so through document reviews and through a deeper exploration of three areas that regional policymakers had prioritised: (i) involvement of African actors in global health governance on financing for health systems; (ii) collaboration in overcoming bottlenecks to local medicine production, including through south–south relationships; and (iii) health worker migration and the implementation of the WHO Global Code of Practice on the International Recruitment of Health Personnel (termed the 'Code') (Loewenson, et al., 2011).

The results of the desk reviews and of the three case studies are reported in full in separate published papers, cited and referenced in this chapter. This chapter synthesises the learning across the whole programme of work on the factors affecting the agency and uptake of African interests in global health diplomacy during the agenda-setting phase, policy selection and negotiations, and implementation.

## Methods

The methods for the reviews and case studies that this chapter draws on are more fully described in separate papers (Loewenson, et al., 2011; Loewenson, et al., 2014; SEATINI and CEHURD, 2014; Barnes, et al., 2014; Dambisya, et al., 2013; Blouin, et al., 2012). The document reviews (Loewenson, et al., 2014; Blouin, et al., 2012) included published and grey literature obtained using key word searches in online databases such as Google Scholar, Google Books, PubMed, Medline, PAIS International, and other political science and foreign policy online libraries. The selected papers were reviewed first as abstracts, then as full papers, and selected based on criteria related to the purpose of the paper (GHD in Africa in the first review and GHD conceptual frameworks and research methods in the second).

The three case studies used document reviews, semi-structured key informant interviews, and observation and thematic analysis of policy dialogue. The first case study investigated how local, national, regional, and global health actors in South Africa, Tanzania, and Zambia participate in decision-making processes related to performance-based financing mechanisms associated with the Global Fund to Fight AIDS, Tuberculosis and Malaria (Global Fund or GFTAM) and World Bank (Barnes, et al., 2014). The second case study explored whether and how cooperation on production of medicines, including cooperation with emergent economies, is addressing the bottlenecks (as identified by African and regional bodies) to pharmaceutical manufacturing, with a focus on Kenya, Uganda, and Zimbabwe (SEATINI and CEHURD, 2014). The third case study explored how the policy interests of African countries informed the Code and how it has been used, implemented, and monitored in ESA countries, particularly in Kenya, Malawi, and South Africa (Dambisya, et al., 2013). The studies obtained ethics clearances/authorisations and permission, and verbal consent from all informants. National and regional diplomatic, policy, and technical personnel in the relevant fields reviewed and validated the findings for all the studies.

We applied a manual thematic content analysis on the text of the reviews and case study reports, focusing on specific content areas within four phases in the policy process:

- Agenda-setting phase: analysing the timing, roles, processes, and expressed interests of African and other actors; the policy content, relative to policy statements within the region, and the policy actors, forums, and processes involved.
- Policy development phase: analysing changes in policy content and their African and other sources and the role of African actors, networks, and alliances.
- Policy selection and negotiation phase: analysing stated factors influencing policy adoption and the role of and communication among African countries, regional and diplomatic actors.
- Policy implementation phase: analysing the factors influencing policy implementation and the use of implementation to raise agendas and negotiation issues.

The analysis identified common and different findings for each thematic area, particularly across the case studies, while the desk reviews were used to triangulate evidence, understand limitations of methods, and interpret findings.

A number of limitations were identified. While the case studies sought to obtain deeper qualitative information, they included a limited number of countries and there were difficulties in accessing evidence not in the public domain, gaps in institutional memory, and sensitivity in discussing some policy issues and processes (SEATINI and CEHURD, 2014; Barnes, et al., 2014; Dambisya, et al., 2013). Many African diplomacy interactions are unrecorded or unavailable, or documented through the lens of northern or global actors (Loewenson, et al., 2014). There are inadequate theoretical or analytic frameworks for this area of work, and much published work is descriptive (Blouin, et al., 2012). Despite these limitations, the case studies yielded valuable information as one of the few empirical research projects on GHD in ESA (Blouin, et al., 2012). The three case studies shared a policy analysis framework developed collectively at the inception, with evidence gathered on process, actors, and policy content. Each study used a stakeholder analysis to locate the main actors at the outset and included new stakeholders identified during interviews, and the majority of key actors/sectors were included in the interviews. The case study interviews were supported and supplemented by other research strategies, including literature reviews and direct engagement with policymakers to review and validate evidence.

## Findings

This section presents the findings of the content analysis on the three case studies, reported within the four focus areas of agenda setting, policy development, policy selection and negotiation, and implementation, and with a focus on the thematic categories outlined in the methods section.

### The agenda-setting phase

The three case studies were selected because they address policy concerns in ESA countries (Loewenson, et al., 2011). However, they show different levels of integration of ESA policy concerns in global or international policy agendas.

Partnership, participation, and agency in global health policy are well-established normative aims at national to global levels, and regional policy bodies have sought to strengthen effective African representation in global bodies (Loewenson, et al., 2011). The research conducted for the case examining performance-based financing (PBF) found divergent views, however, on how far Africans had shaped the PBF measures used by global agencies. On the one hand, the Rwandan government was widely cited as an innovator, whose experience on PBF had informed scale-up of the approach 'south to south' in other ESA countries. On the other hand, interviewees in Africa and in UN bodies reported a perception that external funders, particularly the World Bank and Global Fund, had driven the introduction, design, and in some cases even the targets of PBF (Barnes, et al., 2014). Various factors blurred how and by whom the PBF agenda was defined. This case study also reported that the design was introduced as an expression of existing, rather than new, policy, operationalising existing policy goals like participation, control of corruption, improved health and system outcomes, and value for money. Informal dialogues in both Geneva and within countries were reported to play a role in shaping the design and uptake, as commented on by an interviewee:

> Geneva is a small place and we all know each other. We often chat about what's working and what's not, what needs more attention and what's getting too much. These chats filter into WHO policy and these policies affect the operations of the Global Fund and World Bank.
>
> *Barnes, et al., 2014, p. 26*

These informal interactions made the features applied in the design of PBF appear to already be familiar to those involved by the time they were raised in more formal processes.

Technology transfer and access to medicines have become prominent issues in the current global agenda. The case study on south–south cooperation in overcoming bottlenecks to local medicine production explored these issues as they escalated in profile as a global trade issue. The resulting debates emerged with the intensely contested African Group draft declaration in 2001 on the TRIPS (Trade-Related Aspects of Intellectual Property Rights) Agreement and Public Health, successfully negotiated at the landmark Doha Declaration that protected public health and access to medicines in the interpretation of the TRIPS Agreement (WTO, 2001; Loewenson, et al., 2014). Africans levered support by linking medicines access to a recognised global issue – the AIDS epidemic – with further support and pressure from civil society on access to treatment as a human right.

While the issue of health worker migration was found to be largely brought to the global agenda by health ministers (Dambisya, et al., 2013), international cooperation on local medicine production affects a number of sectors. African plans such as the Pharmaceutical Manufacturing Plan for Africa (PMPA) 2007 were raised at the level of heads of state (SEATINI and CEHURD, 2014), with meetings on the issue between African countries and those in the BRICS (the collective body of Brazil, Russia, India, China, and South Africa) led by ministers of foreign affairs (South Centre, 2009). The health sector played a role in technical cooperation, such as in the African Network for Drugs and Diagnostics Innovation (ANDI) set up in 2009 to support research and development (R&D) on medicines, vaccines, and diagnostics (SEATINI and CEHURD, 2014). Nevertheless, a decade after Doha, Kenya proposed a resolution at the 65th WHA in 2012 that the WHO Director General convene an intergovernmental negotiating body to draft and negotiate a WHO Convention on Research and Development Financing and Co-ordination, again elevating African voice on global negotiations on medicines, this time on technology and skills transfer, in alliance with Brazil and India (WHO, 2012; SEATINI and CEHURD, 2014).

Such south–south alliances appear to have given useful support to African voice in global platforms. A content analysis of policy statements made in high-level meetings of the BRICS, of bilateral forums with Brazil, India, and China, and of the AU, SADC, East African community, and East Central and Southern African Health Community (ECSA-HC) reported shared concern on medicines access in support of such south–south alliances (Brown, et al., 2015). At the same time, the analysis also found divergent interests on how to achieve medicine access and less evidence of operational commitments supporting local production in Africa (Brown, et al., 2015). The evidence suggests that while some alliances may help to raise the issue on policy agendas, others may be needed to support their implementation. This was also found in relation to the Code, discussed later.

Of the three case studies, the global policy agenda and policy articulated in the region were most directly linked in the case of health worker migration and the Code. African actors were at the forefront of raising concerns on health worker migration, with the 2001 Southern African Development Community (SADC) issuing a strongly worded ministerial statement that: 'The active and vigorous recruitment from developing countries … could be seen as looting from these countries … similar to that experienced during the periods of colonisation when all resources, including minerals, were looted to developed countries' (SADC, 2001, cited by Pagett and Padarath, 2007, p. 28).

Similar concerns were articulated in other ESA policy forums between 2003 and 2010. ESA ministers of health escalated the issue to a global level in meetings with global institutions in that decade (WHO, World Bank, UNESCO), with health worker losses blamed as undermining the achievement of the Millennium Development Goals (Dambisya, et al., 2013; Kirigia, et al., 2006). From 2004, when African health ministers raised a resolution at the WHA, they maintained pressure on the issue, with a subsequent WHA resolution in 2005 (tabled by South Africa for the Africa group) urging implementation of the 2004 resolution. This was followed by high-level meetings and processes (described later) that sustained attention on the issue and motivated the drafting first of bilateral and multilateral codes and then the global WHO Code (Dambisya, et al., 2013). The language used – and reference to colonial practices – evoked a liberation ethic, while linking the issue to delivery on the MDGs raised its global relevance and built support from northern actors, backed by evidence on health worker shortfalls to support the arguments (Dambisya, et al., 2013). African voice, particularly that of health ministers and regional organisations, was identified as instrumental in raising health worker migration and recruitment as a global policy issue (Gilson and Erasmus, 2005; Chen and Boufford, 2005; Taylor and Dillon, 2011). Subsequent sections explore how far this agenda was sustained in the course of policy negotiation.

## The policy development phase

The changes that took place as the policies examined were developed are not always reported in the public domain, especially where they were advanced in informal networks. Nevertheless, supported by evidence from key informants, this section presents the findings on how the policies or agreements developed and the roles, processes, and factors that affected this. The three policy areas reported in the case studies are rather different: one (agreements on medicine production) with international cooperation negotiated nationally; one (on PBF) largely negotiated and spread within ESA countries by global finance institutions; and the last (on the Code) negotiated at the global level. This affects the policy development phase.

As noted in the case study on medicine production, bilateral negotiations on local production took place at the executive level of government and generally not in the public domain. How far BRICS positions on fair access to medicines and to innovation reported in the policy content analysis (Brown, et al., 2015) were carried into bilateral negotiations on medicine production thus needs to be inferred from subsequent practice. The case studies on medicines production reported the presence of clear policy statements in the region on the bottlenecks to be addressed in local production that would be expected to inform cooperation on local production. These bottlenecks included shortfalls in capital and public investment, skills, regulation and enforcement capacities, and R&D capacities; disabling tariffs and infrastructures; competition from cheaper imports; and fragmentation of local markets. The case studies also reported limited links and mechanisms for technology transfer and sourcing of active pharmaceutical ingredients (SEATINI and CEHURD, 2014).

An assessment of the cooperation between the Uganda Quality Chemicals International Limited (QCIL) and India's Cipla Limited suggested that some of these bottlenecks were addressed through African influence on the content of the agreements, including establishment of an R&D unit, capital investment, skills training, and some level of technology transfer. The involvement of officials at top levels of government in Uganda facilitated provision in return for favourable tax and tariff measures, infrastructure, and market access. In both cases these provisions were limited to the QCIL plant and not more widely spread in the industry (SEATINI and CEHURD, 2014). A number of international cooperation initiatives were reported in the ESA region, such as on ANDI, on pharmacist recruitment, and on market access. However, the medicines production case study reported that other bilateral agreements between the ESA countries studied and emergent economies had not materialised or had taken significantly longer than planned, thus making it difficult to assess policy development in these cases. Key informants raised concern that despite stated policy intentions on cooperation in south–south forums, the fact that technical partners from countries in BRICS also provide the finance and technology makes them relatively powerful in negotiating agreements. This means that African countries must negotiate mutuality of benefit, as in any other form of international cooperation, notwithstanding shared policy intentions. Hence, for example, China's role in providing active pharmaceutical ingredients for Indian generic production, and the dominance by India of the supply of generic medicines to countries like Kenya 'raises questions about how far there will be real willingness to support local African production' (SEATINI and CEHURD, 2014, p. 37; UNDP, 2013).

Evidence on the process of policy development was more accessible in the other two case studies: first the case considering the involvement of African actors in global health governance on financing for health systems; and the second on the Code. The first, the study on African participation in the design of global financing explored (i) pay for performance (P4P) schemes, where attainment of specific targets resulted in payments, and (ii) older models of aid conditionality, where objectives, indicators, and targets are set by recipients. The case study noted 'the design and conception of PBF [to be] … politically complex' (Barnes, et al., 2014, p. 21). The process built on relatively well-established technical working groups, review meetings, subcommittees, and formal networks, often involving a range of national stakeholders.

The African negotiations were thus less affected by the level of formal participation than by its quality, in terms of negotiators' understanding of and familiarity with the proposals and their access to credible evidence of their impact on the health system. Negotiations were also significantly affected by the relative power of different groups in these forums, particularly given the involvement of external funders. External funder interests were reported to be accepted largely as a reasonable demand of aid delivery, focusing the debate in policy development less on whether PBF should be applied than on the targets and how they would be monitored and evaluated. Even in these areas, some inequality was reported in the negotiations, depending on the economic strength of the recipient country. On the one hand, external funders were seen to be open to concerns. Differences and uncertainties were addressed in part through visits to countries where PBF was being applied, through evaluation of pilot sites, and through brokerage support from other global agencies, such as UNAIDS. On the other hand, some African interviewees raised concerns that highlighting negative impacts was seen to threaten access to new external funding linked to PBF, and that external consultants and accountancy firms had a large influence on design of targets and evaluation of performance. In all the case study countries the 'bottom line' for policy development was an end goal of access to additional health system funding that overrode uncertainties on design. As stated by a Zambian respondent: 'They ask if you want the money, you want the money, so you do the project' (Barnes, et al., 2014, p. 23).

While countries did thus have input to policy development, the compromises made led to a number of concerns over the targets and design fragmenting the system, the targets selected, conditional accounting targets, high administrative and monitoring demands, a lack of confidence in the audit system used by external funders and their local fund agent, and lack of clear, nationally owned arbitration procedures (Barnes, et al., 2014).

The relative power imbalance noted in the two case studies on medicines and financing was less evident in the early years of policy development on the Code. The African political leaders that led this process and their political framing of the issue may have provided some leverage in this power imbalance. African political, technical, and diplomatic actors negotiated bilateral and multilateral codes before the global negotiations, often after dialogue within regional organisations, and the Africa Group facilitated unity across countries in the inputs made in the WHA and on the global Code. Tracking development of the global Code, Taylor and Dhillon (2011) found that many of the issues raised by African countries were integrated into the text. However, the clauses on compensation and mutuality of benefits faced strong opposition from developed countries, many of whom were both external funders and destination countries of health workers from ESA countries. African key informants observed that the final Code fell short in addressing issues of compensation to source countries, support for training health professionals, arrangements for return, thus inadequately addressing the impact of health worker migration on health systems in the region (an issue termed 'mutuality of benefit'). They were also dissatisfied with the soft law nature of the Code (Dambisya, et al., 2013). Taylor and Dhillon (2011) relate these losses in policy content to a loss of African voice in policy development. However, they also noted that when this voice was regained during the final drafting committee process, monitoring and reporting mechanisms that northern countries had initially opposed were reintegrated (Taylor and Dhillon, 2011). At the same time, the case study suggests that perceptions on the issue also shifted within the ESA region, with migration falling as a concern as development aid began funding health workers. While Africa Group positions strengthened unity, the case study reports that there may have been inadequate engagement with individual country views as positions shifted, attenuating African voice in the process (Dambisya, et al., 2013).

## The policy selection and negotiation phase

African states were reported to be actively engaged in the policy selection and negotiation phase in some areas, but less so in others. The processes noted earlier in relation to the Code case study included strong policy statements within the region, and a decade of diplomatic engagement, advocacy, and meetings. Critically, the negotiation of multilateral instruments such as the 2003 Commonwealth Code of Practice on Ethical Recruitment of Health Personnel and bilateral instruments such as the 2003 Memorandum of Understanding between South Africa and the United Kingdom on ethical recruitment of health workers, reinforced the ultimate adoption of the global Code in 2010. On local medicine production, African global engagement on public health protections in intellectual property agreements and on R&D on medicines were supportive of local production, although not directly so (Loewenson, et al., 2014; SEATINI and CEHURD, 2014).

Notwithstanding the positive role model of Rwanda in the work on global financing, in the case study examining PBF, African actors were seen to have weaker influence in designing financing policy than that of external funders: 'The World Bank and Global Fund have a key role in driving (or attempting to drive) forward PBF interventions within African health systems. External funders have invested significant volumes of money in generating knowledge about health sector-oriented PBF' (Barnes, et al., 2014, p. 29). Being less dependent on external funding, as was the case in South Africa, was reported to give countries more power to shape policy and implementation.

Unity of voice; strong regional, national, and international linkages among stakeholders; and multisectoral engagement were also found to strengthen African influence in policy selection. This was evident, for example, in negotiations on the Code (Dambisya, et al., 2013) and in decision-making on the design of PBF (Barnes, et al., 2014). Partnerships, both south–south across countries and public–private within countries, were also reported to facilitate uptake of African policy positions on medicine production (SEATINI and CEHURD, 2014).

Having prior bilateral or multilateral instruments, as with the Code, or positive role models in countries were reported to facilitate and inform policy selection (Dambisya, et al., 2013). Another example is drawn from the case study on medicines production, where the partnership between QCIL and CIPLA Limited on R&D and capacity development enabled processes for compliance with WHO Good Manufacturing Practices (GMP) in the ESA region. Such examples acted as role models, motivating and informing further negotiations and reinforcing policy implementation, discussed further later (SEATINI and CEHURD, 2014).

Policy selection was reported to be enhanced by 'champion' countries and actors: Kenya, Zimbabwe, and Malawi through, amongst other things, engagement at the WHA were mentioned as champions of regional interests on the Code and on intellectual property, medicines access, and R&D (SEATINI and CEHURD, 2014; Dambisya, et al., 2013; Loewenson, et al., 2014). South Africa was noted to have had strong influence in shaping global financing for HIV in line with national system targets 'through internally driven mechanisms' (Barnes, et al., 2014 p. 44; Biesma, et al., 2009). Regional agreements and champions were also supportive, such as the African Union (AU), SADC, and East African Community (EAC)'s pharmaceutical policies; the statement by SADC health ministers on the recruitment of health personnel by developed countries; and various SADC and ECSA-HC resolutions on health worker recruitment (Dambisya, et al., 2013; SEATINI and CEHURD, 2014).

By contrast, competing interests, and especially opposing interests from northern actors, appeared to be a significant barrier to the inclusion of content proposed from African countries in global policies and agreements. Opportunities of external funding were noted earlier to influence positions on PBF design, while a powerful pharmaceutical lobby allied with high-income countries (some of whom fund medicines supplies through development aid), presented a strong opposing lobby in negotiations on patent protection (SEATINI and CEHURD, 2014; Elbeshbishi, 2007).

Influence in policy selection was weakened when ESA countries had conflicting or competing interests and positions or weak domestic policy support, poor communication and coordination across domestic actors, and limited involvement of African civil society (SEATINI and CEHURD, 2014; Dambisya, et al., 2013; Barnes, et al., 2014). For example, the case study on the Code reported that the resistance of many high-income countries to clauses on compensation, mutuality of benefit, or enforceability of agreements became a more influential factor in policy negotiation and selection when some African countries also began to see migration as a source of income or better dealt with through traditional aid approaches, raising competing interests on the issue (Dambisya, et al., 2013; Taylor and Dhillon, 2011).

Communication flows appeared to have a key influence on both policy negotiation and implementation. Dialogue, regular meetings, and communication between capitals and embassies, through the Africa Group at the WHA and through regional organisations in the ESA region, were found to strengthen and coordinate African voice in negotiations on the Code (Taylor and Dhillon, 2011). Conversely, the design of PBF and agreements on pharmaceuticals were noted to be weakened by irregular communication between national organisations and between national and regional actors, weakening national input and 'learning ... generated between national governments and their individual experiences' (Barnes, et al., 2014, p. 56).

## The implementation phase

The presence of specific mandates, leadership, implementation, and the use of monitoring and reporting can increase the likelihood that diplomacy leads to actual change in health systems and supports accountability on policy commitments. As noted earlier, leadership may shift during diplomatic processes, from those who negotiate agreements to a different group of actors who implement them.

Despite strong policy commitments from within the region and some measures being implemented, comprehensive implementation on both the Code and policies for overcoming bottlenecks to medicine production had been slow by the time of the research. The time taken to negotiate the Code made institutional memory critical to translate negotiation into implementation. While it is still early to evaluate the outcome, weaker implementation of the Code was attributed to a decline in concern over health worker out-migration by 2010 compared to internal migration, underfunding, and absolute shortages of health workers (Dambisya, et al., 2013). The lag in implementation was further attributed to a range of factors: turnover and loss of leading national and regional voices, lack of dissemination and awareness of the instrument, poor communication with other sectors affected, and weak follow-up from the WHO with changes in its global secretariat apparently downgrading the issue (Dambisya, et al., 2013). There is also a reported perception that agreements represent the end, rather than the start, of the process. One key informant summed it up as: 'What happened at the WHA in 2010 was it for the Code. We then went back to other things. For the Code, it was mission accomplished, and we didn't have any more energy for it' (Dambisya, et al., 2013, p. 20).

Implementation appears to be more likely when it is synergistic with existing domestic practice. For example, speaking of the Code, a key informant from Malawi stated:

> ... in all honesty, we have not done anything directly related to the Code. But when looking at the Code you can see that we are doing things expected from the Code ... the discussion on support for training, our strategic direction on HR, all those are in the spirit of the Code. Yeah, but not because of the Code, perhaps...
>
> *Dambisya, et al., 2013, p. 26*

Implementation was thus found to depend in part on the existence of appropriately resourced actors and institutions. Overburdened ministry level human resource (HR) departments saw the Code as adding to, rather than supporting, other responsibilities, thus weakening implementation. One key informant put it this way:

> You get back from the World Health Assembly full of morale, many new ideas, but also many tasks generated. As you settle down, you realize that the work you left pending before the WHA is waiting for you. And the work plans do not include the new issues for the remainder of the year.
>
> *Dambisya, et al., 2013, p. 25*

The strength of the monitoring and evaluation frameworks, availability of information, and dissemination of reporting were found to support implementation. Conversely, a lack of dependable information, limited up-to-date data, and weak public reporting on agreements and their implementation meant that policymakers, parliamentarians, and the public were less able to assess whether interventions are working as designed and to build learning for the next round of negotiation (Barnes, et al., 2014; SEATINI and CEHURD, 2014; Dambisya, et al., 2013).

Implementation also depends on enabling policy and legal frameworks. For example, Kenya's national industrialisation policy framework (2010) was reported to encourage procurement of locally manufactured pharmaceutical products (SEATINI and CEHURD, 2014; Government of Kenya, 2010). Other factors affecting implementation of agreements included leadership from a designated authority (as observed in the Code) (Dambisya, et al., 2013) and dissemination of negotiated outcomes to all implementation levels, as found in the work on PBF (Barnes, et al., 2014).

These factors do not depend only on the health sector. In all three case studies, beyond the involvement of foreign affairs in negotiations, the implementation of policy commitments called for other sectors to act, such as to reduce tariffs on imported inputs, provide reliable infrastructures, domestic financing (in PBF), and skills training, and to implement legal reforms on medicine production. In all three case study areas, ministries of foreign affairs, finance, education, labour, planning and national development, immigration, infrastructure, and various regulatory councils needed to be coordinated for implementation (Dambisya, et al., 2013; SEATINI and CEHURD, 2014; Barnes, et al., 2014). Also, in all cases, the weak involvement of civil society was reported to not only weaken leverage of African positions in global negotiations, but also to weaken accountability in implementation (Dambisya et al., 2013).

## Discussion and conclusions

Overall, the research carried out in this project suggests that there is variation in the factors that influence the effectiveness of negotiation of health agreements and cooperation at different phases of the policy process, depending on the issue. Nevertheless, some conclusions may be drawn from the findings within the theme areas of agenda setting, policy development, policy selection and negotiation, and implementation.

### African agency and interests in global policy agendas

On agenda setting, the three cases highlight that there is no 'toolbox' for bringing ESA policy concerns to the global agenda. Some strategies do appear more frequently, including linking the issue to existing global norms (such as fair participation; rights to access treatment), commitments (such as MDGs) or concerns (such as HIV); building and articulating unified positions across African countries through regional bodies and through alliances with other strong actors (including from northern countries, Brazil and India); and linking political, sectoral, and diplomatic leadership to technical and/or civil society support. The findings highlight that the process is complex and that it takes time to build support to push an issue forward. The cases appeared to have limited involvement of civil society or domestic private sector actors, except in the early negotiations on medicine access. It could be argued that weak involvement by non-state actors deprives state actors of support from sustained social pressure, local technical information, and domestic role models of practice, all noted to be contributors to agenda setting and policy selection. The case studies highlight the complexity of advancing health sector policies, such as those medicines and HR, where many other sectors have influence; and suggest these are more easily addressed where there is already multisectoral coordination in countries (Loewenson, et al., 2014).

The successful escalation of the issue of health worker migration from the regional to global level appeared to be due to a strong starting position and clear policy rooted in regional principles and dialogue; sustained and amplified through ministerial, multilateral, and other forums; and consolidated through negotiation of subsidiary instruments, even before it got to the global level. Political and diplomatic actors appeared to be the most influential 'policy innovators' in that issue. This pathway suggests the importance of links between capitals and embassies in the agenda-setting phase, to give a platform in diplomacy to political actors in ESA countries, and also for diplomats to engage more effectively in global-level informal networks and alliances that play a role in shaping agendas. It points to the positive value in building positions, evidence, and support regionally over a sustained period to create and maintain momentum on agenda setting and policy development and selection. It further highlights the value of information across governments, including to and from diplomats, to support political voice with evidence.

## Uptake of African interests in global policy development and selection

The findings highlight that the process of policy development globally is a political one, with technical dimensions that can widen or reduce power imbalances between international actors. While in two cases (medicines and financing instruments) it was crafted as 'cooperation', this did not negate the fact that different interests and levels of power were involved, with mixed outcomes in the policy content a reflection of this power differential across those involved. The findings consistently point to the influence on agenda setting and policy selection of agencies that are both technical partners and funders. These may be global agencies, such as on HR, or emergent economy 'partners', such as on medicines, who bring both funding and technical resources to processes, often to underfunded sectors in ESA countries. The economic status and level of external funding of African health systems appeared to play a significant role in the power relations around policy development in all three areas, with external funders – and the consultants they bring – having leverage beyond the technical arguments and processes.

A number of factors were noted to enable African influence in shaping policy development in this context. Policy selection and negotiation appear to rely on strong, unified positions, effective leaderships, and sound knowledge of the issues, particularly as power imbalances sharpen during negotiations. Hence, for example, in the Code case study, leadership and strong policy statements within the region and a history of diplomatic engagement and advocacy on the issue of health worker migration supported negotiation and adoption of the Code. A unified African position helped promote shared African interests in the final outcome, even in the face of strong opposing positions (Dambisya, et al., 2013). Other factors included having: clear policy positions on the issue, at country and regional levels, shared across sectors and with diplomats; strong political leadership and sufficient public articulation of issues and positions to engage wider stakeholders; clarity and support from technical actors; and alliances across countries within and beyond the region. Strong political leadership, champions and positions, regional and continental unity, and evidence from role models and alliances were also noted in the findings to redress this power imbalance.

Consultants from global agencies appeared to play a more visibly influential role in policy development and selection than local technical personnel. The link between technical and funding power raises an argument, however, for involvement of independent technical brokers, not linked to funding, whether from WHO or from within the ESA countries and regional organisations. Investment in public sector R&D, in the quantity and quality of scientific/technical personnel, collaboration across R&D and technical institutions, and with domestic private sector were noted in India, for example, as contributing to the country's successful capacities in international trade (Lunogelo and Baregu, 2013). Other factors were less clear in their impact: informal networks appeared to play a role in shaping policy development, such as in the dialogue on PBF, but are less transparent and so their role is not as easy to define. African unity at a global level strengthened African voice, as noted earlier, but there was a question in the negotiation on the Code about how far it accommodated or ignored individual country views. Civil society representing affected groups appeared to play a limited role in policy development in all three case study areas reviewed, despite the evident political nature of the process.

Several additional factors affected policy selection. First, the presence of policy and legal frameworks provided parameters for choosing policy. Regional or other agreements or role models; alliances and partnerships on shared positions; champion countries linked to regional networks and exchange and unity of voice, as built in the Africa Group, provided support for African positions in negotiations on the Code and on medicines production. Also in these two areas, making reference to domestic policies and having examples of local practices that demonstrate the policy positions being negotiated were observed to support policy selection and implementation.

## Barriers and facilitators to implementation

At the same time the case studies highlighted shortfalls: in the use by African actors of informal spaces for engagement and regional processes for reviewing and informing policies; in the implementation of domestic policies that align to foreign policy positions (such as in the case of local production); and in domestic capacities and communication on global processes within and across ESA countries.

These shortfalls in communication and wider awareness of the content of global negotiations and cooperation agreements were found to combine with inadequate support from global institutions and limited data to weaken implementation and monitoring of agreements. The Code case study particularly highlights this point. The authors conclude that three years after its adoption, the Code was largely unknown in the region, in part due to an absence of local champions and overburdened HR departments (Dambisya, et al., 2013). The negotiations on PBF were noted to face challenges in the lack of reliable information and effective monitoring frameworks to both set and adequately evaluate the success of targets (Barnes, et al., 2014).

The implementation stage generally brings a new set of actors to translate negotiated agreements/policy into health system change that need to be appropriately informed and resourced. At the same time, as found in the studies, embedding implementation within existing processes so they do not represent additional tasks is important for already overburdened actors. The long time-frames in which many negotiations take place call for mechanisms for institutional continuity, whilst recognising the need to communicate and transfer mandates to different management actors for implementation. The existence of clear and effective monitoring and evaluation frameworks can help increase the likelihood of effective implementation. The findings suggest that cooperation agreements and global negotiations need to include resources, duties and information systems, and support for monitoring and evaluation methods and capacities to facilitate implementation.

## Opportunities, challenges and limitations to diplomacy in health

This chapter began with Fidler's three ways in which health is applied in foreign policy, viz: as regression, as remediation, or as revolution (Fidler, 2005). In the case studies, African actors raised health in the 'revolution' framework, seeking greater global justice on health worker migration, health financing, or medicines access. However, the negotiations themselves evolved more as remediation, with compromises made reflecting more traditional relations. The policy initiative to challenge losses from health worker migration, to strengthen local production or negotiate fairer global measures on innovation and intellectual property represent forms of structural diplomacy, challenging current global norms. However, over time the forms of cooperation around these areas have been shaped more by development aid paradigms than by critiques of global inequality and injustice that are used to influence public perceptions and generate the symbolic capital of public diplomacy in order to advance or protect regional interests (Bustamante and Sweig, 2008).

Proposals to strengthen proactive, political, and policy driven approaches that sustain pressure for public health norms and goals, including through the inclusion of key domestic stakeholders, can play a role in more transformative global health diplomacy. Many measures are domestic, and some call for strengthened regional cooperation as a basis for global engagement, while recognising the different situations of member states in these organisations.

There is, however, also a question of the paradigm of health diplomacy prevailing in Africa, as is suggested by the findings, particularly given the significant interest in African resources. The case studies suggest that there is an opportunity cost in framing health diplomacy in the region within a 'development aid' paradigm, if the compromises agreed to weaken longer-term systems and capacities. As one key informant noted in the case study on medicines access, donations of essential medicines produced outside the country, while important for health services, also raised dependency on donated medicines, reducing the incentive to invest in local pharmaceutical production. Disease-focused aid initiatives can be argued to have led to a dominance of remedial, humanitarian engagement in African international relations on health, with less sustained attention to structural determinants, such as the public health impacts of unfair trade. In such circumstances, as raised in the case study on governance, for health to have a transformative role in foreign policy, countries would need to be willing to say no.

## Acknowledgement

This work was implemented in a research programme of the Regional Network for Equity in Health in East and Southern Africa (EQUINET) on global health diplomacy in east and southern Africa supported by IDRC (Canada). Special thanks to Andreas Papamichail for support with analysis and to the case study teams for their separately published reports. Thanks for permission from the *Journal for Health Diplomacy* for use of this material as a reprint from its publication as an open-access article in the *Journal of Health Diplomacy*, Vol. 1, Issue 3, jointly edited by the Journal with EQUINET (http://media.wix.com/ugd/35c673_015bd4d0defc4b1fb9238be8c10b86ef.pdf). The paper in the *Journal of Health Diplomacy* was distributed under the terms of the Creative Commons Attribution License, which permits unrestricted use, distribution, and reproduction in any medium, provided the original author and source are credited and permission has been given for its reproduction with minor modifications in this text.

## References

Amosu, A. (2007) 'Dangerous times for Africa', *Review of African Political Economy*, 34(114): 711–13.

AU, UNECA (African Union, United Nations Economic Commission for Africa). (2007) 'Accelerating Africa's development through diversification', Ethiopia: AU, UNECA.

Barnes, A., Brown, G., Harman, S., Banda P., Hayes R., and Mulambia C. (2014) 'African participation and partnership in performance-based financing: a case study in global health policy', EQUINET Discussion Paper 102. Harare: EQUINET.

Biesma, R.G., Brugha, R., Harmer, A., Walsh, A., Spicer, N., and Walt, G (2009) 'The effects of global health initiatives on country health systems: a review of the evidence from HIV/AIDS control', *Health Policy and Planning*, 24: 239–52.

Blouin, C., Molenaar-Neufeld, B., and Pearcey, M. (2012) 'Annotated literature review: conceptual frameworks and strategies for research on global health diplomacy', EQUINET Discussion Paper 92. CTPL\EQUINET, July.

Brown, G.B., Loewenson, R., Modisenyane, M., and Papamichail, A. (2015) 'Business as usual? The role of BRICS co-operation in addressing health system priorities in East and Southern Africa', *Journal of Health Diplomacy*, 1(3), available at https://media.wix.com/ugd/35c673_b4cfdbae1f334eb0b07c1656d96d0380.pdf (accessed on 25 January 2015).

Bustamante, M. and Sweig, J. (2008) 'Buena vista solidarity and the axis of aid: Cuban and Venezuelan public diplomacy', *Annals of the American Academy of Political and Social Science*, 616(1): 223–56.

Chen, L.C. and Boufford, J.L. (2005) 'Fatal flows – doctors on the move', *New England Journal of Medicine*, 353: 1850–2.

Dambisya, Y.M., Malema, N., Dulo, C., Matinhure, S., and Kadama, P. (2013) 'The engagement of east and southern African countries on the WHO code of practice on the international recruitment of health personnel and its implementation', EQUINET Discussion Paper 103. Harare: EQUINET.

Elbeshbishi, A.N. (2007) 'TRIPS and public health: what should African countries do?', ATPC Work in progress No. 49. Addis Ababa: Economic Commission for Africa.

Fidler, D. (2005) *Health and Foreign Policy: A conceptual overview*. London: Nuffield Trust.

Gagnon, M.L. (2012) 'Global health diplomacy: understanding how and why health is integrated into foreign policy', Doctoral dissertation, available at: https://ruor.uottawa.ca/handle/10393/23141 (accessed on 21 July 2017)

Gilson, L. and Erasmus, E. (2005) 'Supporting the retention of HRH: SADC policy context', EQUINET Discussion Paper 26. Johannesburg: EQUINET and Health Systems Trust.

Government of Kenya. (2010) *Kenya National Industrialisation Policy Framework*. Nairobi: Ministry of Industrialisation.

Haynes, L., Legge, D., London, L., McCoy, D., Sanders, D., and Schuftan, S. (2013) 'Will the struggle for health equity and social justice be best served by a framework convention on global health', *Health and Human Rights*, 15(1): 111–6.

Hoffman, S.J. (2010) 'Strengthening global health diplomacy in Canada's foreign policy architecture: literature review and key informant interviews', *Canadian Foreign Policy Journal*, 16(3): 17–41.

Kirigia, J.M., Gbary, A.R., Muthuri, L.K., Nyoni, J., and Seddoh, A. (2006) 'The cost of health professionals' brain drain in Kenya', *BMC Health Services Research*, 6: 89.

Lee, K. and Smith, R. (2011) 'What is 'global health diplomacy'? A conceptual review', *Global Health Governance*, V(I), available at: http://blogs.shu.edu/ghg/2011/11/21/what-is-%E2%80%98global-health-diplomacy-a-conceptual-review/.

Loewenson, R., Machemedze, R., and Manyau, E. (2011) 'Research to support strategic leadership in global health diplomacy in east, central and southern Africa', TARSC, SEATINI (EQUINET) and ECSA HC. Discussion Paper 88. Harare: EQUINET and Arusha: ECSA HC.

Loewenson, R., Modisenyane, M., and Pearcey, M. (2014) 'African perspectives in global health diplomacy', *Journal of Health Diplomacy*, 1(2):1–20.

Lunogelo, H.B. and Baregu, S. (2013) 'Indo-Africa relationship: Opportunities for technology transfer between India and African countries', Economic and Social Research Foundation Discussion Paper No. 52. Dar es Salaam.

SADC (Southern Africa Development Community). (2001) 'Statement by SADC health ministers on the recruitment of health personnel by developed countries' [Cited by Pagett, C. & Padarath, A. (2007) 'A review of codes and protocols for the migration of health workers', EQUINET Discussion Paper 50. Harare: EQUINET].

SADC (Southern Africa Development Community). (2009) *Round 9 proposal*. London: HIV Cross Border Initiative.

Southern and Eastern African Trade, Information and Negotiations Institute (SEATINI) and Centre for Human Rights and Development (CEHURD). (2014) 'Medicines production and procurement in east and southern Africa and the role of south-south co-operation', EQUINET Discussion Paper 104. Harare: EQUINET.

South Centre. (2009) 'South-south co-operation principles: an essential element in south-south co-operation', Geneva: South Centre.

Taylor, A. and Dhillon, I. (2011) 'The WHO Global Code of practice on the international recruitment of health personnel: The evolution of global health diplomacy', *Global Health Governance*, 5(1), Georgetown Public Law Research Paper No. 11–140; Georgetown Law and Economics Research Paper No. 11–31, available at SSRN: https://ssrn.com/abstract=1970315 (accessed on 21 July 2017).

UNDP (United Nations Development Programme). (2013) *Intellectual property rights and access to affordable ARVs in China*. Bangkok: UNDP.

WHO (World Health Organisation). (2012) 'Research and development co-ordination and financing report of the expert working group', Geneva: WHO, available at www.who.int/phi/documents/RDFinancingEN.pdf (accessed on 19 August 2015).

WTO (World Trade Organisation) Ministerial. (2001) 'Declaration on the TRIPS agreement and public health. Geneva: WTO. Adopted on 14 November 2001', Doha, available at www.wto.org/english/thewto_e/minist_e/min01_e/mindecl_trips_e.htm (accessed on 19 August 2015).

# 15

# China's role in global health governance

*Jeremy Youde*

## Introduction

When it comes to global health governance, the People's Republic of China occupies a unique position – a uniqueness derived from its ambiguous positioning. Here is one of the world's most populous countries with one of the largest economies and a seeming desire to play a larger role in global governance. At the same time, though, China tends to portray itself as a leader of the Global South and has not taken much of a leadership role on global health governance issues. It is a country that both contributes to and receives aid from global health governance institutions like the Global Fund to Fight AIDS, Tuberculosis, and Malaria and the World Bank. It has explicitly incorporated health into its foreign policy, deploying medical teams to countries around the world to improve access to health care and promote its own soft power, and it actively promoted the candidacy of Margaret Chan for the role of director-general of the World Health Organization (WHO) (Chan, et al., 2009). That has not necessarily translated into a willingness to engage with global health governance's values and norms. It has repeatedly shown a reluctance to collaborate with surveillance systems or engage in other information-sharing activities that are at the heart of contemporary global health governance (Chan, 2011, pp. 2–3).

Such ambivalence actually highlights the importance of figuring out where China fits within global health governance. Huang (2010) notes that China possesses one-fifth of the world's population, contains one-seventh of the world's disease burden, and has been the origin site for a number of prominent international infectious disease pandemics like Severe Acute Respiratory Syndrome (SARS) and the H5N1 and H7N9 influenza strains. The country obviously has an important role to play – not only in keeping its own citizens healthy, but also in protecting people around the world – but its engagement with global health governance architecture remains uncertain. A failure to include China in these structures could undermine global health governance's ability to combat disease outbreaks, but such thinking also assumes that the Chinese government *wants* to engage with global health governance. Former Premier Wen Jiabao has spoken of the need to create 'a model of developing foreign aid with Chinese characteristics', but it is unclear what exactly that means (Clark, 2014, p. 318).

## China and global health governance institutions

There exists an ambiguous relationship between the People's Republic of China and international society within global health governance. On the one hand, the Chinese government recognises the value of participating in global health governance institutions and has taken steps to demonstrate its willingness to embrace some elements of the global health governance system (Jing, et al., 2011). This includes its re-engagement with WHO after the organisation had criticised the Chinese government's response to SARS and its cooperation with UNAIDS. On the other hand, its prioritisation of state sovereignty and nationalism has discouraged more active collaboration with these same institutions. The government has historically had an ambivalent relationship with WHO, and Chan, et al. (2009, p. 4) describe China's traditional approach to health as Westphalian as opposed to globally oriented. Tan, et al. (2012) call this wariness between China and global health governance the twin dynamic of receptivity and resistance.

Many analysts of global health governance lament China's reluctance to take a stronger leadership and financial role within the system. Yoon (2008) argues that China tends to respond to infectious disease outbreaks with policies that emphasise national protection over international cooperation. The government views disease outbreaks as weakening national power and construes national power as a zero-sum game. As such, sharing information about disease outbreaks with others could give them the tools to take advantage of China (Yoon, 2008). Stevenson and Cooper (2009, p. 1380) note, 'Although China aspires to be a global leader, it continues to work to constrain the application of exogenous norms' in global health governance. They argue that global health governance institutions emphasise the notion that health is a human right that should be protected by the state and that public health is key for collective security in a globalising world. The Chinese government, by contrast, makes health-related policy changes solely based on its own selfish political and economic calculations and invokes a sovereign right to self-determination as it sees fits (Stevenson and Cooper, 2009). Lee and Chan (2014, p. 298) echo this view, arguing that China stays on the periphery of global health governance because of its dualistic national identities and its efforts to present different images of itself to different audiences. They ascribe a nearly conspiratorial element to China's attitude, saying that any effort to get China to contribute more financially to these institutions 'is a trap [by the West] to exhaust [China's] limited resources.' This has discouraged Chinese health experts from collaborating with global health governance, which further isolates the government from the larger system. The result is an attitude where the government is simultaneously fearful about being left behind but also unmotivated to reshape global health governance institutions (Lee and Chan, 2014).

Even when there have been conscious efforts to reshape global health governance's institutions within international society, China has tended to be conspicuously absent. During the 1990s and 2000s, WHO undertook a massive effort to fundamentally rewrite the International Health Regulations (IHR). Despite the fact that this was one of the largest global health diplomacy efforts undertaken, China had relatively little involvement. It did not take an active role in the negotiations that produced the final version, and it offered little experience or expertise to inform the debates (Lee, et al., 2012).

What makes China's minor role in these revisions all the more curious is that much of the impetus for overhauling the IHR came from China's experience with Severe Acute Respiratory Syndrome (SARS). When SARS first appeared in Guangdong Province in November 2002, the disease had never been seen before. As the outbreak garnered greater international attention, the Chinese government strenuously denied that there was a problem, blocked investigators from meeting patients, and thwarted WHO's efforts to stop SARS' international spread. It maintained this antagonistic posture until April 2003, when it rapidly shifted its policy to welcome global cooperation and sacked a number of high-ranking officials for their inability to stop SARS' spread (Abraham, 2004). SARS was 'a good example of an "exogenous shock"' to global health governance, demonstrating the need for the system to change (Price-Smith, 2009, p. 15). In this case, the Chinese government's efforts to cover up the extent of SARS' spread, its reluctance to cooperate with international organisations, and its obfuscation to domestic and international audiences provided international society with the final validation that it needed to change its norms and expectations regarding disease surveillance (Davies, et al., 2015).

This reluctance extends to other health-related treaties, too. During the negotiations that crafted the Framework Convention on Tobacco Control, China's involvement was driven largely by industry interests rather than broader public health concerns. This attitude may seem odd, but it is worth remembering that China is both the largest producer and largest consumer of tobacco (Lee, et al., 2012). By promoting the concerns of tobacco companies over larger public health interests, China again demonstrated its ambivalent attitude towards global health governance (though it was not the only country that tried to protect its tobacco industry).

While there certainly is space to criticise China's reluctance to engage with global health governance, it is important to remember that China has not completely shunned these institutions. There is no clearer sign of its interest in engaging with WHO than Margaret Chan. The Chinese government actively promoted Chan's candidacy for WHO Director-General, just a few years after it had been criticised by WHO for its failures in responding to SARS (*People's Daily*, 2006b). China's actions could be perceived as recognition that working with WHO is the best way to help craft the norms and values underlying global health governance. Lo (2010, p. 23) notes, 'The presence of Margaret Chan – a Chinese citizen – as Director-General of WHO could give China even more of an opportunity to become *the* leader in global health governance.' On the other hand, the move could be interpreted as a cynical attempt to block future reforms. China may have feared sanctioning by WHO or being subject to more intrusive surveillance efforts. It may have also feared that the SARS experience could give credence to Taiwan's efforts to join WHO on its own. With one of its own citizens as Director-General, China could theoretically prevent WHO from introducing policies that would challenge its sovereignty (Chan, 2011). While it is impossible to know the Chinese government's exact motivation, it is worth noting that China's increased engagement with WHO is in line with its general trend of joining international organisations and signing on to various treaties and cooperation agreements (Chan, 2011).

China's approach to global health governance has evolved considerably since the 1960s when it started deploying medical teams in developing countries. In the early days, China's approach could be described as largely defensive. The medical teams were an effort to counter both the Soviet Union and the United States and build alliances with potentially friendly states. The country embraced a bilateral approach to global health issues, preferring to work in a one-on-one relationship with recipient states selected specifically because of their real or perceived strategic importance (Huang, 2010). China eschewed the multilateral elements of global health governance because 'it regarded the international system as alien and illegitimate' (Huang, 2010, p. 110). Until the 1980s, then, it would be difficult to argue that China saw much, if any, value within global health governance.

China's attitude towards global health governance institutions starts to shift during the 1990s. Huang (2010) ascribes this change to the government developing a new sense of accountability and commitment to the international system, a desire to promote an image as an internationally responsible citizen, and a recognition of human security and non-traditional approaches to security. He also cites SARS as providing an impetus for further engagement with global health governance. The outbreak undermined the country's long efforts to improve its international image and project an air of legitimacy and competency. As a result, the government showed a willingness to collaborate with WHO and regional ASEAN partners for health assistance because it recognised both that it lacked the necessary expertise to handle outbreaks on its own and that it had demonstrated its vulnerability. 'In an age of globalization', Huang (2010, p. 121) argues, 'it [the Chinese government] can no longer monopolize information or act alone in addressing NTS [non-traditional security] challenges.'

China finds itself in an interesting position within the global economy and global health governance. The sheer size of its economy raises expectations about significant contributions to various international organisations and health campaigns. On a per capita basis, though, China is a middle-income country. It is precisely in these middle-income countries where the bulk of the world's poor live and where the global burden of disease is shifting. While this means that middle-income states are likely to need additional resources in order to address the health concerns of their citizens, their relative wealth means that many of them are no longer eligible for funding from leading global health governance institutions (Glassman, et al., 2013). This may help explain why the Chinese government is contributing funds to leading international health organisations, but not at the level that might be expected given the size of the Chinese economy.

Aside from its financial commitments, the Chinese government has started to participate in global health governance in other ways. One of the most visible is through contributing its medical personnel to United Nations peacekeeping missions in Africa and for global disease outbreak responses. Nearly 900 Chinese medical personnel served on eight UN-sponsored African peacekeeping missions in 2005 (Sutter, 2008). Fung (2016) says that China's contribution of medical teams to peacekeeping missions provides the necessary backbone that makes such operations possible. More recently, the Chinese government turned to the People's Liberation Army to provide assistance in West Africa to combat Ebola. Troops constructed health facilities, military scientists conducted research on Ebola treatments and vaccines, and much of China's aid to combat Ebola was funnelled through the military (Tiezzi, 2014).

## China and health diplomacy in Africa

Despite (or perhaps because of) its increasing prominence in international relations, health diplomacy frequently gets defined in different ways by different audiences. Feldbaum and Michaud (2012) identify a number of usages for the term, ranging from the role of globalisation and non-state actors in global health to using foreign policy programmes to support global health to recognising how the benefits of health interventions can promote a country's foreign policy interests. Katz, et al. (2011) distinguish between health's role in more traditional state-based diplomatic efforts to those programmes that involve a multiplicity of stakeholders or operate through informal means. The World Health Organization (n.d.) describes health diplomacy as being the intersection of public health, foreign policy, and trade to implement more pro-active procedures to address health problems and build health systems capacity. In all of these definitions, though, there is a recognition that health and foreign policy are interrelated and can be harnessed by states for a variety of purposes.

China's health diplomacy efforts go back to the 1960s. Zhou Enlai inaugurated China's efforts to support African health care systems when he dispatched the first Chinese medical teams to Algeria (Eisenman, 2007). These initial programmes provided necessary personnel and supplies, but they also sought to position China vis-à-vis the United States and Soviet Union in the midst of the Cold War. This allowed it to build support among developing countries, particularly newly independent African states.

During the 1970s and 1980s, Chinese health diplomacy in Africa became less prominent. This coincided with Africa's decreased importance to China and the country's economic reforms under Deng Xiaoping (Taylor, 1998). It was not until the late 1990s that China sought to re-engage with Africa in a serious, sustained manner, and those efforts included health diplomacy (Chan, et al., 2011).

This importance of Chinese health diplomacy in Africa became clear at the first Forum on China-Africa Cooperation (FOCAC) in October 2000 in Beijing. Bringing together leaders from 45 African states and top Chinese government officials, the summit was a concrete demonstration of China's renewed commitment to Africa. China forgave US$1.2 billion in foreign debt owed by African states and pledged to increase its aid contributions to the continent in all realms, including health. Three years later, when the FOCAC re-convened in Addis Ababa, the Chinese government made more explicit health diplomacy promises. It specifically highlighted the treatment and prevention of disease as one of its priority areas, pledging additional funds for these efforts. Health also featured prominently at the third FOCAC meeting in November 2006. Not only did the Chinese government pledge to double its aid to Africa by 2009 and offer US$5 billion in preferential loans to the continent, but it also emphasised the prominent role of health and education programmes in its African aid efforts (Sutter, 2008). At this same meeting, the Chinese government pledged to build 30 hospitals in Africa, provide US$37.5 million in grants for anti-malarial drugs developed and manufactured in China, and develop 30 demonstration centres for the treatment and prevention of malaria. It also renewed its commitment to send medical teams to the best of its ability for the next three years (*People's Daily*, 2006a).

After the 2015 FOCAC Summit in Johannesburg, public health and medical care had a prominent place in the final action plan. The representatives of the assembled African governments 'expresse[d] [their] appreciation for China's continued assistance to countries in need … and further appreciate[d] China's continued support to reconstruct public health, economic, and societal systems of the affected countries during the post-Ebola period.' The Chinese government pledged a number of specific steps that it would undertake to support African health systems, including:

1. Assist with improving disease surveillance and epidemiological systems;
2. Strengthen efforts to prevent and treat malaria and other infectious diseases;
3. Support cooperation between 20 Chinese hospitals and 20 African hospitals on demonstration projects;
4. Continue training doctors, nurses, and other health care workers for Africa;
5. Support building an African Union Disease Control Centre and other efforts to enhance the continent's medical research and diagnostic capabilities;
6. Continue sending medical teams from China to African states;
7. Encourage joint medical and pharmaceutical efforts between Chinese and African firms;
8. Improve the continent's health infrastructure;
9. Improve access to maternal and child health and reproductive health services; and
10. Facilitate high-level exchanges between health policymakers.

(Forum on China-Africa Cooperation, 2015a, n.p.)

To support China's ambitious plans for health in Africa, President Xi Jinping announced that his government would make US$60 billion in various funding support programmes (Forum on China-Africa Cooperation, 2015b). This is a tripling of the funding that China has previously made available after FOCAC meetings (Sun, 2015).

Chinese health diplomacy in Africa takes three key forms. First, as it has since 1963, China deploys country medical teams (CMTs) throughout Africa. These CMTs remain an important element of Chinese health diplomacy in Africa today. In 2014, China deployed 43 such teams to 42 different African states at a cost of US$20–40 million (Lin et al., 2016). CMTs generally serve a two-year term in the receiving country, frequently serving in rural, underserved communities. In addition to sending general practitioners, these teams frequently included a broad array of specialists (Hsu, 2008). While the Chinese national government negotiates the agreements to provide medical personnel to African states, the implementation of these agreements falls to individual provinces. Particular Chinese provinces are linked with one or more particular African countries (Thompson, 2005). Shen and Fan (2014) describe this strategy as provincial diplomacy because the provinces are responsible for implementing a larger national foreign policy plan. While this can build longer-term ties, it can also cause unevenness in the scope and quality of deployed medical teams and complicate efforts to craft a coherent national-level health diplomacy strategy. CMTs are also an important element of China's emphasis on building human resources for health. Between 2010 and 2012, the Chinese government says that it trained more than 3,000 medical personnel throughout Africa, either by providing scholarships for them to study in China or by creating training programmes in African states (State Council of the People's Republic of China, 2014).

Second, China has focused on the development of the health care infrastructure in receiving states. In a 2014 white paper on its foreign aid, the Chinese government reported that it had supported the construction of approximately 80 hospitals and health clinics around the world between 2010 and 2012. These efforts 'effectively alleviated the shortage of medical and health facilities in recipient countries' (State Council of the People's Republic of China, 2014, n.p.). Looking at Africa specifically, the Chinese government constructed 30 hospitals and 30 malaria treatment centres, and helped to build the region's health care capacities.

Third, China has emphasised providing equipment, supplies, and drugs. These efforts include approximately US$120 million in medical supplies and equipment between 2010 and 2012, with a particular emphasis on malaria treatments (State Council of the People's Republic of China, 2014). Though HIV and AIDS receive more funding than any other single global health issue from donors, the Chinese government has provided almost no money for the disease. It has instead identified malaria as its top priority among specific health conditions (Grépin, et al., 2014). This is likely connected to its development of artemisinin, an anti-malaria drug created from a plant commonly used in Chinese traditional medicine. Between 2005 and 2014, the number of artemisinin treatment courses for malaria shot up from 11 million to 337 million (World Health Organization, 2016).

These engagement strategies make China an increasingly important global donor for health aid – not just in Africa, but around the world. Understanding just how important, though, is incredibly difficult. China is the most significant foreign aid donor that is not a part of the Development Assistance Committee (DAC) of the Organization for Economic Cooperation and Development (Harman and Williams, 2014). DAC member states are the traditional aid donors, and they are required to have a framework for providing development assistance and engage in monitoring and evaluation activities of their efforts (Organization for Economic Cooperation and Development, 2016). While non-members of DAC play an increasing role in providing aid, there is less transparency for understanding how much and where they are providing aid. This is particularly true with China, where the government does not release its foreign aid figures due to domestic and international political sensitivities (Florini, et al. 2012). As a result, researchers employ a variety of different strategies to try and triangulate information to estimate aid flows.

Drawing on the AidData database, Grépin, et al. (2014) find that China provided approximately US$3 billion in bilateral or regional health aid to African states between 2000 and 2012. If this figure is correct, then it would make China the ninth largest provider of bilateral health aid in Africa during this time period. While the total amount is relatively large, they note that this aid is spread over a dozen years and approximately 50 countries (Grépin, et al., 2014). Using different sources over a shorter period of time, Florini, et al. (2012) estimate that China contributed slightly more than US$300 million in cash and in-kind contributions in development assistance for health overall in 2007 and 2008. They found that most of the funding was distributed bilaterally, but organisations like WHO, United Nations, and the Global Fund to Fight AIDS, Tuberculosis, and Malaria received about US$35 million. Interestingly, during this same time period, China both gave the Global Fund US$2 million and received US$1 billion from the organisation for its own programmes (Florini, et al., 2012).

It is notable that China's development assistance for health overwhelmingly goes through bilateral, as opposed to multilateral, channels. China's preference for bilateral channels likely reflects its relative newness to the development assistance for health realm, the unsettled foreign aid bureaucracy within the country, its interests in increasing the sovereign capacities of its recipient states, and its concerns about the role of civil society organisations and nongovernmental organisations in service delivery (Florini, et al., 2012; Huang, 2010).

## Questions about Chinese health diplomacy

Debates remain about the underlying motivation of Chinese health diplomacy. Other countries like Brazil and India have engaged in health diplomacy efforts premised on building South–South solidarity, but China's programmes are both more extensive and better financed than other efforts. The Chinese government has frequently presented its programmes as altruistic efforts to demonstrate South–South solidarity and provide an alternative model for development (Lin, et al., 2016). China is instead providing health aid with 'no strings attached' in contrast to the West's insistence on conditionality. Others have countered that China wants to use health diplomacy to promote its economic prosperity. The government will target its health aid towards countries that have natural resources that it wants, and it will seek to build new markets for its health and pharmaceutical goods (Thompson, 2005; Youde, 2010). While this is a popular line of argumentation, quantitative studies find little to no correlation between the African states that receive the most Chinese health aid and their economic value to China (Grépin, et al., 2014). A third line of thought suggests that health diplomacy is part of China's larger diplomatic strategy more akin to a 'hearts-and-minds' approach that will make people in other countries feel more favourably inclined towards China and willing to support its international efforts. In particular, China seeks to counter the influence of Taiwan and build support for its positions towards Tibet and the Uyghur people (Chan, et al., 2010). Finally, there is a suggestion that the Chinese government actually lacks a coordinated health diplomacy strategy. Because its efforts are shared among at least 11 different national-level ministries and implemented at the subnational level, health diplomacy is less of a conscious plan and more of a series of ad hoc policies (Shen and Fan, 2014).

The importance of understanding the reasons for China's health diplomacy engagement relate to its continuing and future engagement. China has largely concentrated on bilateral efforts in one region of the world, but it has shown an increased interest in multilateral efforts. If its health diplomacy is largely oriented towards promoting its own political and economic interests, then there is little reason to believe that China will play a major role in global health governance. If, on the other hand, China sees health diplomacy as part of its responsibilities as an increasingly powerful economic and political player in the international system, then global health governance may become a more important element of China's international engagement – and questions will emerge about whether the Chinese government will work within the existing rules of global health governance or seek to change them to better suit its own ideas and preferences. Jing, et al. (2011) argue that China is increasingly interested in playing an active role in multilateral global health governance, though many of the examples they cite include situations in which China is a recipient of assistance rather than the provider of assistance.

## Conclusion

China's engagement with global health governance is evolving. To date, it has focused primarily on its bilateral relationships with African states, but there is evidence that the Chinese government is evincing some interest in engaging with multilateral health organisations to a greater degree. China's health diplomacy in Africa has concentrated primarily on supporting infrastructure, human resources, providing supplies and drugs, and working on anti-malaria efforts. Between its financial support for some intergovernmental organisations working on health issues and its willingness to deploy its soldiers on health-related missions, the country is taking tentative steps towards more sustained engagement. What remains to be seen is whether this engagement will bring with it efforts to change existing global health governance structures.

## References

Abraham, T. (2004) *Twenty-First Century Plague: The story of SARS*, Baltimore, MD: Johns Hopkins University Press.
Chan, G., Lee, P., and Chan, L. (2011) *China Engages Global Governance: A new world order in the making?*, New York: Routledge.
Chan, L. (2011) *China Engages Global Health Governance: Responsible Stakeholder or system-transformer?*, New York: Palgrave Macmillan.
Chan, L., Chen, L., and Xu, J. (2010) 'China's engagement with global health diplomacy: was SARS a watershed moment?', *PLoS Science*, 7: 1–6.
Chan, L., Lee, P., and Chan, G. (2009) 'China engages global health governance: processes and dilemmas', *Global Public Health*, 4: 1–30.

Clark, I. (2014) 'International society and China: the power of norms and the norms of power', *Chinese Journal of International Politics*, 7: 315–40.

Davies, S., Kamradt-Scott, A., and Rushton, S. (2015) *Disease Diplomacy: International norms and global health security*, Baltimore, MD: Johns Hopkins University Press.

Eisenman, J. (2007) 'China's post-Cold War strategy in Africa: examining Beijing's methods and objectives', In: J. Eisenman, E. Heginbotham, and D. Mitchell (Eds.) *China and the Developing World: Beijing's strategy for the twenty-first century*, Armonk, NY: M.E. Sharpe, pp. 29–59.

Feldbaum, H. and Michaud, J. (2012) 'Health diplomacy and the enduring relevance of foreign policy interests', *PLoS Medicine*, 7: 1–6.

Florini, A., Nachiappan, K., Pang, T., and Pilcavage, C. (2012) 'Global health governance: analysing China, India, and Japan as global health aid donors', *Global Policy*, 3: 336–47.

Forum on China-Africa Cooperation (2015a) 'The Forum on China-Africa cooperation Johannesburg action plan (2016–2018)', available at www.focac.org/eng/ltda/dwjbzjjhys_1/t1327961.htm (accessed on 24 January 2017).

Forum on China-Africa Cooperation (2015b) 'Xi announces 10 major China-Africa cooperation plans for coming 3 years', available at www.focac.org/eng/ltda/dwjbzjjhys_1/t1322068.htm (accessed on 24 January 2017).

Fung, C. (2016) 'China's troop contributions to UN peacekeeping', *Peace Brief, United States Institute of Peace*, available at www.usip.org/sites/default/files/PB212-China-s-Troop-Contributions-to-UN-Peacekeeping.pdf (accessed on 26 January 2017).

Glassman, A., Duran, D., and Sumner, A. (2013) 'Global health and the new bottom billion: what do shifts in global poverty and disease burden mean for donor agencies?' *Global Policy*, 4: 1–14.

Grépin, K., Fan, V., Shen, G., and Chen, L. (2014) 'China's role as a global health donor in Africa: what can we learn from studying underreported resource flows?' *Globalization and Health*, 10: 1–11, available at https://globalizationandhealth.biomedcentral.com/articles/10.1186/s12992-014-0084-6 (accessed on 26 January 2017).

Harman, S. and Williams, D. (2014) 'International development in transition', *International Affairs*, 90: 925–41.

Hsu, E. (2008) 'Medicine as business: Chinese medicine in Tanzania', In: C. Alden, D. Large, and R. Soares de Oliveira (Eds.) *China Returns to Africa: A superpower and a continent*, New York: Columbia University Press, pp. 221–35.

Huang, Y. (2010) 'Pursuing health as foreign policy: the case of China', *Indiana Journal of Global Legal Studies*, 17: 105–46.

Jing, X., Peilong, L., and Yan, G. (2011) 'Health diplomacy in China', *Global Health Governance*, 4: 1–12.

Katz, R., Kornblet, S., Arnold, G., Lief, E., and Fischer, J. (2011) 'Defining health diplomacy: changing demands in the era of globalization', *Milbank Quarterly*, 89: 503–23.

Lee, K., Kamradt-Scott, A., Yoon, S., and Xu, J. (2012) 'Asian contributions to three instruments of global health governance', *Global Policy*, 3: 348–61.

Lee, P. and Chan, L. (2014) 'China joins global health governance: new player, more medicines, and new rules?' *Global Governance*, 20: 297–323.

Lin, S., Gao, L., Reyes, M., Cheng, F., Kaufman, J., and El-Sadr, W. (2016) 'China's health assistance to Africa: opportunism or altruism?' *Globalization and Health*, 12: 1–5.

Lo, C. (2010) 'Values to be added to an "Eastphalian order" by emerging China', *Indiana Journal of Global Legal Studies*, 17: 13–25.

Organization for Economic Cooperation and Development (2016) 'DAC members', available at www.oecd.org/dac/dacmembers.htm (accessed on 24 January 2017).

*People's Daily* (2006a) 'China, Africa vow closer cooperation in fighting HIV/AIDS: action plan', 6 November, available at http://english.peopledaily.com.cn/200611/06/eng20061106_318575.html (accessed on 24 January 2017).

*People's Daily* (2006b) 'China throws full support behind Margaret Chan's candidacy for WHO Director-General', 19 September, available at http://en.people.cn/200609/18/eng20060918_303910.html (accessed on 24 January 2017).

Price-Smith, A. (2009) *Contagion and Chaos: Disease, ecology, and national security in the era of globalization*, Cambridge, MA: MIT Press.

Shen, G. and Fan, V. (2014) 'China's provincial diplomacy to Africa: applications to health cooperation', *Contemporary Politics*, 20: 182–208.

State Council of the People's Republic of China (2014) 'China's foreign aid', available at http://english.gov.cn/archive/white_paper/2014/08/23/content_281474982986592.htm (accessed on 26 January 2017).

Stevenson, M. and Cooper, A. (2009) 'Overcoming constraints of state sovereignty: global health governance in Asia', *Third World Quarterly*, 30: 1379–94.

Sun, Y. (2015) 'Xi and the 6th Forum on China Africa Cooperation: major commitments, but with questions', Africa in Focus, 7 December, available at www.brookings.edu/blogs/africa-in-focus/posts/2015/12/07-china-africa-focac-investment-economy-sun (accessed on 24 January 2017).

Sutter, R. (2008) *Chinese Foreign Relations: Power and policy since the Cold War*, Lanham, MD: Rowman and Littlefield.

Tan, Y., Lee, K., and Pang, T. (2012) 'Global health governance and the rise of Asia', *Global Policy*, 3: 324–35.

Taylor, I. (1998) 'China's foreign policy towards Africa in the 1990s', *Journal of Modern African Studies*, 36(3): 443–60.

Thompson, D. (2005) 'China's soft power in Africa: from the "Beijing Consensus" to health diplomacy', *Asia Brief*, 5(21): 1–5.

Tiezzi, S. (2014) 'China's military wages war on Ebola', *The Diplomat*, 31 October, available at http://thediplomat.com/2014/10/chinas-military-wages-war-on-ebola/ (accessed on 24 January 2017).

World Health Organization (n.d.) 'Global health diplomacy', available at www.who.int/trade/diplomacy/en/ (accessed on 20 July 2017).

World Health Organization (2016) 'Q&A on artemisinin resistance', available at http://who.int/malaria/media/artemisinin_resistance_qa/en/ (accessed on 26 January 2017).

Yoon, S. (2008) 'Sovereign dignity, nationalism, and the health of a nation: a study of China's response in combat of epidemics', *Studies in Ethnicity and Nationalism*, 8: 80–100.

Youde, J. (2010) 'China's health diplomacy in Africa', *China: An International Journal*, 8: 151–63.

# 16

# Aiming for synergies between global health security and global health equity, with help from a Framework Convention on Global Health

*Gorik Ooms and Albrecht Jahn*

## Introduction

Most definitions of global health include a reference to equity. For example, Koplan, et al. (2009, p. 1995) define global health as 'an area for study, research, and practice that places a priority on improving health and achieving equity in health for all people worldwide.' Equity means the absence of inequities, and the term inequity, as Whitehead (1992, p. 431) explains, 'refers to differences which are *unnecessary* and *avoidable*, but in addition are considered *unfair* and *unjust*'. In this chapter, we will explore the challenges that come with applying the term inequity at the global level; for now, we can conclude that global health is – or should be – a collective effort to reduce differences in health outcomes between all people worldwide that are unnecessary, avoidable, and unjust.

Wondering whether the politics of global health are also concerned with global health equity, Labonté and Gagnon (2010) analysed governmental foreign policy statements on global health. They concluded that although '[d]evelopment, human rights and ethical/moral arguments for global health assistance, the traditional "low politics" of foreign policy, are present in discourse', 'most states, even when committed to health as a foreign policy goal, still make decisions primarily on the basis of the "high politics" of national security and economic material interests' (Labonté and Gagnon, 2010, p. 1). The preoccupation of the politics of global health with global health security is not new; it has been at the centre of most health-related international cooperation, long before the terms 'global health' and 'global health security' were coined (Ooms and Hammonds, 2016). The eight International Sanitary Conferences, convened between 1851 and 1894, were all about the spread of infectious disease in Europe, not about health equity in Europe (Huber, 2006).

Still, efforts to improve global health security can contribute to global health equity, as many inequalities in health outcomes between all people worldwide are still caused by infectious diseases: infectious disease control reduces health inequalities. Nonetheless, we will argue that preoccupation of the politics of global health with global health security is problematic, as it falls short of the expectations of global health equity, and as it is inefficient in its own purpose (the latter precisely because of the first). International efforts to promote global health security in isolation are perceived as an *unfair offer* from the wealthiest to the poorer countries, and the governments of poorer countries are becoming reluctant to lend their support. To improve both global health security and global health equity, a clearer allocation of common but differentiated responsibilities (CBDR) at national and international levels is needed. A Framework Convention on Global Health (FCGH) would allow to clearly articulate the responsibilities of states, domestically and internationally, to improve global health security as well as to promote global health equity.

## Global health equity

While most people would agree intuitively that the present situation of health outcomes in the world is problematic – for example, the finding that under-5 mortality is about eight times higher in Africa than in Europe (World Health Organization, 2017, p. 92) – we have no widely accepted definition or description of global health equity. When we transfer accepted definitions of health equity that were developed for the national level to the global level, we run into problems.

As mentioned earlier, for Whitehead (1992), the term inequity refers to inequalities that are *unnecessary* and *avoidable*, and also *unfair* and *unjust*. She adds that 'in order to describe a certain situation as inequitable, the *cause* has to be examined and *judged* to be unfair in the *context* of what is going on in the rest of society' (Whitehead, 1992, p. 431). While Whitehead's definition or description of health equity remains widely accepted, several scholars have added, and emphasised, the importance of a fair and inclusive process to decide the magnitude of resources society should allocate to tackle inequalities and how to distribute them: 'If we have no consensus on principles capable of resolving disputes about resource allocation for health and health care, then we must find a fair process whose outcomes we can accept as just or fair' (Daniels, 2008, p. 109).

With these principles only, it is difficult to describe what global health equity means. It is relatively easy to identify health inequalities between countries, for example the huge difference in under-5 mortality between Africa and Europe mentioned previously. This stark *inequality* is probably avoidable, at least to some extent, through international assistance and other means. It also seems unfair and unjust, certainly from the African perspective. However, confirming that it is unfair and unjust requires at least a rough account of what justice and fairness would demand. What exactly should the international community do to reduce this inequality, not as a matter of charity or compassion, but as a matter of fairness and justice? This inequality has multiple causes, but an obvious one is the inequality in wealth and economic product, leading to an equally obvious inequality in available and accessible water, nutrition, and health care. International assistance can mitigate the latter and is part of 'what is going on' in the world; part of the context that we need to consider when deciding whether inequalities are also inequities. Can we argue that insufficient international assistance causes the inequality?

Not everyone would agree that fairness and justice demand greater international assistance, or redistribution of resources across borders. Some of the proponents of so-called 'statist' accounts of global justice argue that we simply do not have the international institutions required for a fair redistribution of resources across borders (Nagel, 2005); others argue that we do not and should not have such institutions, for the sake of allowing every nation to take its own decisions (Miller, 2007). The proponents of so-called 'cosmopolitan' accounts of global justice start from a different premise. Moellendorf (2002, p. 49), for example, emphasises the principle of equal opportunity: 'If equality of opportunity were realized, a child growing up in rural Mozambique would be statistically as likely as the child of a senior executive at a Swiss bank to reach the position of the latter's parent.' In the absence of agreement on these principles, we cannot agree on which global health inequalities are avoidable. Returning to the example of the difference in under-5 mortality between Africa and Europe, those who side with 'statist' accounts of global justice are likely to focus on the in-country inequalities – which do account for almost half of the global inequality (Amouzou, et al., 2014) – and consider the remaining inequality as unavoidable (i.e., not an inequity). Those who side with the 'cosmopolitan' accounts of global justice would probably qualify (or classify) a much wider scope of the existing inequality as an inequity.

At this point, we have to start looking for a fair and inclusive process. But we do not have that, at the global level, at least not the global equivalent of the processes we have at the national level, like parliaments agreeing on budgets and ministries of health deciding on the allocation of agreed budget envelopes; unless we consider the combination of international law, United Nations' agencies, and collective deliberations and resolutions – such as the Millennium Development Goals (MDGs) and now the Sustainable Development Goals (SDGs) – as a somewhat fair and somewhat inclusive process. After all, no nation has been forced to ratify a human rights treaty, or to endorse the MDGs or SDGs. Then the right to health as enshrined in the International Covenant on Economic, Social and Cultural Rights – including a provision about international obligations to provide assistance – provides a benchmark for assessing which health inequalities between countries are unjust (and therefore, inequities), at least for the 164 states that ratified it. Furthermore, the health SDG – including the goal of universal health coverage – provides an additional benchmark for all United Nations' members and SDG 10 (reduced inequalities) calls for social protection policies, in order to achieve greater equality. This approach allows us to judge health inequalities between countries that are, first, incompatible with the right to health as enshrined in the International Covenant on Economic, Social and Cultural Rights or with the health SDG, and, second, remediable through increased international cooperation, as global health inequities.

## Global health security

Global health security is – much like global health equity – a frequently used but ill-defined expression. As Aldis (2008, p. 369) explains,

> [p]olicymakers in industrialized countries emphasize protection of their populations especially against external threats, for example terrorism and pandemics; while health workers and policymakers in developing countries and within the United Nations system understand the term in a broader public health context.

In this chapter, we will use 'narrowly defined health security' as shorthand for health security that emphasises infectious disease control, and 'broadly defined health security' as shorthand for health security that rests on strong and effective health systems.

This difference in approaches could be explained by a different understanding of the importance of health systems for health security: wealthier countries think it is possible to improve health security without strengthening health systems; poorer countries think that stronger health systems are required to improve health security. If that were the main cause of the difference, empirical evidence should be able to resolve it. But we would argue that the difference in approaches is essentially a normative one: poorer countries think the narrow definition of health security is unfair, and that is the main reason why they oppose it. They link health security with the concept of human security, which is a much broader (and more demanding) concept: 'to protect the vital core of all human lives in ways that enhance human freedoms and human fulfillment' (Ogata and Sen, 2003, p. 4).

Furthermore, as Rushton (2011, p. 779) argues, 'there is in fact a good deal more consensus than we are often led to believe' on the meaning of health security:

> In particular there is a high level of agreement evident over what the major threats to 'health security' are and what should be done about them. These are a particular set of health risks which are primarily seen as major threats by Western developed nations, and contemporary global responses – often couched in the language of global health security – have a tendency to focus on containment rather than prevention.
>
> *Rushton, 2011, p. 779*

In other words, the consensus in practice is on narrowly defined health security. This explains the increasing discontentment among the poorer countries, who feel that the global health security agenda 'predicates Western, high-income countries' interests above others' (Kamradt-Scott, 2015, p. 153).

We agree with Aldis (2008, p. 369) that the difference in approaches to global health security is setting 'the stage for breakdown in global cooperation'. Aldis' primary reference is 'the crisis that followed Indonesia's refusal to share virus isolates from human cases of H5N1 influenza A infection (avian influenza), on the grounds that Indonesia was unlikely to receive any benefits including vaccines or technology transfer' (Aldis, 2008, p. 372) and the following 'failure of a major international nego-tiation, the Intergovernmental Meeting on Influenza Viruses and Benefit Sharing in November 2007' (Aldis, 2008, p. 373). In 2011, however, after many years of negotiation, an international agreement on a pandemic influenza preparedness (PIP) framework for the sharing of influenza viruses and access to vaccines was reached (Fidler and Gostin, 2011), and we are not aware of any similar crisis since then. Case closed? We do not think so. Aldis' (2008, p. 373) point that the '[s]trengthening of surveillance for epidemic-prone diseases brings little benefit to any country which lacks the public health infrastruc-ture necessary for an effective response' remains valid. And while we cannot exclude that crises like Indonesia's refusal to share virus samples will occur again, we think it is quite plausible – and indeed, already occurring – that developing countries are loathing to strengthen disease surveillance in a way they know will not protect their own people but merely allow rapid containment of disease outbreaks. One should not expect reluctantly implemented disease surveillance to be highly effective disease surveillance. Thus, global health security's narrow focus on 'health risks which are primarily seen as major threats by Western developed nations', and global responses aiming for 'containment rather than prevention' (Rushton, 2011, p. 779) may be a self-defeating approach: it undermines the necessary cooperation, rather than fostering it.

## Synergies and tensions

Considering the discontentment about the global health security agenda, can there be synergies between that agenda and the goal of global health equity? We think there can be. At a practical level: if we take the right to health and the health SDG as benchmarks for judging whether health inequalities between countries are also health inequities (unfair, unjust), then we cannot deny that both the right to health and the health SDG include effective infectious disease control. Article 12 of the International Covenant on Economic, Social and Cultural Rights has two sections. The first defines the right to health in general, and the second breaks it down into more concrete steps for states to take; one of these steps (article 12.1(c)) is '[t]he prevention, treatment and control of epidemic, endemic, occupational and other diseases'. Several targets of the health SDG are about or require infectious disease control. Thus, efforts to improve global health security contribute to global health equity, albeit only to a part of global health equity. For example, they do not contribute to '[t]he creation of conditions which would assure access to all medical service and medical attention in the event of sickness' (article 12.1.(d) of the International Covenant on Economic, Social and Cultural Rights) if the sickness has a non-communicable cause.

Still at a practical level, efforts to improve global health equity would also contribute to global health security. Disease surveillance and early intervention are essential for global health security. To ensure that a new epidemic is detected rapidly, and followed by appropriate intervention, it is essential that people who feel sick go to a health facility. If they are reluctant to do so – because they know they will have to pay user fees they cannot afford, because they know that in many cases the health facility cannot provide the appropriate diagnosis or treatment, or because they know that there is a high probability that the under-paid health worker will be rather unfriendly – new epidemics can spread widely before anyone is aware of them. Thus, the realisation of all elements of the right to health and the health SDG would contribute to global health security.

At a more conceptual level, it is quite difficult to think of global health equity without having a sizeable envelope of financial and technical resources to share across borders. If there are no funds allocated to (re)distribute across borders, then every country is left to its own devices, and health inequalities between countries would be unavoidable (and therefore not health inequities). As mentioned earlier, the history of health-related international cooperation started with efforts to improve health security: the International Sanitary Conferences of the nineteenth century were about health security, not about health equity. Solidarity did not drive this cooperation, enlightened self-interest did. However, now that we have a practice of international assistance, we can start discussing whether it is allocated to the right priorities: we can start questioning its fairness and push it towards more equity.

We would argue that discussion about health equity at the national level followed a similar pattern. The first societal efforts to improve public health at a national scale were probably more driven by the enlightened self-interest of the wealthier citizens – who had to agree to pay for such efforts – than by solidarity. The Sanitary Movement in nineteenth-century England was born out of fear of infectious disease: 'Without being his brother's keeper, anyone who valued his life felt it eminently desirable not to have virulent diseases and the conditions that fostered them too close at hand' (Rosen, 1993, p. 184). Then, '[a] second wave of public health, roughly spanning 1890–1950, was partly precipitated by the discovery of poor health in Boer War recruits' (Hanlon, et al., 2011, p. 31). While some may argue that ensuring young men's fitness to become soldiers is a kind of solidarity, we would rather qualify this as enlightened self-interest. In any case, these efforts created the institutions and the budgets that could then be criticised for not being equitable, for not focusing on the right priorities, for valuing some lives over others. And that is what is happening now, at the global level: institutions and budgets that may have been created with the primary intention to protect the citizens of wealthier states against disease threats emerging from poorer corners of the world are being criticised for 'misfinancing global health' (Sridhar and Rudan, 2015, p. 151).

## Allocating national and international responsibilities: a Framework Convention on Global Health

According to Nagel (2005, p. 146), '[w]e are unlikely to see the spread of global justice in the long run unless we first create strong supranational institutions that do not aim at justice but that pursue common interests and reflect the inequalities of bargaining power among existing states'. With some reluctance, we tend to agree with this statement. The question then becomes: at what point are supranational institutions strong enough to be improved, rather than undermined, by critiques about their unfairness? For example, at what point can we criticise the Global Fund to fight AIDS, Tuberculosis and Malaria for ignoring all other health issues, without risking that some wealthier states will use that as an alibi to withdraw their commitment to global health overall? Another important question arises at the same time: what is the bargaining power of poorer states, when it comes to global health equity and global health security? They could withdraw from global health security cooperation as a way to force wealthier states to invest more in global health equity, but if such a strategy backfires, it would lead to less global health security and less global health equity.

In our opinion, one of the crucial elements to escape from this conundrum is a process that allows for negotiation – and regular renegotiation – of the national and international responsibilities of states, for global health security and for global health equity. A Framework Convention on Global Health (FCGH) could provide exactly that.

Several papers have been written on the idea of a FCGH since Gostin (2007) launched his bold idea in 2007, and different people are starting to have different ideas on what it should include. We will focus on Gostin's 2012 paper in the *Journal of the American Medical Association* to summarise the key features. Like the Framework Convention on Tobacco Control (or indeed other framework conventions), it would have a single binding treaty 'using an incremental process whereby states negotiate a framework with key normative standards' (Gostin, 2012, p. 2088), and several protocols to subsequently agree on more detailed obligations. Gostin's paper mentions different *objectives* – e.g., 'Define state responsibilities for the health of their domestic populations', 'Define international responsibilities to provide sustainable funding' – and different *modalities* – e.g., 'Establish domestic funding targets covering health care, public health, and social determinants of health, with timelines for compliance', 'Establish a global health financing framework to ensure reliable funding' (Gostin, 2012, p. 2089). One could also imagine protocols that are candid about the tension between global health security and global health equity; for example, one protocol on shared responsibilities for the implementation of the International Health Regulations – which are focused on global health security – and another protocol on shared responsibilities for universal health coverage – which, according to the World Health Organization (WHO), is a 'practical expression of the concern for health equity and the right to health' (WHO, 2012, p. 3).

Hoffman and Røttingen (2013, p. 117) question the feasibility of a FCGH, and argue that 'any proposal for new international law must be fully evaluated and compared with benefits and competing alternatives to ensure adoption will not create more problems than solutions'. While we agree with the importance of a deep evaluation, the alternatives they propose – interestingly, but somewhat confusingly, as 'options for strengthening the FCGH proposal' (Hoffman and Røttingen, 2013, p. 127) – do not convince us, but rather highlight the unique (potential) advantages of a FCGH. The alternatives to (or options for strengthening) the FCGH proposal proposed by Hoffman and Røttingen are:

1. Abandoning international law as the primary commitment mechanism and instead pursuing agreement towards a less formal 'framework for global health' which has fewer costs and can better engage non-state actors as appropriate;
2. Seeking fundamental constitutional reform of WHO to address weaknesses in its architecture and broader gaps in global governance for health;
3. Mobilising for a separate political platform through which states can negotiate global health issues that completely bypasses WHO and encourages it to specialise into a purely technical agency; or
4. Narrowing the scope of sought changes to one particular governance issue, such as financing for global health needs, and seeking more precise binding commitments for domestic and external financing.

Each of these options entails the risk of divorcing global health security from global health equity. The first option would rely on voluntary cooperation that can be revoked – partially and integrally – at any time. The second option – a stronger WHO – would certainly help a FCGH, and vice versa: a FCGH would strengthen WHO. However, a WHO that continues to rely on earmarked funding from wealthier states will continue to prioritise the issues that matter most for wealthier states, and that is likely to be global health security rather than global health equity. The third option – a separate political platform, bypassing WHO – is one we do not fully understand. Should WHO then focus on global health equity and a separate political platform on global health security? This may already be happening with the creation of the Global Health Security Agenda (Ooms, et al., 2017). Or should it be the other way around: WHO focusing on global health security and another platform of global health equity? In both cases, global health security would be divorced from global health equity. The fourth option – an FCGH focusing on financing – would arguably not separate global health security from global health equity. However, it would separate commitments about financial efforts from commitments about other efforts, and that seems untenable in the long run.

If, at the national level, in many countries, health security evolved into health equity – and enlightened self-interest evolved into solidarity – it is because health security efforts where governed by institutions that were accountable to their constituencies, because these constituencies claimed equity for all, instead of security for some, and because the institutions had the power to make the dissenting members of their constituencies align. At the global level, we do not have these institutions.

A binding framework treaty, under which cooperation for global health security is linked with cooperation for global health equity, is probably the closest we can get to a fair and inclusive process at the global level.

## References

Aldis, W. (2008) 'Health security as a public health concept: a critical analysis', *Health Policy and Planning*, 23(6): 369–75.

Amouzou, A., Kozuki, N., Gwatkin, and D.R. (2014) 'Where is the gap? The contribution of disparities within developing countries to global inequalities in under-five mortality', *BMC Public Health*, 14(1): 216.

Daniels, N. (2008) *Just Health: Meeting health needs fairly*, Cambridge: Cambridge University Press.

Fidler, D.P. and Gostin, L.O. (2011) 'The WHO pandemic influenza preparedness framework: a milestone in global governance for health', *JAMA*, 306(2): 200–1.

Gostin, L.O. (2007) 'A proposal for a framework convention on global health', *Journal of International Economic Law*, 10(4): 989–1008.

Gostin, L.O. (2012) 'A framework convention on global health: health for all, justice for all', *JAMA*, 307(19): 2087–92.

Hanlon, P., Carlisle, S., Hannah, M., Reilly, D., and Lyon, A. (2011) 'Making the case for a "fifth wave" in public health', *Public health*, 125(1): 30–6.

Hoffman, S.J. and Røttingen, J.A. (2013) 'Dark sides of the proposed Framework Convention on Global Health's many virtues: a systematic review and critical analysis', *Health and Human Rights Journal*, 15(1): 117–34.

Huber, V. (2006) 'The unification of the globe by disease? The international sanitary conferences on cholera, 1851–1894', *The Historical Journal*, 49(2): 453–76.

Kamradt-Scott, A. (2015) *Managing Global Health Security: The World Health Organization and disease outbreak control*, Basingstoke: Palgrave MacMillan.

Koplan, J.P., Bond, T.C., Merson, M.H., Reddy, K.S., Rodriguez, M.H., Sewankambo, N.K., and Wasserheit, J.N. (2009) 'Towards a common definition of global health', *The Lancet*, 373(9679): 1993–5.

Labonté, R. and Gagnon, M.L. (2010) 'Framing health and foreign policy: lessons for global health diplomacy', *Globalization and Health*, 6(1):14.

Miller, D. (2007) *National Responsibility and Global Justice*, Oxford: Oxford University Press.

Moellendorf, D. (2002) *Cosmopolitan Justice*, Boulder, CO: Westview Press.

Nagel, T. (2005) 'The problem of global justice', *Philosophy & Public Affairs*, 33(2): 113–47.

Ogata, S. and Sen, A. (2003) 'Human security now. New York: Commission on Human Security', available at www.un.org/humansecurity/sites/www.un.org.humansecurity/files/chs_final_report_-_english.pdf (accessed on 14 June 2017).

Ooms, G. and Hammonds, R. (2016) 'Global constitutionalism, applied to global health governance: uncovering legitimacy deficits and suggesting remedies', Globalization and *Health*, 12(1): 84.

Ooms, G., Beiersmann, C., Flores, W., Hanefeld, J., Müller, O., Mulumba, M., Ottersen, T., Sarker, M., and Jahn, A. (2017) 'Synergies and tensions between universal health coverage and global health security: why we need a second "Maximizing Positive Synergies" initiative'. *BMJ Global Health*, 2(1): e000217.

Rosen, G. (1993) *A History of Public Health*, expanded edition, Baltimore, MD: Johns Hopkins University Press.

Rushton, S. (2011) 'Global health security: security for whom? Security from what?' *Political Studies*, 59(4): 779–96.

Sridhar, D. and Rudan, I. (2015) *Healthy Ideas: Improving global health and development in the 21st century*. Edinburgh, JoGH.

Whitehead, M. (1992) 'The concepts and principles of equity and health', *International journal of health services*, 22(3): 429–45.

World Health Organization. (2012) 'Positioning health in the post-2015 development agenda', available at www.who.int/topics/millennium_development_goals/post2015/WHOdiscussionpaper_October2012.pdf (accessed on 14 June 2017).

World Health Organization. (2017) 'World health statistics 2017', available at http://apps.who.int/iris/bitstream/10665/255336/1/9789241565486-eng.pdf (accessed on 14 June 2017).

# 17

# Health and global governance

## The case of development cooperation on

*Håkan Thörn*

## Introduction

The 'global governance' literature emphasises the de-centralised character of contemporary global political processes. For example, Held and McGrew (2002, p. 9) have argued that global governance 'is defined by diverse sources of rule-making, political authority and power'. Global health governance is a case in point, as it appears as an extremely complex phenomenon. Considering the multiplicity of institutions, actors, and projects that are currently involved, including national, regional, and international political institutions; private–public partnerships; corporations; civil society organisations; private foundations; and even social movements, it has even been argued that global health governance is a 'confusing phenomenon' (Harman, 2012, p. 2). Discussing the case of development partnerships with civil society in the field of HIV/AIDS, I will, however, argue that beyond the surface of a confusing appearance, 'global health governance' is defined by particular and unequal power relations and involves rationalities and techniques that harmonise policy interventions and standardise their design, implementation, and evaluation. The argument is based on a research project on development cooperation with civil society on HIV/AIDS in sub-Saharan Africa (Follér, et. al., 2013; Thörn, 2016).

I will show how 'global health governance' involves new forms of power operating at the scale of *transnational* population through strategies of governance that particularly target civil society. In doing so, I draw on Rose and Miller's (2008) notion of 'advanced liberalism' as a mode of governance which, inspired by neoliberal philosophy, began to take shape in the 1970s:

> It entailed the development of new technologies of governing from a centre through powerful means of governing at a distance: these appeared to enhance the autonomy of zones, persons, entities, but enwrapped them in a new form of regulation – audits, budgets, standards, risk management, targets [...]
> *Miller and Rose, 2008, p. 18*

Building on this, I use 'advanced liberal *engineering*' (Larsson, et al., 2012) to further underscore the use of a perspective that is contrary to ideas about (neo)liberal governance as fundamentally being about *de*-regulations. Advanced liberal engineering refers first and foremost to a form of governance that introduces *new regulations* to support market mechanisms and entrepreneurship through various techniques of responsibilisation. In this chapter, responsibilisation refers to a transfer of responsibilities from government agencies to 'partners'. This means governing them at a distance 'through the instrumentalisation of a regulated autonomy' (Miller and Rose, 2008, p. 213). Such regulated self-regulation is practiced through certain administrative procedures. From the perspective of governance, this means imposing a cluster of techniques, which I call *a package of responsibilisation* (Thörn, 2016) on the 'partners'. These methods are not unique to HIV/AIDS-assistance but can be found in donor policies in other health areas as well. Further, in terms of power relations, this package involves ambivalence: it treats organisations and communities as autonomous actors while at the same prescribes techniques designed to lead and control them at a distance.

## Development partnerships with civil society in the field of HIV/AIDS as a case of global health governance

The case of international development cooperation on HIV/AIDS work between donors and civil society organisations (CSOs) in sub-Saharan Africa has a more general relevance in several respects. First, as one of 'the big three' (with tuberculosis and malaria), HIV/AIDS is a major policy field in the context of 'global health governance' more generally (Harman, 2012; Hein, et al., 2007). Second, HIV/AIDS is a major issue in the field of international development aid. Third, sub-Saharan Africa is the most important region in this context, receiving the greatest share of global AIDS spending (Kates, et al., 2013, p. 2), something that should be seen in relation both to the degree of poverty and the prevalence of the disease in sub-Saharan Africa.

During the last decade, donors have put significant emphasis on support to CSOs when addressing the HIV/AIDS issue in the global South. This involves taking a distance from 'old style conditionality' in development aid, instead emphasising 'partnership' with civil society. Such aid, however, still comes with conditions, which today more often concern the *formal aspects* than *the content* of the AIDS-related work that donors support (Thörn, 2011, 2016).

International aid for HIV/AIDS is part of the overall development cooperation established with the Millennium Development Goals (MDGs) and the 2005 Paris Declaration. The research that this chapter is based on studied a wide range of donors. Most importantly, this included government donors, such as PEPFAR/USAID; international organisations such as UNAIDS and WHO; foundations such as the Global Fund and Bill & Melinda Gates Foundation; and INGOs, such as Doctors Without Borders, Family Health International, and OXFAM. However, I have focused on the two donor organisations that have become dominant in the context of HIV/AIDS governance in the 2000s. First, The Global Fund to Fight AIDS, Tuberculosis and Malaria (GF), established in 2001 to increase global funding for fighting the three diseases. The GF was set up after a decision taken at the G8 Meeting in Genoa in 2001, as a response to calls made at two African conferences in 2000 and an appeal from UN General Secretary Kofi Annan. Over the years the GF has achieved a status of a 'global policy driver' in the field of HIV/AIDS. It is formally defined as a 'public–private partnership' and has a status as a foundation under Swiss law. GF relies on both public and private contributions and even after the economic crisis in 2008, the GF has continued to distribute significant funding. Second, PEPFAR (the US President's Emergency Plan for AIDS Relief), which was launched in 2003 as a five-year initiative to fight HIV/AIDS (with a total of US$15 billion) and has been continued after 2008.

## Why civil society? – Development cooperation on HIV/AIDS as advanced liberal engineering

In the 2000s, international development cooperation on health policy has increasingly focused on strategies for governing populations at a distance through civil society. According to a World Bank Study this has presented a 'dramatic strategic shift' in the 2000s, based on the following assumption:

A belief that small NGOs [non-governmental organizations] and CBOs [community-based organizations] might be able to 'engineer' changes in knowledge and behavior at the local level, as the factors that influence the norms and practice of sexual behavior are more likely to be better understood by CBOs than by public sector entities.

*Bonnel, et al., 2013, p. 6*

In our study on development partnerships on HIV/AIDS with civil society in sub-Saharan Africa, we analysed the programmes of the major donors in the field – and of the problematisations that they involved – meaning how they constitute certain conditions as a 'problem' to be addressed and acted upon (Miller and Rose, 2008, p. 16). There were striking similarities between the different policy documents: they presented similar pictures of 'the situation' that made support to civil society 'necessary' and suggested the same principles for its implementation. According to our analysis, the most important programmatic themes were:

- *A strong emphasis on the need to support and involve civil society.* For example, the GF argues that CSOs can play an important role where states are insensitive to the needs of populations and/or lack capacity to act and reach out. The GF argues that CSOs provide 'insight into the need and experiences of communities'. They are further 'effective' in working with 'hard-to-reach communities'. Even more importantly, they are *efficient* as implementers of GF grants, performing 'equally [...] well, if not better, than all other types of implementing agencies' (Global Fund, 2006, p. 24).
- *An emphasis on business models and market principles in development partnerships.* The GF declares that it 'is not an implementing entity; it is a financial instrument [...] with funds allocated on strict performance criteria'. Further, it represents a 'unique business model' (Global Fund, 2006 p. 33).
- *A quantitative and scientific approach to assessment, evaluation, and other forms of knowledge production*, with a strong emphasis on scientific claims in the form of so-called 'evidence-based methods'. This practice puts pressure on donors as well as CSOs to conform to certain dominant standards of evaluation.

As is made clear in the quotes listed, the 'improvements' to increase aid efficiency and effectiveness involve an implicit problematisation of previous development aid programmes, in which the state was the main recipient, or in terms of the more recent discourse, 'development partner'. The state is still an important actor in contemporary development partnerships on HIV/AIDS – but as *one of several partners*, in accordance with the policy of 'good governance' that prescribes public–private partnerships. Accordingly, in order for a government to receive GF funding, a 'multisectoral' Country Coordinating Mechanism (CCM) needs to be set up, and must include representatives not only from the government, but also from the business sector and civil society.

As will be evident in the following analysis of the programmes, problematisations, and techniques defining development cooperation in HIIV/AIDS, governance in this field is performed through a mix of regulatory and disciplinary techniques. A key role in the politics of responsibilisation is played by *the intermediary organisation*, who is ascribed the role of channelling funds from donors, government institutions, or international non-governmental organisations (INGOs) to local CBOs. This task also involves taking care of reporting and control of funds for the latter, something which makes the position of the intermediaries defined by fundamental ambivalence. They are selected by donors because on one hand they are part of locally anchored networks; and on the other hand, because they have the capacity to take responsibility for applications, audits, evaluation, and reporting. This puts them in a position of control, and potentially in an antagonist relation to CBOs and community populations.

## Responsibilisation in the practices of development partnerships on HIV/AIDS

By considering the programmatic themes recounted previously, as well as the practices analysed in the following sections, there are three key *rationalities* in the governance of civil society: *marketisation*, *scientisation*, and *standardisation*. I will demonstrate how these rationalities work through what I call a package of responsibilisation, which refers to a cluster of techniques, meaning practices that function as instruments for regulation of self-regulation. In terms of power relations, this package treats organisations and communities as autonomous actors while at the same time prescribing techniques designed to lead and control them at a distance. In this case it refers to the process by which donors assign CSOs responsibilities to carry out certain tasks, while at the same time controlling them by introducing procedures for self-monitoring and reporting.

## Marketisation

Marketisation refers to the introduction of regulations and techniques supporting market principles and business models in order to facilitate competition and entrepreneurship amongst CSOs. An important function of marketisation is to shift certain responsibilities from donor to recipient by making CSOs self-reliant in accordance with the advanced liberal sense of agency: as a self-interested and competitive actor in a market (e.g., Thörn, 2016; Abrahamsen, 2004). In the context of international development cooperation with civil society, the rationality of marketisation is at work in a re-organisation of CSOs and their relationships in line with 'the new managerialism', that involves the notion that the legitimacy of an organisation and its activities depends on its efficiency in a market (Abrahamsen, 2004; Fitzsimons, 1999). In practice this involves the promotion of a culture of competition and entrepreneurship in the context of health policy in civil societies in the global South – practised through the introduction of *techniques* such as entrepreneurship training, systematic under-funding, and formalised processes of competitive tendering, through which donors 'choose' their partners in civil society. This means that the 'partnership' between donor and recipient is constituted as a contractual buyer–seller relationship and that CSOs primarily become service providers. This also involves entrepreneurship training, often provided by donors, to facilitate the creation of subject capabilities functional to such relationships. Such training often comes in the form of workshops, as part of what in donor discourse is termed 'capacity building', organised by donors themselves or by INGOs functioning as intermediaries between donors and local CSOs.

And as we found that donors tend to systematically underfund the activities they support, forcing even salaried staff to do extensive voluntary work, some local organisations set up to fight poverty and disease responded by partly turning into small businesses to compensate.

An overall effect of marketisation is thus a commodification of civil society, affecting and reshaping the social relations between, and the capacities and subjectivities of, organisations, communities, and individuals.

## Scientisation

Scientisation refers to the introduction of regulations and techniques that support management methods based on scientific claims. Scientisation has an important function to legitimise the forms of management that are introduced with the package of responsibilisation. The rationalities of standardisation and scientisation overlap in the introduction of *techniques* to be applied by CSOs in their performance, (self-) monitoring and evaluation (M&E) and – importantly – reporting of their activities. This includes results-based management, evidence-based work, auditing, monitoring, and evaluation; and the use of indicators, reporting tools, templates, and standardised operating procedures.

The 'science part' of the package of responsibilisation primarily comes in the form of evidence-based methods (EBM). These have their origins in medical science, and involve an emphasis on making various practices evaluable through their 'definition, measurement and enumeration' (Winch, et al., 2002, p. 158). When introduced in a number of policy areas, including international aid, they have mainly been used to measure the effectiveness of policies in addressing the needs of target groups (Seckenelgin, 2007; Thörn, 2011).

Another set of techniques claimed to have a scientific status is result-based management (RBM), emphasising the need to shape activities in a way that they produce measurable results, or in the language of RBM discourse, 'outcomes'. RBM's key role in international development cooperation on HIV/AIDS has been highlighted and heavily criticised by a former employee of PEPFAR, Andrew Natsios (2010), who describes RBM as an 'obsessive measurement disorder'.

An overall effect of scientisation is a depoliticisation of 'development partnerships'. When certain practices are presented as science-based solutions to problems of efficiency, administration, and regulation, it means their rootedness in the *political* discourse of advanced liberal engineering becomes concealed. Such an approach ignores the fact that the way in which scientific questions are posed, or scientific problems are constructed and dealt with, are value-laden and politically informed; what constitutes legitimate and desirable effectiveness and results is not a matter of scientific objectivity, but of politics. Ultimately, such a technocratic, problem-solving approach to politics suppresses conflicts between interacting agents who are in positions of unequal dependency (Thörn and Svenberg, 2016).

## Standardisation

Standardisation refers to the introduction of regulations and techniques to support the introduction of certain standardised methods of organisation, involving a formalisation to make categories compatible and facilitate measurability. Standardisation has an important function in allowing donors to stay in control while responsibilising CSOs by enforcing the use of *formalised techniques* as part of their contracts. Various forms of training implement such techniques. What this standardisation basically means in the context of everyday work is that every activity needs to be designed in such a way that it produces the measurable results that the donors require. One effect of such standardisation is that projects that are not designed to produce quantitative results are not likely to get funding. This clearly impacts on activists' and organisations' perceptions of what is possible for them to do.

## Effects of marketisation, standardisation, and scientisation

I have argued that the package of responsibilisation is designed by donors in order to introduce 'self-government' amongst CSOs in the field of HIV/AIDS, while at the same time controlling them at a distance. Put another way, the rationalities of marketisation, scientisation, and standardisation are at work through a cluster of techniques that have the effect of responsibilising CSOs in certain ways, while actually de-responsibilising them in other ways. Marketisation promotes 'economic self-reliance' through techniques that steer CSOs into becoming small businesses and service providers that compete in a service market. Through the technique of tendering, CSOs are made responsible to shape and present themselves as self-sufficient, competitive actors. The transition from grant agreements to service contracts is in a sense reversing the distribution of responsibility between the 'development partners'. What in previous development discourses was defined as a moral responsibility of the donor is now a performance-based contractual responsibility of the CSO (and its sub-contractors). Scientisation and standardisation are at work in the training of CSOs to take responsibility for managing their activities, and in the provision of information about them, according to principles of standardisation and scientific ideals of 'evidence', 'efficiency', and 'effectiveness'. The techniques of scientisation and standardisation involve a complex interplay between responsibilisation and de-responsibilisation. On one hand, donors make CSOs responsible for conducting themselves according to scientific ideals. At the same time, donors fend off responsibility by referring to the external authorities of 'scientific evidence' and 'standardised methods'. This also involves a de-responsibilisation of CSOs, since their everyday work is to be guided by certain pre-defined standards and the external knowledge authority of 'scientific evidence', rather than by considerations based on their knowledge and experience of the local context and its particular circumstances.

## Resistance and coercive discipline

We found that when responsibilisation fails in the sense that agents do not take on the responsibilities imposed on them, new and harsh coercive disciplinary techniques may be used. Our study thus provides further support for those analyses that have highlighted how advanced liberal governance not just shapes subjectivities through new forms of self-discipline, but also involves coercive disciplinary measures as an important element (Death, 2013; Abrahamsen, 2004; Knutsson, 2014). In Abrahamsen's (2004, p. 1454) words, 'the power of partnerships is voluntary and coercive at the same time, producing both new forms of agency and new forms of discipline'. The most common technique is delaying payments – or even terminating contracts. I am not referring to occasions of proven 'financial irregularities', but to cases in all three countries where payments have been withheld by donors because CSOs' reports are not up to standard or not handed in according to schedule. The point is that this marks a change in relation to previous practice, when delayed or incomplete reports did not result in immediate sanctions.

Responsibilisation can also fail because local actors refuse to take on responsibilities imposed on them. Regarding political agency in the form of social movements addressing the AIDS issue, the most significant example in sub-Saharan Africa is the broad-based mobilisation led by TAC (Treatment Action Campaign), which also included labour unions. As this involved international cooperation that organised efforts to fight HIV/AIDS in spite of the government's denialism, it provides an example of how resistance to sovereignty can be performed by circumventing sovereign power centres. South African activists who took part in that struggle suggested to us that responsibilisation is more difficult to resist than the AIDS politics of the Mbeki government, or the old imperialist-style conditionality that was applied by PEPFAR under the Bush administration, when it prohibited their CSO partners from distributing condoms. In that case, some organisations took the money and distributed them anyway, confident that the donor was unable to enforce control at the grassroots level (Thörn, 2011, p. 440).

It may be argued that the resistance of the social movement led by TAC in fact had more wide-reaching and long-term effects, since it involved significant attempts to create a counter-culture, as the movement's practices involved strategies to fight the disease not just by providing treatment, but by constructing alternative sexual identities and counter-knowledge, involving attempts to fuse elements of modern science with the cosmology of 'traditional' African medicine (Robins, 2006; Mbali, 2008).

Compared to this, the field of HIV/AIDS activities in sub-Saharan civil society in the 2010s has, however, been rather de-politicised. This does not mean that acts of resistance in the present context are absent. If the creation of a culture of competition through techniques such as competitive tendering seems very effective, we also found examples where *marketisation techniques were resisted* by acts of solidarity in the form of information sharing regarding funding opportunities, and even by coordination amongst CSOs. When donors, as part of the 'ownership' discourse, invited CSOs to round-table discussions, CSOs in some cases organised pre-meetings to agree on a common strategy so that they could use the round-table to put collective pressure on donors. There were also attempts of resisting techniques of scientisation and standardisation by counter-knowledge production. The forms of such counter-knowledge production could vary, involving on one hand elements of the previously mentioned traditional medicine, or the use of scholarly analysis in a re-framing of donors' demands of reporting by producing evaluation reports providing critical analysis of donors' and governments' prevention programmes in Southern Africa. However, in order to challenge responsibilisation in a more fundamental way, CSOs might have to refuse to 'play the game' by not entering partnerships. Considering the lack of resources among CSOs, it is, of course, difficult to find alternative ways to do important work. Such an alternative strategy would presuppose the mobilisation of significant numbers of supporters and activists and the emergence of a social movement organisation, as in the case of TAC in South Africa (which for a time was able to take a relatively independent position in relation to donors).

## Conclusion

The analysis of programmes for 'development partnerships' on HIV/AIDS in this chapter has highlighted how donors emphasise the need to support and 'strengthen' civil society because it makes possible the penetration of government functions into what, in donor discourse terms, are called 'hard-to-reach communities'. An important effect of this strategy for 'strengthening' civil society, which in different respects may both responsibilise and de-responsibilise CSOs at the same time, is the creation of a particular form of civil society, in which CSOs are steered in the direction of being service providers rather than political actors. In this sense, (de-)responsibilisation has de-politicising effects (Jaeger, 2007; Thörn, 2016).

I have also highlighted how, when (de-)responsibilisation fails, new and harsher disciplinary measures may be introduced. This does not mean that tension, conflict, and even resistance are completely absent. While advanced liberal governance, as exercised in current development partnerships on HIV/AIDS, seems to be very difficult to resist, I argue that the term *politics of responsibilisation* is useful to highlight that there is always a *possibility* that subjects may engage in resistance and even transformative collective action. I have also provided examples of such resistance in the field of HIV/AIDS politics in sub-Saharan Africa, indicating that the new forms of power discussed in this chapter may have not shaped local civil societies as profoundly as assumed by donor programmes.

## References

Abrahamsen, R. (2004) 'The power of partnerships in global governance', *Third World Quarterly*, 25(8): 1453–67.

Bonnel, R., Rodriguez-Garcia, R., and Olivier, J. (2013) *Funding Mechanisms for Civil Society: The experience of the AIDS response*, Washington, DC: World Bank.

Death, C. (2013) 'Governmentality at the limits of the international: African politics and Foucauldian theory', *Review of International Studies*, 39(3): 763–87.

Fitzsimons, P. (1999) 'Managerialism and education', Encyclopedia of Educational Philisophy and Theory, available at http://eepat.net/doku.php?id=managerialism_and_education (accessed on 31 March 2014).

Follér, M.-L., Haug, C., Knutsson, B., and Thörn, H. (2013) *Who is Responsible? Donor-civil society partnerships and the case of HIV/AIDS work*, Uppsala: Nordic Africa Institute.

Global Fund (2006) *Annual Report*, Geneva: The Global Fund.

Harman, S. (2012) *Global Health Governance*, Abingdon: Routledge.

Hein, W., Bartsch S., and Kohlmorgen, L. (Eds.) (2007) *Global Health Governance and the Fight against HIV/AIDS*, Basingstoke: Palgrave.

Held, D. and McGrew, A. (2002) *Governing Globalization: Power, authority and global governance*, London: Polity Press.

Jaeger, H.-M. (2007) '"Global civil society" and the political depoliticization of governance', *International Political Sociology*, 1(3): 257–77.

Kates, J., Michaud, J., Wexter, A., and Valentine, A. (2013) 'Mapping the donor landscape in global health: HIV/AIDS', available at http://kaiserfamilyfoundation.files.wordpress.com (accessed on 13 September 2013).

Knutsson, B. (2014) 'Smooth machinery: global governmentality and civil society HIV/AIDS work in Rwanda', *Globalizations*, 11(6): 793–807.

Larsson, B., Letell, M., and Thörn, H. (Eds.) (2012) *Transformations of the Swedish Welfare State: From social engineering to governance?*, Basingstoke: Palgrave Macmillan.

Mbali, M. (2008) 'Gender, sexuality and global linkages in the history of South African AIDS activism, 1982–94', In: M.-L. Follér and H. Håkan Thörn (Eds.) *The Politics of AIDS: Globalization, the state and civil society*, Basingstoke: Palgrave/Macmillan, pp. 177–98.

Miller, P. and Rose, N. (2008) *Governing the Present*, Cambridge: Polity Press.

Natsios, A. (2010) *The Clash of the Counter-bureaucracy and Development*, Washington, DC: Center for Global Development, available at www.cgdev.org/content/publications/detail/1424271 (accessed on 10 January 2012).

Robins, S. (2006) 'From rights to "ritual": AIDS activism and treatment testimonies in South Africa', *American Anthropologist*, 108(2): 312–23.

Seckenelgin, H. (2007) 'Evidence-based policy for HIV/AIDS interventions: questions of external validity, or relevance for use' *Development and Change*, 38(6): 1219–34.

Thörn, H. (2011) 'AID(S) politics and power: a critique of global governance', *Politikon*, 38(3): 433–52.

Thörn, H. (2016) 'Politics of responsibility: governing distant populations through civil society in Mozambique, Rwanda and South Africa', *Third World Quarterly*, 37(8): 1505–23.

Thörn, H. and Svenberg, S. (2016) 'We feel the responsibility that you shirk: the politics of responsibility and the case of the Swedish environmental movement', *Social Movement Studies*, 15(6): 593–609.

Winch, S., Creedy, D., and Chaboyer, W. (2002) 'Governing nursing conduct: the rise of evidence-based practice', *Nursing Inquiry*, 9(3): 156–61.

# Part IV
# Development assistance and the politics of global health

# 18

# Global health challenges in the era of the Sustainable Development Goals

*Nana Poku and Jim Whitman*

## Introduction

After the partial, but still impressive health-related outcomes of the Millennium Development Goals (MDGs), it might be supposed that the Sustainable Development Goals (SDGs) from 2015 would consolidate and extend those achievements. However, the compass and substance of the SDGs reflect a rapidly changing world in which human health – and the single health issue which predominated the period of the MDGs, HIV and AIDS – are now sited within a greatly enlarged arena of urgent and costly imperatives as well as rising costs set against diminished resources. These conditions will present developing countries with difficult challenges at a time of rising expectations. The forward momentum of the MDGs is by no means assured; nor are the health-related particularities of the SDGs likely to regain the status or support they enjoyed prior to 2015.

The MDGs were conceived with simplicity and clarity in keeping with the idealism and determination behind them. Yet the gap between the high aspirations of its eight goals and its 22 targets revealed a more realistic assessment of the practical possibilities across its 15-year time-span. For example, beneath Goal 1 – 'eradicate extreme poverty and hunger' – was Target 1.C – 'Halve, between 1990 and 2015, the proportion of people who suffer from hunger '(United Nations, 2000, n.p.). So:

> the continuance of the MDGs in some form beyond 2015 [was] implicit not only in the nature and scale of the normative commitment, but also in the gap between the ideal and the practical targets that [were] set and agreed.
>
> *Poku and Whitman, 2011, p. 182*

The limited number of MDG targets and the focus in half of them on women and children – (achieve universal primary education; promote gender equality and empower women; reduce child mortality; and improve maternal health) – directly and indirectly ensured many notable advances. As the *UN Millennium Development Goals 2015 Report* noted (albeit using 1990 as a baseline), the global under-5 mortality rate has declined by more than half, dropping from 90 to 43 deaths per 1,000 live births; and the maternal mortality ratio has declined by 45 per cent worldwide, with most of the reduction having occurred since 2000 (United Nations, 2015a).

By far the most impressive health outcomes of the MDGs were in dealing with the HIV/AIDS epidemic. The international community had been galvanised to confront the AIDS epidemic in the years preceding the MDGs to the extent that it found expression as Goal 6, 'Combat HIV/AIDS, malaria and other diseases'. The inclusion of malaria (with TB also listed in the targets) was not nominal, but by 2000, the concerted international struggle against HIV and AIDS was already under way. The progress made against HIV and AIDS during the course of the MDGs has rightly been hailed as an unprecedented, extended expression of global solidarity; as a first-order organisational and political achievement (UNAIDS and Lancet Commission, 2015); and as a unique programme combining bio-medical and behavioural interventions; sustained, in-country innovations in prevention; an astonishing marshalling of financial resources; and feats of consensus-building and coordination against all manner of national, organisational, and cultural divides – not least overcoming the corporate and national opposition to the production of affordable, generic anti-retroviral medicines (Thoen, 2002). New HIV infections have fallen by 35 per cent since 2000 (and by 58 per cent among children); AIDS-related deaths have fallen by 42 per cent since the peak in 2004; and 30 million new HIV infections and nearly eight million AIDS-related deaths have been averted since 2000, when the MDGs were set. By mid-2015, the number of people accessing antiretroviral therapy reached nearly 16 million – double the number of just five years earlier – a truly remarkable achievement compared to fewer than 1 per cent of people living with HIV in low- and middle-income countries who had access to treatment in 2001.

It is important that the headline statistics from the conclusion of MDG 6 receive the widest possible circulation; and expressions of satisfaction and gratitude not only have their place, but are also norm-strengthening at the start of another 15 years of effort. However, although ending the AIDS epidemic is possible, it is by no means in sight, or assured; and nor is securing UNAIDS' 2030 goals (UNAIDS, 2014) largely a matter of 'one final push'. Without in any way discounting the very considerable political, med-ical, logistical, and other related challenges that continue to be encountered, once generic antiretrovirals (ARVs) were made affordable, the key indicators were almost certain to be very impressive – such was the scale of both the epidemic itself and the ARV roll-out. But these programmes generate another range of challenges, including an expanding cohort of patients with co-morbidities; treatment failures; trans-missible drug resistance; and the as-yet unmet costs of second- and third-line treatments. Most tellingly, recruitment onto ARV programmes is not keeping pace with the rate of new infections (UNAIDS, 2011).

By 2014, 36.9 million people were living with HIV, and that number continues to increase, in large part because more people globally are accessing antiretroviral therapy and as a result are living longer, healthier lives. As WHO launched the new 2015 AIDS treatment Guidelines shifting to 'Test and Start', the number of HIV-infected people who will need treatment will considerably increase, and so will the funding needs. At the same time, even though new HIV infections have declined, there is still an unacceptably high number of new HIV infections and AIDS-related deaths occurring each year. In 2014, around two million people were newly infected with HIV and 1.2 million people died of AIDS-related illnesses. Incidence among young women in Africa is persistently high.

According to UNAIDS (UNAIDS, 2016), at the end of 2014, US$19.2 billion was invested in the AIDS response in low- and middle-income countries, of which domestic resources constituted 57 per cent. The most recent estimates indicate that US$26.2 billion will be required for the AIDS response in 2020. So, the consequences and costs of the AIDS epidemic will continue to shape global health challenges throughout the period of the SDGs and beyond, but the conditions which facilitated the scale and consistency of the global response to HIV and AIDS during the MDGs are no longer in place. This has implications which extend across the full span of large-scale health issues.

## The health-related aspects of the Sustainable Development Goals

The Sustainable Development Goals retain the form of the MDGs, but on a scale which privileges inclu-siveness over actionable priority-setting. However well integrated the post-2015 SDGs and targets are thematically, the programmatic difficulties entailed in 17 goals and 169 targets spread across nearly every important aspect of planetary sustainability and human equity are likely to create a range of imperatives that cannot be reconciled, politically or economically, even in the absence of unforeseen setbacks such as the financial turbulence the world experienced in 2008. More fundamentally, the Third International Conference on Financing for Development (2015) did not specify costs for any of the listed aspirations; and aside from the creation of new institutions, gave little indication where the financing will come from, aside from asserting the centrality of the Monterey Consensus (International Conference on Financial Development, 2002) as a broadening and enabling means. This is despite the fact that a year earlier, the Report on the Intergovernmental Committee of Experts on Sustainable Development Financing (United Nations General Assembly, 2014) did offer some indicative costs – for example, US$66 billion for a global safety net to eradicate extreme poverty; and a global cost of between US$5 and 7 billion annually to meet infrastructural needs in water, agriculture, forestry, telecoms, power, transport, and buildings (Greenhill and Ali, 2013). Notably, neither HIV and AIDS nor other health issues were included in the indicative costings.

The SDGs replace the disease-specific focus of MDG 6 with the remarkably inclusive SDG 3: 'Ensure healthy lives and promote wellbeing for all at all ages.' There is some virtue in enlarging the compass of global health targets to include matters ranging from substance abuse and motor vehicle accidents to maternal health and vaccines, but there is also a danger of the SDGs failing to secure a clear sense of priorities and programmatic coherence, particularly in view of the incomplete costings and the all but inevitable competition for resources. This certainly applies to health issues: the one mention of HIV and AIDS in the SDGs is embedded in a single target (3.3), 'By 2030, end the epidemics of AIDS, tuberculosis, malaria and neglected tropical diseases and combat hepatitis, water-borne diseases and other communicable diseases.' It is difficult to regard this as a meaningful target; and one need not be dismissive of aspiration on this scale in order to see that the sheer breadth and comprehensiveness of the SDGs – including a fair approximation of the costs of achieving them – will entail a good deal of regretful prioritisation and some very hard choices, either considered or by default. Two things are already clear: HIV and AIDS are no longer perceived as uniquely large and urgent global issues; and the resources available for the steeply rising costs of the epidemic are stagnant, at best. An expansive sustainable development agenda creates still further pressure points for many other global health issues.

## The changing donor–recipient landscape

Overseas Development Assistance (ODA) provides the most compelling indicator of the nature of the current financial uncertainties. After a noticeable decline during the 1990s, total ODA financing increased substantially from US$53.6 billion in 2000 to US$87.1 billion in 2008 (in constant 2002 USD) (World Bank, 2010). The increase was entirely driven by new global commitments to fight HIV, TB, and malaria (Institute of Health Metrics Evaluation, 2010). As a result of the market collapse of 2008, global commitment to ODA declined by 13 per cent during 2009–10, though there was a modest rebound of 8 per cent in 2012 over 2011 (Kaiser Family Foundation/UNAIDS, 2013). But the days of abundant funding for developing country health initiatives appear to have ended. Although the fifth replenishment of the Global Fund for AIDS, TB, and malaria successfully raised US$12.9 billion in 2016, the UNAIDS five-year 'Fast Track' initiative – which requires the front-loading of an additional US$7 billion in the years to 2020 – has not made any significant headway.

The stagnation and/or decline in broader ODA also has both direct and indirect impacts on the conditions which create, sustain, or exacerbate ill-health on a large scale, most notably poverty and its multiple impacts. At the height of the global financial crisis, a World Bank background paper observed:

> The challenge facing developing countries is how, with fewer resources, to pursue policies that can protect or expand critical expenditures, including on social safety nets, human development

and critical infrastructure. This will be especially difficult for LICs [Low-Income Countries]: the slowdown in growth will likely deepen the degree of deprivation of the existing poor, since large numbers of people are clustered just above the poverty line and particularly vulnerable to economic volatility and temporary slowdowns. Many of the most affected LICs are heavily dependent on official concessional flows, which will be under pressure in donor countries facing their own fiscal challenges.

*World Bank, 2009, p. 1*

Given the scale and time-span of the SDGs, a continued emphasis on extending the sources of funding as widely as possible is unavoidable; in the case of needed efficiencies and the mobilisation of domestic resources, highly desirable; and in any event, a broad consensus around diversifying funding has been in place since the launch of the MDGs. However, even on an assumption that we will not again suffer financial turbulence and its aftermath of the kind the world has endured from 2008–9, the diversity and more routine volatilities of global finance, the necessary incentives required for some forms of financing, provision for large-scale emergencies, and other factors are likely to make both cost estimates and possible funding sources highly provisional. Moreover, the expansion of global health priority areas to encompass diseases of affluence (such as heart disease, obesity, and diabetes) will move prioritisation for development in a geographical sense (North/South or developed/less developed) to thematic issues, which are global and applicable to all countries. The implication is that, more so than usual, donors will need to balance their international commitments with domestic priorities under conditions of restrained fiscal budgets for both arenas. The substantive transition from geographical space to thematic issues will also embolden civil societies in donor countries to ask for larger support from governments on issues that are pertinent to their own immediate and growing needs, especially those occasioned by the ageing of their populations.

Work on identifying the sources and sustainability of finance will obviously feature largely, if not predominate deliberation over, the full range of SDG priorities; and understanding the multiple sources of extant and projected declines in donor funding need to be grasped in detail to frame appropriate responses. A number of the SDGs are 'big ticket' issues: key among these are climate change, sustainable cities and human settlements, and demanding funding commitments of a size and duration that will inevitably have an impact on the sums available for health. And in addition to HIV/AIDS, TB, and malaria, other costly and enduring health and health system demands are also growing in urgency, including Universal Health Coverage (UHC) and Sexual and Reproductive Health and Rights (SRHR) along with maternal health (United Nations, 2015b).

The cost/benefit calculus of ODA is changing, with less room for fiscal manoeuvre and more sharply defined and politically sensitive concerns to the fore. There is in addition the substantial risk of a 'fiscal cliff' for countries that received support being unable to maintain their previous achievements in health. That threatens the substantial progress made to date in many health issues areas, and risks sparking domestic frustration. It may also have international repercussions, including a resurgence of disease in poorer neighbouring countries.

## Enduring and emerging health issues in the era of the Sustainable Development Goals

Although it is no longer perceived as the largest – and for some, the most urgent – issue confronting us, ending the AIDS epidemic is critical for achieving the SDGs. AIDS remains an epidemic, and the gains made throughout the course of the MDGs are not irreversible. Additionally, there are two other considerable health issue areas which have myriad links with HIV and AIDS. The prospects for diminishing the relational pathways to HIV infections, dealing with AIDS, and meeting the considerable and growing health needs of developing nations must be considered.

The first is Sexual and Reproductive Health Rights (SRHR). Although the many issues entwined with SRHR are prevalent throughout the world, they are particularly entrenched in the developing world – and in Africa in particular, where their intersection with HIV and AIDS gives them particular salience. The demography of Africa critically shapes the prospects for promoting and securing a healthy future for its peoples, in line with Goal 5 of the SDGs and the broader aspirations of *Africa 2063: The Future We Want* (African Union Commission, 2015). That is because Africa has a very young age profile, with about two-fifths of its population in the 0–14 age bracket and nearly one-fifth (19 per cent) in the 15–24 age bracket. This means that the current 'demographic bulge' of sexually active young adults will grow still further and persist for decades as the generation of 0–14-year-olds also become sexually active. Against that background, the right to accessible, high-quality SRHR services is clearly fundamental. In addition, the obvious health vulnerabilities of adolescents and young adults arising from risky behaviours are shaped and amplified by the discriminatory and often pernicious ways in which gender relations are structured. Hence SDG 5 targets including the elimination of all forms of discrimination against women and girls, including all forms of gender violence in the public and private spheres as well as harmful practices such as child, early, and forced marriage, and female genital mutilation.

A reorientation of social norms on this scale requires dedicated, consistent effort across many dimensions of social relations; it cannot be accomplished by declaratory and legal means alone – and in this situation, regional efforts might be particularly efficacious. At the same time, issue-specific matters, particularly those which fall under the aegis of SRHR, can be addressed programmatically – and they can serve as powerful catalysts for larger changes in gender relations. Education also has a key role to play in disseminating knowledge about sexual and reproductive matters, diminishing stigmas, and exposing all aspects of gender relations to deliberation and choice.

For the purpose of determining linkages between the global and national levels of the SDGs, the 'connective tissue' between them extends considerably beyond the addition of mid-level arenas – that is, regional or sub-regional intergovernmental organisations – important though these are. Although both politics and geography demarcate a hierarchy of levels for conceiving, agreeing, and enacting SRHR initiatives, these levels are highly permeable and interactive – and they need to be. That is because advances in SRHR cannot be 'delivered' as so many other health requisites are; they are largely relational – and while they range from forms of interpersonal adjustment and training to the alteration of social norms, statistically significant advances in SRHR cannot be expected to cascade downward from the global level, from high principle to on-the-ground enactment. After all, even with a global human rights regime, what counts as a health 'right' in particular social contexts, with their politico-legal, historical religious, ethnic, class, and legal fixtures and dynamics can be highly contested (Standing, et al., 2011).

The strongly relational quality of SRHR is not only an essential aspect of the way in which they are often enacted and/or contested; it also points to the larger SDG agenda in which they are framed:

> Tangible indicators, such as the reduction in the numbers of people living in poverty or the reduction in women dying from pregnancy-related causes, provide information on outcomes that could be a result of any number of complex interventions. A maternal death for instance, is as much an outcome of poverty, rights violations, poor access, poor human resources for health and non-existent transport infrastructure as it is an outcome of postpartum haemorrhage or eclampsia. An exclusive focus on clinical interventions, critical though these are, would certainly reduce deaths from cases that report successfully to the health services, but will do very little to prevent those cases that never reached the health services. It has been much easier, therefore to concentrate resources on the concrete interventions that have a tangible and short-term impact than to invest in the translation and

operationalization of complex social phenomena such as changes in societal attitudes, values and protection of human rights. The critical point is that the focus on the endpoint has been at the cost of the importance of the route taken during the journey.

*Allotey and Reidpath, 2015, p. 152*

So, the linkages between processes, be they political, programmatic, or normative, are what will give impetus to the advancement of SRHR under the aegis of the SDGs. But those processes require institutional homes because there is no escape from politics or from the kinds of authoritative, concerted marshalling of resources that governments and intergovernmental institutions can marshal and sustain.

Second is Universal Health Coverage (UHC). The expansion of the post-MDG agenda will inevitably mean that financing for HIV and AIDS programming and support activities will decline. Early signs of this are already evident with the current review of PEPFAR preceded by a signal from the US government that it expects recipient countries to assume a larger share of the fiscal burden going forward. More worrying still, there has been no new specific commitment for the epidemic by any significant donor since 2008. In real terms, financing for the epidemic actually declined by 15 per cent during 2009–13 (Kaiser Family Foundation/UNAIDS, 2013). And as the thematic priorities expand, there will be enormous pressure to collapse the generally vertical HIV and AIDS programmes into the broader health sector of affected countries (Nigatu, 2012). The argument will be that doing so will not only ensure the long-term sustainability of the HIV and AIDS response, but will also enable the much-needed strengthening of health systems to be initiated. This is a central though not sole driver of the campaign for UHC (Poku, 2016). However, accommodating the HIV and AIDS response into the governance of health in countries which already struggle with the strength, reach, and coherence of their health systems will present a formidable challenge to Ministries of Health and Finance.

But while both national and international expectation of UHC is intensifying (Universal Health Coverage Coalition, 2016), there is no precise, agreed understanding of what it should or might best comprise – and on what basis (such as full state provision; mixed public/private; insurance-based). Quite aside from ever-present budgetary constraints, neither universal coverage nor a transformation of the strength, coherence, and accessibility of existing systems can be conjured. As the WHO/World Bank First Global Monitoring Report on Universal Health Coverage has outlined:

We face three main challenges in tracking UHC: first, sourcing reliable data on a broad set of health service coverage and financial protection indicators; second, disaggregating data to expose coverage inequities; third, measuring effective coverage, which not only includes whether people receive the services they need but also takes into account the quality of services provided and the ultimate impact on health. [...Because] health system strengthening is the main means by which countries can progress towards UHC, UHC monitoring needs to be integrated into broader health systems performance assessment, and because UHC includes health services and financial protection coverage, it is essential that UHC monitoring of both aspects takes place side by side. Many countries with weak health systems score strongly on financial protection coverage simply because citizens forgo needed health services. It is only by evaluating the coverage of health services and financial protection jointly that we can reach appropriate conclusions as to how effectively the health system is providing coverage.

*WHO/World Bank, 2015, p. 1*

And whether even the most viable of developing world health systems will be able to absorb the pressures of a retrenchment of funding on the scale already underway – for HIV and AIDS most clearly, but not only for those – remains to be seen. It is not difficult to abstract any of the SDGs' targets from their context; and while it is easy to foresee that progress in many will be meagre at best, it seems unlikely that any large and sustainable human betterment will be possible without a truly concerted effort to secure the mainstays of the largest and closely inter-connected global health challenges which are set to persist.

## References

African Union Commission. (2015) 'Africa 2063: the Africa we want', available at www.un.org/en/africa/osaa/pdf/au/agenda2063.pdf (accessed on 21 August 2017).

Allotey, P. and Reidpath, D.D. (2015) 'Sexual and reproductive health and rights post 2015-challenges and opportunities', *BJOG: An International Journal of Obstetrics and Gynaecology*, 122(2): 152–5.

Greenhill, R. and Ali, A. (2013) 'Paying for progress: how will emerging post-2015 goals be financed in the new aid landscape?' ODI Working Paper Number 366 (April), available at www.odi.org/sites/odi.org.uk/files/odi-assets/publications-opinion-files/8319.pdf (accessed on 12 July 2017).

Institute of Health Metrics Evaluation. (2010) 'Financing global health 2010: development assistance and country spending in economic uncertainty', available at www.healthmetricsandevaluation.org/publications/policy-report/financing_global_health_2010_IHME (accessed on 1 August 2017).

International Conference on Financing for Development. (2002) 'Report of the International Conference on Financing for Development, Monterrey, Mexico, 18–22 March 2002', available at www.un.org/esa/ffd/monterrey/MonterreyConsensus.pdf (accessed on 4 June 2017).

International Conference on Financing for Development. (2015) 'Outcome document of the Third International Conference on Financing for Development: Addis Ababa Action Agenda (13–16 July 2015)', available at www.uneca.org/sites/default/files/uploaded-documents/FFD3-2015/outcome-document.pdf (accessed on 3 August 2017).

Kaiser Family Foundation/UNAIDS. (2013) 'Financing the response to HIV in low- and middle-income countries', available at www.unaids.org/en/media/unaids/contentassets/documents/document/2013/09/20130923_KFF_UNAIDS_Financing.pdf (accessed 12 August 2017).

Nigatu, T. (2012) 'Integration of HIV and noncommunicable diseases in health care delivery in low- and middle-income countries', *CDC – Preventing Chronic Disease*, 9: 1545–51.

Poku, N. (2016) 'How should the post-2015 response to AIDS relate to the drive for Universal Health Coverage?' *Global Public Health*, available at: http://dx.doi.org/10.1080/17441692.2016.1215486

Poku, N. and Whitman, J. (2011) 'The Millennium Development Goals and development after 2015', *Third World Quarterly*, 32(1): 181–98.

Standing, H., Oronje, R.N., and Hawkins, K. (Eds.) (2011) *BMC International Health and Human Rights*, 11 (Suppl.3), available at: www.ncbi.nlm.nih.gov/pmc/issues/205987/ (accessed on 28 July 2017).

Thoen, E. (2002) 'TRIPS, pharmaceutical patents and access to essential medicines: a long way from Seattle to Doha', *Chicago Journal of International Law*, 3(1): 27–68.

United Nations. (2000) 'We can end poverty: Millennium Development Goals and beyond 2015', available at www.un.org/millenniumgoals/poverty.shtml (accessed on 28 July 2017).

United Nations. (2015a) 'The Millennium Development Goals report 2015', available at www.un.org/millenniumgoals/2015_MDG_Report/pdf/MDG%202015%20rev%20(July%201).pdf (accessed on 28 July 2017).

United Nations. (2015b) 'The Addis Ababa action agenda of the Third International Conference on Financing for Development', available at www.un.org/esa/ffd/ffd3/wp-content/uploads/sites/2/2015/07/Addis-Ababa-Action-Agenda-Draft-Outcome-Document-7-July-2015.pdf (accessed on 29 July 2017).

United Nations General Assembly. (2014) 'Report of the Intergovernmental Committee of Experts on sustainable development financing (15 August 2014)', A/69/315, available at www.un.org/ga/search/view_doc.asp?symbol=A/69/315&Lang=E (accessed on 4 August 2017).

UNAIDS. (2011) 'AIDS at 30: nations at a crossroads', available at http://reliefweb.int/sites/reliefweb.int/files/resources/aids-at-30.pdf (accessed on 4 August 2017).

UNAIDS. (2014) 'Fast-track: ending the AIDS epidemic by 2030', available at www.unaids.org/en/resources/documents/2014/JC2686_WAD2014report (accessed on 5 August 2017).

UNAIDS. (2016) 'Fact sheet – latest statistics on the status of the AIDS epidemic', available at www.unaids.org/en/resources/fact-sheet (accessed on 3 August 2017).

UNAIDS and Lancet Commission. (2015) 'Defeating AIDS, advancing global health', *The Lancet*, 25 June, available at http://thelancet.com/commissions/defeating-aids-advancing-global-health (accessed on 3 August 2017).

Universal Health Coverage Coalition. (2016) available at http://universalhealthcoverageday.org/welcome/ (accessed on 1 August 2017).

WHO/World Bank. (2015) 'Tracking Universal Health Coverage: first Global Monitoring Report' available at http://apps.who.int/iris/bitstream/10665/174536/1/9789241564977_eng.pdf (accessed on 15 July 2017).

World Bank. (2009) 'Swimming against the tide: how developing countries are coping with the global crisis', Background Paper prepared by World Bank Staff for the G20 Finance Ministers and Central Bank Governors Meeting, Horsham, United Kingdom on 13–14 March, 2009, available at www.un.org/ga/president/63/PDFs/WorldBankreport.pdf (accessed on 17 September 2016).

World Bank. (2010) 'Global monitoring report 2010: the MDGs after the crisis', available at https://openknowledge.worldbank.org/handle/10986/2444 (accessed on 4 May 2015).

# 19

# Disrupting global health

## The Gates Foundation and the vaccine business

*Jacob Levich*

Recent critiques of the Bill & Melinda Gates Foundation (BMGF) acknowledge, to varying degrees, the malign effects of 'philanthrocapitalism' on the people's health (Aschoff, 2016; McGoey, 2015). Yet these effects are typically portrayed as the unintentional consequences of misguided benevolence. The multibillionaires mean well, it is suggested, but are somehow too naïve to recognise the inherent limitations of market-based solutions to health crises.

It is more realistic to assume that Bill Gates and his ilk are highly sophisticated capitalists who know what they want and how best to get it. While critics are correct in pointing out that BMGF has failed to deliver the public health miracles it promises, this line of argument may be missing the point. BMGF is only secondarily concerned, if at all, with saving lives; primarily, it is devoted to expanding worldwide markets and facilitating commerce on behalf of Western capitalism. The Foundation's embrace of the practices and organisational norms of corporate capitalism is neither accidental nor misguided, but is central to a deliberate strategy for bringing 'disruptive innovation' to the public health field.

The concept of disruptive innovation entered management theory in the late 1990s at a time when global capital, liberated by the fall of the Soviet Union, had set about tearing down old monopolies in order to make room for new ones (Lepore, 2014). The term is flattering to entrepreneurs, because it connotes bold, original thinking, but in reality it describes a process as old as capitalism itself: the more or less ruthless restructuring of existing systems and norms to create space for even more profitable replacements.

Originally associated with high-tech startups, the concept soon became central to business ideology and is now applied to neoliberal 'reforms' in every sector: workforce reductions made possible by automation and digital outsourcing, union-busting measures aimed at the privatisation of public schools, the substitution of private health insurance markets for health care entitlements, etc. Newly minted philanthrocapitalists were naturally inclined to impose familiar business practices on their charitable endeavours; hence, 'disruption' has become a watchword and a guiding principle throughout the field of philanthropy. For Bill Gates, who became the world's richest human being through notoriously anti-competitive business practices (Gavil and First, 2014), the public health field offered a global laboratory for further experimentation with disruptive strategies.

## Vaccines and the pharma business

BMGF's style of disruption is nowhere more evident than in the area of vaccines, Bill Gates's particular focus and historically the central business of his foundation. When Seth Berkeley, CEO of the Gates-controlled vaccine consortium GAVI, advised a conference of pharmaceutical entrepreneurs that 'GAVI is a disruptive instrument', he was not merely mouthing a management shibboleth. He was describing, in a rare moment of frankness, the true business of the Gates Foundation. Today, traditional systems of vaccine procurement and distribution are rapidly giving way to vast public–private supply chains, steered and substantially funded by the Gates Foundation in collaboration with the pharmaceutical industry (Gates, 2013).

The symbiosis between the world's most powerful charitable enterprise and Big Pharma, infamous for its cynicism and criminality, arises from the particular requirements of pharmaceutical capital. Despite annual revenues approaching US$1 trillion, the industry has been unable to reverse a declining rate of profit and finds itself in a perpetual state of crisis. The search for exploitable new molecules is becoming increasingly frantic and expensive (Roy, 2012). Advertising costs, meanwhile, are skyrocketing as the industry attempts to wring revenue from wary and financially strapped customers (Dobrow, 2015).

Industry publicists like to frame the business as a noble quest to meet society's relentless demand for new cures. In reality, Big Pharma manufactures and shapes demand, not vice versa. The nature of the drug business, like every industry under capitalism, is conditioned by the need to dispose of surplus profitably: 'In order to absorb potential economic output and forestall excess capacity, business interests must continuously search for new markets to exploit …' (Wrenn, 2016, p. 63).

Market pressures are particularly acute in the pharma business because of unusually high development costs and a narrow patent window. Pharmaceutical firms rely on high-reward 'blockbuster drugs' – those with annual sales of US$1 billion or more – to boost stock prices and generate sometimes astonishing profit margins (Anderson, 2014). However, US and EU patent protections grant pharmaceutical firms a 20-year period of exclusive rights to new drugs.

Consequently, Big Pharma must take exceedingly aggressive measures to maximise profits as the so-called 'patent cliff' approaches. The ostensible market for newly developed drugs – i.e., people who actually suffer from the conditions that the medications are meant to treat – is rapidly saturated. New buyers must then be found, or manufactured. Multi-million-dollar advertising campaigns are devised to push treatments for dubious conditions such as 'restless leg syndrome' or 'female sexual dysfunction' (Allen, 2009). Doctors are pressured to write off-label prescriptions that permit the dispensing of medications for unapproved uses (Stafford, 2008). These unethical but technically legal tactics are supplemented with a wide range of criminal activities, including falsifying the results of clinical trials, suppressing information about side effects, and paying kickbacks to health care professionals (Groeger, 2014; Srinivasan, 2010b). Such practices are so common in the industry that massive criminal fines are considered merely 'the cost of doing business' (Tozzi, 2015).

Big Pharma's well-deserved notoriety is not due to exceptional wickedness on the part of executives and shareholders. Rather, it reflects a logical response to imperatives that shape every facet of the pharmaceutical industry:

- The largest possible markets for approved 'blockbuster drugs' must be found, expanded, and ruthlessly exploited. Where no market exists, it is necessary to create one – or many.
- The scramble for new blockbusters is ceaseless and fraught. Factors that hinder rapid commercialisation of new drugs – e.g., safety testing requirements or national regulatory regimes – must be ameliorated, subverted, or outflanked.
- The substantial capital investment required to bring drugs to market – i.e, R&D, safety testing, and marketing – must be reduced or defrayed wherever possible. Subsidies from government and charitable institutions that support high drug prices must be pursued energetically.

- Investment must be steered towards products targeting large worldwide markets, like vaccines, in pursuit of an attractive risk–return tradeoff. A drug of dubious efficacy that targets a large population may be more profitable than a highly efficacious drug targeting a rare disease.

This state of affairs has serious implications for the health and well-being of the world's poorest billions. Increasingly, Big Pharma seeks to supplement declining sales in wealthy Western countries by exploiting largely untapped 'pharmerging markets' (Smedley, 2015, n.p.). Since 70 per cent of the world's population lives in countries so designated, profits are potentially enormous.

The growing number of sick people in the South offers unprecedented scope for selling putatively therapeutic medicines; vaccines, by contrast, promise revenue because they can be sold to vast numbers of *healthy* people. Revisions to national immunisation calendars can expand the addressable population for patented vaccines by hundreds of millions. No wonder emerging markets are seen as 'the next big growth engine in Pharma' (Mooraj, 2013, n.p.).

For these reasons, manufacturing new channels of demand in poor countries is a business necessity. Barriers to entry – price controls, regulatory regimes, lack of health care infrastructure – must be outflanked by innovative tactics. Extensive collaboration with Western NGOs, PPPs, foundations, and private firms is considered essential to overcoming such obstacles, both in 'top-tier' markets (i.e., BRICS) and in the poorest nations of the global South (Badoria, et al., 2012; Levy, 2015). Hence the requirement for 'disruptive innovation': existing mechanisms of health care delivery must be restructured or even destroyed in order to make way for a profit-directed value chain.

In another sense the people of the South figure prominently in Big Pharma's business strategies. Cost-cutting on the development side is seen as an answer to declining revenues; offshoring is an effective expedient. Hence the relocation of clinical trials to emerging markets, where drug safety testing is seen as relatively cheap, speedy, and lax. GlaxoSmithKline CEO Jean-Pierre Garnier has frankly characterised this process as 'massive arbitrage' facilitated by globalisation: 'arbitrage in labour cost, in financial cost, but also in pools of skilled employees and in regulatory and administrative hurdles' (Petryna, 2009, p. 82).

According to anthropologist Adriana Petryna, 'the geography of clinical testing is changing dramatically. In 2005, 40 percent of all trials were carried out in emerging markets, up from 10 percent in 1991' (Petryna, 2009, p. 13). In India in 2011 more than 150,000 people were involved in at least 1,600 clinical trials, conducted on behalf of British, American, and European firms (Buncombe and Lakhani, 2011). R&D offshoring is now so widespread in the global South that clinical trials are considered a 'normal part of healthcare delivery' (Petryna, 2007, p. 22). As a South African newspaper declared, 'We are guinea pigs for the drugmakers' (Child, 2013).

Thus the imperatives of the pharmaceutical business have created a perfect storm centering on the people of the South. It is in this context that BMGF's interventions are critical to the industry. With its worldwide organisation, resources, and muscle, BMGF is ideally situated to facilitate profitable connections between Big Pharma, the global health bureaucracy, and state health ministries. It functions as an essential link in a pharmaceutical value chain that extends all the way from BMGF's US$500 million headquarters in Seattle to the poorest villages of Africa and South Asia.

## Enter the Gates Foundation

The Gates Foundation's ties with the pharmaceutical industry are intimate, complex, and longstanding. Soon after its founding, BMGF invested US$205 million in pharmaceutical companies, including Merck & Co., Pfizer Inc., Johnson & Johnson, and GlaxoSmithKline (Colorni, 2013). The relationship has grown in subsequent years, creating a revolving door that now routinely shuttles executives between BMGF, Gates-controlled NGOs, and pharma's big five (Herper, 2011a). The leadership team for BMGF's Global Health Division includes former executives of AstraZeneca, Baxter International Healthcare Corp., Eli-Lilly,

Novartis, Parke-Davis, Pfizer, and Wyeth (BMGF, 2017c). PATH, described by *The Lancet* as virtually an 'agent of the Foundation' (Global Justice Now, 2016, p. 21), functions openly as a facilitator for more than 60 corporate partners, creating 'market-based solutions' for pharmaceutical companies such as Merck and Sanofi.

It is unsurprising, then, that BMGF's goals align closely with the needs of the pharmaceutical industry. The Foundation is openly committed to supporting R&D strategies tailored to the realities of the developing world, where '[t]o speed the translation of scientific discovery into implementable solutions, we seek better ways to evaluate and refine potential interventions – such as vaccine candidates – before they enter costly and time-consuming clinical trials' (BMGF, 2017a, n.p.). In plain language, BMGF promises to assist Big Pharma in its efforts to circumvent Western regulatory regimes by sponsoring cut-rate drug trials in the periphery. At the same time, BMGF steers the budgets of sovereign nations towards investments that create markets for Western transnational corporations (TNCs), even when such investments require radical reallocations of funds away from traditional public health programmes. The goal, as frankly stated in a USAID report, is to 'leverage market actors and dynamics to stimulate demand' (USAID, 2014, p. 51).

BMGF entered the field in 1999 with a US$50 million contribution establishing the Malaria Vaccine Initiative. Here Bill Gates saw an opportunity for his fledgling foundation to dominate, instantly and decisively, an entire field of charitable endeavour: 'With one grant ... we became the biggest private funder of malaria research. It just sort of blows the mind' (Strouse, 2000, n.p.). Since then, BMGF's involvement in vaccine production and delivery has been transformative, integrating private corporations and investment capital into a field where, until quite recently, the profit motive had played a relatively minor role.

State-sponsored immunisation programmes spread widely during the twentieth century and doubtless saved millions of lives, especially in countries that were able to integrate vaccine administration into robust public health programmes. For the pharmaceutical industry, vaccines became a source of steady but meager profits. The most widely administered vaccines were not patented: when Jonas Salk was asked who owned the patent on his polio vaccine, he replied 'the people', adding, 'There is no patent. Could you patent the sun?' (Hiltzik, 2014, n.p.). Although Big Pharma spokesmen were happy to take credit for immunisation successes, vaccines were in fact a 'neglected corner of the drugs business' (The Economist, 2010, n.p.); industry involvement was a matter of manufacturing doses and selling them in a buyer's market shaped by government procurement programmes that tended to depress prices. Margins were so slim that by the mid-2000s many firms contemplated exiting the business altogether (The Economist, 2010).

Countries in the non-socialist periphery, meanwhile, found it difficult or impossible to emulate the immunisation successes of the first and second world. Relying on financial and technical support from UN institutions, limited national immunisation programmes developed unevenly across the global South during the postwar era, but these were severely hampered by lack of resources and infrastructure (Miller and Sentz, 2006). Austerity regimes imposed by the West after the fall of socialism were further devastating to the national public health apparatus required for effective vaccine distribution. In business terms, the addressable market remained immense, but the supply chain was dysfunctional and the buyer base was small, concentrated, and increasingly cash-poor. By the late 1990s, money for procurement was scarce or nonexistent, and Western pharmaceutical firms had little incentive to pursue profits in low-income countries.

This bleak business landscape was radically altered by the intervention of the Gates Foundation. Working in close collaboration with pharma, BMGF and its subsidiary organisations disrupted and revitalised the industry with novel schemes to pry open emerging markets. Within a decade of BMGF's initial investments, vaccines were no longer a neglected sector but had become the cornerstone of Big Pharma's prodigious revenues – indeed, the global vaccine market was recently projected to reach US$77.5 billion by 2024 (Grand View Research, 2016). In an encomium to the vaccine strategies of 'one of history's greatest business visionaries', *Forbes* praised Bill Gates for demonstrating 'how power and capital – both literal and political – can be spent to maximize positive impact on the world.' He had done so, the article conceded in less grandiloquent terms, by 'creat[ing] a lasting market for big pharma that wouldn't cost them their shirts' (Herper, 2011b, n.p.).

BMGF's philosophy holds that charitable endeavours need to be evaluated in much the same terms as business deals (BMGF, 2017d). Vaccines offered an irresistible opportunity to 'meet the needs of the poor in ways that generate profits and recognition for business' (Gates, 2008, n.p.) by employing commercial strategies adapted from Microsoft and Wall Street. These can best be summarised in the language of business theory, part of the ideology that structures the thinking of contemporary capitalists:

- First mover advantage: As the first significant occupant of a neglected market segment, BMGF could create the business conditions that would make the rules for subsequent players, ensuring its continued ascendancy in the field.
- The vertical market: A problem that might be addressed via 'vertical' health initiatives (programmes aimed at particular diseases as opposed to broad-based public health efforts) was readily adaptable to Microsoft's vertical marketing strategies and would be congenial to the Foundation's preference for benchmark-friendly quick fixes over infrastructural investments.
- Actionable measurement: By applying the simplistic business math that Gates sees as the solution to society's ills, a field traditionally entrusted to public authorities could be more effectively managed via the supposedly superior wisdom of the private sector. Vertical programmes, due to their narrow scope and goals, would lend themselves naturally to numerical data analysis aimed at 'optimizing scarce resources for maximum impact' (BMGF, 2017b, n.p.).
- Value Unlocking: Partial privatisation of vaccine administration could be said to liberate the value of public capital, resulting in a projected $100 billion in economic benefits for poor countries (Lee, et al., 2013). At the same time, new forms of development funding aimed at harnessing the profit motive could be touted as unlocking the value of private markets.
- Leverage: A pre-existing but underfunded and feeble institutional apparatus (e.g., WHO's immunisation department; state public health ministries) could easily be subordinated and steered by strategic investments. In combination with public–private partnerships founded and ultimately controlled by BMGF, the Foundation could wield vast resources with relatively little investment of its own.

In sum, Bill Gates found in the vaccine market conditions that would facilitate his wholesale appropriation of a key public health sector. Almost overnight, BMGF became the originator and final arbiter of global vaccine policy, ensuring that decisions affecting lives and health of the underdeveloped world would be centralised in Seattle. According to Melinda Gates, Bill's partner in all things philanthropic, the choice was clear: 'Where's the place you can have the biggest impact with the money?' (Herper, 2011b, n.p.).

## GAVI

BMGF's raid on the immunisation field commenced with the creation of GAVI, the Global Alliance for Vaccines and Immunization, perhaps the most influential 'public–private partnership' in public health. Launched by BMGF in 2000 with the 'explicit goal to shape vaccine markets' (GAVI Alliance, 2017b, n.p.), GAVI is a consortium connecting major international institutions (WHO, UNICEF, the World Bank) with the big powers of the pharmaceutical industry (Janssen, GSK, Merck, Sanofi Pasteur, Pfizer, et al.) – all mediated and steered by the Gates Foundation.

GAVI supplied the leverage Gates needed to direct global policy. BMGF seeded the organisation, holds a permanent seat on its board of directors, and has contributed more than US$4 billion to its operations (GAVI Alliance, 2017a). Vividly described as a '900 pound gorilla' (Kingah, 2001, p. 132), GAVI sets the agenda for all players in the vaccine field: its approval is both a necessary and a sufficient condition for the launch of vaccine-related initiatives.

From the outset GAVI promised to: (a) accelerate introduction of new vaccines, (b) expand the use of 'existing cost effective vaccines'; and (c) fast-track R&D for new vaccines 'relevant to developing countries' (BMGF, 1999, n.p.). Notably, however, GAVI funds have rarely been used to support the distribution to global South countries of vaccines traditionally deemed necessary for Western children – diphtheria, mumps, pertussis, tetanus, et al.[1] Instead, GAVI has consistently focused on promoting precisely the new and expensive 'blockbuster vaccines' that pad Big Pharma's profit margins. The bulk of its early investments were geared towards immunisation against pneumococcal disease (with a vaccine developed by Pfizer), hepatitis B (GlaxoSmithKline and Merck), and the flu-like bacterial infection Hib (Merck and Sanofi). As of 2012, four of the five top-selling vaccine products – Pfizer's Prevnar-13, Sanofi's PENTAct-HIB, GSK's Cervarix and hepatitis vaccine franchise – had been heavily subsidised and promoted by GAVI (EvaluatePharma, 2012).

In 2009 GAVI pioneered the use of a new type of development financing, the Advance Market Commitment (AMC), as a means of subsidising the sale of Pfizer's new pneumococcal vaccine, Prevnar, to low-income countries (GAVI Alliance, 2009). Through GAVI, BMGF and five wealthy countries – Italy, the United Kingdom, Canada, Norway, and Russia – offered a contract guaranteeing a viable market for the drug, committing to buy new vaccines at a negotiated high price purporting to cover development costs. The pilot country was ravaged Rwanda, which was converted overnight into a market for 1.6 million doses of the patented vaccine (Sheikh and Ngoboka, 2009). As a condition of the deal, Rwanda agreed to add Prevnar to its routine national immunisation programme, though it was unclear how the country might hope to finance its commitment to future purchases once GAVI subsidies lapsed. Soon thereafter, Benin, Central African Republic, and Cameroon were also enlisted, expanding the market by further millions. AMC financing proved so lucrative that by 2012 Prevnar had become the world's leading vaccine product, with projected 2018 sales of US$6.7 billion (EvaluatePharma, 2012). GAVI, meanwhile, had demonstrated 'proof of concept' of an elaborate neoliberal scheme that transferred public funds to private coffers.

A more recent addition to GAVI's array of services is 'innovative development financing', a debt-based mechanism that taps capital markets to subsidise vaccine buyers and manufacturers. Through an intermediary, the International Finance Facility for Immunisation (IFFIm), GAVI floats bonds on the Japanese *urudashi* market. The bonds are secured by the promise of government donors to buy millions of doses of vaccines at a set price over periods as long as 20 years. The system is hailed in development circles as a neoliberal 'win-win': although capitalists take a cut at every stage of the value chain, poor countries are said to benefit from access to vaccines that might not otherwise be affordable. Bondholders receive a tax-free guaranteed return on investment, suited to an era of ultra-low interest rates. For GAVI, this 'organizational form without country presence' offers a powerful means of steering peripheral vaccine markets from the core while outflanking the political inconveniences of traditional development aid. Hence IFFIm now annually supplies as much as 39 per cent of GAVI's cash (EvaluatePharma, 2012).

Pharmaceutical firms, meanwhile, are able to peddle expensive vaccines at subsidised prices in a cash-poor but vast and risk-free market: 'by creating a predictable demand pull, IFFIm addresses a major constraint to immunisation scale-up: the scarcity of stable, predictable, and coordinated cash flows for an extended period' (Atun, et al., 2012, p. 2045). Although GAVI's involvement in vaccine pricing is typically praised as though the organisation is dedicated to setting price ceilings, in fact it acts invariably to raise the floor.

Occasionally criticised but seemingly irresistible is GAVI's role in blurring the distinctions between private enterprise and public policy. In some cases BMGF/GAVI has effectively annexed the health ministries of poor countries (Ghosh, 2016, n.p.). The organisation seems entirely unabashed by its role in reconstituting what some have called 'pharmaceutical colonialism'. In Sri Lanka, for example, GAVI intervened in 2002, offering to subsidise a high-priced vaccine supplied by Crucell, a subsidiary of Johnson & Johnson. The vaccine, known as pentavalent Hib, was a cocktail adding Haemophilus influenzae type b immunity to the traditional DTwP shot; it was this new formula that made the drug patentable and thus profitable. The voices of critics, who argued that 'new, "relatively useless" vaccines were being allowed to piggy-back on standard essential vaccines like DPT', went unheard (Bindu, 2016, n.p.).

Since the sticker price for pentavalent Hib was nearly 20 times greater than the drugs it replaced, GAVI offered Sri Lanka temporary subsidies, so long as the country committed to adding the vaccine to its national immunisation schedule.

Within three months of the vaccine's introduction, 24 adverse reactions including four deaths were reported, leading Sri Lanka to suspend use of the vaccine (WHO, 2013). Subsequently 21 infants died from adverse reactions in India. Critics pointed out that Hib is a minor public health issue in South Asia, and that adverse reactions could be projected to cause the deaths of 3,125 children for every 350 lives saved by the vaccine (Kalyanam, 2013). Thus the customary argument in favour of new vaccines – that the significance of a few drug-related deaths is far outweighed by the number of lives saved – was flipped on its head. Nevertheless, WHO, a GAVI partner, promptly stepped in to declare the vaccine safe – whereupon Sri Lanka reversed the suspension (Narendran, 2011).

Once pentavalent vaccine was firmly ensconced in Sri Lanka's national immunisation programme, GAVI began to phase out its financial support. In effect, GAVI secured Sri Lanka's legal commitment to buy patented vaccines on an ongoing basis, using subsidised prices as a loss leader, and then left the country on the hook with a perpetual obligation to buy. GAVI calls this process 'graduation' (Saxenian, et al., 2014). In a write-up appearing on GAVI's promotional website, Sri Lankan health minister Ananda Amarasinghe purported to reveal 'the secrets behind the country's immunisation success story.' Collaboration with GAVI has been effective, Dr. Amarasinghe suggests, because 'our *colonial masters* [emphasis added] established a good foundation' (Endean, 2015, n.p.). Evidently no irony was intended.

## PATH

GAVI would serve to steer the overall direction of global vaccine policy, but BMGF required another subsidiary to assist in the development of new vaccines at every stage of the value chain, 'from initial discovery through clinical trials and licensure' (Boslego, 2012, p.700). In keeping with the principle of leverage, Gates declined to create a new organisation *ex nihilo*, but instead commandeered an existing entity. This was the Program for Appropriate Technology in Health (PATH), a Seattle-based population control NGO to which the Foundation was already connected through Gates's father. BMGF showered the organisation with funds, installed representatives on the board of directors, and was soon in a position to name as its CEO Steve Davis, a Microsoft alumnus and former law partner of Bill Gates Sr. (Barker, 2008). The process by which BMGF remolded PATH for its own purposes resembled what is known in the business world as a friendly takeover.

Although PATH continued to boost contraceptives, supporting the development and distribution of vaccines soon became its central mission. At the back end of the value chain, PATH acts to defray pharma's development expenses by funding research. In particular, PATH acts to connect scientists in the non-profit field with vaccine manufacturers and biotech firms, ensuring that the public and private spheres are blended throughout the process (PATH, 2017). Since PATH's grant-making reflects the aims of BMGF and the commercial interests of Big Pharma, academic research is inevitably steered in directions regarded by the industry as potentially profitable, e.g., rotavirus, malaria, HIV/AIDS, and influenza. PATH also sometimes collaborates with BRICS-based drug firms such as the Serum Institute of India, owned by billionaire 'vaccine king' Cyrus Poonawalla. The partnerships arranged by PATH in this context help to ensure that local industries do not develop independently of the requirements of Western pharmaceutical capital.

PATH is heavily involved in orchestrating and funding clinical trials necessary to bring branded vaccines to market. To manage the trials, PATH hires Contract Research Organisations (CROs), which in turn recruit local organisations to carry out operations cheaply on the ground, exploiting core/periphery wage differentials. In this Taylorised offshoring system, pressure to achieve speedy, favourable results is immense and ethical violations are rife (Elliott, 2012).

A review of the literature reveals a disturbing pattern in PATH-sponsored trials, which nearly always raise ethical questions but evidently never fail to secure the desired approvals. In 2010, for example, PATH organised a Phase III trial of Mosquirix, a malaria vaccine developed by GlacoSmithKline (GSK), and administered the experimental treatment to thousands of African infants across seven countries. GSK and BMGF declared the trials a smashing success, and their publicity was uncritically reproduced by the popular press (Boseley, 2011). In fact the vaccine was only narrowly efficacious, apparently reducing malaria rates in a range from 18 per cent to 36 per cent. The study's fine print revealed that the trials resulted in 151 deaths and caused 'serious adverse effects' (e.g., paralysis, seizures, febrile convulsions) in 1,049 of 5,949 children aged 5–17 months (RTS,S Clinical Trials Partnership, 2011). The results should have raised serious questions about whether the limited benefits outweighed the serious risks. Instead, WHO moved forward with a sweeping pilot programme targeting sub-Saharan Africa, anticipating universal implementation in the near future (WHO, 2016).

Other PATH-sponsored vaccine trials in the global South revealed a similar pattern of dubious efficacy, ethical violations, and widespread deaths and injuries (e.g., GSK's rotavirus vaccine, tested in India in 2011 [Carome, 2004], and the BMGF-financed MenAfriVac meningitis vaccine, tested in Chad in 2011–12 [*Suna Times*, 2013]). In these cases, too, the approval of relevant health ministries was swiftly secured.

In one highly publicised case, however, popular outrage appeared to have thwarted PATH's designs, at least temporarily. In 2010 seven adolescent tribal girls in Gujarat and Andhra Pradesh died after receiving injections of HPV (Human Papilloma Virus) vaccines as part of a large-scale 'demonstrational study' funded by the Gates Foundation and administered by PATH (Srinivasan, 2010a). The vaccines, developed by GSK and Merck, were given to approximately 23,000 girls between 10 and 14 years of age, ostensibly to guard against cervical cancers they might develop in old age.

Extrapolating from trial data, Indian physicians later estimated that at least 1,200 girls experienced severe side effects or developed auto-immune disorders as a result of the injections (Mehta, et al., 2013). No follow-up examinations or medical care were offered to the victims. Further investigations revealed pervasive violations of ethical norms: vulnerable village girls were virtually press-ganged into the trials, their parents bullied into signing consent forms they could not read by PATH representatives who made false claims about the safety and efficacy of the drugs. In many cases signatures were simply forged (Dhar, 2013).

An Indian Parliamentary Committee found that PATH had 'violated all laws and regulations laid down for clinical trials by the government' in a 'clear-cut violation of human rights and a case of child abuse' (Parliament of India, 2013). In the months following release of the committee report, no action was taken: the government declined to act on its recommendations; a lawsuit on behalf of the victims remained 'stuck in limbo' before the Indian Supreme Court (Mittal, 2016). PATH, evidently unperturbed, steamed forward with trials of a new flavour of HPV vaccine, Merck's Gardasil 9, with typical consequences including reports of coercion, lack of informed consent, and paralysing injuries (Chamberlain, 2015). Meanwhile, India's state and local health ministries experienced increasing pressure from the highest levels of the global public health apparatus to embrace HPV vaccines (Narayanan, 2018).

PATH-endorsed vaccine development resembles a juggernaut that rolls irresistibly forward despite hazardous clinical trials, unsatisfactory results, or resistance from the people. According to public health journalist Sandhya Srinivasan, 'PATH's research agenda is to look for ways to introduce the vaccine into the national immunisation programme. The question is not "whether" but "when" and "how"' (Srinivasan, 2011).

## Buying WHO

Coopting the health ministries of poor countries was no great challenge for an organisation as powerful as BMGF, but the creation of a genuinely global vaccine market would require steering and investment on an international scale. To that end, BMGF needed to ensure the collaboration of the World Health Organization. WHO is empowered to marshal and allocate financial commitments from UN member nations (securing, for example, the cash GAVI needs to raise the floor for drug prices); additionally, the agency figures prominently in the regulatory process by which underdeveloped countries issue approvals for new vaccines and other drugs. In order to assimilate WHO's authority, BMGF employed yet another business strategy: it took an ownership stake.

BMGF's contributions to WHO started early and rose steadily; by 2016, BMGF was investing US$227 million annually, underwriting fully 11 per cent of the agency's annual budget – more than any member state with the exception of the US (Global Justice Now, 2016). GAVI and PATH together added US$75 million to the total (WHO, 2017). Here BMGF's strategy emulated the cross-ownership deals by which business firms routinely seek to disrupt or neutralise competitors. Gates saw no need to fund a majority of WHO's budget; rather, his Foundation invested just heavily enough that the agency would be unable to function without BMGF's ongoing participation.

Exploiting this financial leverage, BMGF was able effectively to seize control of the global health agenda: According to public health insiders, 'Gates' priorities have become the WHO's' (Huet, et al., 2017). Bill Gates was widely understood to have been the kingmaker in the 2017 choice of Tedros Adhanom Ghebreyesus to succeed Margaret Chan as director-general of WHO, where Gates is now treated 'like a head of state' (Huet, et al., 2017). In the same year, despite a letter of protest signed by 30 health advocacy groups, BMGF secured appointment as a non-voting member of WHO's governing board, solemnising what had become a de facto partnership between a once-prestigious multilateral institution and one of the world's most powerful capitalists (Kadama, et al., 2017).

The arrangement with WHO consolidated BMGF's disruptive project, securing the long-term global interests of Western capital. Longstanding structures of health care delivery had been deliberately dismantled, subordinating public health to the ruthless imperatives of profit-seeking. The Gates model seemed likely to spread, offering a template for Mark Zuckerberg, Jeff Bezos, and other billionaires embarking on large-scale and systematic interventions in various sectors of philanthropy. As Melinda Gates informed a 2013 Gates-organised conference on 'Positive Disruption', the couple's endeavours are ultimately intended 'to give more people the courage to be disruptive and in doing so, unlock the potential of many others all over the world' (Anderson, et al., 2013). A plausible translation of this thinly coded language might read: 'to be disruptive [is to] unlock potential profits from the people of the global South.'

## Note

1   An exception is polio vaccine, which GAVI consistently supports in keeping with Bill Gates' frequently stated commitment to ridding the world of polio. Although polio is no longer a major public health threat – only 48 cases were reported in 2015 – its final eradication appears to be of tremendous symbolic importance to Gates.

## References

Allen, T.J. (2009) 'Restless vagina syndrome', In These Times, available at http://inthesetimes.com/article/5016/restless_vagina_syndrome/ (accessed on 12 November 2017).

Anderson, C., et al. (2013) 'Positive disruption Q&A: Melinda Gates and Chris Anderson on TEDx as a force for change', Impatient Optimists, available at www.impatientoptimists.org/Posts/2013/03/Positive-Disruption-QampA-Melinda-Gates-and-Chris-Anderson-on-TEDxChange-as-a-Force-for-Change (accessed on 12 March 2018).

Anderson, R. (2014) 'Pharmaceutical industry gets high on fat profits', BBC News, available at www.bbc.com/news/business-28212223 (accessed on 12 November 2017).

Aschoff, N. (2016) The New Prophets of Capital, London: Verso.

Atun, R., et al. (2012) 'Innovative financing for health: what is truly innovative?', The Lancet, 380(9858): 2044–9.

Badoria, V. et al. (2012) Transforming India's Vaccine Market: Saving lives, creating value, Mumbai: McKinsey & Co., 15 September, p. 34.

Barker, M. (2008) 'The Gates Foundation: Microsoft's "charity"', available at https://zcomm.org/znetarticle/the-gates-foundation-microsoft-s-charity-part-2-of-3-by-michael-barker/ (accessed on 29 November 2017).

Bindu, S. (2016) 'Unhealthy reporting', Himal, available at http://himalmag.com/unhealthy-reporting/ (accessed on 29 November 2017).

BMGF. (1999) 'Bill & Melinda Gates Foundation announces $750 million gift to speed delivery of life-saving vaccines', available at www.gatesfoundation.org/Media-Center/Press-Releases/1999/11/Global-Alliance-for-Vaccines-and-Immunization (accessed on 29 November 2017).

BMGF. (2017a) 'Discovery and translational sciences strategy overview', available at www.gatesfoundation.org/What-We-Do/Global-Health/Discovery-and-Translational-Sciences (accessed on 12 November 2017).

BMGF. (2017b) 'Evaluation policy', available at www.gatesfoundation.org/How-We-Work/General-Information/Evaluation-Policy (accessed on 29 November 2017).

BMGF. (2017c) 'Global health leadership', available at www.gatesfoundation.org/Who-We-Are/General-Information/Leadership/Global-Health (accessed on 12 November 2017).

BMGF. (2017d) 'How we work', available at www.gatesfoundation.org/How-We-Work (accessed on 29 November 2017).

Boseley, S. (2011) 'Malaria vaccine could save millions of children's lives', The Guardian, available at www.theguardian.com/society/2011/oct/18/malaria-vaccine-save-millions-children (accessed on 29 November 2017).

Boslego, J.W. (2012) 'PATH's vaccine development global program', Human Vaccines, 8(6): 700.

Buncombe, A. and Lakhani, N. (2011) 'Without consent: how drug companies exploit Indian "guinea pigs"', Independent, available at www.independent.co.uk/news/world/asia/without-consent-how-drugs-companies-exploit-indian-guinea-pigs-6261919.html (accessed on 12 November 2017).

Carome, M. (2004) 'Unethical clinical trials still being conducted in developing countries', Huffington Post, available at www.huffingtonpost.com/michael-carome-md/unethical-clinical-trials_b_5927660.html (accessed on 29 November 2017).

Chamberlain, G. (2015) 'Judges demand answers after children die in controversial cancer vaccine trial in India', Daily Mail, available at www.dailymail.co.uk/news/article-2908963/Judges-demand-answers-children-die-controversial-cancer-vaccine-trial-India.html (accessed on 29 November 2017).

Child, K. (2013) 'We are guinea pigs for the drugmakers', available at www.timeslive.co.za/news/2013/07/25/we-are-guinea-pigs-for-the-drugmakers (accessed on 12 November 2017).

Colorni, R.R. (2013) 'Bill Gates, Big Pharma, bogus philanthropy', available at http://newsjunkiepost.com/2013/06/07/bill-gates-big-pharma-bogus-philanthropy/ (accessed on 12 November 2017).

Dhar, A. (2013) 'It's a PATH of violations, all the way to vaccine trials: House panel', The Hindu, available at www.thehindu.com/news/national/its-a-path-of-violations-all-the-way-to-vaccine-trials-house-panel/article5083151.ece (accessed on 29 November 2017).

Dobrow, L. (2015) 'Pharma DTC spending jumps almost 21% in 2014', Medical Marketing & Media, available at www.mmm-online.com/agency/pharma-dtc-spending-jumps-almost-21-in-2014/article/404922/ (accessed on 10 November 2017).

Elliott, C. (2012) 'What happens when profit margins drive clinical research', available at www.motherjones.com/environment/2010/09/clinical-trials-contact-research-organizations (accessed on 29 November 2017).

Endean, C. (2015) 'Sri Lanka: five steps to vaccine success', available at www.vaccineswork.org/post/133290012222/sri-lanka-five-steps-to-vaccine-success (accessed on 29 November 2017).

EvaluatePharma. (2012) 'World preview 2018: embracing the patent cliff', available at http://download.bioon.com.cn/view/upload/201207/04104656_3288.pdf (accessed on 29 November 2017).

Gates, B. (2008) 'Creative capitalism', remarks at the 2008 Davos World Economic Forum, available at www.gatesfoundation.org/media-center/speeches/2008/01/bill-gates-2008-world-economic-forum (accessed on 29 November 2017).

Gates, B. (2013) 'Innovation, disruption, and progress: what do vaccines, software, and shipping containers have in common?', available at www.gatesnotes.com/Books/The-Box (accessed on 10 November 2017).

GAVI Alliance. (2009) 'GAVI partners fulfill promise to fight pneumococcal disease', available at www.gavi.org/library/news/press-releases/2009/gavi-partners-fulfill-promise-to-fight-pneumococcal-disease/ (accessed on 29 November 2017).

GAVI Alliance. (2017a) 'The Bill & Melinda Gates Foundation', available at www.gavi.org/about/partners/bmgf/ (accessed on 29 November 2017).

GAVI Alliance. (2017b) 'Vaccine supply and procurement', available at www.gavi.org/about/gavis-business-model/vaccine-supply-and-procurement/ (accessed on 29 November 2017).

Gavil, A. and First, H. (2014) The Microsoft Antitrust Cases: Competition policy for the 21st century, Cambridge, MA: MIT Press.

Ghosh, A. (2016) '"Conflict of interest": NHM panel raises questions on Bill Gates Foundation', Indian Express, available at http://indianexpress.com/article/india/india-news-india/conflict-of-interest-nhm-panel-raises-questions-on-bill-gates-foundation/ (accessed on 29 November 2017).

Global Justice Now. (2016) 'Gated development: is the Gates Foundation always a force for good?', available at www.globaljustice.org.uk/sites/default/files/files/resources/gjn_gates_report_june_2016_web_final_version_2.pdf (accessed on 12 November 2017).

Grand View Research. (2016) 'Vaccine market analysis by type', available at www.grandviewresearch.com/industry-analysis/vaccine-market (accessed on 29 November 2017).

Groeger, L. (2014) 'Big Pharma's big fines', Pro Publica, available at http://projects.propublica.org/graphics/bigpharma (accessed on 12 November 2017).

Herper, M. (2011a) 'What Bill Gates says about drug companies', Forbes, available at www.forbes.com/sites/matthewherper/2011/11/10/what-bill-gates-says-about-drug-companies-2/#10932e874412 (accessed on 12 November 2017).

Herper, M. (2011b) 'With vaccines, Bill Gates changes the world again', Forbes, available at www.forbes.com/sites/matthewherper/2011/11/02/the-second-coming-of-bill-gates (accessed on 29 November 2017).

Hiltzik, M. (2014) 'On Jonas Salk's 100th birthday, a celebration of his polio vaccine', L.A. Times, available at www.latimes.com/business/hiltzik/la-fi-mh-polio-vaccine-20141028-column.html (accessed on 12 November 2017).

Huet, N., et al. (2017) 'Meet the world's most powerful doctor', Politico, available at www.politico.eu/article/bill-gates-who-most-powerful-doctor (accessed on 10 March 2018).

Kadama, P.Y., et al. (2017) 'Open Letter to the Executive Board of the World Health Oranization', available at http://healthscienceandlaw.ca/wp-content/uploads/2017/01/Public-Interest-Position.WHO_.FENSAGates.Jan2017.pdf (accessed on 10 March 2017).

Kalyanam, S. (2013) 'Medical experts divided over use of Pentavalent vaccine on children', Indian Express, available at www.newindianexpress.com/cities/bengaluru/Medical-experts-divided-over-use-of-pentavalent-vaccine-on-Children/2013/07/29/article1707186.ece (accessed on 29 November 2017).

Kingah, S. (2001) Access to Medicines and Vaccines in the South, Brussels: Brussels University Press.

Lee, L., et al. (2013) 'The estimated mortality impact of vaccinations forecast to be administered during 2011–2020 in 73 countries supported by the GAVI Alliance', Vaccine, 31(2): B61–72.

Lepore, J. (2014) 'The disruption machine', The New Yorker, available at www.newyorker.com/magazine/2014/06/23/the-disruption-machine (accessed on 10 November 2017).

Levy, J. (2015) 'How can pharma succeed in emerging markets?', Pharmafile, available at www.pharmafile.com/news/499479/how-can-pharma-succeed-emerging-markets (accessed on 12 November 2017).

McGoey, L. (2015) No Such Thing as a Free Gift: The Gates Foundation and the price of philanthropy, London: Verso.

Mehta, K., Bhanot, N., and Rao, V.R. (2013) 'Supreme Court pulls up government of India over licensing and trials with "cervical cancer" vaccines', Countercurrents, available at www.countercurrents.org/mehta070113.htm (accessed on 29 November 2017).

Miller, M.A. and Sentz, J.T. (2006) 'Vaccine-preventable diseases', In: D.T. Jamison, et al. (Eds.) Disease and Mortality in Sub-Saharan Africa, 2d edn, Washington, DC: World Bank, pp. 163–77.

Mittal, P. (2016) 'Legal updates: Supreme Court to continue hearing tax entry case', LiveMint, available at www.livemint.com/Politics/yX18YC3JwYnCeS3Sl54FBK/Legal-updates-Supreme-Court-to-continue-hearing-entry-tax-c.html (accessed on 29 November 2017).

Mooraj, H. (2013) 'How Big Pharma can win in emerging markets', Industry Week, available at www.industryweek.com/emerging-markets/how-big-pharma-can-win-emerging-markets (accessed on 12 November 2017).

Narayanan, N. (2018), 'Efficacy, safety, cost: India's decade-old debate on the cervical cancer vaccine erupts again, Scroll.in, available at https://scroll.in/pulse/865284/efficacy-safety-cost-indias-decade-old-debate-on-the-cervical-cancer-vaccine-erupts-again (accessed on 11 March 2018).

Narendran, R. (2011) 'WHO expert clears doubts on pentavalent vaccine', Indian Express, available at www.newindianexpress.com/states/kerala/article363437.ece (accessed on 29 November 2017).

Parliament of India. (2013) '72nd report on alleged irregularities in the conduct of studies using Human Papilloma Virus (HPV) vaccine by PATH in India, sec. II', available at www.pharmamedtechbi.com/~/media/Supporting%20Documents/Pharmasia%20News/2013/September/HPV%20Vaccines%20Parliameetnary%20Report%20%20Aug%2031%202013.pdf (accessed on 29 November 2017).

PATH. (2017) 'Our strategy: vaccines for the world's underserved populations', available at http://sites.path.org/vaccinedevelopment/our-strategy/ (accessed on 29 November 2017).

Petryna, A. (2007) 'Clinical trials offshored: on private sector science and public health', BioSocieties, 2.

Petryna, A. (2009) *When Experiments Travel: Clinical trials and the global search for human subjects*, Princeton, NJ: Princeton University Press.

Roy, A. (2012) 'Stifling new cures: the true cost of lengthy clinical drug trials', available at www.manhattan-institute. org/html/stifling-new-cures-true-cost-lengthy-clinical-drug-trials-6013.html (accessed on 10 November 2017).

RTS,S Clinical Trials Partnership. (2011) 'First results of phase 3 trial of RTS,S/AS01 malaria vaccine in African children', *New England Journal of Medicine*, 365(20): 1863–75.

Saxenian, H., et al. (2014) 'Overcoming challenges to sustainable immunization financing: early experience from GAVI graduating countries', *Health Policy and Planning*, 30(2): 197–205.

Sheikh, M. and Ngoboka, C. (2009) 'Historic pneumococcal vaccine shipment arrives in Rwanda', available at www2. unicef.org:60090/immunization/rwanda_48945.html (accessed on 29 November 2017).

Smedley, T. (2015) 'Big Pharma attempts to cast off bad reputation by targeting the poor', The Guardian, available at www.theguardian.com/sustainable-business/2015/jun/25/big-pharma-attempts-to-cast-off-bad-reputation-by-targeting-the-poor (accessed on 12 November 2017).

Srinivasan, S. (2010a) 'A vaccine for every ailment', Infochange, available at http://infochangeindia.org/public-health/healthcare-markets-and-you/a-vaccine-for-every-ailment.html (accessed on 29 November 2017).

Srinivasan, S. (2010b) 'Disease-mongering: any which way to find a market', Infochange, available at http://infochangeindia.org/agenda/medical-technology-ethics/disease-mongering-any-which-way-to-find-a-market.html (accessed on 12 November 2017).

Srinivasan, S. (2011) 'HPV vaccine trial and sleeping watchdogs', available at www.issuesinmedicalethics.org/index.php/ijme/article/view/143/231 (accessed on 29 November 2017).

Stafford, R.S. (2008) 'Regulating off-label drug use – rethinking the role of the FDA', *NEJM*, 358: 1427–9.

Strouse, J. (2000) 'How to give away $21.8 billion', The New York Times, available at www.nytimes.com/2000/04/16/magazine/how-to-give-away-21.8-billion.html (accessed on 12 November 2012).

*Suna Times*. (2013) 'The plight of the Tibu children and the Chad vaccination case', available at http://sunatimes.com/articles/2554/The-Plight-of-the-Tibu-Children-and-the-Chad-Vaccination-Case (accessed on 29 November 2017).

The Economist. (2010) 'A smarter jab', available at www.economist.com/node/17258858 (accessed on 29 November 2017).

Tozzi, J. (2015) 'Bill Ackman's right: Big Pharma gets fined all the time', Bloomberg, available at www.bloomberg.com/news/articles/2015-10-30/bill-ackman-s-valeant-defense-fines-are-cost-of-doing-business (accessed on 12 November 2017).

USAID. (2014) 'Healthy markets for global health: a market-shaping primer', available at www.usaid.gov/sites/default/files/documents/1864/healthymarkets_primer.pdf (accessed on 12 November 2017).

WHO. (2013) 'Pentavalent vaccine in Asian countries', available at www.who.int/vaccine_safety/committee/topics/pentavalent_vaccine/Jul_2013/en/ (accessed on 29 November 2017).

WHO. (2016) 'Malaria vaccine: WHO position paper', Weekly Epidemiological Record, available at www.who.int/wer/2016/wer9104.pdf (accessed on 29 November 2017).

WHO. (2017) 'Voluntary contributions by fund and by contributor, 2016', available at www.who.int/about/finances-accountability/reports/A70_INF4-en.pdf (accessed on 10 March 2018).

Wrenn, M.V. (2016) 'Surplus absorption and waste in neoliberal monopoly capitalism', *Monthly Review*, 68(3): 63.

# 20

# National influence in global health governance

## The case of the United Kingdom's Department for International Development

*Daniel E. Esser*

Despite the rise of private foundations, multi-donor initiatives and transnational advocacy networks in development assistant for health (DAH) (MacLean and MacLean, 2009; Fidler, 2010), national governments remain important agenda setters in global health governance. While a realist perspective on international relations would expect national agencies to focus on implementing independent policy priorities of their governments, 'bandwagoning' (Wezel and Saka-Helmhout, 2005), i.e., the adoption or imitation of certain agencies' agendas by other aid organisations (DiMaggio and Powell, 1983), is in fact widespread. Why, then, are some national donors looked to by their international peers for prioritising issues and developing practices in global health? In contrast to donor–recipient dynamics in DAH, which have been documented in detail (Hunsmann, 2012; Esser, 2014), inter-organisational influence between DAH donors has received limited attention to date (Siddiqi, et al., 2009; Jones, et al., 2017). In response, this chapter offers a case-based neo-institutionalist interpretation of the United Kingdom's (UK) Department for International Development (DFID)'s influence on DAH. By foregrounding systemic and managerial determinants at the national scale, it challenges not only realist theories of international relations, but also constructivist explanations of global policies as resulting mainly from ideational convergence (Kraatz, 1998; Shiffman, et al., 2016).

The chapter begins with a brief overview of neo-institutionalist theory and then situates DFID in the context of global health governance. Heeding to calls for 'open[ing] the black box of organizational routines' (Pentland and Feldman, 2009, p. 300), it then synthesises qualitative data from 16 interviews with aid experts working on DAH both within and outside of DFID. Themes arising from these interviews illustrate a complex interplay of structural and agentic forces anchored in the UK's national political economy. Agency-specific approaches to building in-house knowledge, a track record of evidence-based aid allocation, and a macro-level perspective on multilateralism are found to be influential in creating political influence in global health governance. At the same time, domestic governance frameworks and electoral dynamics in donor countries are credited with affecting an agency's ability to adhere to evidence-based programming, which in turn co-determines its clout in transnational global health networks.

In international studies, neo-institutionalism sits in-between theories of structural dominance on the one hand, and individual – or organisational – agency (Wendt, 1987; Schneider, 1991; Greenwood and

Hinings, 1996; Pierson, 2003) on the other. The theory is comparable to the sociological concept of structuration (Giddens, 1984), which posits that structures frame agency, which in turn alters structures. Neo-institutionalism thus regards institutions not merely as rules providing firm sets of incentives for rational actors, but as 'cognitive scripts' (Hall and Taylor, 1996) that shape practices of political life and that are at the same time susceptible to political challenge and resulting change. At the analytical level of globally active organisations, this theoretical proposition implies that these organisations and their leaders are certainly not free agents, but neither are they perfectly beholden to frameworks inherited from past governing arrangements (Moe, 2005).

From a neo-institutionalist perspective, a given organisation's performance is determined by how well it conforms with existing institutions, while instantaneously challenging the limitations of these institutions in ways that benefit its unique set of competitive advantages. Herein, deliberate actions using internal capacity allow organisations to maximise their *efficiency* (March and Sutton, 1997; Horowitz, 2007; Bersch, et al., 2016). In contrast, their *effectiveness* tends to increase with greater structural autonomy (Tendler and Freedheim, 1994; Evans, 1995; Carpenter, 2001), over which most organisations have no direct control. In essence, then, neither agentic nor structural factors alone can provide an exhaustive explanation of organisational impact; it is their interaction that determines specific (and ultimately also systemic) outcomes. Organisations can and do act as 'norm entrepreneurs' (Sunstein, 1996), but they still have to take into account existing practices (Bourdieu, 1977; Guler, et al., 2002; Adler and Pouliot, 2011) since the latter reflect past compromises – explicit as well as tacit – between relevant stakeholders (Moe, 2005; Rasche and Esser, 2006).

At the turn of the millennium, the World Health Organization (WHO), which for decades had served as the main convener of national health agencies, was drawing fierce criticism from constituents for its bloated bureaucracy, waning expertise, and ineffective programmes (Levine, 2006; Youde, 2012). This pressure exacerbated the already weak structural position of the WHO relative to the agenda-setting power of other UN organisations focusing on other salient global issues, such as environmental change or the plight of refugees (Mooney, 2012). The resulting proliferation of alternative hubs of DAH coordination, which had already begun with the HIV crisis during the 1980s, fuelled concerns that global health governance could eventually become unmanageable (Prah Ruger, 2004; McColl, 2008; Sridhar, 2010; Wood Pallas and Prah Ruger, 2017). Indeed, writing shortly after the close of global health governance's first decade (2000–9), Youde (2012, p. 5) diagnosed 'a serious lack of global health leadership', creating a situation in which 'responses to health concerns may be rather ad hoc and fragmented' (ibid.). He concluded, 'there exists no single global health governance hierarchy [in] a highly chaotic system' (Youde, 2012, pp. 3–5).

As much as this depiction of contemporary global health governance captures the multitude of interests and stakeholders present, it risks overlooking the historical role of some organisations in shaping the field's approaches and practices. In the following section, this chapter argues that DFID can be characterised as a norm entrepreneur not just broadly with regard to poverty reduction (Mawdsley, 2015, p. 343), but also more specifically in the area of global health. Although the department's role never amounted to that of a lead agency as envisioned by Youde (2012), this reading of organisational entrepreneurship counters the representation of global health governance as a 'highly chaotic system' (ibid.). Even where formal hierarchies are absent, leadership does occur.

Replacing the UK's Overseas Development Administration in 1997, DFID was created as an independent government department to underscore the 'UK's claim to an international leadership role' in global development cooperation (Mawdsley, 2015, p. 348). Under the direction of Clare Short as the country's first cabinet-level Secretary of State for International Development, DFID swiftly gained a reputation for research-driven programming (Mawdsley, 2012). During Short's tenure, DAH was one of the department's focus areas, and would remain so for the following decade. Although the United States (US) ran the largest budget for global health between 1995 and 2007, the UK led in terms of the percentage of aid earmarked for health interventions abroad, hovering around 15 per cent between 1995 and 2007 (Stepping, 2016).

Although total funding amounts do of course matter, country-level DAH allocations often bear no logical connection to recipient countries' population sizes or actual disease burdens (Esser and Keating Bench, 2011). It is therefore important to note that during the period from 1995 until 2007, the UK was the only donor country that disbursed more DAH to countries with larger populations, *ceteris paribus* (Stepping, 2016). In addition, DAH flows from the UK were also the only ones among all health donors to respond to relatively higher immunisation rates in recipient countries (ibid.). Unsurprisingly then, DFID forged a reputation as the world's most transparent and efficient DAH donor (Duran and Glassman, 2012) while being recognised as an international ringleader with substantial 'political fire power' in global health governance (Buse, 2005, p. 23).

DFID complemented such targeting practices with strategic innovations. For instance, it was among the first donors to implement a maternal health strategy, a move that allowed it to play an influencer role in multi-stakeholder networks (ICAI, 2018) leading up to the formulation and adoption of the 2015 Sustainable Development Goals (SDGs). It was also successful at counterbalancing the centrality of poverty reduction in global development discourses by highlighting the importance of not just reducing poverty, but also addressing inequality (Esser and Williams, 2014).

In order to better understand how this international leadership position came about, in-depth interviews were conducted with DFID staffers as well as senior global health stakeholders outside of the agency. Following Tansey's (2007) approach to elite interviewing, informants were selected based on personal references and subsequent snowballing. This technique allowed for the identification of policy-making participants with knowledge of DFID's internal workings and the department's standing among global health stakeholders. Forty-four potential informants were contacted via e-mail and invited to participate. Table 20.1 summarises the sample's key characteristics. Data are presented in a way that ensures anonymity, as requested by most informants.

The resulting 16 interviews were carried out over a period of five months (June until November 2012) either in person in London and Washington, DC, or via Voice over Internet Protocol (VoIP). Interviews lasted between 35 minutes and over two hours. The high number of declined interview requests from within DFID resulted from the first two interviews with informants in the department being conducted with staff members whom many of their colleagues regarded as 'representative', thus – in the latter's view – rendering additional input 'redundant'. The experience highlights a regrettable flaw in the research design, i.e., interviewing senior bureaucratic personnel *before* documenting the views of less senior staffers. Nonetheless, qualitative data saturation was reached for the whole sample after a dozen interviews, suggesting that no critically relevant data were missed (Guest, et al., 2006; Francis, et al., 2010).

Thematic clustering of the raw data then produced six overarching themes, listed in the following in their order of salience, represented parenthetically by the number of interviews in which each theme was evoked: 'political structures' (16), 'strategies of cooperation' (15), 'organisational management' (14), 'political dynamics' (14), 'organisational structures' (13), and 'organisational culture, diversity, and idiosyncrasies' (9). The six themes contain a total of 235 textual references to the interview transcripts. These references are distributed roughly equally except for the least salient theme ('organisational culture, diversity, and idiosyncrasies'), which only contains 13 references.

## Political structure

The 'political structure' within which DFID has been operating since 1997 was singled out in all interviews. The department's status as a separate ministry that is 'not a part of the foreign office' (Int #15) has created 'a high level of political autonomy' (ibid.). This relative 'structural independence' (Int #4) was argued to have 'given [DFID] more of a free reign to be less inhibited, and to champion […] what they perceive as aid effectiveness or as the most effective, or most aid-effective approach' (Int #1). A DFID staffer (Int #10) linked this structurally advantageous position to the department's parliamentary backing of its mandate through the UK's International Development Act:

Table 20.1 Potential and actual informants, June–November 2012

| Organisational affiliation | Invited, but declined to be interviewed | Interviewed |
| --- | --- | --- |
| DFID | (14) | Interim Head of Department; Team Leader; Program and Policy Manager; Health Economist (4) |
| WHO | (2) | Senior Advisor to the Assistant Director General; Director (2) |
| Organisation for Economic Co-operation and Development | (0) | Deputy Director; Senior Health Economist (2) |
| World Bank | (1) | Senior Manager (1) |
| UNAIDS | (1) | |
| United States Agency for International Development (USAID) | (0) | Senior Advisor (1) |
| Save the Children UK | (2) | Head of Unit (1) |
| Oxfam UK | (1) | |
| Gavi, the Vaccine Alliance | (1) | |
| Marie Stopes International | (0) | Consultant (1) |
| Bill & Melinda Gates Foundation | (1) | |
| Children's Investment Fund Foundation | (0) | Director (1) |
| Brookings Institution | (0) | Fellow (1) |
| Center for Global Development | (1) | |
| Chatham House | (1) | |
| Overseas Development Institute | (0) | Senior Research Associate (1) |
| London School of Health and Tropical Medicine | (1) | Professor (1) |
| London School of Economics and Political Science | (1) | |
| Network of International Consultants in Health and Development | (1) | |
| Total (44) | 28 | 16 |

We have a different political and constitutional framework the way that DFID operates. [...] By that, I mean having a development agency which is actually a government department and which is headed by a cabinet-level minister. I think also the legal framework that we operate under, which restricts very carefully what we can spend our budget on, so it has to go towards poverty reduction [...], and that's legally safeguarded which, I think, does a certain amount to protect DFID's budget against potential other uses of the funds. We have that actually enshrined in law, which is helpful.

A similar point was made by another DFID staffer who argued that the International Development Act 'sort of shielded DFID from all sorts of influences and actually allowed freedom to really think through, "how do we best do this?"' (Int #3). Another informant used the same rationale to point to a 'critical difference between DFID and USAID [being] the role that parliament plays in assigning budgets. [...] USAID colleagues can do nothing without Congress's agreement' (Int #2). This was echoed by another interviewee who argued that UK ministers 'have a lot of space to, within the legal framework, within the policy frame-work, to get on with things and do things – you compare that to the US where, with the earmarks and daily reporting, that's very difficult'. This contrast also came up in the account of a US-based informant who stressed 'the freedom that DFID has to allocate its resources' (Int #7). Meanwhile, he argued, the US 'Congress is, particularly in health, pretty clear about the categories of assistance that are acceptable' (ibid.).

According to several internal DFID sources, the department's relatively independent political position and legally protected mandate resulted in an 'overwhelming amount of [UK] development assistance [being] controlled by DIFD' (Int #9) and in 'other donors know[ing] that we can take a little more risk than quite a few others, and we're flexible in how we give out, not only how we give out aid, but in terms of what we do' (Int #6). In addition, informants also underlined generally higher public support, whether for the government as a whole ('there is in the UK [...] a respect for government, unlike in the case of the US'; Int #12) or its commitment to foreign aid (e.g., 'public perception of the importance of foreign assistance in Britain'; Int #7) by the UK electorate. Finally, DFID's embeddedness in a strong national research environment was stressed as a complementary structural advantage (Int #14).

DFID's position in the UK's governance structure thus emerged as an important factor in co-determining the department's perceived influence in global health governance. This was compounded by concurrent 'political dynamics'. Illustrating the influence of singular political actors, one informant (Int #3; also Int #5) quipped, 'Sometimes the Secretary of State decides this is what we're going to do, and then we're going to do it'. Beginning with the department's first secretary, Clare Short, almost all informants raised the UK's political climate leading into the first decade of the new millennium as highly conducive to both efficiency and effectiveness. One of them (Int #16) circumscribed Short's vision for DFID by stressing its 'very clear anti-poverty remit. It was about development, not about aid. It was about trying to change the structure in countries so that there would be less poverty'. Others concurred, crediting Short for providing 'clarity of goals' (Int #4; also Int #11) from the outset. One of them (Int #15) explained,

Going back to 1997 and the New Labour government, when DFID came into being, that was a turning point. There can be no question about that in terms of the level of political commitment given to development, a level of ambition, if you like, that Clare Short had about what the UK should be trying to do. [...] And I think there was also at that time quite a lot of, I would say possibly more so than now [2012], a lot of like-mindedness among a group of European donors that also, I guess, the Netherlands, the Swedes, the Nordics, to some extent Germany, where there was a time there was a kind of commonality in the politics. There was a moment when all these development ministers were female. There was this close-knit grouping. And health was something that was seen very much as one of the areas where this grouping could be working closely together on.

Such political support for global health persisted beyond Short's resignation over the US-led invasion of Iraq in May 2003. 'I think during [Chancellor and later Prime Minister Gordon] Brown['s] government', one interviewee (Int #11; also Int #9, Int #10) intimated, 'Brown was very close to [billionaire Bill] Gates, and so there was a lot of interaction at a very high level'. This sentiment was echoed by another informant who suggested, 'The kind of policy leadership that Gordon Brown provided and the interest that he took in development, that's not something you find in other places'. Another DFID staffer (Int #10) stated, 'We've also had, for some years now, cross party support for the development budget, which is fantastic and has been maintained by the present [Conservative] government as well, so we had really favourable political conditions'. Such 'cross-party political consensus' (Int #4; also #14, #15) was pointed to repeatedly, not least because it had resulted in 'having the backing from the Treasury' (Int #3; also Int #5, Int #10) as well. In sum, 'a level of political leadership – goal setting, organisation, the bureaucracy, and clear messaging, and powerful leadership internationally – is part of the story about what has made DFID a relatively good development institution in global health' (Int

#4). In fact, top-level political clout was considered so central by some (Int #3) that its loss could mean that 'we become another USAID'.

## Organisational structures

The critical importance of highest-level backing does not suggest, however, that DFID's internal 'organisational structures' and management practices were negligible. Exercising influence in transnational network governance requires competence and presence, for which bureaucratic capacity is a precondition (Kahler, 1999). Moreover, capable staff members can also exercise considerable influence over political practices internally (Chwieroth, 2013). For DFID, both of these prerequisites were in place. 'Historically', one informant (Int #14) confirmed, 'DFID had strong chief advisor positions across a range of sectors, Chief Health Advisor […] and so on'. In combination with 'quite large numbers of health advisors and professional staff' (Int #1) and 'a lot of technical staff in country' (Int #2), this made for a 'health cadre [of] a very significant size' (Int #15). One of the interviewees (Int #12) not affiliated with the department explained this as follows: 'Whenever I have worked on a policy issue, DFID has had more people, and serious people, who are working on it, than say the Dutch, or the Swedes, or the Germans'. This quote also illustrates that even among like-minded donors, capacity differed.

This positive impact of staff quantity was amplified by increasing staff quality. 'Over the last 10 years or so, with the emphasis on increasing British aid', some informants (Int #14; also Int #2, Int #5) argued, 'the quality of the civil servants within DFID has increased very considerably'. This widely held perception of 'high flying graduates wanting to go into DFID, in part because of the nature of the work and its reputation' (Int #15) is also echoed in the scholarly literature (Distler, 2016, p. 106). This dynamic rendered a 'very high level of technical competence among [DFID's] staff' (Int #7).

It is the combination of quantity and quality that had a direct bearing on the department's international clout. One informant (Int #11) exemplified this interaction follows:

> [I]n order to influence a multilateral, you have to go to all the board meetings and staff them, and prepare papers for it, and be strategic. Civil servants, people at DFID, they're good at that sort of staffing, that sort of influencing multilaterals; it's sort of a natural fit with the skill set that a lot of the DFID people have, because DFID has advisors and administrators and the administrators are sort of traditional civil servants and basically they do well in bureaucratic situations like that.

Another informant (Int #7) also credited DFID's in-house expertise with the department's ability 'to swim in the same sort of waters as the Bill & Melinda Gates Foundation, perhaps to a higher degree than other official donors'. At the same time, 'simpler' (Int #2) internal decision-making and reporting structures were stressed as contributing significantly to DFID's efficiency. 'Heads of office [at headquarters] have more freedom in deciding how to spend their budget than other bilateral heads of agency in each [recipient] country' (Int #10). Indeed, several informants stressed that DFID's 'country offices have a huge amount of autonomy' (Int #2; also Int #6).

## Learning culture

Fuelled by a 'strong learning culture' (Int #1; also Int #15), there was also a 'growing sense that [DFID's] policy decisions need[ed] to be evidence-based' (Int #5) to the extent that 'every business case [for a new aid program] ha[d] to be littered with evidence about cost effectiveness of the approaches' (Int #6). At a personal level, informants stated that DFID was 'considered a good place to work, quite different from the US' (Int #12); a department where 'pretty young smart people are given a high level of responsibility, and I think that that has been a characteristic particularly of DFID' (Int #15). The department's staff quality was such that – in contrast to a concern outlined earlier – some informants even felt confident that its cadre could withstand and contain the detrimental effects of poor leadership (Int #2).

It seems, then, that DFID's competent bureaucratic cadre working in an efficient decision-making and reporting structure gradually forged a hallmark *modus operandi*, as several informants attested. 'DFID's working method is through short, sharp, frequently well-documented and argued positions that are subject to sequential decisions and iteration by ministers, rather than long, involved, bureaucratic, encyclopaedic sector studies', said one of them (Int #9). Underlying this approach was a 'belief in a political strategy [...] that [the UK] can achieve greater impact through shaping the 95 per cent of the world's development resources that are not ours' (Int #4). 'DFID staff are judged on their ability to form and maintain and deepen partnerships', another informant (Int #2) explained.

In order to translate this valorisation of multilateralism into practice, DFID took the decision to support recipient countries' sectors rather than fund specific projects. Often referred to as a 'systems-oriented approach' (Int #4; also Int #13), over time it thus nurtured 'a codification of the set of rules, with budget support and sector-wide approaches emerging as preferred instruments within DFID' (ibid.). This tactic marked another contrast to the practices by the world's most financially committed health donor, the United States, as one informant (Int #2) noted: 'DFID will put millions of pounds into countries behind country-led processes and trust their people in those countries to get the best value for money out of those funds; US systems aren't set up to do that' (ibid.).

DFID's strategic focus on systems rather than specific problems equally informed the department's negotiations in the context of global health governance forums. One of the interviewees (Int #14) explained, 'DFID has been very strategic in not just worrying about specific programs of assistance or projects, but also about the broader aid environment and broader engagement within countries'. Through general budget support,

> you don't need so many people to actually manage specific projects and what you have to do is engage in policy dialogue within countries because you need to be in the game of influencing of all government decision making rather than choosing particular projects.
>
> *ibid.; also Int #6, Int #16*

In addition to DFID's relatively larger quantity of technical staff, its overarching strategy thus allowed it to be present and proactively offer input at crucial decision-making points in global health governance, with the effect that 'other donors started to get on board' (Int #6). Moreover, the department also upheld 'a very active policy of placing their own staff in other institutions' (Int #3), with decisions by other DAH agencies often co-formulated by staff on loan from DFID.

As a result of this focus on multilateralism through coalitions that 'engage others' (Int #8) and 'bind in partners' (Int #15), and leveraging the fact that British aid remained untied (Int #2, Int #11) during the period of study, DFID succeeded at expanding its role as a 'critical friend' (Int #1) with 'a hard hat' (Int #12) to the WHO, whose convening powers continued to wane. In 2011, in an exercise of 'wielding its global power' (Int #13), the department then carried out its first comprehensive multilateral aid review. This comparative study of UN agencies' performance was remarkable not only for its open criticism of the WHO's lack of efficiency and effectiveness, but also for spurring an international coalition of DAH donors urging that the 2005 Paris goals on aid effectiveness should finally be translated into organisational reforms. The move elevated DFID's role from a contributor of DAH to that of an evaluator of multilateral cooperation, notably in the absence of any official international mandate.

## Conclusion

The qualitative analysis offered in this chapter suggests that DFID's ascendancy an influential national actor in global health governance is the result of a combination of systemic and agentic factors coinciding at the beginning of the new millennium and reaching well into its first decade. Using a neo-institutionalist lens allows us to recognise DFID's advantageous structural position while simultaneously shedding light on the importance of strategic leadership and bureaucratic practices. For DFID to become an efficient and effective player in global health in transnational networks comprising both state and non-state actors, it had to mobilise structural capital, namely its position in the UK's governance structure, by securing lasting political support while shielding itself from mission creep. At the same time, DFID took advantage of a structural opening in global health governance by exploiting the demise of the WHO's expertise and convening power through new strategic partnerships beyond the realm of national governments as the most established stakeholders in the international system. This strategy focused on attaining a *primus inter pares* ('first among equals') status in global multilateral forums through presence and expertise, while prioritising collaboration with one particular non-state actor, the Bill & Melinda Gates Foundation. The latter's technocratic approach to DAH, coupled with its rootedness in forging innovation and lean corporate management practices, proved to be highly complementary to the political weight and vision of one of the world's leading national donor agencies. The Foundation has since topped the list of single-donor contributions to the WHO, thus consolidating the dyad's influence over the UN body and bolstering DFID's position as a global health agenda setter.

As much as electoral dynamics and committed political leadership creating and defending spaces for experimentation and risk-taking are to be credited when explaining DFID's international impact, more recent political trends and resulting policy changes in the UK do not bode well for the department's future role in global health governance. Scandals aside, such as the *Daily Mail*'s cover stories on allegedly squandered funds (*Daily Mail*, 2017) or the dismissal of DFID's Secretary after she had attempted to open an independent foreign policy channel with the Government of Israel (*The Guardian*, 2017), the successive Conservative cabinets of Prime Ministers Cameron and May have put a premium on British aid's attributability by seeking to demonstrate its impact first and foremost to domestic voters rather than to local beneficiaries or international partners. As a consequence, the UK has reversed its stance on multilateral state and non-state collaboration and instead returned to bilateral control as the primary mode of international assistance. With the country preparing for Brexit amid increasingly shrill nationalism, this might seem like a logical approach, but it risks DFID's credibility as a leading voice on DAH. If one agrees that the analysis presented in this chapter makes a case for the virtues of national influence in global health governance, then the outlook for DFID is sombre.

## Acknowledgement

Funding in support of this research was provided by American University's International Travel Award for Faculty and is gratefully acknowledged. Participants at the April 2015 Center on Health, Risk & Society (CHRS) seminar at American University offered useful comments on an earlier version of this chapter. Nico von der Goltz at the World Bank assisted with initial contacts in DFID, and Jonathan Fox shared many helpful documents detailing DFID's strategic direction. Anne J. Kantel provided invaluable assistance through reviewing background literature and preparing the qualitative data analysis; the chapter in its final form would not have materialised without her.

## References

Adler, E. and Pouliot, V. (2011) 'International practices: introduction and framework', In: E. Adler and V. Pouliot (Eds.) *International Practices*, New York, NY: Cambridge University Press, pp. 3–35.

Bersch, K., Praça, S., and Taylor, M.M. (2016) 'Bureaucratic capacity and political autonomy within national states: mapping the archipelago of excellence in Brazil', In: M.A. Centeno, A. Kohli, and D.J. Yashar (Eds.), *States in the Developing World*, New York, NY: Cambridge University Press, pp. 157–83.

Bourdieu, P. (1977) *Outline of a Theory of Practice*, New York, NY: Cambridge University Press.

Buse, K. (2005) *Global Health Partnerships: Increasing their impact by improved governance*, London: DFID Health Resource Centre.

Carpenter, D. (2001) *The Forging of Bureaucratic Autonomy: Reputations, networks, and policy innovation in executive agencies, 1862–1928*, Princeton, NJ: Princeton University Press.

Chwieroth, J.M. (2013) '"The silent revolution": how the staff exercise informal governance over IMF lending', *Review of International Organizations*, 8(2): 265–90.

*Daily Mail* (2017) 'Foreign aid fat cats who misused taxpayers' money will FINALLY be investigated by watchdog probing £1billion-a-year industry', 24 June, available online: www.dailymail.co.uk/news/article-4636482/Foreign-aid-fat-cats-FINALLY-investigated.html (accessed on 24 January 2018).

DiMaggio, P.J. and Powell, W.W. (1983) 'The iron cage revisited: institutional isomorphism and collective rationality in organizational fields', *American Sociological Review*, 48(2): 147–60.

Distler, L.K. (2016) 'The third channel: new development aid financing in global health', PhD dissertation, Munich: Ludwig-Maximilians-Universität München.

Duran, D. and Glassman, A.L. (2012) 'An Index of the Quality of Official Development assistance in health', working paper # 287, Washington, DC: Center for Global Development.

Esser, D.E. (2014) 'Elusive accountabilities in the HIV scale-up: "ownership" as a functional tautology', *Global Public Health*, 9(1–2): 43–56.

Esser, D.E. and Keating Bench, K. (2011) 'Does global health funding respond to recipients' needs? Comparing public and private donors' allocations in 2005–2007', *World Development*, 39(8): 1271–80.

Esser, D.E. and Williams, B.J. (2014) 'Tracing poverty and inequality in international development discourses: an algorithmic and visual analysis of agencies' annual reports and occasional white papers, 1978–2010', *Journal of Social Policy*, 43(1): 173–200.

Evans, P.B. (1995) *Embedded Autonomy: States and industrial transformation*, Princeton, NJ: Princeton University Press.

Fidler, D.P. (2010) 'The challenge of global health governance', working paper, New York, NY: Council on Foreign Relations.

Francis, J.J., Johnston, M., Robertson, C., Glidewell, L., Entwistle, V., Eccles, M.P., and Grimshaw, J.M. (2010) 'What is an adequate sample size? Operationalising data saturation for theory-based interview studies', *Psychology & Health*, 25(10): 1229–45.

Giddens, A. (1984) *The Constitution of Society: Outline of a theory of structuration*, Berkeley, CA: University of California Press.

Greenwood, R. and Hinings, C.R. (1996) 'Understanding radical organizational change: bringing together the old and the new institutionalism', *The Academy of Management Review*, 21(4): 1022–54.

Guest, G., Bunce, A., and Johnson, L. (2006) 'How many interviews are enough? an experiment with data saturation and variability', *Field Methods*, 18(1): 59–82.

Guler, I., Guillén, M.F., and Macpherson, J.M. (2002) 'Global competition, institutions, and the diffusion of organizational practices: the international spread of ISO 9000 quality certificates', *Administrative Science Quarterly*, 47(2): 207–32.

Hall, P.A. and Taylor, R.R. (1996) 'Political science and the three new institutionalisms', *Political Studies*, XLIV: 936–57.

Horowitz, M.C. (2007) *The Diffusion of Military Power: Causes and consequences for international politics*, Princeton, NJ: Princeton University Press.

Hunsmann, M. (2012) 'Limits to evidence-based health policymaking: Policy hurdles to structural HIV prevention in Tanzania', *Social Science & Medicine*, 74(10): 1477–85.

ICAI (2018) 'DFID's contribution to improving maternal health: An impact review approach paper', London: Independent Commission for Aid Impact, January.

Jones, C.M., Clavier, C., and Potvin, L. (2017) 'Adapting public policy theory for public health research: a framework to understand the development of national policies on global health', *Social Science & Medicine*, 177: 69–77.

Kahler, M. (1999) 'Evolution, choice, and international change', In: D.A. Lake and R. Powell (Eds.) *Strategic Choice and International Relations*, Princeton, NJ: Princeton University Press, pp. 165–96.

Kraatz, M.S. (1998) 'Learning by association? Interorganizational networks and adaptation to environmental change', *Academy of Management Journal*, 41(6): 621–43.

Levine, R. (2006) 'Open letter to the incoming director general of the World Health Organization', *British Medical Journal*, 333(7576): 1015–7.

MacLean, S.J. and MacLean, D.R. (2009) 'The political economy of global health research', In: S.J. MacLean, S.A. Brown, and P. Fourie (Eds.) *Health for Some: The political economy of global health governance*, New York, NY: Springer, pp. 165–82.

March, J.G. and Sutton, R.I. (1997) 'Organizational performance as a dependent variable', *Organization Science*, 8(6): 698–706.

Mawdsley, E. (2012) *From Recipients to Donors: Emerging powers and the changing development landscape*, London: Zed Books.

Mawdsley, E. (2015) 'DFID, the private sector and the re-centring of an economic growth agenda in international development', *Global Society*, 29(3): 339–58.

McColl, K. (2008) 'Europe told to deliver more aid for health', *The Lancet*, 37 (9630): 2072–3.

Moe, T. (2005) 'Power and political institutions', *Perspectives on Politics*, 3(2): 215–33.

Mooney, G. (2012) *The Health of Nations: Towards a new political economy*, London: Zed Books.

Pentland, B.T. and Feldman, M.S. (2009) 'Issues in empirical field studies of organizational routines', In: M.C. Becker (Ed.) *Handbook of Organizational Routines*, Cheltenham: Edward Elgar, pp. 281–300.

Pierson, P. (2003) 'Big, slow-moving, and… invisible', In: J. Mahoney and D. Rueschemeyer (Eds.) *Comparative Historical Analysis in the Social Sciences*, New York, NY: Cambridge University Press, pp. 177–207.

Prah Ruger, J. (2004) 'The changing role of the World Bank in public health', *American Journal of Public Health*, 95(1): 60–70.

Rasche, A, and Esser, D.E. (2006) 'From stakeholder management to stakeholder accountability: applying habermasian discourse ethics to accountability research', *Journal of Business Ethics*, 65(3): 251–67.

Schneider, B.R. (1991) *Politics within the State: Elite bureaucrats and industrial policy in authoritarian Brazil*, Pittsburgh, PA: University of Pittsburgh Press.

Shiffman, J., Schmitz, H.P., Berlan, D., Smith, S.L., Quissell, K., Gneiting, U. and Pelletier, D. (2016) 'The emergence and effectiveness of global health networks: findings and future research', *Health Policy and Planning*, 31: i110-23.

Siddiqi, S., Masid, T.I., Nishtar, S., Peters, D.H., Sabri, B., Bile, K.M. and Jama, M.A. (2009) 'Framework for assessing governance of the health system in developing countries: gateway to good governance', *Health Policy*, 90(1): 13–25.

Sridhar, D. (2010) 'Seven challenges in international development assistance for health and ways forward', *Journal of Law, Medicine, and Ethics*, 38(3): 459–69.

Stepping, K.M.K. (2016) 'Do health conditions determine the flow of external health resources? Evidence from panel data', *European Journal of Development Research*, 28(2): 270–93.

Sunstein, C.R. (1996) 'Social norms and social roles', *Columbia Law Review*, 96(4): 903–68.

Tansey, O. (2007) 'Process tracing and elite interviewing: a case for non-probability sampling', *PS: Political Science & Politics*, 40(4): 765–72.

Tendler, J. and Freedheim, S. (1994) 'Trust in a rent-seeking world: health and government transformed in NE Brazil', *World Development*, 22(12): 1771–91.

*The Guardian* (2017) 'Priti Patel forced to resign over meetings with Israeli officials', 8 November, available at www.theguardian.com/politics/live/2017/nov/08/priti-patel-secret-israel-meetings-politics-live (accessed on 24 January 2018).

Wendt, A.E. (1987) 'The agent-structure problem in international relations theory', *International Organization*, 41(3): 335–70.

Wezel, F.C. and Saka-Helmhout, A. (2005) 'Antecedents and consequences of organizational change: "institutionalizing" the behavioral theory of the firm', *Organization Studies*, 27(2): 265–86.

Wood Pallas, S. and Prah Ruger, J. (2017) 'Effects of donor proliferation in development aid for health on health program performance: a conceptual framework', *Social Science & Medicine*, 175: 177–86.

Youde, J. (2012) *Global Health Governance*, Cambridge: Polity Press.

# 21

# The crossroads of development assistance and national development agendas in the countries of South Eastern Europe

*Neda Milevska Kostova, Elizabeth J. King, and Kristefer Stojanovski*

Upon gaining independence in the early 1990s, the countries of South Eastern Europe (SEE) have embarked on political and economic transformations. SEE is made up of the countries located in the Balkan Peninsula (also commonly referred to as the Western Balkans). This chapter will focus on the following countries: Albania, Bosnia and Herzegovina, Bulgaria, Croatia, Kosovo, Macedonia, Montenegro, Romania, Serbia, and Slovenia. The former Yugoslavia, a socialist federation, which ceased to exist in 1991, faced a series of conflicts and wars, including the rise of ethnic nationalism and in some instances extending to ethnic cleansing and rape as a tool of war. Yugoslavia dissolved into the following successor states: Bosnia and Herzegovina, Croatia, Kosovo, Macedonia, Montenegro, Serbia, and Slovenia. Some countries have fared better in terms of economic and political stability – and both Slovenia and Croatia are already members of the European Union (EU) – while others have taken longer to overcome the hardships of the political and economic transition and post-war rebuilding. Macedonia, Montenegro, and Serbia are currently EU candidates, while Bosnia and Herzegovina and Kosovo have yet to achieve candidate status. Of the others, Albania is an EU candidate country and Bulgaria and Romania already joined the EU. According to the World Bank classification, Kosovo is classified as a lower-middle-income country and all of the other SEE countries are either upper-middle-income or high-income countries.

## Brief historical overview of development assistance in SEE

The international donor community has played a key role in economic development and democratic and rule of law processes, with considerable official development assistance being extended since the 1990s (Kekic, 2001; Karajkov, 2009; Kurze, 2009). The development assistance landscape was quite diversified and ever changing. Initially, dominated by the UN family of organisations and bilateral donor agencies from high-income countries (Parker and Sommer, 2011, p. 2), it also soon became a place for the EU foreign and security policy, due to the geographical positioning and aspirations of these countries to join the EU.

In the 1990s, during the break-up of Yugoslavia and fall of communism, international aid poured in for humanitarian and conflict resolution purposes with a strategic approach focused on rebuilding the war-torn Balkan states. With the wars ending, humanitarian assistance ceased, and donors directed interests and funds to building functional welfare societies with delivering economies and operative systems (Kekic, 2001). After the post-conflict emergency assistance, the dominating efforts were placed on pluralism, consolidation of democratic deficit, and liberalisation (Anastasiakis, 2013). In addition, poverty reduction, social inclusion, and social cohesion – all fairly new concepts introduced by the international community (IMF, 2016) – were also of interest, but which the countries had neither the experience with nor capacities to co-opt and institutionalise on their own.

Thus, the most prominent approach was absorption of donor-driven initiatives and projects, mainly due to the lack of strategic forward-thinking capacity in the countries for conceptualisation of needed reforms and desired outcomes. Coupled with their ideal of becoming part of the desired 'West', this deficiency fit well with the donor agendas of fixing the 'troubled Balkans' and finally making it a suitable partner at the table. The explicit Westernisation aspirations often gave a 'carte blanche' to the foreign assistance patterns, taking them as an overall useful approach without a real alternative (Schmunk, 2010). The milieu of multiple, sometimes conflicting, priorities and the democratic deficit gave way to the opportunity of fulfilling daily political agendas coated as participatory democracy, at the expense of well-planned and well-communicated political, social, and health thorough reforms.

This chapter examines the intended outcomes and unintended consequences of donor-driven assistance and development in SEE, explores lessons learned, and also serves as an example of the need to align donor agendas with national priorities that global health leaders and national stakeholders must consider in the field of health and development.

## International aid and national health agendas

In parallel with the post-conflict emergency assistance, health became a point of interest in the late 1990s, as part of the reconstruction and reform activities. Although health came into focus, it was to a large extent put on the backburner of the broader regional peace building, conflict resolution, and other national development agendas. However, the health sector was one of the sectors much affected by the transition and deemed as needing improvement. At the time, the assistance of UN agencies was aimed mostly at social stability and ensuring access to a minimum of basic social and health services in line with the Millennium Development Goals (MDGs) (Kickbusch and Brindley, 2013, p.11). Health-related assistance then was mostly concerned with provision of emergency medicine supplies, health technologies, and training for their use. Between 1991 and 2010, the majority of support from the EU had been allocated to humanitarian assistance, socio-economic development, and towards fulfilment of political conditionality in the EU accession processes (Grimm and Mathis, 2015), while its support for health came mostly through bilateral programmes from EU member states.

The major donor concerned with health during the mid- to late-1990s was the World Bank. It was the largest single source of external funding in health during the 1990s (World Bank, 1993, pp. 165–6), which significantly influenced and stewarded the national health agendas of the SEE countries. With their dominant focus on infrastructure and resource efficiency, the main discourse was an understanding of health as health care.

## Health as health care

In SEE, since times before independence, health has been considered an expenditure sector, and not a contributor to the economic development and growth. Thus, many of the SEE countries have not particularly considered health as a key aspect in their national development agendas. The donor assistance in SEE focused on tackling health through reestablishment of health insurance, sustainability of health financing, and fighting corruption.

As noted earlier, the key player of such health reforms was the World Bank. In line with their definition for post–conflict reconstruction and enabling conditions for a functioning peacetime society (World Bank, 1998, p.14), the main focus in the Bank's lending portfolio was health systems' restructuring (World Bank, 2017) mainly oriented at reduction of the vast health infrastructure and improvement of the health care system's inefficiency of past decades. The World Bank's roadmap included cutting down what was thought to be an abundant health care infrastructure and workforce inherited from socialism alongside health market liberalisation and privatisation of primary care services. Rushing into abandonment of the past, the governments of SEE countries shaped their health systems' reforms around this idea, with a rather segmented approach and without assessing outcomes, developing contingency plans or creating longer-term vision for the health as a public good. And while such an approach might have been justified as a starting point of health reform, it did not move towards a broader understanding of health outside of the health care system despite the World Development Report of 1993 reinforcing that health is not just an expenditure sector but a key component to healthy economic growth and societal development (World Bank, 1993).

The cost containment strategies prevailed, bringing decreases in salaries and benefits for the health professionals, reduced supplies, and retirement of equipment that was already obsolete. This also led to an impoverished quality of health services in the public sector, which acted as an additional boost to the development of private sector services and out-of-pocket payments. The flaw of the pathway taken – intentionally or not – was the lack of understanding of how to manage the spill over of high quality human resources to the better-paid private providers. As governments were not equipped to regulate the health market or negotiate purchase of services with public funding, user side health care expenditures have dramatically increased, from nearly zero to high percentages, and in some of these countries this issue still remains (see Figure 21.1).

In this respect, according to WHO data, the foreign aid failed to provide assistance to address rapidly increasing private payments and catastrophic costs for health (WHO, 2016). Furthermore, the pathway chosen, and limited rule of law, did not prevent the interference of political interests and power in making merit-based decisions in relation to health. Most of these projects were concerned with the inputs rather than outputs of health care, and as such were considered successful by achieved indicators of reduced number of beds in the public sector, ensuring essential hospital services (of limited quality), and completed privatisation of services. Simultaneously, health systems' strengthening and improved pharmaceutical supply was the dominant focus of the assistance provided by the multilateral donors (e.g., Project HOPE, USAID, WHO), and several bilateral assistance programmes (e.g., Norway, Switzerland, Sweden) committed their assistance to fighting corruption and inefficient use of public funds, both highly present in the health sector (USAID, 2016). And, while these are all essential to improved health sector as a precondition to better health, it is only one side of the input–output coin. If donors' and national governments' sincere intentions were to address the health and economic well-being of communities, then scoping beyond the health system and structure would have been necessary and should have started earlier.

Additionally, the aid designated for health sector reform had scarce, if any, assessments as to whether and to what extent these investments have contributed to the improvement of the health status of the population; or what the economic return was associated with health outcomes; what have been the economic consequences of out-of-pocket expenditures for the worse-off; or what measures would have alleviated their further impoverishment, and so forth. This is particularly relevant, as data from low-middle-income countries have shown a private–public sector divide in quality of care. This is, particularly important for populations who have been marginalised and who receive poorer care in general, and even more so in the private sector (Das and Gertler, 2007). Exceptions were the infant mortality indicators, which have been long before defined as a gauge for the broader social determinants of health, such as education of the mother, for example (Caldwell and McDonald, 1982). However, use of quantified indicators such as the MDGs of reduced infant mortality and 'adequate prenatal care' as four or more prenatal visits, the desired measure by international donors, did little to truly measure how donor-driven health system changes

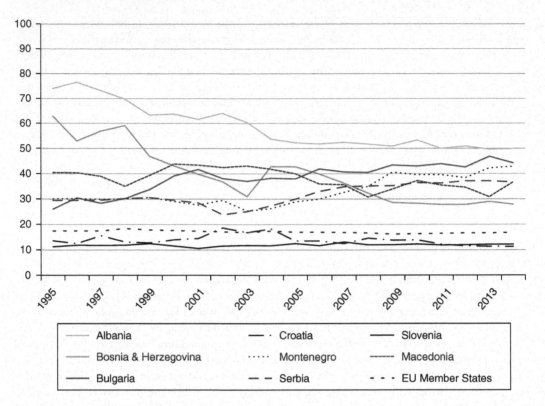

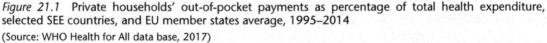

*Figure 21.1* Private households' out-of-pocket payments as percentage of total health expenditure, selected SEE countries, and EU member states average, 1995–2014
(Source: WHO Health for All data base, 2017)

also may have inadvertently decreased the *quality* of care received, particularly by populations that have been marginalised during the wars, post-conflict, and in contemporary times in the region (Hodgins and D'Agostino, 2014).

The focus on input-side of the health system restructuring and the lack of attention to the societal and other factors influencing health resulted in further medicalisation of the society and increased demand for specialised care (particularly in the private sector), at the expense of the already existing public health and prevention, which also needed attention and modernisation to respond to the changing epidemiologic profile of the economically advancing SEE societies.

## Public health

Overall, during the first decades of development assistance to the SEE countries, the health infrastructure and inefficiency downsizing were approached from the health systems' perspective. A focus on public health on the part of the donors was almost absent during and post-conflict; preventive public health measures were put at the margins of health investments, in large part due to their long-term return of investment. The attention to public health has increased during the 2000s, however, mainly to strengthening what SEE countries considered low hanging fruits.

Governments focused on traditional public health functions such as immunisation and sanitary-hygienic practices for improving community health. Although health data and management are necessary functions for adequate and comprehensive epidemiology measurement, subsequent interventions, and public health functions in general, these were still invested in modestly. Therefore, public health approaches remained confined to the most basic functions such as hygiene and immunisation.

While at the country-level, funding focused on the more medical public health interventions, global donor assistance helped to boost attention to the more complex structural and social public health issues affecting the region. For example, development assistance from UNICEF, the Global Fund to Fight AIDS, Tuberculosis and Malaria (Global Fund) and the WHO, addressed immunisation, tuberculosis, and HIV/AIDS (e.g., Romania, Macedonia, Serbia, Moldova), introducing breakthrough activities such as issues of stigma, creating resilient communities, and human rights in health care, as first attempts for scoping beyond the health sector. Although donor organisations recognised the need for work on the social determinants of health and the implementation of human rights-based approaches to health, diffusion into national initiatives and implementation strategies was not forthcoming, even today. At the verge of 2010s, the prevailing priorities in development plans were still in health system restructuring and sustainable health financing (Government of Macedonia, 2007; Government of Serbia, 2007), despite the push for wider understanding coming through in health policies (e.g., HIV/AIDS strategies of Macedonia and Serbia). The holistic social determinant and human rights-based approaches to the understanding of health vs. health- and medical-care are still lacking in the SEE countries (albeit changing).

## Paradigm shift: health as an investment

In the attempt to improve health and not just health care, and to expand the understanding of health beyond health system, SEE countries began to change the rhetoric in their development plans and the respective national agendas. The international community has played a major role in pushing for this paradigm shift. Initiation of the MDGs and the subsequent post-2015 agenda have acted as catalyst for the shift in focusing the health agendas away from bilateral project and fragmented attention, to a wider angle understanding and response to global health agenda reflected in the national circumstances.

### Post-2015 agenda

However, the international community has recognised that MDGs achievement timeframe was too ambitious. The new global development agenda was set to follow up on what the MDGs initiative was unable to accomplish. The Sustainable Development Goals (SDGs) are designed to be far more comprehensive, far-sighted and globally relevant, intending to leave no one behind (UN, 2015). SDGs not only put special focus on health through SDG 3, but also emphasise its interrelatedness with other goals across all societal, economic, and environmental determinants. Preceding the 2030 Agenda was the endorsement of the European policy framework for health and well-being Health2020 (WHO, 2013), founded on the same premise of health as key asset to economic growth and social development. These two globally and regionally relevant health policies have influenced the national strategic approaches in many countries including SEE.

With donors' assistance, SEE countries are beginning to grasp and acknowledge the importance of investment in health. The prevailing priorities focused on health infrastructure are increasingly being accompanied with considerations for human rights-based approaches to health and in some instances social determinants of health (Stillo and Turusbekova, 2017). More importantly, 'health' was terminologically emerging in its wider meaning, i.e., outside of the boundaries of health care and health protection that for decades was used in its medicalised and clinical understanding. The global health agenda through MDGs, and later SDGs, and Health2020 rather than the individual donors have played a crucial role in shaping this new development policy landscape that began to include health as one of the key priorities.

In terms of improvement in health and development, the effects of the considerable amounts of international assistance in the Balkans have not been extensively assessed, and there have been inconclusive general results on the overall impact of foreign aid on growth (Kekic, 2001). In parallel, the global health arena experienced declining health aid as a share of total development assistance (World Bank, 1993, Kickbusch and Brindley, 2013). It also became clear that health exceeds boundaries of the health system, and that the next step in global health development would be a renewed attention to the social determinants of health (Kickbusch and Brindley, 2013, p. 11). Such global developments resonated with the apparent lag in achieving the desired health outcomes in SEE countries, yet required new skills and experience for negotiating and partnering in development assistance, still not mastered in the region. The political elites once again reached out to donor assistance for incorporating concepts of health in all policies, and intersectoral approaches to health. In widening the understanding, some countries have renamed their ministry from 'health care' to 'health' (e.g., Croatia, Serbia), and in others, the appointed ministers or heads of health insurance funds were not medical professionals, something that was once an unquestionable stance (e.g., Macedonia, Albania, Serbia). These more recent developments are indicative of the slow but emerging paradigm shift of health understanding in the region.

Global and regional policies have offered a new approach for the countries of SEE to take in understanding health and its value in economic development. New entry points are identified and beginning to be employed in addressing health and health equity, such as environment, education, employment, social inclusion, and so forth. Comprehensive national mechanisms, such as United Nations Development Assistance Framework (UNDAF), and regional initiatives such as the Roma Decade and the European Environment and Health process, acknowledged health as an investment in economic growth and societal development, and were finding ways for measuring the impact health had on the growth, and vice versa. However, these processes too are supported, if not driven, by the international community, with significant technical and financial assistance and have not yet been fully accepted or meaningfully absorbed into national agendas or priorities.

## Paradigm shift is still shifting

Although great efforts have been made to shift to a new approach to health, initiatives developed did not fully penetrate the communities at the level required to improve the health indicators of the populations they were tailored to. For example, the Decade of Roma Inclusion was a multi- and inter-national (founded by the World Bank, UNDP, Open Society Institute, and Council of Europe) effort to improve the social inclusion and health of Roma populations in many SEE countries between 2005 and 2015. The approach towards public health work with Roma communities in the SEE countries depicts fragmentation even with basic functions – although immunisation rates are over 80 per cent in the general child population, rates among Roma children are 20–50 per cent lower depending on the country (Stojanovski, 2016).

Although an applauded effort, the Decade saw limited health improvements on a limited number of indicators, while overall differential morbidity and mortality continues to grow between Roma and non-Roma (European Union, 2014). Moreover, social inclusion, which was a main desired outcome, has failed due to lack of an overall strategy and Decade countries not fully recognising the contribution of Roma to society, but rather as ways of securing funds from donors (Jovanovic, 2015; Skenderi, 2016). In addition, the aid provided has seen inequitable funds' distribution, with many countries of SEE experiencing urban–rural gaps and continued burden of disease in this and other marginalised populations.

Although health is recognised as an important determinant to invest in, this recognition has not been enough to deter from changes and subsequent loss in funding. Countries in the region have experienced 'economic growth' according to international organisations such as World Bank, which has changed the economic development level of countries from low-middle-income countries to middle-high-income countries. Despite such definitional changes, the economic reality on the ground for many of the populations, and particularly those who are marginalized, has not been an experience of improvement (Slay, et al., 2014). Subsequently, a consequence of the national economic upward mobility has resulted in loss of eligibility for funds such as HIV and AIDS prevention and treatment funding provided by the Global Fund. Although the goal of the Global Fund is to have national governments take over financing as their economic prospects improve, governments of SEE have not yet committed to funding the newly created gap (Ibisevic and Bakh, 2015; Summers and Streifel, 2015; *The Lancet HIV*, 2016). This issue is also related to SEE not fully absorbing the paradigm shift into their national agendas, nor have they or the international donors critically evaluated sustainability of the much-needed programmes and funding. However, the more recent developments are indicative of the slowly occurring shift in health, which could be meaningfully operationalised into tangible results towards desired health equity.

## Discussion

### Unintended consequences of development assistance in health

While it can be argued that the development assistance was largely successful in stopping or preventing further conflict, humanitarian assistance, and strengthening state institutions (Huliaras, 2011), it has not been as successful in promoting development (Kekic, 2001) or sustainability (*The Guardian*, 2015; Kopinak, 2013). One of the most significant downsides of the process is that the SEE countries became and remain dependent on foreign aid and technical assistance (Gligorov, 2007). This reliance is seen in a multitude of spheres such as providing basic public health functions, particularly to marginalised populations, to prevention and treatment of HIV, and at a higher level to development and implementation of national health policies to create and deliver on the vision for the better health of each country's population.

The priorities of the international community have been imposed and accepted by the recipient countries – as Karajkov (2009) mentions, nobody has ever denied the strong role of donor self-interest in development aid, such as promoting national interests (Schraeder, et al., 1998), protecting national security (Radelet, 2006), or using it as a tool of foreign policy (Hook, 1995). At first justified as lack of capacity and strategic vision, but the continuation of such – in many cases – submissive attitude shows the inertia and continuous lacking on the part of these countries to consider, construct, and maintain sustainable realities for their citizens. There is still present promotion of possibly conflicting goals, which can serve to undermine sustainable development objectives (Huliaras, 2011). Understandably so, under certain circumstances, foreign aid has a catalytic effect on development, not only boosting recipients' consumption and investment in the short term, but also helping to create conditions for sustainable long-term growth (Kekic, 2001).

However, recipients of donor funds must also fully commit to meeting the goals of the projects. As can be seen by the Roma Decade example earlier, governments signed onto the initiative, but the efforts and Decade were never fully absorbed into national agendas or strategies, particularly around issues of social inclusion of Roma, as in the example of segregated schools for Roma children in Hungary and Slovakia during the Decade. Despite the huge investments made through international development, the concept of poverty reduction had not shown much improvement to date; the countries of SEE are still among the poorest in Europe (DiVirgilio, 2013). Additionally, data shows that the equity gap widens with populations that are marginalised, such as Roma, living in higher levels of abject poverty compared to non-Roma in all countries of South Eastern Europe (Slay, et al., 2014).

During the first two decades after the break-up of Yugoslavia, development assistance to the SEE countries, the health infrastructure, and inefficiency downsizing were approached from the core health-systems' perspective. Although appropriate for the purpose, it did not take into consideration the public value of health and its interrelatedness to other societal factors. The input–output analysis of foreign assistance was a convenient approach, although both governments and development agencies recognised that it can only be a starting point, beyond which the organisational rationality and absorption capacities had to be considered so as to ensure sustainability of the impact (Kurze, 2009). As Tendler described, the necessity to reach beyond the mere measurement of inputs and outputs calls for applying the institutional theory that points to the inevitability to understand and factor in the contextual factors in defining the content and scope of the development assistance (1975, p. 2). In order to ensure effective global health development, donor agencies must truly hold nation-states accountable to the commitments made and must help create not only political buy-in, but also community-level support to the initiatives being undertaken. Global health professionals should be mindful of the need for community-level and bottom-up approaches to fully achieve the desired changes to improve population health and equity and ensure sustainable development.

## Opportunities of development assistance in health

Although a paradigm shift is emerging under the pressing international and regional commitments of the governments to deliver upon promises to promote health and well-being of their citizens, much still needs to be done for breaking the sectoral silos. In addition, the culture of pointing fingers at the health sector for stagnation in improvement of health status or life expectancy prevails, in the same way in which the laurels for reduced infant mortality are still mainly attributed solely to the health sector.

While environment is increasingly present in the vocabulary of the health policies, and vice versa, other contributing policies of taxation, education, or employment continue to treat health in a rhetorical or declarative manner, without strong commitment to measuring their actual impact on health of individuals or communities. The 2030 Agenda aims to continue providing strategic templates for addressing health in a comprehensive manner. And, similar to the MDGs agenda, setting the SDGs has raised the bar in requesting countries to commit to contributing towards the global indicators and targets through various facets that are affected by or can contribute to health.

The role of international and regional policies can be crucial in this paradigm shift, but the autonomy of national priority setting for responding to these commitments, which are still largely confined within the traditional economic sphere, raises concerns and calls for changing the approaches of the donor assistance. It is also important to think more broadly about donor-driven prerogatives and their influence on health in the region. For example, the UK Department of International Development has been active in SEE focusing on supporting good governance and economic reform (Government of the United Kingdom, 2015). Such foci, although not directly related to health, have health implications and recently rule of law has been considered an important social determinant to health (Dingake, 2017). The role of international donors in global health and development is also contingent upon the changing geopolitical realities on the ground. The 'frozen' integration of the Balkans into the EU, pressure regarding 'good neighbourly relations', and autonomy in decision-making are all important factors for absorption of donor-driven initiatives into national and regional agendas and policies in SEE (Flessenkemper and Reljic, 2017). In addition, the United Kingdom exit from the EU and its implications on the future of the EU raises concerns about the Balkans' stability and future foreign aid patterns ensuing from diverse new agendas coming from both the West and the East (Ker-Lindsay, 2015; Butler, 2016).

In addition, future efforts should be performed in collaboration not only with national governments, but with local authorities as well, so that political will at the national level may be fortified by, but also built from, these grassroot efforts. Furthermore, additional oversight of donor-provided funding is needed in order to minimise corruption and inefficiency that to date remains a tripping stone in SEE.

## Conclusions

The lack of strategic direction made way for donor-driven agendas, which were oriented to investments in privatisation, health technology, and medicalisation of health in the region. These agendas focused on and nurtured the clinical aspects of health; although, SEE countries already had vast infrastructure in health care buildings, hospital beds, and health care personnel. A paradigm shift began to emerge in the early 2000s with the EU accession processes occurring in several of the SEE countries and the emerging global demands for improved well-being of populations. This shift in the conceptualisation of health imposed a more upstream approach to health in the SEE region. Investments in preventive and primary care services were increasingly requested by foreign donor assistance, alongside investments in other social, environmental, and political determinants of health. Nearly two decades later, despite the paradigm shift, misalignment of development assistance and strategic vision of governments remain areas of concern. However, as SEE countries continue joining the EU and experiencing economic growth, their reliance on international donor assistance will dwindle and the countries themselves will have more autonomy in shaping how health and development are conceptualised for their people. This could have both positive and negative impacts on population health, especially for populations vulnerable to exclusion and marginalisation. Signs of a paradigm shift from how health was viewed during socialism, then during wartime and in the post-conflict rebuilding, and more recently with the pressures of EU and NATO accession are evident. Some of this shift has come from within the countries themselves, though the role of international donors' agendas has been significant. Undoubtedly, the SEE countries will continue to be places where global and local agendas for health play out, sometimes in tandem and in other ways in discordance, with consequences for public health and development.

## References

Anastasiakis, O. (2013) 'Post-1989 political change in the Balkan States: a legacy of the early illiberal transition years', *Perceptions*, 18(2): 91–112.

Butler, E. (2016) 'Brexit and the Balkans: implications for future EU enlargement', European Futures academic blog, available at www.europeanfutures.ed.ac.uk/article-3981 (accessed 8 October 2017).

Caldwell, J. and McDonald, P. (1982) 'Influence of maternal education on infant and child mortality: levels and causes', *Health Policy Education*, 2(3–4): 251–67.

Das, J. and Gertler, P. (2007) 'Variations in practice quality in five low-income countries: a conceptual overview', *Health Affairs*, 26: 296–309.

Dingake, O.B.K. (2017) 'Letter to the editor: the rule of law as a social determinant to health', *Health and Human Rights Journal*, available at www.hhrjournal.org/2017/09/letter-to-the-editor-the-rule-of-law-as-a-social-determinant-of-health/ (accessed on 27 September 2017).

DiVirgilio, A. (2013) 'The 10 most poverty ridden countries in Europe', The Richest, 24 October, available at www.therichest.com/rich-list/poorest-list/the-10-most-poverty-ridden-countries-in-europe/ (accessed on 8 June 2017).

European Union (2014) 'Roma health report', available at http://ec.europa.eu/health//sites/health/files/social_determinants/docs/2014_roma_health_report_es_en.pdf (accessed on 12 July 2017).

Flessenkemper, T. and Reljic, D. (2017) 'EU enlargement: a six percent target for the Western Balkans', German Institute for International and Security Affairs, available at www.swp-berlin.org/en/point-of-view/eu-enlargement-a-six-percent-target-for-the-western-balkans/ (accessed on 25 September 2017).

Gligorov, V. (2007) 'Transition, integration and development in Southeast Europe', *Ekonomski Pregled*, 58(5–6): 259–304.

Government of Macedonia (2007) 'National development plan of the Republic of Macedonia 2007–2009', available at www.esiweb.org/pdf/macedonia_National_Development_Plan_2007-2009.pdf (accessed on 20 May 2017).

Government of Serbia (2007) 'National sustainable development strategy of Serbia 2007', available at www.un.org/esa/agenda21/natlinfo/countr/serbia/nsds_serbia.pdf (accessed on 23 May 2017).

Government of the United Kingdom (2015) 'Stability in the Western Balkans', available at www.gov.uk/government/news/new-uk-funding-to-help-build-stronger-and-more-democratic-nations-in-the-eastern-neighbourhood-and-balkans (accessed on 27 September 2017).

Grimm, S. and Mathis, O.L. (2015). 'Stability first, development second, democracy third: the European Union's policy towards the post-conflict Western Balkans, 1991–2010', *Europe-Asia Studies*, 67(6): 916–47.

Hodgins, S. and D'Agostino, A. (2014) 'The quality-coverage gap in antenatal care: toward better measurement of effective coverage', *Global Health, Science, and Practice*, 2: 173–81.

Hook, S.W. (1995) *National Interest and Foreign Aid*, Boulder, CO: Lynne Rienner Publishers.

Huliaras, A. (2011) 'Foreign aid to the Balkans (1990–2010): the dynamics of the "silent" human security agenda', *Southeast European and Black Sea Studies*, 11(4): 421–34, DOI: 10.1080/14683857.2011.632543.

Ibisevic, S. and Bakh, U. (2015) 'Seeking solutions for the danger of the Global Fund withdrawal from the Balkan Countries', Association PROI, available at www.slideshare.net/UlianaBakh/seeking-solutions-for-the-danger-of-the-global-fund-withdrawal-from-the-balkan-countries (accessed on 12 July 2017).

IMF. (2016) 'Database of poverty reduction strategy papers of all countries', available at: www.imf.org/external/np/prsp/prsp.aspx (accessed on 13 May 2017).

Jovanovic, Z. (2015) 'Why Europe's "Roma Decade" didn't lead to inclusion', Open Society Foundation, available at www.opensocietyfoundations.org/voices/why-europe-s-roma-decade-didn-t-lead-inclusion (accessed on 25 September 2017).

Karajkov, R. (2009) 'Foreign aid to the Balkans 1990–2005: who gave aid, to whom, and why: disaggregation of foreign assistance flows to the region of the Balkans in the period of transition', PhD dissertation.

Kekic, L. (2001) 'Aid to the Balkans: addicts and pushers', *Southeast European and Black Sea Studies*, 1(1): 20–40.

Ker-Lindsay, J. (2015) 'Britain, "Brexit" and the Balkans'. *The RUSI Journal*, 160(5): 24–9.

Kickbusch, I. and Brindley, C. (2013) *Health in the Post-2015 Development Agenda*, Geneva: Graduate Institute.

Kopinak, J.K. (2013). 'Humanitarian aid: are effectiveness and sustainability impossible dreams?', *The Journal of Humanitarian Assistance*, available at https://sites.tufts.edu/jha/archives/1935 (accessed on 8 June 2017).

Kurze, A. (2009) 'EU politics of foreign aid in the Balkans: development, integration, and reform in perspective', *Global Studies Review*, 5(1), available at www.globality-gmu.net/archives/53 (accessed on 25 September 2017).

Parker, R. and Sommer, M. (Eds.) (2011) *Routledge Handbook of Global Public Health*, New York: Routledge.

Radelet S. (2006) 'A primer on foreign aid', Working Paper, No. 92, Center for Global Development, available at www.cgdev.org/sites/default/files/8846_file_WP92.pdf (accessed on 25 September 2017).

Schmunk, M. (2010) '15 Years of peace-, state- and nation-building: basic lessons from the Balkan lab', In: *15 Years of Peace-Building in the Western Balkans – Lessons Learnt and Current Challenges* – 20th Workshop of the Study Group 'Regional Stability in South East Europe' proceedings, Vienna: National Defence Academy and Bureau for Security Policy.

Schraeder P.J., Hook S.W., and Taylor B. (1998) 'Clarifying the foreign aid puzzle: a comparison of American, Japanese, French, and Swedish aid flows'. *World Politics*, 50(2): 294–323.

Skenderi, S. (2016) 'The flaws of the decade of Roma inclusion 2005–2015', Politheor, available at http://politheor.net/the-flaws-of-the-decade-of-roma-inclusion-2005–2015/ (accessed on 16 February 2016).

Slay, B., Danilova-Cross, E., Papa, J., Peleah, M., Marnie, S., and Henrich, C. (2014) *Poverty, Inequality, and Vulnerability in the Transition and Developing Economies and Central Asia*, New York: United Nations Development Programme.

Stillo, J. and Turusbekova, N. (2017) 'Romanian integrated community support services for tuberculosis', Stockholm: ECDC, available at http://stop-tb.ro/wp-content/uploads/2017/05/Romania-Integrated-Community-Based-TB-Support-Services-FINAL-2.pdf (accessed on 31 May 2017).

Stojanovski, K. (2016) 'Immunization among Roma children in Central and Eastern Europe: what are the true vaccination rates and barriers to coverage?' World Health Organization Roma Researchers Meeting, Debrecen, Hungary.

Summers, T. and Streifel, C. (2015) 'Key populations and the next Global Fund strategy: a focus on upper-middle income countries', Centre for Strategic and International Studies (CSIS), available at http://csis.org/files/publication/151117_Summers_KeyPopulations_Web.pdf (accessed on 8 June 2017).

Tendler, J. (1975) *Inside Foreign Aid*, Baltimore, MD: Johns Hopkins University Press.

*The Guardian* (2015) 'NGOs in Malawi: what happens when donors leave?', The Guardian, 28 September 2015, available at www.theguardian.com/global-development-professionals-network/2015/sep/28/ngos-in-malawi-what-happens-when-donors-leave (accessed on 8 June 2017).

*The Lancet HIV* (2016) 'HIV on the fast-track to sustainability', *The Lancet HIV*, 3(1): e1.

UN. (2015) Transforming Our World: The 2030 Agenda for Sustainable Development, New York: UN, available at www.un.org/ga/search/view_doc.asp?symbol=A/RES/70/1&Lang=E (accessed on 8 June 2017).

USAID. (2016) 'Zero Corruption project in Serbia 2013–2016', available at www.usaid.gov/results-data/success-stories/healing-healthcare-system-transparency-and-integrity (accessed on 12 July 2017).

WHO. (2013) 'Health 2020. A European policy framework and strategy for the 21st century', available at www.euro.who.int/__data/assets/pdf_file/0011/199532/Health2020-Long.pdf?ua=1 (accessed on 8 June 2017).

WHO. (2016) 'WHO Health For All database' available at https://gateway.euro.who.int/en/datasets/european-health-for-all-database/ (accessed on 8 June 2017).

World Bank. (1993) *World Development Report 1993: Investing in health*, New York: Oxford University Press.

World Bank. (1998) *Post-Conflict Reconstruction: The role of the World Bank*, Washington, DC: World Bank.

World Bank. (2017) 'World Bank project database', available at http://projects.worldbank.org/?lang=en (accessed on 1 June 2017).

# 22

# On the life history of HIV interventions in India

## Avahan, organic intellectuals, and the fate of community mobilisation

*Robert Lorway, Shamshad Khan, Monika Doshi,*
*Sundar Sundararaman, and Sushena-Reza Paul*

## Introduction

Critical scholars characterise the historical emergence of global health as occurring around the intensification of standardised measurement practices that pivot on neoliberal logics of efficiency and accountability. Scholars raise a number of important questions that confront the rise of evidence-based medicine in global health, and the evidentiary regimes that tend to distance us from a closer attention to on-the-ground lived realities (Adams, 2016; Erikson, 2012; Lorway and Khan, 2014). In the global response to the HIV pandemic, the prime value accorded to positivistic knowledge that is assumed to be verifiable and universally comparable is especially reflected in the public health literature that pertains to sex workers; it is replete with interpretations of data generated from prefixed quantitative indicators that are biological, behavioural, and spatial in nature (Lorway and Khan, 2014). We ask, within these terrains of measurement, what forms of sociopolitical awareness emerge among sex workers?

To begin to explore this question, we examine HIV Initiatives in India, focusing in particular upon the Bill & Melinda Gates-funded HIV initiative known as Avahan and the period following its transition to the public system (Rao, 2010). Many leaders from the sex work community in India draw a sharp distinction between the former Avahan programme and the current government programme. Yet, how do we understand this distinction when both programmes have employed similar enumerative techniques to govern the health of sex workers? In this chapter, we illustrate how sex work leaders – who have experienced more than a decade of transformation around HIV initiatives – employ a form of 'critical nostalgia' (Cashman, 2006) as a way to construct a history of the present that expresses opposition to reigning forms of health governance. What is important to note in their versions of history and change is how the lauding (and perhaps idealisation) of Avahan's technical approach to HIV prevention enables leaders to express their dissent towards the current governmental health regime in highly precision-oriented technical terms.

A transnational consortium of business managers, health scientists, programme planners, and NGOs orchestrated the implementation of the Avahan programme in six of India's so-called high prevalence states between 2003 and 2010. Avahan has been hailed as a success given the estimated number of HIV infections averted and the statistically significant reduction of curable STIs and HIV incidence recorded (Pickles, et al., 2013). These results have been associated with 'community mobilisation' (CM) (Reza-Paul, et al., 2008) – a word that conjures up notions of solidarity and social justice. In practice CM gets put to multiple uses in global health projects that strive to improve the uptake of health services.

The emphasis placed on community participation in global health discourse can be associated with the triumphs and tribulations of the primary health care movement of the 1960s and 1970s – an era in international health that celebrated the 'barefoot doctor' movement in China and the rural Ayurvedic practitioners of India (Farmer, et al., 2013, p. 76). For current large-scale interventions that focus on the HIV global pandemic and poor maternal, newborn, and child health (MNCH) outcomes in low-resource settings, the goal of 'success' often hinges on the participation of communities and local community-based social service and health workers. The centrality of community participation is vividly exemplified by the global policy integration of greater/meaningful involvement of people with HIV and AIDS, a set of principles which has profoundly shaped the global landscape of HIV responses (Mykhalovskiy, et al., 2009). Similarly, global health specialists who aim to strengthen government service delivery in MNCH commonly work through networks of local community health workers (Gopalan, et al., 2012). This process intensifies local engagement in on-the-ground programme coverage tracking activities, and binds community participation in a relation of accountability to foreign expertise. Furthermore, as Elsa Fan (2014, p. 85) notes with respect to China, important health services are commonly outsourced to community-based organisations (CBOs) which 'come to rely on outsourcing as a long-term funding base' to keep their organisations afloat. Although community mobilisation schemes often cast community health workers as 'agents of social change', CBOs are often forced to confront an avalanche of paperwork and bureaucratic reporting procedures required by funders and governments as evidence of progress and success (Lorway 2017). How do local community groups contend with and realise their own political priorities within the context of such 'audit cultures' (Strathern, 2000, pp. 2–5)?

Under the first two phases of Avahan, CM schemes were cultivated within a culture of management expertise. Intervention planners and implementers emphasised the business logics of 'flexibility' and 'innovation', which permitted field-level 'problem solving' with community leaders and opened up a communicative interface between sex workers and programme experts, thereby engaging sex workers directly in discussions of measurement. The value of flexibility is clearly articulated in the Avahan business model advanced by Alexander and Ramakrisnan,

> Flexibility: Market solutions are constantly evolving and lasting business adapt with them. Avahan is trying things for the first time, placing large and small bets. Avahan trusts its own judgment, take reasonable risks, check results, and make technically appropriate changes as the realities on the ground demand.
>
> *Ramakrishana and Alexander, 2006, p. 58*

Such entrepreneurial logics encouraged interveners to take calculated risks to address on-the-ground challenges. However, following the transition of the Avahan programme to the public system between 2010 and 2012, sex workers describe intensely rigid reporting procedures, overtly coercive financial regulatory mechanisms and funding cuts, and unrealistic outreach targets – all of which point towards the demise of CM.

## The technical and the political

We treat CM as a technological formation that, on the one hand, enables policymakers, scientists, and community members alike to accomplish very practical and arbitrary tasks like linking people to health services, determining programme coverage targets, and establishing the precise terms of funding allocations.

We also view CM, from the perspective of sex workers themselves, as an *ethico-political technology* given how its reiteration in different localities quickly sparks moral reflections on the meaning and value of collective life, giving rise to political perspectives.

Our attempt to bring out sex workers' perspectives on transformations arising from Avahan's transfer to the public system is not intended to interrogate the governmental motives behind particular policy changes, per se. For sure, it could be argued that the techniques, resources, and network of services furnished under the lavishly funded Avahan programme are simply unsustainable given governmental funding structures and human resource capacities. Instead, taking as our starting point Gramsci's notion of 'organic intellectuals', we attempt to illuminate how a form of organic leadership has emerged within a political field cultivated by Avahan and brought into profound conflict under the current governmental policy regime change. Underpinned by a chimera of 'immaterial' (Hardt and Negri, 2005) concerns for evidence and more material class-based realities, organic leadership among sex workers neither calls for the dismissal of enumerative practices nor the overthrow of 'the numbers'; rather it renders a political account of how measurement practices and evidence production need not be at odds with the fine-grain social justice work that is vital for the transformation of social conditions that underpin sex workers' oppression and vulnerability to illness.

Our findings draw upon the narratives generated during focus groups discussions and key informant interviews conducted as part of a larger, more extensive qualitative study that attempts to reconstruct the life history of HIV interventions in India. Our interpretations of these recent findings build on our long-term experience of working on HIV interventions in India, stretching back more than ten years. During this period, we have participated in various forms of ethnographic, participatory, and applied public health research. The narratives we analyse here were generated by female and male sex work (FSW and MSW) leaders who have been directly engaged in community-based HIV epidemic responses in three different States of India, since the earliest days of the Avahan programme.

## Remembering dystopias

Participants' narratives depicted changes in the history of HIV interventions following a similar story-line: they positioned Avahan as ushering in an era of enlightenment and salvation, doing so by contrasting and temporalising it against a dystopic past:

> Before this project started here, that is before 2004, we did not have any awareness about either STI or HIV. There were a few organisations working at that time who were distributing condoms, but we did not have any knowledge of how to use the condoms.
>
> *Karnataka, MSW*

> Sex workers who stood on the road soliciting clients faced many problems both from the police and the public.... Four thugs took a woman away forcibly, police would beat us or have free sex with us and warn us not to tell it to anyone or else the action against us the next day would be different – the situation was like that.
>
> *Maharashtra, FSW*

> There was no programme in place before that; we did not even know what HIV is. It all started only when Gates Foundation came and funded [names an NGO] directly. No condoms were available before that, so clients who visited brothels would have unsafe sex and could possibly be infecting sex workers there. Only after [the Avahan-funded NGO] came in we started learning about condoms, distributing them and it helped save a lot of women from HIV.
>
> *Andhra Pradesh, FSW*

241

Such narratives of dystopia remember the social suffering of sex workers prior to Avahan as a period of fear, discrimination, violence, a weak sense of social solidarity, poor access to health services, and a general lack of understanding regarding the sexual health problems facing their community. The theme of everyday forms of violence committed by partners, gang members, and police officers recurred in these dystopic narratives. As another participant further explains,

> The reason we could not mobilise at that time [prior to the Avahan programme] was because we had accepted violence as part of our life; if we faced problems from boyfriends we accepted it and were even happy about it. We felt it was right; that we give him money and he beat us. If police harassed us we tolerated because we thought we were doing 'bad' work. We had accepted violence as part of our life. Only when the technical team came and we started discussing with them we understood we are also human beings with equal rights and any form of violence is wrong. Individually we all had talent and skill but no one recognised it and we also did not understand what we could do if all of us joined together.
>
> *Karnataka, FSW*

Articulating such portrayals of 'ordinary' violence in the pre-Avahan era enabled participants to make sense of the collective transformations that occurred as the lives of sex workers became drawn into Avahan,

> In February 2002, I tested positive. But there was no platform then to seek advice, where do I go, whom should I speak to, what should I ask? Then I felt that we should all come together and talk about HIV. I started searching for groups who were discussing about it. I found state level networks, I went and tried to join them, but at that time they did not allow me in…. In December 2003 this [technical] team came here … then I got my platform and I joined here and started mobilising community. About 16 of us joined then and from there we have become so many now. There was nothing in terms of mobilisation before that.
>
> *Karnataka, FSW*

Although the following two participants claimed to have had some prior access to health resources through a local NGO, they insisted that a sense of control over their sexual health destinies was not realised until the introduction of the Avahan project,

> R2: Earlier we would do outreach clinics where a doctor would go, examine women and give medicines, but when [Avahan-funded NGO] came, we could do this in a more organised manner. We could plan how many clinics, where, how many women need to be examined, how much of medicines to take along with us etc.
>
> *Andra Pradesh, FSW*

> R1: Let me give an example of a TV remote. Previously the remote was controlled by others and so we had to watch those channels they switched on to. After [the Avahan-funded NGO] came in, the remote was handed to us and we could decide which channel to watch. It made such a difference.
>
> *Karnataka, MSW*

As the previous discussion suggests, Avahan's technical approach enhanced a sense of collective responsibility, ownership, and control over the intervention process among sex workers. Moreover, new techniques for reaching 'the community' extended the influence of local leaders, reflected in their ability to gather greater numbers of their peers around the project of community health and epidemic prevention.

## Technical learning

According to the participants, the technical knowledge they received from programme specialists imparted tactics that were crucial to the development of an effective outreach programme. Initially, however, distrust plagued the formation of sex workers' relationships with technical teams:

> In the beginning a technical team had come here to meet us, but we also used to run away from them unwilling to meet them. We knew they were outsiders and there were rumours that time that people would kidnap you and sell your eyes or kidneys, so we were scared of them. The same way that the technical team never gave up, were with us in the field throughout the day and were addressing our issues and won our trust, in a similar manner we did so with our community to win their trust.
>
> *Karnataka, MSW*

Guided by experts on particular techniques to link sex workers to health services, participants claimed to have learned how to build rapport with peers to overcome initial distrust:

> At that time we got this project from the Bill & Melinda Gates Foundation through Avahan. Our journey started from there. Initially we were 10 to 12 people who joined the project and we were given awareness about condoms, STI and HIV. Then we went to the field and met our friends there and gave them this information. Initially ... no one was interested in listening, then the non-community [technical] staff taught us how to talk and approach the community and then we started talking to the community about their needs and the problems and issues they faced and tried to help them. By befriending them we won their trust and this enabled us to give the information to them.
>
> *Karnataka, FSW*

Although the technical team imparted specific outreach techniques to community members, this practical knowledge was not imposed on them as a set of directives; rather, it engaged and inspired sex work leaders to cultivate their own intervention tactics for reaching their peers:

> The technical team also did not give us solutions but showed ways of solving the problems ourselves. Similarly we also helped our community members by showing them a path to solve their problems. For instance if a community woman wanted a house we could not provide one, but we could assist her in linking her to people who could help her out. This way we won their trust.
>
> *Karnataka, MSW*

Another participant describes the beginning of her involvement in the Avahan programme. Although she received training from programme experts, the refinement of her intervention techniques took place in the practical and concrete realm of 'the field', where technical knowledge became grounded in lived experience. There, she and other outreach workers engaged in problem solving to gain access to harder-to-reach networks of sex workers:

> Initially an organisation called [names an NGO funded by Avahan] approached us asking us if we could work for them. ... [W]e joined as outreach workers in the organization, [the Avahan-funded NGO]. They did not pay us salary immediately ... so we worked voluntarily ... I was able to bring women from villages for testing, I used to accompany them to these places ... In the morning we used to have review meetings during which they would provide us tea, snacks and Biriyani for lunch and tea and snacks again in the evening, take us out to picnics.... [W]e faced some problems, especially meeting women in the brothels and the bus stands. In fact it would take us at least a week of observing in the

bus stand before we could ascertain a woman standing there was a sex worker, and then we would take her for testing. Despite the difficulties faced we were happy to work for [the Avahan-funded NGO] because they were providing us snacks and lunch and taking us for a picnic once a week.

*Andra Pradesh, FSW*

The social significance of the reference to eating should not be lost here, given the cultural politics around sharing food in India. The refusal of food from people of a 'lower caste' indeed is one important way that the legacy of the caste system, although outlawed, survives today. Thus the sharing of food and social space together, although seemingly mundane, profoundly affected the bonding and relations of trust that formed between technical staff and the sex workers, as it unsettled caste boundaries (even if it did not entirely do away with them).

As the next narrative suggests, technical training was particularly effective in reinforcing notions of collective existence and empowerment. Enacting a form of 'moral citizenship' (Schinkel, 2010), technical staff 'responsibilised' (Ilcan and Basok, 2004) groups of sex workers by venerating 'the community' as a source of political unity and protective fortitude:

The same staff from MSPSS approached us and asked us if we are willing to work for the project. They told us we will get Rs. 100/- for it and also training to do the work. They said you are all together here and if you feel you should work for each other, then you can come to us. Then they trained us on STIs, putting condoms on and also about HIV. This carried on for a year ... Then they selected a few of us to work as peer educator for different spots ... It was stressed upon us that we should all be united and only then our voices will be heard. Then we were also trained on forming our own organisation giving the example of how it is easy to break a stick but difficult to break a bunch of sticks that are tied together. They also gave the example of how a tiger would pick up a goat from a herd but if the herd is strong then they can chase the tiger away. For a year they trained us on forming our organisation.

*Maharashtra, FSW*

In this way, participants viewed the early training process itself as transcending the ability to complete a set of routinised tasks, such as meeting programme enrolment targets. Instead they regarded the technical guidance they received as giving rise to an important moment in the lives of sex workers – a moment in which a vital collective consciousness emerged:

When we were discussing about mobilisation the word 'organisation' cropped up, our own organisation. When we started discussing it, the possibilities opened up when we thought if we are together we could fight for our rights, get our collective voices heard, get things done for ourselves, so the word 'together' kept coming up and we realised being together is beneficial for us and for this mobilisation is a must. Whether it is for services, fight for our rights, addressing violence or any other thing, having our organisation is important.

*Karnataka, MSW*

The numbers produced and utilised by the technical team to set up programme coverage targets held a particular ontological status in the birth of 'the community'. Participants viewed the enumerative procedures employed in the early days of Avahan as calling 'the community' into being. For instance, when asked about how the community began to form at the beginning of Avahan, one participant discussed the results of an extensive baseline monitoring and evaluation process as though it were an important milestone in how the community began to unite around the project of HIV prevention:

At that time we also did an IBBA, Integrated Behavioral and Biological Assessment, and it revealed that 26 per cent of sex workers in [names a state district] were infected. When we disseminated this to the community we all were in tears because we did not know who was infected and who wasn't. A sample of 425 women was tested and 26 per cent were found with HIV. Then through a small skit we gave the results of the assessment to the community and we started giving more HIV related information to our community at the field level because we were sharing clients and anyone could become positive.

*Karnataka, FSW*

Others echoed the importance of enumerative procedures in bringing about a sense of being part of a larger collective:

In fact the first time when we did capture-recapture [a method for enumerating a population] and so many women came to the DIC [drop-in centre] to be part of it; we felt we were not alone and there are so many of us. For the first time we felt it was not just 'I' or 'we' but 'us'; that was a good feeling.

*Karnataka, FSW*

According to the account of participants, the emergence of CM through the technical guidance of experts hinged on distinctive social and political realities: solidarity between sex workers and the technical team; a sense of responsibility and belonging to a community; and a growing awareness of the more forceful political position that comes with a unity found in counting and being counted among others with 'similar experiences'.

## Transition to techno-bureaucracy

Across the discussions, participants repeatedly made reference to numbers, targets, sizes, proportions, and percentages to index the changing political positionality of sex workers in the HIV response over time. With respect to the transition to the public system, sex workers recounted precise details pertaining to the new governmental constraints placed on their work. New policies abruptly placed a cap on programme coverage targets, thereby contrasting with Avahan's approach that encouraged outreach to as many members of the community who might be in need. One participant tells how the government's restrictive coverage target affected their intervention work:

During the [Avahan era] the board was concentrating on how to increase the membership of the organisation from 1000 to 1500 or 2000. We were very motivated to do so. Now we simply ask the programme team whether they finished their target or not; just targets and nothing else.

*Maharashtra, FSW*

The new government outreach target sizes were based more arbitrarily on the logics of funding allocation, efficiency, and fiscal conservativeness. Reductions in the coverage size were also accompanied by higher contact-to-outreach worker ratios:

[The State AIDS Control Society (SACS)] … has created problems. Previously an outreach worker had 100 contacts and she along with the concerned peer educator would look after them. Now the government has fixed a target that an outreach worker has to cover 300 sex workers. They did increase the salaries of peers and outreach workers but the target is very stiff. People who had tested before come repeatedly for testing, getting newer women including some college students who do casual sex work is a challenge and we are trying to address this.

*Andhra Pradesh, FSW*

The new calculus of risk – tied to a cost-benefit analysis more than the on-the-ground exigencies – was accompanied by a swift policy shift towards targeting younger sex workers (sometimes referred to by participants as 'new sex workers'), as indicated earlier. Older sex workers who fell outside the new age targets, therefore, were dropped from the programme:

I have seen a 60-year-old woman who tested positive recently. Why should she? She says if I listen to your words I will have to starve to death. I have my daughter-in-law and grandchildren to look after, so if a client is willing to pay high I have sex without condom. Why should she be made so vulnerable? [The SACS] says address young women because they are at high risk; women above the age of 40 are also at high risk. [The SACS] should understand this.

*Maharashtra, FSW*

The new focus on reaching younger sex workers and the resultant exclusion of older sex workers meant that many long-time members of the programme who had found a profound sense of belonging in the programme came to suffer exclusion from 'the community' – a source of considerable social support and political legitimacy.

Participant narratives thus paint a picture of the government as enacting a particularly coercive mode of rule in contrast to the more democratic and collaborative approach of Avahan, which valued sex workers' experiences and insight, and engaged sex work leaders in crucial decision-making exercises. Under the governmental intervention regime, 'the field' received diminished importance within the monitoring and evaluation system:

Another thing is when we got information of a visit from Avahan we were enthused because we could present to them what we have done so far and also *take them to the field and show it*. They could easily measure whether we have done what we said we had…. But when government people come they don't bother about anything else but records. They don't care what is happening in the field or how we are addressing issues there.

*Karnataka, MSW*

Participants interpreted the diminished attention accorded to 'the field' as signaling the disinterest of government health officials towards the on-the-ground lived realities of sex workers. The strong reaction of many participants to this deletion suggests the moral and epistemological value attached to 'the field' in comprising the project of caring for the community.

## Flexibility

Some participants contrasted the rigidity of the governmental system to Avahan's 'flexibility', a notion that can be traced to the legacy of Avahan and the re-assertion of its business model in promoting cultures of innovation. They portrayed Avahan's flexible approach as upholding a concern for the care of the community and collaborative decision-making, while the governmental programme was characterised as being more technocratically driven:

Another thing in the TI is they have guidelines. They have to understand that guidelines are meant to show a path or direction and should have flexibility on how it is implemented. There should be community consultation and based on what and how they think a thing should be done it should be accordingly. But the government thinks community must just follow what they say. That will not produce good results because when community take the lead they will also take responsibility, government should keep that in their minds and act accordingly. When Avahan gave us the flexibility as community we showed how we can reduce the incidence of HIV.

*Karnataka, MSW*

Another participant discusses how flexibility supported community cohesiveness and unity; a reality that they saw as threatened under the government's enforcement of more restrictive programme targets:

If for a program budget has been prepared for 100 women and 150 turned up, there was flexibility to include them and feed them also. Even our staff would take lunch. There was flexibility then. Now if we do a programme we have to tell the staff to get their lunch boxes. We feel bad, still we try to share our food with them. We don't have the flexibility to do a program as per the needs of the community with the result many are leaving.

*Maharashtra, FSW*

## From 'vertical' to 'horizontal' health service delivery

Further governmental modifications that troubled participants related to the delivery locations where sex workers received clinical services. Under Avahan, a network of specialised clinical services was tied to sex worker drop-in centres, in places that sex workers regarded as safe spaces for them to access and utilise these resources. Located there, these clinics fostered a sense of ownership over health services (Dixon, et al., 2012).

Criticism of such specialised, disease-based 'vertical services' occupies considerable debate in the global health literature (Béhague and Storeng, 2008). In an effort to provide more sustainable health services, the government reduced community-based clinical services delivered in sex worker organisations, shifting towards a more 'horizontal approach' that aimed at integrating with the government system. However, participants reported mistreatment at the hands of health professionals, which ultimately undermined the health seeking norms fostered by CM:

R2: We used to have our own doctor who would spend so much time with each community member, but now all have to be referred to the government hospital....When we were running a clinic, women were happy that the doctor gave attention and gave good medicines and good counselling was available. In the government hospital we don't get any attention, on the other hand we have to face abusive language. Our women also complain to us about this frequently.

*Karnataka, FSW*

Moreover, when clinical services were delivered in spaces managed by sex work organisations, identity disclosure was often not required as health seekers were personally known to the community and health professional staff, thus affording them easy access to nondiscriminatory health services:

The counsellor in the ICTC [Integrated Counselling and Testing Centre (government facility)] now asks for *Aadhar* card [identity card based on biometric and demographic data], why does he need it? He says he wants to know whether the woman has given the correct name. How does it matter? Sex workers will have over 10 different names, why insist on her true name? She will never give it in the government hospital....

*Maharashtra, FSW*

As explained by a participant, additionally, the health promotion work around regular HIV testing became more challenging with the shift to the public system. When community representatives accompanied their peers to government hospitals, to support the referral process (and meet their outreach targets), their presence was not always welcomed by health professionals:

> Previously we had our own doctor and clinic and testing was easier. Now everyone has to be referred to the government hospital which is far off. So women are reluctant to come all the way for the test and keep deferring it. That's the problem we are facing now. Moreover, even if we convince them and take them all the way the doctor may not be available, or the counsellor or the lab technician.… So one after another we are given problems at the ICTC.
>
> *Karnataka, FSW*

The various accounts of mistreatment faced by community members in government facilities raises important questions about (1) the sustainability of 'enabling environments' created under Avahan as part of its approach to structural interventions, and (2) the lack of readiness to handle the specific health needs of sex workers within the public system.

The next participant further describes the obstacles posed by delivering health services to sex workers in conjunction with the government system when community-assisted referrals are no longer funded:

> They ask for data and whatever we have done we show them. If 100 women have come for health check-up they ask why these women have not gone for ICTC. Where is the money for them to travel to another place? Previously [the Avahan-funded NGO] used to give us a vehicle and also provide tea or snacks to the community who come. Nothing is available now. On the other hand community accuse us now saying you are getting money from the government and you are eating it yourself and not giving anything to us.… We used to distribute condoms, do STI examination through speculum and treatment, syphilis tests were done, ICTC once in six months, all services were made available then, now nothing is there. [The State AIDS Control Society] asks us for data and whatever we have done we report truthfully online once a week and once a month. They don't have the guts to ask us why we have done so low because they have not given us the funds.
>
> *Karnataka, FSW*

As this participant indicates, a metric-based system of programme evaluation, one that is dislodged from the messier lived realities of programme implementation, leaves little room to understand the contextual nature of 'low performance'.

## Funding cuts and delays

The defunding of HIV programmes in India coincided with the rise to power of Narendra Modi of the conservative Bharatiya Janata Party (BJP), who formed the new government of India in May 2014. The National AIDS Control Organization (NACO) was previously unencumbered by bureaucracy during the Avahan era, as it directly reported to the health ministry. However, by August 2014 NACO was merged with the Department of Health & Family Welfare, which effectively mired the HIV division in a system in which the goal of helping the poor is continually 'subverted by the very procedures of the bureaucracy' (Gupta, 2012, p. 23).

All participants recounted how CBOs struggled to function amid government initiated funding reductions. They were especially concerned with unexpected cuts, partial payment transfers, and delays in receiving funds necessary to run their programmes, as one participant explains,

We get funds once in six months and [then] we only get two month's funds. We are unable to pay salaries. Still people are working in the field.... They are distributing condoms and if they don't have money to give to the preferred provider they take the women to the government hospital. But funds are released only once in six months and that took two or three month's money. Money is delayed and not given fully but work has to be done 101 per cent.

*Maharashtra, FSW*

It was argued that funding delays and cuts, without advanced notice, diverted the community's attention away from the goals of HIV prevention work and towards sex work in order to make up the difference from income loss. The defunding of community boards, which played a crucial role in the self-governance of sex work collectives during Avahan, occupied another significant area of frustration:

Previously under [the Avahan-funded NGO] we board members were also working as peer educators and so used to get salaries. We were also in the field till late in the night working as well as doing sex work. So it was not a problem to come to the board meeting. Now there is no money for the board nor do we have any TI [targeted interventions]. So if we call any board member for a meeting she says she doesn't have money to travel to the office for the meeting, they make some excuses not to come.

*Maharashtra, FSW*

Despite widespread disruption to funding flows, community members claimed to uphold a sense of responsibility over the well-being of the community, even paying out of pocket to cover expenses not covered by the programme. However, sex work leaders were often left holding the bill when delayed funding was only partially paid by the government:

Last week I was returning from [names a state district] when I got news that there was a raid on a brothel and women were arrested. I called our programme manager to come to the police station and I also reached there late in the night. They were all there. The police were trying to foist a case of pimping and we spoke to them to stop it. Many had left sex work but had to do it because of delay in disbursement of funds. There is a delay of at least six months. Then they release only for a quarter. One of the women was trying to get her daughter married and needed the money. Money came for three months but many of us have spent our monies for five months on the project. Then we had to pay money to get the women bail and none had any money for it. I paid Rs. 22,000/- and got them out. It becomes very difficult to do such things.

*Maharashtra, FSW*

In general, participants commonly regarded delays and partial funding as an intentional punitive measure on the part of the state for 'poor performance' in meeting programme targets. Rather than troubleshooting with the community, as had been the case during Avahan, according to participants, government health officials often chastised and demeaned them for not meeting their targets, and did so without probing more deeply into the underlying reasons for their 'underperformance'.

## Conclusion

The discussion of Avahan presented in this chapter is telling of how funding received from global humanitarian organisations like the Gates Foundation transforms the expectations of local grassroots actors, thereby sparking tensions with national and state-level governments that might not otherwise have existed.

Through a critical theoretical lens, one could argue that sex work communities in India 'consent' to their own exploitation by adopting, in the first place, Avahan's technological rendition of their social and health problems. From the perspective of governmentality theory, sex workers appear to be subjugated through a form of 'governing through community' (Rose, 2000) – a process whereby experts (1) construct CM as an ethical object *for* sex workers, (2) guide them on the 'correct' course to becoming 'empowered', and (3) inspire them to assume moral responsibility over their own health problems. An ironic form of political domination is exercised, here, as sex workers' political energies, practices, and subjectivities are simultaneously liberated in and subsumed beneath the 'will to empower' (Cruikshank, 1999). Furthermore, we might regard Avahan as enacting a form of hegemony in the Gramscian sense: sex workers take on the perspectives of those who hold power over them, buying into a set of neoliberal ideologies disseminated through Avahan's culture of innovation and efficiency. We might also arrive at the conclusion that Avahan invented and prepared the community to be handed over to the government by implanting logics of enumeration in the very ways that marginalised people come together to form 'communities'.

However, in this chapter we have attempted to illuminate a form of collective consciousness that suggests far more than the idea that sex workers became incited into numerical accounts that depoliticise their struggles; rather, their employment of numerical references enables them to articulate 'the political' through an appeal to the politics of measurement itself. With respect to Gramsci's notion of organic intellectuals, Kate Crehan notes that 'as a class becomes a self-conscious entity, as it moves from being merely a class-in-itself to being a class-for-itself, it brings into being its own intellectuals' (2002, p. 137). Unlike traditional intellectuals that locate expertise in 'the intrinsic nature of intellectual activities' (Gramsci, 2010, p. 263), organic intellectualism, as conceived by Gramsci, shifts our attention to the structural, economic, and social conditions that instill particular ways of knowing in individuals and groups whose role it is to 'help subalterns to understand their oppression and mobilize to change it' (Li, 2007, p. 124). From this vantage point, our participants' perspectives, although entangled in technical and governmental preoccupations, need not be viewed as standing in opposition to seemingly 'purer' ethical and theoretical perspectives than some traditional intellectuals might espouse. In the words of Zimmerman (2017), 'The eloquence employed by organic intellectuals need not be synonymous with the rhetoric of traditional scholarship. Instead, arguments rooted in technical, personal, and practical matters are also powerful vehicles for ideological revolution.'

We have tried to orient the reader towards a more grounded way of thinking about the interrelatedness of 'the technical' and 'the political' with respect to sex worker mobilisations for global health. The birth of a collective consciousness was indeed mediated through an engagement with particular intervention techniques, emerging within a field of social relations forming between sex workers, programme planners, researchers, and managers. A sense of belonging to a 'wider collective' among sex workers came into being through the realm of praxis, through practical and technical learning *in the field*. Therefore, the SACS inattention to 'the field', in favour of a more removed technocratic rendition of evidence, enacts a form of epistemological dispossession. Denying the relevance of 'the field' dislocates sex worker legitimacy from a vital experiential ground of knowledge production, authority, and moral citizenship. At the same time, the various criticisms launched against the current governmental regime are themselves only possible by these leaders' very entanglements in the technical project of governing community health. Their specific reference to targets, population sizes, ratios, coverage, and disease prevalence, funding gaps, paints a precise (and certainly damning) portrait of the consequences of the technocratic approach deployed by the government. But more than a mere demonstration of attention to detail and politics, the participants articulate a host of social relations that are crucial to making 'the numbers' matter in the lives of sex workers, in ways that confront stigma and exclusion within the health system, and, more vitally, open up greater democratic possibilities for them to realise their own visions and priorities within the field of global health.

# References

Adams, V. (2016) *Metrics: What counts in global health*, Durham, NC: Duke University Press.

Béhague, D.P. and Storeng, K.T. (2008) 'Collapsing the vertical–horizontal divide: an ethnographic study of evidence-based policymaking in maternal health', *American Journal of Public Health*, 98(4): 644–9.

Cashman, R. (2006) 'Critical nostalgia and material culture in Northern Ireland', *Journal of American Folklore*, 119(472): 137–60.

Crehan, K.A. (2002) *Gramsci, Culture and Anthropology*, Berkeley, CA: University of California Press.

Cruikshank, B. (1999) *The Will to Empower: Democratic citizens and other subjects*, Ithaca, NY: Cornell University Press.

Dixon, V., Reza-Paul, S., D'Souza, F.M., O'Neil, J., O'Brien, N., and Lorway, R. (2012) 'Increasing access and ownership of clinical services at an HIV prevention project for sex workers in Mysore, India', *Global Public Health*, 7(7): 779–91.

Erikson, S.L. (2012) 'Global health business: the production and performativity of statistics in Sierra Leone and Germany', *Medical Anthropology*, 31(4): 367–84.

Fan, E.L. (2014) 'HIV testing as prevention among MSM in China: the business of scaling-up', *Global Public Health*, 9(1–2): 85–97.

Farmer, P., Kim, J.Y., Kleinman, A., and Basilico, M. (2013) *Reimagining Global Health: An introduction*, Berkeley, CA: University of California Press.

Gopalan, S.S., Mohanty, S., and Das, A. (2012) 'Assessing community health workers' performance motivation: a mixed-methods approach on India's Accredited Social Health Activists (ASHA) programme', *BMJ Open*, 2(5): e001557.

Gramsci, A. (2010) 'Intellectuals and hegemony', In: C.C. Lemert (Ed.) *Social Theory: The multicultural and classic readings*, Boulder, CO: Westview Press, pp. 263–5.

Gupta, A. (2012) *Red Tape: Bureaucracy, structural violence, and poverty in India*, Durham, NC: Duke University Press.

Hardt, M. and Negri, A. (2005) *Multitude: War and democracy in the age of empire*, London: Penguin Books.

Ilcan, S. and Basok, T. (2004) 'Community government: voluntary agencies, social justice, and the responsibilization of citizens', *Citizenship Studies*, 8(2): 129–44.

Li, T.M. (2007) *The Will to Improve: Governmentality, development, and the practice of politics*, Durham, NC: Duke University Press.

Lorway, R. (2017) 'Making global health knowledge: documents, standards, and evidentiary sovereignty in HIV interventions in South India', *Critical Public Health*, 27(2): 177–92.

Lorway, R. and Khan, S. (2014) 'Reassembling epidemiology: mapping, monitoring and making-up people in the context of HIV prevention in India', *Social Science & Medicine*, 112: 51–62.

Mykhalovskiy, E., Patten, S., Sanders, C., Bailey, M., and Taylor, D. (2009) 'Beyond buzzwords: toward a community-based model of the integration of HIV treatment and prevention', *AIDS care*, 21(1): 25–30.

Pickles, M., Boily, M.C., Vickerman, P., Lowndes, C.M., Moses, S., Blanchard, J.F., Deering, K.N., Bradley, J., Ramesh, B.M., Washington, R., and Adhikary, R. (2013) 'Assessment of the population-level effectiveness of the Avahan HIV-prevention programme in South India: a preplanned, causal-pathway-based modelling analysis', *The Lancet Global Health*, 1(5): e289–99.

Ramakrishnan, A. and Alexander, A. (2006) 'Practicing theory: management in HIV intervention', *Harvard International Review*, 28(2): 58.

Rao, P.J. (2010) 'Avahan: the transition to a publicly funded programme as a next stage', *Sexually Transmitted Infections*, 86(Suppl.1): i7.

Reza-Paul, S., Beattie, T., Syed, H.U.R., Venukumar, K.T., Venugopal, M.S., Fathima, M.P., Raghavendra, H.R., Akram, P., Manjula, R., Lakshmi, M., and Isac, S. (2008) 'Declines in risk behaviour and sexually transmitted infection prevalence following a community-led HIV preventive intervention among FSWs in Mysore, India, *AIDS*, 22: S91–100.

Rose, N. (2000) 'Community, citizenship, and the third way', *American Behavioral Scientist*, 43(9): 1395–411.

Schinkel, W. (2010) 'The virtualization of citizenship', *Critical Sociology*, 36(2): 265–83.

Strathern, M. (Ed.) (2000) *Audit Cultures: Anthropological studies in accountability, ethics, and the academy*, Hove, UK: Psychology Press.

Zimmerman, A. (2017) 'The role of organic intellectuals in the era of a Trump presidency', available at www.berkeleyreviewofeducation.com/cfc2016-blog/the-role-of-organic-intellectuals-in-the-era-of-a-trump-presidency (accessed on 6 October 2017).

# Part V

# Scale-up, scale-down, and the sustainability of global health programmes

# 23

# Scaling-up and losing the signal
## The global HIV and AIDS epidemic

*Alan Whiteside*

## Introduction

The Acquired Immunodeficiency Syndrome (AIDS) caused by the Human Immuno-Deficiency Virus (HIV) is the disease that tested global health responses and subsequently framed and drove them from 1981 up to about 2014. This chapter traces the history of the epidemic and the extensive responses which included civil society, especially activists; public health officials, governments; national and international non-governmental organisations; and international funders.

While the initial reaction was exemplary and sustained, this has changed. The AIDS epidemic provides the first example of global scale-up in response to a very real global threat followed by, if not a scale-down, then global stagnation in interest and allocation of resources. The consequences of this will be increased mortality and new 'mini HIV epidemics' in certain settings. The pattern of 'scale-up' and 'scale-down' holds the lessons for global health advocates and practitioners, not just for HIV, but also for other health challenges.

The history of the HIV epidemic has been extensively and comprehensively documented (Shilts, 1987; Timberg and Halperin, 2014; Seeley, 2015; Whiteside, 2016). The early years of the HIV and AIDS epidemic, from 1981 to 1990, were a period of great concern as the scale and trend of the disease were not clear. By 1991, in the US, AIDS was the leading cause of death for adults aged 25 to 44 and rates reached close to 40 deaths per 100,000 by 1995. In 1991, it was estimated about 10 million people were infected worldwide. In 1995 alone, there were an estimated 4.7 million new HIV infections (AVERT, 2017).

The importance of the disease led to the creation of the Joint United Nations Programme on AIDS (UNAIDS) which began operations in 1996. This agency was established to advocate for global action on the epidemic and coordinate the response to HIV and AIDS across the UN. In part its establishment was because the World Health Organization (WHO) had proven to be completely ineffective in mounting and leading a response to the epidemic. At this time most donor agencies and multilateral organisations established desks or divisions to look at, and develop reactions to, the new health threat.

## Epidemiology

By the end of the 1990s, it was apparent that the magnitude of the HIV epidemic and its impact would vary. This was also the decade when HIV began its rapid spread in Southern Africa and prevalence reached unprecedented levels. UNAIDS and the WHO categorised four epidemiological scenarios:

(1) Low-level: where HIV has not spread to significant levels in any sub-population. This included Western nations, much of the Americas, and parts of the Middle East and North Africa.

(2) Concentrated: where prevalence is high enough in one or more sub-populations, such as men who have sex with men (MSM), injection drug users (IDUs), or sex workers and clients to maintain the epidemic, but it is not in the general population. Countries include those of Eastern Europe, Asia, and some Caribbean nations.

(3) Generalised: where HIV prevalence is between 1 and 5 per cent in pregnant women attending ante-natal clinics. The presence of HIV in the general population is sufficient for sexual networking to drive the epidemic. The majority of these countries are in Africa.

(4) Hyper-endemic: HIV is above 15 per cent in adults in the general population, driven through extensive heterosexual, multiple concurrent partner relations, with low and inconsistent condom use. All sexually active persons are at risk. This epidemic is located primarily in Southern Africa.

Many countries with concentrated epidemics have already seen a 'unique' kind of scaling-up and scaling-down. The epidemics here were among marginal groups, ones which national governments chose to ignore, such as drug users. In various of these settings the response was led by international donors, both governments and NGOs. For example, Ukraine's HIV epidemic was closely associated with IDU, which increased in the mid-1990s, during the socio-economic crisis following the break-up of the Soviet Union.

It is in the third and fourth categories that the most significant scaling-up took place and where (premature and potentially damaging) scaling-down is occurring. Global adult prevalence in 2015 is shown in Figure 23.1. The worst affected nations, with adult prevalence above 10 per cent, are Botswana, Lesotho, Mozambique, Namibia, South Africa, Swaziland, Zambia, and Zimbabwe. There are three countries with prevalence between 5 and 10 per cent: Kenya, Malawi, and Uganda.

There was rapid identification of the causes of AIDS, the human immuno-deficiency virus, or HIV. The challenge became to find ways to prevent its transmission and provide treatments for those who were infected. In the absence of treatment, after a period of eight to ten years for most people, HIV-infected people began to experience periods of illness that increased in frequency, severity, and duration until they died. The first drug, AZT, was approved in 1987, but the virus quickly mutated and became resistant, with the result that lives were extended by only a matter of months. AZT was, however, found to be effective in preventing HIV transmission from mother to child. The result was that while infants could be kept HIV-free, the outlook for their mothers, and indeed all infected adults, was bleak.

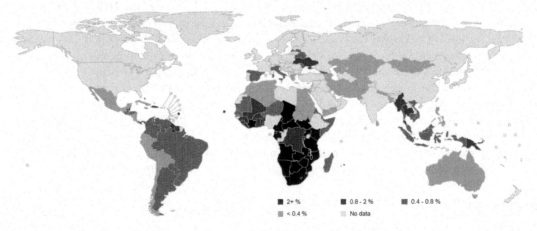

*Figure 23.1* 2015 adult HIV prevalence
(Source: UNAIDS)

Up to 1996, despite the best efforts of the scientific community, attempts to develop treatment were unsuccessful. In that year it was announced, at the International AIDS Conference (IAC) in Vancouver, that new treatments were available (Maugh, 1996). The breakthrough was the finding that antiretroviral therapies (ART) should be taken in a combination of three drugs. These acted at different points in the infection cycle and reduced the viral load allowing people's immune systems to recover. The early treatment regimens were extremely complex – numerous pills to be taken at prescribed times in a day, and were eye wateringly expensive – US$10,000 per person per year (pppy). Despite advances – to the point where a patient may only have to take one pill a day – there is no cure. The drugs have to be taken consistently, for life, and if people miss enough doses then the virus will develop resistance and the patient will begin to fall ill again.

At the end of the millennium, just under 20 years into the epidemic, there was a large, growing and untreated epidemic in East and Southern Africa. In Asia, the Caribbean and Latin America, Eastern Europe, and North Africa the epidemic was contained and mainly located in specific population groups – known at one point as most at risk populations or MARPs. These groups included men who had sex with men, intravenous drug users, and commercial sex workers. In the West the epidemic was concentrated and contained. The first 30 odd years of AIDS was a story of scaling up; the next several years were of stagnation and we are now entering the scaling-down phase.

## Scaling-up

### Prevention and advocacy

The first scaling-up was in prevention. The initial lack of treatment meant the emphasis had to be on keeping people uninfected. Obviously, the best way to avoid (any) infection is to not be exposed to the pathogen, in this case a virus. A number of the initial transmissions were due to people receiving contaminated blood or blood products. As soon as there was a test, it was possible to provide safe blood and blood products. The majority of infections were, and are, through sexual contact, most as a result of heterosexual intercourse. This could be addressed through behaviour modification: at the most extreme avoiding all sexual intercourse. Other strategies included reducing the number of partners or sticking to one partner (and expecting them to be faithful as well). It was appreciated, early in the epidemic, that due to biological and social reasons women and adolescent girls were at greater risk of infection, and so there was a gendered element to prevention efforts and messages.

If people were going to engage in risky behaviours, the most obvious intervention was to use a barrier (condom) to prevent virus transmission, although getting people to use the condoms involved behaviour change. The use of AZT to prevent transmission to infants was rapidly and effectively rolled out. The importance of reducing infections among intravenous drug users (IDU) led to needle exchange programmes and opioid substitution in affected communities. In many, particularly East European countries, these initiatives were led by local civil society as the government ignored the epidemics, which took off very rapidly.

In Ukraine, between 1987 and 1994, there were a mere 398 cases of AIDS of whom only three were identified as being infected through IDU. In 1995 alone, there were 1,489 cases of which 1,021 were IDUs. The first response was from civil society organisations supported by international NGOs such as the International AIDS Alliance and the Open Society; development assistance programmes such as the UK's Department for International Development and British Council; and USAID and foreign governments. In 1997, I and Professor Tony Barnett were invited to Ukraine by the British Council, to carry out a study on 'The Social and Economic Impact of HIV/AIDS in Ukraine'. The report was written up for publication (Barnett, et al., 2000). The expectation was that, in the long-term, government would take over programmes.

Scaling-up involved major efforts in advocacy to put the epidemic on the global agenda. One of the key features of AIDS was it rapidly gained attention across the world. This was undoubtedly helped by the early location of the disease and consequent activism in the gay male population of the US. Horrified by illnesses and deaths among friends, they mobilised and in 1987 formed the AIDS Coalition to Unleash Power (ACT-UP) to protest high drug prices and inadequate response from the various levels of government in the US (Shilts, 1987). This activism was mirrored in other Western countries. In the UK, the Terrence Higgins Trust was formed in 1982 to personalise and humanise AIDS. Famously as early as the mid-1980s Princess Diana was photographed visiting, shaking hands, and hugging AIDS patients.

There was community activism in a number of hard-hit developing countries: in Uganda in 1987, Noerine Kaleeba and colleagues set up The AIDS Support Organization (TASO), to provide care, support, and counselling, and mobilise communities and neighbourhood care for people with HIV and AIDS and their families. In the same year the Family AIDS Caring Trust (FACT), a Christian national development NGO based in Mutare, Zimbabwe was established. In general, though, the organisations in developing countries set out to provide services rather than get involved in the politics of response. The exception was the Treatment Action Campaign (TAC), founded in South Africa in 1998, which sought to do both.

By 2000, globally the potential political, economic, and social impact of AIDS was being acknowledged. A key individual in placing the disease on the international agenda was Richard Holbrooke, who served as the 22nd US Ambassador to the United Nations from 1999 to 2001. In January 2000, when the United States held rotating presidency of the UN Security Council, Holbrooke called a meeting of the Security Council to discuss AIDS in Africa, with Vice President Al Gore presiding. It declared AIDS was a security threat to all nations. This marked the first time a health issue was discussed as a threat to peace and security.

Following the Millennium Summit of the United Nations, in 2000 the Millennium Development Goals (MDGs) were adopted. The sixth of the eight goals was to combat HIV/AIDS, malaria, and other diseases. The first United Nation's General Assembly Special Session on AIDS was held in 2001, and Secretary General Kofi Annan called for the creation of a global fund to combat the spread of HIV. The perceived importance of the disease was growing and the response was scaling-up.

Despite this, the reality in 2000 was a huge gap in the way people were being treated in the West and the options open to AIDS patients in the developing world. In the developed nations treatment was available, although it was extremely expensive. It was generally subsidised by the state. In the developing nations, the only people who were lucky enough to get treatment were either extremely wealthy, or those who had been placed on clinical trials.

## Scaling-up treatment

The inequality in access to treatment caused international outrage. In 2000, President Clinton issued an Executive Order to 'assist developing countries in importing and producing generic HIV treatments' (Executive Order 13155, 2000). In 2000, the IAC was held in Durban with a theme of 'Breaking the Silence'. This encompassed the need to break the silence on equal access to treatment and care. In July, UNAIDS, WHO, and other global health groups announced a joint initiative with five major pharmaceutical manufacturers to negotiate reduced prices for HIV/AIDS drugs in developing countries (Whiteside and Lee, 2005). Indian pharmaceutical companies began producing and marketing generic drugs and prices fell dramatically.

Despite the fall in price, treatment remained beyond the reach of low-income, high-burden countries, especially those in Africa. In order for treatment to be scaled up there had to be increased funding and this happened with three major initiatives. The Global Fund to Fight AIDS, Tuberculosis and Malaria (GFATM) was established in Geneva in 2002 – the year UNAIDS reported AIDS was the leading cause of death in sub-Saharan Africa. The GFATM had its roots in the UN's Special Sessions on AIDS; it was discussed at a

G8 summit in Okinawa, Japan, in 2000, as well as at the African Union summit in April 2001; and it was finally endorsed by the G8 summit in July 2001.

In 2003, the US President George W. Bush announced the creation of President's Emergency Plan for AIDS Relief (PEPFAR) in his State of the Union address. The first round of PEPFAR funding was US$15 billion for five years, primarily for countries with a high burden of infections. Between 2004 and 2015, PEPFAR committed a staggering US$65,921 million, and in 2016 the funding request was for US$6,542 million. PEPFAR data show, in 2014, they were supporting 7.7 million people on ART.

In the same year the WHO announced the '3 by 5' initiative to bring HIV treatment to three million people by 2005. This did not bring new money to the table but endorsed the roll-out of treatment. It was clear the international community was stepping up to the plate in a big way, and the response, especially in treatment, was being scaled up. Provision of ART was helped by the dramatic falls in prices of drugs, easier dosing regimens, and the expansion of health services, although HIV care tended to be provided in silos.

With the falls in price, increased funding available, and the new initiatives, the numbers of people on treatment began to grow rapidly. In 2000, at the time of the IAC in Durban, a basic antiretroviral (ARV) regimen cost over US$10,000 pppy. In 2017, first line ART cost approximately US$100 pppy for the lowest-priced, generic drugs. The lowest-priced generic second line regimen, zidovudine/lamivudine (AZT/3TC) and atazanavir/r (ATV/r) is US$286 pppy. In 2000, an estimated 773,257 people were receiving drugs out of 28,900,000 people living with HIV. The numbers for Africa were just 6,161 on treatment out of 21,700,000 infections. By 2015 there were 17,023,200 people on treatment out of 36,700,000 infected (the African figures were 12,091,100 and 25,500,000 respectively) (WHO, 2017).

There has also been a change in the guidelines as to who should be treated and when. Initially treatment was recommended for those whose CD4 cell count had fallen below 200 per cubic millimetre of blood. This gradually increased over time, to a CD4 count of 350, then 500. By 2015, WHO guidelines were unequivocal: ART should be initiated in all HIV-positive people no matter what their CD4 cell count is. There was an additional reason for this; data showed that HIV infected people who took the drugs consistently would achieve viral suppression, and so would be very many times less likely to infect others. Treatment acted as prevention. This has given rise to a switch of resources from slower acting community-based prevention methods such as provision of condoms and information and education to the immediacy of providing treatment. Oberth et al. (2017) analysed recent global fund grants to see what percentage of countries were requesting the UNAIDS benchmark of 26 per cent for prevention in their grant applications. Of the 23 countries only ten requested a quarter for prevention, and only two had signed grants with at least 25 per cent allocated for prevention. It is unclear how this will play out in the years ahead.

## Financing the response

From the beginning of the epidemic in the 1980s, responses to the disease in the developing world were largely funded by international organisations, NGOs, and foreign governments. There were good reasons for this dominance of international funding. The bulk of the science emanated from laboratories in the US, UK, and France. Grassroots activism – which characterised the response to HIV – had its origins in the US and UK. Finally, as the early spread of HIV was silent – indeed, prevalence levels in most Southern African countries were below 5 per cent in 1990 – governments were not dealing with cases (i.e., of visibly sick people requiring care), but with invisible HIV infections. The epidemic was imperceptible.

In 2011, UNAIDS proposed an investment framework to reduce new infections and deaths in low- and middle-income countries (LMICs) by 2015. This faltered, was revisited, and resulted in the 2015 document, 'UNAIDS 2016–2021 Strategy: On the Fast-Track to end AIDS', which seeks a rapid scale-up of effective intervention and treatment programmes. The UNAIDS targets are that by 2020, 90 per cent of all people living with HIV know their HIV status; 90 per cent of all people with diagnosed HIV infection receive sustained ARV therapy; and 90 per cent of all people receiving ART have viral suppression.

*Table 23.1* Selected country data for HIV and currencies

| Country | HIV prevalence (% of population ages 15–49) (2015) | People living with HIV (2015) | Percent of people receiving ART (2015) | HIV spending all sources (US$ millions) | Percent HIV spending (domestic sources) | GNI per capita (2015) | World Bank ranking (2014) |
|---|---|---|---|---|---|---|---|
| Botswana | 22.2 | 350000 | 78 | $390 (2011) | 76.7 | $6510 | Upper middle income |
| Lesotho | 22.7 | 310000 | 42 | $94.20 (2013) | 27.5 | $1330 (2014) | Lower middle income |
| Malawi | 9.1 | 980000 | 61 | $145 (2012) | 8.2 | $350 | Low income |
| Mozambique | 10.5 | 1500000 | 53 | $352 (2014) | 3.5 | $580 | Low income |
| Namibia | 13.3 | 210000 | 69 | $211 (2013) | 64.7 | $5210 | Upper middle income |
| South Africa | 19.2 | 7000000 | 48 | $1880 (2014) | 79.4 | $6050 | Upper middle income |
| Swaziland | 28.8 | 220000 | 67 | $96.90 (2013) | 34.2 | $3230 | Lower middle income |
| Zambia | 12.9 | 1200000 | 63 | $279 (2012) | 5.7 | $1500 | Lower middle income |
| Zimbabwe | 14.7 | 1400000 | 62 | $253 (2013) | 13.6 | $850 | Low income |

To pay for this UNAIDS proposed the funding target of at least US$30 billion for LMICs. It recommends:

> From 2014 to 2020, the share of HIV investment from domestic public sources is proposed to increase from 10% to 12% in 31 low-income countries, from 22% to 45% in 43 lower-middle-income countries and from 84% to 95% in 42 upper-middle-income countries.
>
> *UNAIDS, 2016, p. 12*

This marks a clear shift away from a world where HIV and AIDS funding primarily came from international donors. However, this shift in funding may prove difficult for some countries to achieve. For example, as is shown in Table 23.1, only 3.5 per cent of the money for HIV and AIDS came from domestic funding in Mozambique; in Zambia, the proportion was just 5.7 per cent.

## Scaling-down the response

### Priorities

From 2008 onward, a number of major shifts occurred in the global responses. HIV and AIDS no longer held the status as the premier global threat to health. In part, this was due to the success of expansion of treatment. Infected people were living longer, more productive lives as a result of cheaper ART. HIV and AIDS policy had become normalised, shifting away from an emergency state of response to a mode characterised by increased accountability for results and an emphasis on cost-effectiveness (Smith and Whiteside, 2010).

The financial crisis of 2008 rocked global economies. It was generally expected that the international community would reduce DAH, and although, as shown in Figure 23.2, there was a period when the funding plateaued, it remained remarkably robust and began to rise again. There is, however, a sense that this changed in 2016–17, as will be discussed later.

The MDGs came to an end in 2015 and were replaced by the Sustainable Development Goals (SDGs). AIDS was specifically mentioned in one of the MDGs, but it is only a sub-clause in the SDGs (UNDP, 2017). SDG 3 is to: 'Ensure healthy lives and promote well-being for all at all ages.' The HIV and AIDS specific target is to end the epidemics of AIDS, tuberculosis, malaria, and neglected tropical diseases and combat hepatitis, water-borne diseases, and other communicable diseases by 2030. The UN has set a target of less than 500,000 new HIV infections annually, less than 500,000 AIDS-related deaths annually, and the elimination of HIV-related discrimination by 2020.

## Funding needs

It has been clear that human and financial resources for HIV and AIDS need to increase. Despite scientific advances, treatment is relatively costly and labour intensive. Improvements in treatment mean people infected with HIV can have close to normal life expectancy and AIDS deaths are decreasing. At the same time, prevention efforts have not been universally successful; the number of infected people requiring medicines and care continues to rise. The need is even greater due to the global consensus that HIV-infected individuals should commence treatment as early as possible (WHO, 2015).

By the end of 2015, UNAIDS estimated that about US$19 billion was invested in LMICs in that year. There is no evidence of major new investments, despite the fact that UNAIDS believes US$26.2 billion will be required for the HIV and AIDS response by 2020 in order to meet their fast track targets. What this means is, despite a significant amount of money – allocated by a range of donors and the growing mobilisation and increase in domestic funding – there is still a major need for more and continued financing. This was confirmed in a 2016 modelling paper by Stover et al. (2016). The question of where the money should come from is increasingly important. Two potential sources that have been mooted are increased domestic resource mobilisation and innovative financing schemes: neither can fill the gap, however.

The concept of an 'AIDS transition', developed by Mead Over at the Centre of Global Development in Washington, is blindingly simple (Over, 2011). The AIDS transition suggests that until the number of new infections falls below the number of deaths of HIV-infected people, from whatever cause, the need for treatment will rise. If the lines do not cross, this number will grow indefinitely, as will the costs of combatting the epidemic. This idea is shown in Figure 23.2. When data are applied to a number of countries including South Africa, which has the largest epidemic in the world (about seven million infections in 2017), it is evident that the 'AIDS transition' is not in sight. The implication of this is either that there will need to be ever more donor support or that the country will have to increase the domestic resources allocated for the disease. South Africa can find more money internally. This is not the case for a number of the other countries in the region, such as Lesotho and Malawi. They simply do not have the resources to provide treatment, especially drugs, to their infected populations.

## Funding sources

Although there are increasing quantities of domestic resources going into the AIDS response, international DAH remains important and indeed it is critical in a number of countries. By far the largest amount of money comes directly from the US. When the US contribution to multilateral organisations such as the GFATM is taken into account, it is clear that the dependency on one country's generosity is considerable. The UK has been a major player in global health; although the amounts of money are significantly smaller,

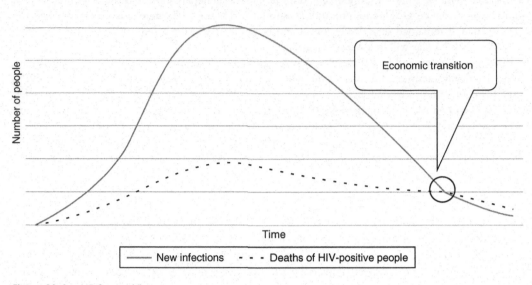

*Figure 23.2* AIDS transition

it has been an influential donor and has contributed significantly to policy. The status of both these funders is in some doubt.

There are clear indications that the US administration under President Trump is likely to reduce its commitments to global health, as well as much of the UN system (Garrett, 2017). During the World Health Assembly, in May 2017, the White House released its proposed 2018 budget with enormous cuts in health and science. Laurie Garrett (2017), a noted commentator at the New York-based Council for Foreign Relations, reported these cuts as:

- 26 per cent of State Department and US Agency for International Development (USAID) global health spending;
- 20 per cent of Centers for Disease Control and Prevention (CDC) global health spending;
- 11 per cent of US President's Emergency Plan for AIDS Relief (PEPFAR) spending on overseas HIV programs;
- 18 per cent of all agency spending on HIV/AIDS overseas;
- 100 per cent of funding for international family planning;
- 44 per cent of overseas malaria spending;
- 26 per cent of tuberculosis spending; and
- 25 per cent of spending on neglected tropical diseases.

The situation in the UK is somewhat different, but certainly more complicated. The British government undertook to meet the UN target of spending 0.7 per cent of the gross national product on aid. This was confirmed by the Conservative government under David Cameron and then reaffirmed under Theresa May's leadership. All the major parties (Conservative, Labour, Liberal Democrat, and Scottish Nationalist) have affirmed this commitment. There are three caveats that need to be discussed.

The first is how development assistance is counted. There has been lobbying to change the definition of aid as set by the Organisation for Economic Co-operation and Development (OECD):

> The rules for what counts as development assistance matter when a country sets out a spending target like the U.K. does. Such a change to the rules aimed at including more kinds of "aid" … would allow the government to meet its spending commitment without really increasing spending on development assistance.
>
> *Humanosphere, 2017, n.p.*

The Cameron government released a plan in late 2015 to cut the proportion of aid money spent by the Department for International Development (DFID) from 86 per cent to 70 per cent. At the same time, they lobbied the OECD to change its rules for what counts as development assistance to include peace and security programmes – some of which are military programmes (Humanosphere, 2017, n.p.).

The second caveat was the British political situation. This article was completed after the 8th June 2017 election. The Prime Minister went to the country to get a clear mandate for the Brexit negotiations and, she thought, increase her majority. In fact, the Conservatives lost so many seats that they had to enter a coalition in order to establish a government. This and the Brexit process do not bode well for international issues including development assistance; attention will be focussed on domestic matters for some time to come and new elections may be necessary.

The third factor concerns the value of the pound. Since the Brexit vote in June 2016 the pound has steadily lost value against the dollar. The value of the pound fell from a peak of £1 = US$1.71 in July 2014 to a low of £1 = US$1.19 on 15 January 2017. Predictions suggest that the pound may stabilise at lower levels. The dollar value of the British contribution to multilateral agencies will therefore be lower. An example is that DFID, the second largest donor to the GFATM, committed £1.1 billion to the fifth replenishment in September 2016. It is not clear what this will be worth in US dollars, the currency of the Fund in 2017 or 2018. For bilateral contributions, the fall in the value of most recipients' currencies' values should offset the fall in the pound. Where contributions are counted or spent in dollars if the pound falls in value, the UK will have to either increase the amount of money they give or their contribution will be worth less.

The US and the UK are both, albeit for different reasons, retreating from the world stage. This is of concern and points to the continued scaling-down in allocations of international funding to HIV which began in 2015. There was a move by a number of European countries to plug the gap left by the US application of the global gag rule. In March 2017,

> about 50 governments are attending the hastily convened She Decides conference in Brussels on Thursday, with early pledges closing in on $100m (£80m). Sweden promised $22m and Finland $21m to compensate for the reinstated "global gag rule", which bans US funding for NGOs that provide abortion or information on the procedure to women in developing countries.
>
> *Rankin, 2017, n.p.*

However, the amount that will be raised remains to be seen.

## Conclusion

What have we learnt from the scaling-up and scaling-down of the response to HIV?

Perhaps the most important lesson is that global resources can be mobilised for urgent health issues (as was seen for the Ebola outbreak), but that it is hard to maintain momentum: the exceptional becomes normalised and attention switches to the next issue. This happened too soon for the AIDS epidemic; there are still new infections and in a number of countries the AIDS transition has not been achieved. The costs of treatment mean some nations cannot afford to treat the infected people in their populations and they remain dependent on the donor community.

It is clear that AIDS did not have the same priority globally in 2015 as it did in 2000. In some settings the view was that at-risk populations were 'not worthy' of attention, or that they somehow deserved their fate. In Africa the influx of donor money led to governments taking the back seat and arguing that, 'if the donors saw HIV as a problem, then it was up to them to deal with it'.

The scientific response was unexpected and astonishing. It has allowed many medical and other fields to make rapid progress, and these gains will benefit future generations. Technology has an important role to play in the development of new and better drugs, and in increasing the availability of and speed of testing. In the United States testing in community pharmacies has been piloted (Weidle, et al., 2014). In Malawi, a feasibility study showed self-testing, where a person can use a rapid diagnostic kit and get the result in private, was successful. Three-quarters of people who were given a kit used it and 76 per cent of these then had access to a counsellor to talk about the results (London School of Hygiene and Tropical Medicine, 2015). This enabled those who were infected to be put on care and provided an incentive to those who were not infected to stay that way.

The spotlight on adolescent girls and younger women is to be welcomed. In Africa, the majority of infections are among this group. The challenges are many: patriarchal, exploitative, and disrespectful attitudes towards young women and girls are a major issue. Intimate partner violence and lack of access to opportunities help drive the epidemic. Poverty and food insecurity may lead to higher levels of transactional sex. It is not enough to provide prevention technology such as condoms or microbicides; these women need to be empowered to make decisions about their own health.

The structural barriers have to be addressed. There have been, and continue to be, pilot projects looking at conditional cash transfers which might, among other things, keep girls in school. This is known to be protective against HIV transmission. In Botswana, the length of schooling was increased by one year in 1996, which increased the likelihood of young women remaining HIV-negative. The challenge is to move from pilot projects to national ones. AIDS was the most serious disease to emerge in the last century. The consequences, responses, and lessons place the global health community in a stronger position to face the inevitable new pathogens and epidemics.

# References

AVERT. (2017) 'Global HIV and AIDS statistics', available at www.avert.org/global-hiv-and-aids-statistics (accessed on 19 September 2017).

Barnett, T., Kruglov, Y., Steshenko, V., and Khodakevick, L. (2000) 'The social and economic impact of HIV/AIDS in Ukraine', *Social Science and Medicine*, 51(9): 1–17.

Executive Order 13155 (2000) 'Access to HIV/AIDS pharmaceuticals and medical technologies', 10 May, available at www.gpo.gov/fdsys/pkg/FR-2000-05-12/pdf/00-12177.pdf (accessed on 26 September 2017).

Garrett, L. (2017) 'Garrett on global health', available at www.cfr.org/about/newsletters/archive/newsletter/n4591 (accessed on 19 September 2017).

Humanosphere. (2017) 'Where Britain stands on foreign aid-development and why it matters worldwide', available at www.humanosphere.org/world-politics/2017/06/u-k-decides-major-parties-stand-foreign-aid-development (accessed on 19 September 2017).

London School of Hygiene and Tropical Medicine. (2015) 'HIV self-testing found safe, acceptable, and accurate in Malawi study' available at www.lshtm.ac.uk/newsevents/news/2015/hiv_self_testing.html (accessed on 9 September 2015).

Maugh, T.H. (1996) 'Studies of combined HIV drugs promising health: experts at AIDS conference unveil early results showing treatment involving certain medications reduces virus to undetectable levels', available at http://articles.latimes.com/1996-07-12/news/mn-23350_1_aids-drugs (accessed on 26 September 2017).

Oberth, G., Torres, M.A., Mumba, O., and O'Conner, M. (2017) 'A quarter for prevention? Global Fund investments in HIV prevention interventions in generalised African epidemics', *Universal Journal of Public Health*, 5(5): 231–41

Over, M. (2011) 'Achieving an AIDS transition: preventing infections to sustain treatment', Washington, DC: Center for Global Development, available at www.cgdev.org/sites/default/files/achieving-an-aids-transition-web.pdf (accessed on 19 September 2017).

Rankin, J. (2017) 'Countries pledge millions to plug hole left by US "global gag rule"', available at www.theguardian.com/global-development/2017/mar/02/countries-to-join-forces-to-raise-funds--safe-abortions-trump-order-conference-global-gag-rule (accessed on 19 September 2017).

Seeley, J. (2015) *HIV and East Africa: Thirty years in the shadow of an epidemic*, Abingdon: Routledge.

Shilts, R. (1987) *And the Band Played On: Politics, people and the AIDS epidemic*, New York: St. Martin's Press.

Smith, J. and Whiteside, A. (2010) 'The history of AIDS exceptionalism', *Journal of the International AIDS Society*, 13: 47.

Stover, J., Bollinger, L., Izazola, J.A., Loures, L., DeLay, P., Ghys, P.D., and Fast Track Modeling Working Group (2016) 'Correction: what is required to end the AIDS epidemic as a public health threat by 2030? The cost and impact of the fast-track approach', *PloS one*, 11(6): e0158253.

Timberg, C. and Halperin, D. (2014) *Tinderbox*, London: Penguin Books.

UNAIDS. (2016) 'Fast-track update on investments neede in the AIDS response', available at www.unaids.org/sites/default/files/media_asset/UNAIDS_Reference_FastTrack_Update_on_investments_en.pdf (accessed on 19 September 2017).

UNDP. (2017) 'Sustainable development goals', available at www.undp.org/content/undp/en/home/sustainable-development-goals.html (accessed on 19 September 2017).

Weidle, P.J., Lecher, S., Botts, L.W., Jones, L., Spach, D.H., Alvarez, J., Jones, R., and Thomas, V. (2014) 'HIV testing in community pharmacies and retail clinics: a model to expand access to screening for HIV infection', *Journal of the American Pharmacists Association*, 54(5): 486–92.

Whiteside, A. (2016) *HIV and AIDS: A very short introduction*, Oxford: Oxford University Press.

Whiteside, A. and Lee, S. (2005) 'The "Free by 5" campaign for universal, free antiretroviral therapy', *PLoS Med*, 2(8): e227.

WHO. (2015) *Guideline on When to Start Antiretroviral Therapy and on Pre-Exposure Prophylaxis for HIV*, Geneva: WHO.

WHO. (2017) 'ART table 2000–2015', available at www.who.int/hiv/data/art_table_2000_2015.png?ua=1 (accessed on 19 September 2017).

# 24

# Brazil and the changing meanings of 'universal access' to antiretrovirals during the early twenty-first century

*Marcos Cueto*

## Introduction

In the mid-1990s, antiretrovirals (ARVs) and Highly Active Antiretroviral Therapy (HAART) revolutionised the history of AIDS treatment. They were not a cure but could turn the disease into a manageable chronic condition. However, they were expensive (about US$12,000 per person per year). Global health organisations, including the World Bank, discouraged these treatments in developing countries as 'non-cost-effective' interventions. Brazilians disagreed. Dozens of Brazilians, including members of NGOs and officers of the Ministry of Health, participated in the 1996 International AIDS meeting in Vancouver where ARVs were announced, and upon their return home demanded their use in Brazil's strong public health system (Nunn, 2009).

In November 1996, President Fernando Henrique Cardoso signed a law that provided free access to generic AIDS medication (drugs identical to brand-name medicines) and to all drugs necessary for treatment (Fonseca, 2015). These decisions interacted with programmes for counselling and testing, and campaigns against homophobia, and were supported by activists and NGOs. Furthermore, the government slashed the tariff on imported condoms lowering their price, promoted local production of condoms, and worked with sex workers to engage them in the programme. In 1999, Brazil's president decreed that his government could license patents because AIDS was a national emergency (in 'compulsory licenses', namely when a government authorises the domestic production of a drug without the consent of the patent owner) (see also Vieira and Di Giano, Chapter 31 in this volume). In a few years, an ambitious Brazilian business of generic medicine produced six of the approximately 12 drugs used in the country. Despite the severe financial crisis and devaluation of the currency, the government persisted in its AIDS policy. In the late 1990s, Jose Serra, Brazilian Minister of Health, kept threatening to issue compulsory licenses for anti-AIDS drugs that certainly were instrumental for obtaining price reductions from pharmaceuticals. By 2001, Brazil estimated that between 1996 and 2001, its programme had reduced AIDS mortality rates by nearly 50 per cent and opportunistic infections by 60–80 per cent; preventing about 360,000 hospital admissions and saving US$1 billion of federal money. The results contradicted the World Bank that predicted in the mid-1990s that 1.2 million Brazilians would have HIV by 2000; only half that figure existed in 2001 (Rosenberg, 2001).

Brazilian generic companies produced drugs with patents that recently expired. Despite its threats, the Brazilian government did not produce copycat versions of drugs protected by patents until 2007. This occurred because Cardoso was a centre-right politician convinced that the country should stick to the rules of the neoliberal international market, which involved accepting the hegemony of the US and the authority of the recently created World Trade Organization (WTO) and its Agreement on Trade-Related Aspects of Intellectual Property Rights (TRIPS). Nevertheless, the Brazilian government would retain its ability to negotiate a reduction of prices of brand-name medicines and use its own global health diplomacy in international meetings.

## The international impact of Brazil's programme

Brazil's fight against AIDS was soon praised as a success story and an example. Thailand, South Africa, and Senegal, among other governments of developing countries, followed Brazil, and international organisations, such as Médicins San Frontières (MSF), Partners in Health, and UNAIDS, launched pilot programmes providing ARVs in developing nations. Pharmaceutical companies considered the production of generic drugs, and compulsory licenses, to be acts of piracy against WTO intellectual property laws. American pharmaceutical companies asked the trade body to intervene and requested that the US government place Brazil on a watch list – a typical first step towards sanctions (Chartrand, 2001).

The net result was a growing reputation of pharmaceuticals as ruthless and evil enterprises that use their monopoly to deny life-saving drugs. A 2001 article in *The New York Times* used a telling title: 'Look at Brazil: Patent laws are malleable. Patients are educable. Drug companies are vincible. The world's AIDS crisis is solvable'. It is important to reproduce one of its strongest statements:

> Brazil is showing that no one who dies of AIDS dies of natural causes. Those who die have been failed – by feckless leaders who see weapons as more alluring purchases than medicines, … and by the multinational drug companies who have kept the price of antiretroviral drugs needlessly out of reach of the vast majority of the world's population.
>
> *Rosenberg, 2001, n.p.*

In addition, the Oxfam report *Drug Companies vs. Brazil: The Threat to Public Health* adamantly criticised the US government and the pharmaceutical industries for undermining Brazil's efforts (Oxfam, 2001).

Since the late 1990s, CEOs of these companies became convinced that they had to repair their image. This occurred when the US Congress and the G8 (the meeting of the richest industrialised countries) construed AIDS as a global security issue that could not be controlled by strict immigration rules and might destabilise several countries in the world (HOR, 2003). Following the Okinawa G8 summit of July 2000, a series of meetings of health experts and diplomats discussed new financial mechanisms to pay for ARVs drugs for developing nations. In February 2001, a preparatory discussion for a United Nations General Assembly Special Session on HIV/AIDS (UNGASS) called for new global mechanisms to assist the purchase of ARV medicines. In the same month, the Indian generic company CIPLA launched its ARV treatment for a few hundred dollars, consequently putting pressure on pharmaceutics to cut prices. Important developments also occurred at the World Health Organization (WHO). In March 2001, the WHO established the Prequalification of Medicines Programme to approve and suggest good-quality low-cost medicines, especially ARVs, for member countries.

In April 2001, Kofi Annan made a dramatic plea at the Organization of African Unity Summit in Abuja requesting US$7–10 billion annually for the establishment of a 'war chest' against AIDS (McLellan, 2001). However, in the following months the funds provided by the Bush administration and the governments of other industrialised nations were smaller than expected. The US, the UK, and Japan initially contributed US$200 million each for the future fund, France committed 127 million over three years, and the Gates Foundation provided 100 million. Annan remained hopeful that donations would increase in the coming years as the fund established a good record of accomplishment. Others were more critical. Oxfam and Health Gap (Global Access Project) Coalition criticised the amount provided by rich countries as too little and worried that the bulk of 'new' financial resources would come out of development assistance funds, which already existed. Also criticised was the significant contrast between the funds donated and the large expenses incurred by military programmes. Later that year, the initial amount approved by the US Congress was US$79 billion to pay for the first phase of the war in Iraq (DeYoung, 2001).

Greater legitimacy for the future fund was born at the UNGASS meeting in June 2001 in which Brazilians and UNAIDS had an active role. It took place in New York and its sole goal was to discuss AIDS. Its main result was a declaration that called for 'the establishment on an urgent basis of a global HIV/AIDS and Health Fund' (United Nations, 2001, p. 41). Before the meeting, the United States Trade Representative (USTR) at the WTO abandoned the trade dispute with Brazil (initiated in January of 2001 by President Clinton).[1] Initially, the fund was called 'the International Fund for HIV/AIDS' or 'Global Fund for AIDS and Health'. The supporters of the name, mainly UNAIDS, believed that the response to AIDS went beyond the health sector, articulated different actors and organisations which were not always related to medicine, and required a political response.

At the same time, changes in pharmaceuticals became visible. Drug companies were willing to supply some products at no profit and make donations to countries on a case by case basis, but were not willing to give away patents; the linchpin of the industry. They also demanded that the UN have a clear position in favour of patents and help to guarantee that lower-priced medicines would not be diverted to higher-priced markets (a claim considered an exaggeration by activists because the US and Japan had strict border controls against smuggling).

In July 2001, 70 representatives of developed and developing countries, and leaders of pharmaceuticals and NGOs, attended a meeting in Brussels to implement the UNGASS Declaration. A member of Health Gap complained about references made to 'balanced approaches' between generic and brand-name drugs and about the fact that bulk purchases [of ARVs] 'are being pushed off the table' (Davis, 2001, p. 1). The G8 summit that took place in Genoa, also in July 2001, made clear that it was going to be a Global Fund focused on HIV/AIDS, malaria, and TB (not a UN agency or an organisation dealing with the political dimensions of HIV/AIDS). The decision reflected the criticism of private donors and bilateral agencies against the UN, regarded as politicised, overly bureaucratic, and unaccountable. It also reflected the G8 organisation of the Millennium Development Goals that gave priority to treatment activities in the three previously mentioned diseases (DFID, 2001). Tragic developments in the US favoured the use of generics by the Fund. After the 2001 terrorist attacks on 11 September 2001 and the anthrax mail attacks that followed shortly thereafter, the Bush government was ready to issue a compulsory license for the generic Ciprofloxacin Hydrochloride, produced in Canada and India (after it became clear that Bayer did not have sufficient quantities of Cipro, the same brand name, antibiotic) (Charatan, 2001).

The organisers of the Fund validated the new financial mechanism after 11 September 2001. It was not only as a response to the three major diseases, but also a means to correct the social inequalities produced by economic globalisation and to secure the stability of the world. The Genoa summit and the meeting in Brussels designed two bodies for the future Fund: first, a Transitional Working Group (TWG) as a consultative body comprising 40 representatives – including Brazil – that worked to have the Fund ready by early 2002; and second, a Technical Support Secretariat (TSS) that was crucial in terms of day-to-day operations. The TSS defined the Global Fund's legal status, structure, governance, eligibility criteria, methods of disbursing funds, and communication strategies. The Fund was designed as a 'technical agency' focused in efficiency and 'good management' (rather than a political actor that would engage with activists); a design that was congruent to the global neoliberal health policies of the industrialised countries. Moreover, it shaped new and old code terms like 'evidence-based decision', 'business-like grant-making process', 'culture of performance', 'business plans', 'cost effectiveness', and the euphemism 'protection to commodities' (which meant protection for intellectual property laws and regulations). These were instrumental to weaken the proposals of favouring generics over brand-name medicines and to make the goal of universal access to ARVs seem more 'practical'. In November 2001, the important Fourth Ministerial Conference of the

WTO took place in Doha, Qatar. The meeting approved a declaration that clarified that nothing in the TRIPS agreement prevented governments from issuing compulsory licenses in health emergencies (World Trade Organization, 2001). During the meeting, the US, Japan, Canada, and some European countries tried to water down the declaration and Zimbabwe, Brazil, and India defended the principle that essential medicines – especially ARVs – were a universal human right. For Brazilians the Declaration was a triumph of an alliance of Brazilian health officers and diplomats and launched a campaign in US journals. Health leaders, like Paulo Teixeira – the architect of the Sao Paulo and Brazil's national anti-AIDS programme – testified before the WTO panel and Brazilian diplomats lobbied politicians in Washington, DC.

All of the events described helped to launch the Global Fund to fight AIDS, Tuberculosis, and Malaria in late January of 2002. It had more resources than the initial donations, US$1.9 billion. However, the amount was short of Annan's 'war chest' call in Abuja. It had the mandate to become the main financial mechanism – not an operation agency – in developing countries and the major public–private partnership (PPP); a type of organisation that crowded global-health activities since the early twenty-first century (Walgate, 2002). The architecture of the Fund in its Geneva headquarters was a Secretariat, an Executive Board, a Technical Review Panel, and Partnership Forum. In these units that met only a few times during the year, Brazil, developing countries, and eventually NGOs and people living with AIDS were given representation. Country Coordinating Mechanisms (CCMs) (conceived as local PPPs) were important in recipient countries. From 2002 to 2007, Richard Feachem, former Director of Health, Nutrition, and Population at the World Bank and professor at the University of California-San Francisco, became Executive Director. He had the goal of making the Global Fund an example that a public institution could use good practices from the private sector. At the same time, the WHO and Indian generic companies moved forward. In March 2002, CIPLA's products became part of WHO's coveted list of approved drugs for HIV and were used by the Fund, despite the criticism of pharmaceutical companies against WHO's Prequalification unit for not being a formal regulatory agency like the FDA (D'Adesky, 2002). In April 2002, the Global Fund approved its first round of grants totalling US$600 million (most of its donations went towards AIDS rather than tuberculosis or malaria).

In the final months of 2002, more developments had an impact in global health responses to AIDS. The first was a change in leadership. In late August of that year, Gro Harlem Brundtland, WHO's director-general who made a number of important reforms but did not launch a radical fight for generics, announced suddenly that she would not run for re-election. A disorganised scramble for the position began with favourites Pascoal Mocumbi, former Minister of Health of Mozambique, Peter Piot, a Belgian well known for his leadership as head of UNAIDS, and Julio Frenk from Mexico, who had worked closely with Brundtland (informally supported by the US but not supported by the Brazilians). In a surprising result, a dark horse insider who had worked for over 20 years at the agency won the election: the Korean Lee Jong-Wook (hereafter Lee) (Vogel, 2003).

## The WHO and universal access to ARVS

More bewildering than Lee's unexpected appointment as director-general of WHO was his decision to make the WHO a champion of ARV treatment. Lee made an alliance with UNAIDS – overcoming any personal animosities with Piot from the recent election process – to launch a major programme called the 3 by 5 initiative to ameliorate the dramatic situation of developing countries, where only about 400,000 people living with HIV received HAART (a small percentage of the people in the world living with HIV). The programme meant a global effort to scale-up successful ARV experiences like the one conducted by Brazil. Previously, a *Science* article and the 2002 Barcelona International AIDS Conference explained that the target was sound and achievable (WHO, 2004; Schwartländer, et al., 2001; Susman, 2002). The American medical doctor and diplomat Jack Chow, who was WHO's assistant director-general in charge of AIDS, tuberculosis, and malaria since the beginning of Lee's term, initially directed the programme. The

Brazilian Paulo Teixeira was director of WHO's HIV/AIDS Department between July 2003 and April 2004 and assisted Chow (previously, between 1996 and 2000, Teixeira was Senior Consultant with UNAIDS for Latin America and the Caribbean but worked in Brazil). Teixeira was part of a small group of Brazilians who worked on AIDS at the WHO but did not stay long in the agency because of health reasons (but he remained in Geneva a few months after April 2004 as special consultant to the WHO to ease the transition of the AIDS programme). Jim Yong Kim, a Korean–American physician and medical anthropologist, who since 2003 was special adviser to Lee, replaced Teixeira as director of WHO's HIV/AIDS department. Also, Chow left the health agency at the same time. In mid-2004, Kim became head of the 3 by 5 programme, a prominent position he would keep in 2005 and 2006. Kim, who had an activist-oriented approach, played an important role in making 3 by 5 WHO's flagship programme.

Initially, there was only a modest increase in the number of people treated and the WHO sent experts to countries such as Brazil to learn how to achieve rapid results. By the end of 2004, WHO officers declared some progress: 700,000 people received ARV in poor and middle-income countries (World Health Organization and UNAIDS, 2004). Another good indicator was that by December of 2004, ten countries had drug coverage rates exceeding 50 per cent (Lee and Piot, 2004). Notwithstanding, in early 2005 it became clear that the programme would not reach its target. A new meaning began to evolve among agency leaders: the aim was not to reach five million people but to be an 'interim step' towards a general goal of universal access to HIV. By the end of 2005, the 3 by 5 programme recognised that only about 1.6 million people were receiving HAART. In April of 2006, less than a quarter of the seven million people in need of ARV therapy received it. In the following months, the programme languished (WHO, 2006a; WHO, 2006b).[2]

The legacy of the programme was controversial (Petryna, et al., 2007). It is argued that 3 by 5 had prevented an estimated 300,000 deaths by mid-2005 and demonstrated that adherence to strict drug regimes in developing countries was good, reversing early scepticism. Data from mid-2005 suggests that some regions of the world, like Latin America, with advanced AIDS programmes benefited the most from the programme. In contrast, in sub-Saharan Africa and in the Middle East less than one-fifth of individuals needing the drugs received them by June of 2005 (World Health Organization and UNAIDS, 2005). According to critics, the 3 by 5 programme failed because the deadline was too short and unrealistic, the political commitment and mobilisation of civil society insufficient, the coordination between international agencies deficient, the technical challenges of the programme not fully anticipated, and the funds needed underestimated (Gutierrez, et al., 2004). In addition, the lack of work with discriminated groups like incarcerated individuals, and an open discussion of sexual diversity, were serious shortfalls. In several developing countries, stigma and violence persisted against people living with AIDS, gays, and women; in many countries sex work, drug use, and homosexuality were crimes. The programme did little in terms of eliminating homophobia.

The problems encountered by the programme were also political and related to US unilateralism. After the lawyer Tommy G. Thompson, the US Secretary of Health and Human Services, became Chairman of the Global Fund's board in January 2003, the US made clear it had done enough for the Fund and that it was up to European governments to increase their contributions. He also disliked the UN and WHO's 3 by 5 programme which he regarded as having no clear 'business plan' (UNAIDS, 2004). As a result of a series of technical factors like the crisis of WHO's Prequalification Process, the relationship between the WHO and the US also deteriorated. Problems in some Indian generic drugs' bioequivalence found in late 2004 resulted in retiring products from the programme and an erosion of the confidence in the process conducted in Geneva (Weekly Epidemiological Record, 2004).

The unilateralism of the US was more evident between 2003 and 2005 with the bilateral programme PEPFAR (President's Emergency Plan for AIDS Relief). Just months before ordering the invasion of Iraq, President Bush announced PEPFAR in his State of the Union discourse. The focus of the programme was to work on 15 developing countries (mainly in Africa) with the unprecedented budget of US$15 billion. Initially, the programme relied on brand-name drugs instead of more affordable generics, mainly because Randall Tobias, a former CEO of Lily, was head of PEPFAR and raised doubts about the quality and efficacy of generics. Tobias and Bush touted Uganda – not Brazil – and referred to the Ugandan AIDS programme as the model for PEPFAR's 'ABC' preventive dimensions (Abstinence, Be faithful – in mutually monogamous relationships – and, if these approaches fail, use Condoms). PEPFAR's approach thus downplayed the effectiveness of condoms and ignored that, for many poor women, abstinence was not an option.

Some AIDS activists believed PEPFAR was 'too little too late' and others – more critical – were irked by its prevention policies and its preference for brand-name drugs (Act Up, 2004). Most UN agencies made mild criticisms of PEPFAR's prevention recommendations and hoped to change the bilateral agency's recommendations. They also hoped to circumvent PEPFAR recommendations by getting other donors, like the European countries, to support the prevention programmes considered controversial by the US administration (Okediji, 2004; Piot, 2013). PEPFAR's constrictions changed a little after an assessment of the US General Accounting Office signalled that more drugs would have been bought if generics had been used and if the FDA had sped up the approval process of generic drugs for AIDS. It began to change in 2006 when physician Mark Dybul succeeded Tobias as head of PEPFAR and even more after 2009 when Barack Obama became the US President (for example the abstinence recommendation was not enforced (GAO, 2004)).

PEPFAR and the UN agencies did little to oppose a new surreptitious attack on the meanings of the 2001 Doha Declaration. Slowly but surely, pharmaceutical companies and governments of industrialised nations pressured developing countries to accept 'TRIPS-plus' provisions and bilateral Free Trade Agreements (FTA) with stringed protection of patents, restrictions on the use of generics, and limits on compulsory licenses. Meanwhile the WTO, with the support of the US and pharmaceuticals, opposed several decisions of compulsory licenses, arguing that it was not completely clear in the Doha Declaration in which conditions countries could make use of them (Muzaka, 2009; see also Vieira and Di Giano, Chapter 31, in this volume).

Paulo Teixeira, a former Director of the Brazilian AIDS programme, who had worked at the WHO at the beginning of the 3 by 5 campaign, wrote an open letter to the participants of the International AIDS Conference in Toronto in 2006. He asked for 'extreme measures' to keep up the struggle because of the ambiguity of UN agencies and donors in relationship to the continuity of the goal of universal access to ARVs. He also made a call to 'resume and intensify the political mobilization and international activism that triggered' the 3 by 5 programme (Teixeira, 2006, p. 1).[3]

## The AIDS backlash and Brazil

In May 2005, President Lula rejected US$40 million from USAID in protest of the requirement to sign a pledge against prostitution and sex trafficking – demanded by USAID and subscribed by PEPFAR. Brazilian authorities believed that the pledge was interference in domestic affairs and that discrimination against sex workers was counterproductive. A conservative congressional representative and an article in the *Wall Street Journal* argued that Brazil's real intention was to enhance its confrontation with the US to disguise the support to its generic drug industry that 'stole' private property of pharmaceutical companies (Fenney, 2005; O'Grady, 2005).

Towards the end of the first half of the first decade of the century, it became clear that scaling up HIV treatment from the few successful developing countries was a complex process and that the crucial alliance between activism and political commitment had been overlooked. No less important was that few governments were committed to negotiate the prices of medicines or rely on generics, and too many feared reappraisals from industrialised countries and transnational pharmaceutical companies. In Brazil, the cost of treatment increased significantly creating a problem of sustainability for the Brazilian AIDS programme.

Costs for 17 drugs to treat about 180,000 individuals in 2006 reached US$400 million and was increasing steeply (Greco and Simão, 2007; D'Adesky, 2002; Hacker, et al., 2007).

At the same time, the Brazilian government became complacent of its internationally praised AIDS programme (for example, in 2003 the country received the Gates Award for Global Health, administered by the Global Health Council, with a US$1 million prize [Bill & Melinda Gates Foundation, 2003]), and tolerated that the epidemic was increasingly concentrated in a few key populations in the country. Complacency also ensued because Brazil was regarded as a leader among middle-income countries, and the largest and strongest economy in Latin America. A false perception spread; the epidemic had reached a zenith. In the final years of President Lula and the government of President Dilma (inaugurated in 2011) less attention was devoted to its health diplomacy. Renowned scientists attacked the Brazilian AIDS policy. Robert Gallo, director of the University of Maryland Institute of Human Virology, was in Brazil in May 2005 and gave an interview to a newspaper arguing that the government should not use a compulsory license against Abbott because Brazil was not a poor developing country entitled to special treatment (Terra, 2005).

Although some Brazilians realised that only one element of Brazil's AIDS programme, namely access to drugs, was coopted by the WHO and UNAIDS in its 3 by 5 programme, little was done to redress the manipulation of the Brazilian experience. Another problem was the insidious persistence of a short-sighted public health tradition that gave priority to treatment over prevention. Treatment with little or incomplete prevention programmes was convenient for politicians because most avoided to get involved in long-term social programmes. Unfortunately, treatment without strong prevention programmes became a mending patch and contributed to the obliteration of the goal of universal access to HIV drugs. As a result, ARVs and medical treatment became part of an understanding of public health in terms of the culture of survival, where the sick who were poor and/or gay received some paternalistic assistance from the state, but little official attention was paid to full treatment or to the reduction of poverty and prejudice (ABIA, 2016).

AIDS programmes faced more problems with the alliance of conservative evangelicals and the Partido dos Trabalhadores (PT), which grew stronger over time as Lula and Dilma sought to gain votes in Congress and to consolidate their political position (Lehmann, 2004; Vianna, 2015). The alliance was detrimental for the fight against AIDS because most evangelicals glorified the ABC prescription and attacked Brazil's tolerant sexual culture. As early as August 2004, the Brazilian network of NGOs *Articulação Nacional de Luta contra AIDS* organised nationwide protests under the motto 'where is the best AIDS programme in the world?' (Beloqui, 2006). Some reaction still existed in the government. In May 2007, Brazil crossed a threshold when, for the first time, it broke the patent of a drug. The government stopped price negotiations with Merck over Efavirenz, used by over 70,000 Brazilians, and imported a generic version from India; arguing it was saving some US$236 million. It is interesting to note that the government did not repeat the move during the following years.

Changes also occurred in the WHO and UNAIDS. After Lee died in 2006, the WHO did not continue to be a leader for accessible ARVs. In March 2006, Kevin De Cock, Professor at the London School of Hygiene and Tropical Medicine, replaced Kim as head of the HIV/AIDS office in the WHO and began to push for policies that would move the AIDS programme in new directions. In the following years, AIDS work at the WHO became part of different units until it was subsumed in a broader Cluster for HIV, TB, Malaria, and Neglected Tropical Diseases (HTM). The new director-general, Margaret Chan, deemphasised compulsory licensing and the use of generics, and sought to emphasise other largely undefined goals for AIDS that would include the collaboration of private companies and bilateral agencies. In late 2008, Piot stepped down as executive director of UNAIDS and the agency faced new and difficult challenges in maintaining its leadership role in coordinating a global and holistic response to the epidemic. In 2011, the Global Fund appointed banker Gabriel Jaramillo to the new position of General Manager; he consequently reduced the staff and the grants of an agency that was under the accusations of waste, fraud, and corruption.

## Final remarks

After the economic crisis of 2008, the funds and political commitment for AIDS began to decline. The concept of universal access to ARVs and the empowerment of developing nations that in the late 1990s came to represent activists' motto 'lives matter more than profits' was obliterated. The aspiration to use treatment as an entry point to reinforce health systems became a distant objective. A new meaning became hegemonic: 'universal access' was an ideal goal to be sought progressively and without major changes in health systems. It was separated from the promotion of the gender-based human rights in developing countries. Universal access became a term meaning selective treatment for marginalised individuals and in 'resource-poor setting contexts' (a euphemism for poor countries). Articles against the original meaning of the term appeared with a criticism of the 'disproportionate' amounts devoted to AIDS (in relationship to the declining morbidity and mortality in developing countries) and the misuse of the AIDS funds (England, 2006, 2007).

The celebration of Brazil and the few countries that gave full access to ARVs became isolated examples of a distant ideal. The portrayal of Brazil as a country that had achieved middle-income country status obliterated its acute inequalities and was instrumental in order to argue that it no longer was entitled to obtain help from abroad. External adulation and domestic complacency converged and combined with serious local religious and economic challenges producing a stagnation of the Brazilian AIDS programme. The relationship of Brazil with the changing meanings of universal access to ARVs is a cautionary tale for the challenges of sustaining global health organisation initiatives coming from developing countries and from activists.

## Notes

1  The original American WTO trade dispute against Brazil initiated in early 2000 cited article 68 of Brazil's 1996 industrial property law, which required foreign companies to produce their patented products in Brazil within three years or else be subject to compulsory license. The US claimed that the Brazilian law was protectionist and in violation of the TRIPS.
2  After 2005, the G8 countries, the UN, and the WHO announced the goals of universal access to prevention, care, support and treating programmes for ten million people by 2010 (WHO, 2006a). Later the goal was to reach 15 million people living with HIV with ARV drugs in 2015 (WHO, 2006b).
3  Paulo Teixeira is currently senior adviser of the São Paulo STD/AIDS state programme, former director of the HIV/AIDS Department of the WHO, and Former Coordinator of the Brazilian STD/AIDS programme.

## Acknowledgement

This article was possible thanks to the support of the Gerda Henkel Foundation.

## References

ABIA. (2016) *Myth vs. Reality: Evaluating the Brazilian response to HIV in 2016*, Rio de Janeiro: ABIA (Brazilian Interdisciplinary AIDS Association).

Act Up. (2004) 'Global AIDS Coordinator Tobias defends US policy not to use generic fixed-dose combination antiretroviral drugs', 29 April, available at www.actupny.org/reports/genericszap.html (accessed on 2 April 2017).

Beloqui, J. (2006) 'Ativismo contra o retrocesso', *Boletim ABIA (Associação Brasileira Interdisciplinar de AIDS)*, 54, August–October, p. 3 available at http://abiaids.org.br/_img/media/bol%20abia%2054.pdf (accessed on 4 April 2017).

Bill & Melinda Gates Foundation. (2003) 'Gates award for global health – Brazilian National AIDS Program, 2003', available at www.gatesfoundation.org/Media-Center/Press-Releases/2003/05/Brazilian-National-AIDS-Program (accessed on 28 October 2017).

Charatan, F. (2001) 'Bayer cuts price of ciprofloxacin after Bush threatens to buy generics', *British Medical Journal*, 3 November, 323(7320): 1023.

Chartrand, D. (2001) 'Patents, in health emergencies, Brazil allows the copying of drugs, to the dismay of American companies', The New York Times, 18 February, available at www.nytimes.com/2001/02/19/business/patents-health-emergencies-brazil-allows-copying-drugs-dismay-american-companies.html (accessed on 5 April 2017).

D'Adesky, A.C. (2002) Moving Mountains: The race to treat global AIDS, London: Verso, p. 67.

Davis, P. (2001) Paul Davis email to Peter Piot, 20 November. BG 0908 PIOT/5/2/7/2 Global Fund Establishment 2001, File 3. London School of Hygiene and Tropical Medicine Archives, London.

DeYoung, K. (2001) 'U.S. to Give to Global AIDS Fund', The Washington Post, 11 May, available at www.washingtonpost.com/archive/politics/2001/05/11/us-to-give-to-global-aids-fund/fcc0c453-9432-4075-9b41-892795502919/?utm_term=.951bac18ec5e (accessed on 2 April 2017).

DFID. (2001) 'Department for International Development, DFID, view on the creation of GHF, draft 8-10-2001'. GB 0809 PIOT/5/2/7/2 Global Fund Establishment, 2001, File 3. London School of Hygiene and Tropical Medicine.

England, R. (2006) 'World spends too much in the fight against Aids', Financial Times, 14 August, available at www.ft.com/content/c2fb7574-2bbd-11db-a7e1-0000779e2340 (accessed on 4 April 2017).

England, R. (2007) 'Are we spending too much on HIV?', British Medical Journal, 15 February, 334(7589): 344.

Fenney, T. (2005) 'Brazil to seize American pharmaceutical patents', Intervention in the House of Representatives 30 June 2005. Congressional Record 1 July, p. 1435, available at www.gpo.gov/fdsys/pkg/CREC-2005-07-01/pdf/CREC-2005-07-01-pt1-PgE1435.pdf (accessed on 4 April 2017).

Fonseca, E.M. (2015) The Politics of Pharmaceutical Policy Reform: A study of generic drug regulation in Brazil, New York: Springer.

GAO. (2004) 'General Accounting Office US AIDS coordinator addressing some key challenges to expanding treatment but others remain', Washington, DC, Government Printing Office, July, available at https://digital.library.unt.edu/ark:/67531/metadc299539/m2/1/high_res_d/243351.pdf (accessed on 4 April 2017).

Greco, D.B. and Simão, M. (2007) 'Brazilian policy of universal access to AIDS treatment: sustainability challenges and perspectives', AIDS, 21(Suppl 4): S37–45.

Gutierrez, J.P., Johns, B., Adam, T., Bertozzi, S.M., Tan-Torres Edejer, T., Greener, R., Hankins, C., and Evans, D.B. (2004) 'Achieving the WHO/UNAIDS antiretroviral treatment 3 by 5 goal: what will it cost?', The Lancet, 9428: 363–4.

Hacker, M.A., Kaida, A., Hogg, R.S., and Bastos, F.I. (2007) 'The first ten years: achievements and challenges of the Brazilian program of universal access to HIV/AIDS comprehensive management and care, 1996–2006', Cadernos de Saúde Pública, 23(3): S345–59.

HOR. (2003) 'Global access to HIV/AIDS prevention, awareness, education and Treatment act of 2001', in Report on the activity of the committee on financial services for the 107th congress, available at www.congress.gov/107/crpt/hrpt798/CRPT-107hrpt798.pdf (accessed on 2 April 2017).

Lee, J.W. and Piot, P. (2004) '3 by 5 Progress report', December, available at www.who.int/3by5/pr_en.pdf?ua=1 (accessed on 4 April 2017).

Lehmann, D. (2004) Struggle for the Spirit, Religious Transformations and Popular Culture in Brazil and Latin America, Cambridge: Polity Press.

McLellan, F. (2001) 'Annan calls for action on AIDS at UN meeting', The Lancet, 357(9274): 2107.

Muzaka, V. (2009) 'Dealing with public health and intellectual property for pharmaceuticals at the world trade organization' In: S. McLean, P. Fourie, and S. Brown (Eds.) Health for Some: The political economy of health governance, Basingstoke: Palgrave, pp. 182–95.

Nunn, A. (2009) The Politics and History of AIDS Treatment in Brazil, New York: Springer.

O'Grady, A. (2005) 'Brazil mulls drug patent theft as an AIDS antidote', The Wall Street Journal, 4 June, available at www.wsj.com/articles/SB111957486659368376 (accessed on 4 April 2017).

Okediji, R.L. (2004) 'Back to bilateralism? Pendulum swing in international intellectual property protection', University of Ottawa Law and Technology Journal, 1: 125–47, available at www.uoltj.ca/articles/vol1.1-2/2003-2004.1.1-2.uoltj.Okediji.125–147.pdf (accessed on 4 April 2017).

Oxfam. (2001) 'Drug companies vs. Brazil: the threat to public health', available at http://oxfamilibrary.openrepository.com/oxfam/bitstream/10546/114469/1/bp-drug-companies-vs-brazil-010501-en.pdf (accessed on 2 April 2017).

Petryna, A., Lakoff, A., and Kleinman, A. (Eds.) (2007) Global Pharmaceuticals: Ethics, markets, practices, Durham, NC: Duke University Press.

Piot, P. (2013) No Time to Lose, a Life in Pursuit of Deadly Viruses, London: Norton.

Rosenberg, T. (2001) 'Look at Brazil', New York Times Magazine, 28 January, available at www.nytimes.com/2001/01/28/magazine/look-at-brazil.html (accessed on 5 April 2017).

Schwartländer, B., Stover, J., Walker, N., Bollinger, L., Gutierrez, J.P., McGreevey, W., Opuni, M., Forsythe, S., Kumaranayake, L., Watts, C., and Bertozzi, S. (2001). 'AIDS, resource needs for HIV/AIDS', Science, 292(5526): 2434–6.

Susman, E. (2002) 'Notes from the XIV International AIDS Conference in Barcelona, Spain', AIDS, 8 November, 16(16): N11–3.

Teixeira, P. (2006) 'Paulo Teixeira's Letter, São Paulo, August 17 2006', GB 0809 PIOT/5/2/6. File 6. London School of Hygiene and Tropical Medicine Archives.

Terra (2005) 'Pesquisador critica oferta de remédios contra a AIDS', Terra: Ciências, 26 July, available at http://noticias.terra.com.br/ciencia/noticias/0,,OI604736-EI298,00-Pesquisador+critica+oferta+de+remedios+contra+aids.html (accessed on 4 April 2017).

United Nations. (2001) 'Declaration on commitment on AIDS, United Nations General Assembly, Special Session on HIV/AIDS, 25–27 June 2001, New York, United Nations', available at www.unaids.org/sites/default/files/sub_landing/files/aidsdeclaration_en_0.pdf (accessed on 29 October 2017).

UNAIDS (2004) 'UNAIDS executive office, meeting with Secretary Thompson 18 March 2004', Briefing Notes Dr. Peter Piot GB 0809 PIOT/5/6, UNAIDS/Correspondence, 1998–2008, no file. London School of Hygiene and Tropical Medicine Archives.

Vianna, C.P. (2015) 'The LGBT movement and the gender and sexual diversity education policies: losses, gains and challenges', Educação e Pesquisa, 41: 791–806.

Vogel, G. (2003) 'World Health Organization Health body taps a consummate insider and disease fighter', Science, 299(5608): 809.

Walgate, R. (2002) 'Global Fund for AIDS, TB and malaria opens shop', Bulletin of the World Health Organization, 80(3): 259.

Weekly Epidemiological Record. (2004) 'Two AIDS medicines back on WHO prequalification list', WER, 79(50): 449–50.

World Health Organization (WHO). (2004) 'The World Wealth Report 2004: Changing history', Geneva: The World Health Organization.

World Health Organization (WHO). (2006a) 'Towards universal access by 2010: how WHO is working with countries to scale-up HIV prevention, treatment, care and support, World Health Organization', Geneva: WHO Department of HIV/AIDS.

World Health Organization (WHO). (2006b) 'Resolution: implementation by WHO of the recommendations of the Global Task Team on Improving AIDS Coordination among Multilateral Institutions and International Donors', Fifty-Ninth World Health Assembly, 27 May, WHA59.12, available at http://apps.who.int/iris/bitstream/10665/21437/1/A59_R12-en.pdf (accessed on 4 April 2017).

World Health Organization and UNAIDS. (2004) '"3 by 5" progress report', December, available at www.who.int/3by5/pr_en.pdf (accessed on 16 September 2018).

World Health Organization and UNAIDS. (2005) 'Progress on global access to HIV antiretroviral therapy, an update on "3 by 5"', June, p. 13, available at www.who.int/hiv/pub/progressreports/3by5%20Progress%20Report_E_light.pdf (accessed on 4 April 2017).

World Trade Organization. (2001) 'Ministerial conference, fourth session Doha, (9–14 November 2001), Declaration on the TRIPS Agreement and Public Health', available at www.who.int/medicines/areas/policy/tripshealth.pdf (accessed on 30 October 2014).

# 25

# 'Ending AIDS' or scaling down the HIV response?

*Nora Kenworthy, Matthew Thomann, and Richard Parker*

## Introduction

If the decade following the first Durban AIDS Conference in 2000 was marked by discourses about an epidemic 'out of control' (Bhattacharya, 2003; Simbanda, 2000), and a politics of emergency that justified exceptional activism and action (Benton, 2015; Piot, 2003), the decade of AIDS responses beginning in 2010 has been distinctly framed by declarations that the end of AIDS is not only possible, but imminent. Crafted in the wake of the 2008 financial crisis and honed by years of funding plateaus and programme retrenchments, the prominence of an 'End of AIDS' discourse was further reinforced in the summer of 2016, first at the UNAIDS High-Level Meeting on Ending AIDS in June, and subsequently at the 21st International AIDS conference in Durban, South Africa. Questioning the feasibility of an end to AIDS without renewed long-term financial commitments and highlighting the persistent and frustrating challenges of sustaining effective treatment and prevention programmes, detractors were quick to question the optimism of this new campaign. 'Although the ... strategy is carefully delineated and politically endorsed, it is financially unsecured; and hard choices await', wrote Nana Poku (2016b, p. 743), highlighting the urgency of a 'strategic reckoning of expanding needs and diminishing means'. Nevertheless, the 2017 UNAIDS report on the status of the global epidemic, while taking a more tempered tone and warning that specific populations and regions were 'lagging behind' in reaching targets, continued to heavily promote the notion of 'progress' towards the achievable goal of 'ending AIDS' (UNAIDS, 2017).

In this chapter, we highlight the contested social terrain surrounding the 'End of AIDS' discourse. We ask what this 'End of AIDS' signifies, and for whom? We question who stands to benefit from a triumphalism that few believe but many endorse. Most importantly, what kinds of AIDS response does this discourse promote, and what forms of knowledge is it rooted in? We argue that the irony of this discourse is that, even though it aims to elicit further commitments to the HIV/AIDS fight, it may result in complacency among donors and governments, who could perceive it as 'minimizing the challenges that remain' (El-Sadr, et al., 2014, p. 166). 'Ending AIDS' may thus provide a timely exit strategy for donors fatigued by the long-term, hard work necessary to feasibly make inroads against AIDS. As a result, the 'End of AIDS' may in fact herald – and justify – two notable shifts in HIV policy: first, the 'scale-down' of donor support for long-term treatment; and second, a pronounced embrace of technical, often short-term, fixes – a 'biomedical turn' that has significant impacts on civil society, health systems, and the real futures of the epidemic (Kenworthy, et al., 2018).

## Building the 'End of AIDS' narrative

As a result of the 2007–8 financial crisis, a series of important donor withdrawals marked the beginning of a shift from 'scale-up' to 'scale-down' that is increasingly visible today (Kaiser Family Foundation (KFF) and UNAIDS, 2017; Zaracostas, 2012). These funding shortfalls have resulted in distinct barriers in access to treatment and services that have been woefully under-reported (Geng, et al., 2010; Mugyenyi, 2009). In the wake of this shift, donors' fear of long-term treatment commitments, and of the resource-intensive work to ensure programme successes, took form in new discourses of sustainability, accountability, and country ownership – which served as both prelude and justification for scale-down (Amaya, et al., 2014; Esser, 2014). Governments and agencies such as the US President's Emergency Plan for AIDS Relief (PEPFAR) redirected aid from earlier priorities (the 'general' population and treatment scale-up) towards a new set of targets ('key' populations and biomedical prevention technologies and techniques) (PEPFAR, 2012). Simultaneously, the financial crisis initiated a reassessment of donor commitments that would later become visible in the failure to fully fund The Global Fund to Fight AIDS, Tuberculosis and Malaria, and other aid shortages (Kates, et al., 2016).

The politics of shifting priorities and slogans in the definition of HIV response strategies is hardly new. It is important to remember that just prior to the emergence of 'End of AIDS' discourses, the so-called 'AIDS Backlash' was in full swing (Nattrass and Gonsalves, 2009). Even in the US, patient groups and members of Congress began questioning 'special' funding allocations for AIDS, in terms of how it received disproportionately more money than diseases with higher death rates, such as heart disease and Alzheimer's (Kaiser, 2015). Furthermore, while disease-specific funding streams allowed HIV programming to operate independently of other health services and drew attention away from other priorities, so-called vertical funding also marginalised alternative forms of care and put HIV-positive individuals in a situation in which they had to compete for limited resources (Benton, 2015). Many in the global AIDS industry became champions of 'health system strengthening' as a way of defending their funding streams and averting attacks on scale-up as a vertical undertaking (Hafner and Shiffman, 2013; Marchal, et al., 2009). Nonetheless, health system strengthening began to give way to talk of 'Ending AIDS' as the third decade of the epidemic graduated into the fourth (Kenworthy, et al., 2018).

Something resembling what would later become the 'End of AIDS' began to be constructed in a 2010 UNAIDS document announcing the 2011–16 'getting to zero' strategy (zero new infections, zero AIDS-related deaths, and zero discrimination) (UNAIDS, 2010). That strategy was formally adopted by the UN General Assembly in its 2011 UNGASS declaration (UN General Assembly, 2011). By December of 2011, UNAIDS Executive Director Michael Sidibe wrote, 'Just a few years ago, talking about ending the AIDS epidemic in the near term seemed impossible, but science, political support and community responses are starting to deliver clear and tangible results' (UNAIDS, 2011, n.p.). Subsequently, the UNAIDS Fast Track Strategy was issued in 2014, with the goal of 90-90-90 (90 per cent of people with HIV diagnosed, 90 per cent of diagnosed people on treatment, and 90 per cent of treated people with fully suppressed viral load) by 2020 (UNAIDS, 2014a). To our knowledge, this is the first explicit articulation of the goal to end AIDS by 2030. Finally, the 2016 UN General Assembly High Level Meeting on Ending AIDS officially adopted the 'Political Declaration on HIV and AIDS: On the Fast-Track to Accelerate the Fight against HIV and to End the AIDS Epidemic by 2030' (UN General Assembly, 2016). So while the concept of ending the epidemic began to be floated by global AIDS administrators as early as 2010, it then took roughly five years of sloganeering and bureaucratic work before it became an official policy declaration adopted by the General Assembly (Kenworthy, et al., 2018).

Not wanting to be left out of the game, over roughly the same time period, the US State Department developed its own version of this goal, most clearly articulated in US Secretary of State Hillary Clinton's 2011 speech at the NIH, which initiated the US/PEPFAR push for 'an AIDS-free generation' (Clinton,

2011). As Clinton (2011, n.p.) made clear, this agenda was based in fiscal pessimism and biomedical optimism: acknowledging 'these difficult budget times', Clinton urged the audience, 'We need to let science guide our efforts'. This goal quickly became the official US discourse, and was at least partially reflected in shifts in funding priorities and allocations at the NIH and other institutions (Green, 2016). It also became an organising call for the 2012 International AIDS Conference in Washington, DC (Havlir and Beyrer, 2012; Porter, 2012).

Starting in 2014, most other major donor agencies began to endorse the UNAIDS Fast Track Strategy (UNAIDS, 2014b; UN News Centre, 2014). This strategy was pushed along by the 'success story' that had been heralded by the global scientific community at the Melbourne AIDS conference in 2014 (*The Economist*, 2014). As soon as the Fast Track Strategy was issued, other major players (The Global Fund, PEPFAR, USAID, etc.) issued statements that articulated 'the end of AIDS in 2030' goal (The Global Fund, 2014; The Office of the U.S. Global AIDS Coordinator, 2014; UNICEF, 2015). The ubiquity of this policy embrace began to make the goal seem like a fait accompli. By 2015 and 2016, private donor buy-in was evident in statements released by emissaries such as Elton John and David Furnish for the Elton John AIDS Foundation (Furnish, 2015; *The Guardian*, 2015). Civil society organisations also rallied around the slogan: for example, UNAIDS sponsored a large CSO meeting in Bangkok in 2015 which aimed to get universal support for the '90-90-90 by 2020' and 'the end of AIDS by 2030' goals (Equal Eyes, 2015; amFAR, 2015). Tellingly, all this was happening at precisely the same time as the elaboration of the post-2015 development goals, in which HIV largely fell from the list of primary development concerns (Poku, 2016a; Interagency Coalition on AIDS and Development, 2015). Indeed, in perhaps the ultimate expression of the apparent 'success' of the 'End of AIDS' story line, by the time of the first-ever meeting of the Ministers of Health of the G20 in Berlin, Germany, in May 2017, the resulting 'Berlin Declaration of G20 Health Ministers' included no emphasis on HIV and AIDS as a global health priority (Berlin Declaration of G20 Health Ministers, 2017).

## The political impacts of the biomedical turn

These events have developed in tandem with what might be described as a 'biomedical turn': an increasingly powerful biomedical triumphalism regarding HIV treatment and prevention, whereby privatised, technological, and, at least in some instances, (allegedly) more cost-effective interventions are promoted, to the deficit of long-term support for lifetime antiretroviral treatment (David, et al., 2015; Kenworthy, et al., 2018). Entities like the Bill & Melinda Gates Foundation have consistently embraced technological advances as a means for achieving new eradication and elimination goals (Birn, 2014; Packard, 2016; Storeng, 2014). This trend clearly moves in multiple directions at the same time. These directions range from large-scale biomedical prevention research trials, such as the iPrEX studies (Cohen, 2010a, 2010b), to the International AIDS Society (IAS)-sponsored 'Towards an HIV Cure Initiative' (International AIDS Society Scientific Working Group on HIV Cure, 2011; International AIDS Society, 2017). But in all of these efforts, biomedical advances become the 'scientific' justification for an 'End of AIDS' discourse. They play a key role in ensuring that the biomedical community will endorse the 'End of AIDS' story line, just as they substantiate, with scientific validity, the feasibility of policymakers' claims that we really can end the epidemic by 2030. These narratives thus become key sources of mutual reinforcement that sustain a vision of the 'End of AIDS' that brings together policy making, diplomacy, programme implementation, and science in the articulation of an 'End of AIDS' narrative.

Defining what 'Ending AIDS' will entail in practice has elicited a powerful chorus of voices defending not one, but many, heavily biomedical programmatic initiatives: from treatment as prevention (TasP) and test and treat initiatives, to pre-exposure prophylaxis (PrEP) and post-exposure prophylaxis (PEP), to microbicides, and to renewed enthusiasm about vaccine and HIV cure research (Fauci and Marston, 2013; Vella, 2015). These biomedical strategies are based in declarations of faith in the power of bench science, big data, population targeting, implementation science, and 'smart investments' (Fauci and Marston, 2013; PEPFAR, 2012). The smooth ending of AIDS is expected to be demonstrated through a modern suite of biotechnological 'tools' that include computer simulations, supply chain calculators, forecasting 'nets', and approaches to data capture that make face-to-face research seem primitive and obsolete (Adams, 2016). Such initiatives encrypt and occlude a neoliberal policy agenda that favours cutting costs (particularly long-term financial commitments) by limiting broad-based scale-up efforts and instead promoting targeted prevention and biomedical treatment expansion. As treatment expansion efforts struggle to meet their goals and funding either plateaus or declines (Geng, et al., 2010; Mugyenyi, 2009; UNAIDS, 2017), patients are routinely lost to follow-up because of the socio-economic challenges that remain unacknowledged by biomedical approaches and feel that treatment options grossly neglect to recognise their broader social suffering (Kenworthy, 2017; Moyer, 2015). Yet donors and experts are doubling-down on a technical, biomedical turn (Coburn, et al., 2017). 'Rather than seizing [the opportunity for reduced transmission and better illness management created by treatment expansion] by demedicalizing the provision of ART', argues MSF's Tom Ellman, 'programs are medicalizing HIV infection in the healthy' (2015, p. 304).

What is most troubling is that the 'End of AIDS' discourse has managed to discredit and open the door to de-funding the very interventions and investments that have the potential to make treatment and prevention more successful. This includes interventions rooted in health systems strengthening, community-based provision, and an embrace of the right to health, as well as those which attend to the broader social inequities and socio-economic constraints that threaten the success of solely biomedical interventions (Packard, 2016). The recent decade of increasingly technocratic scale-ups of HIV treatment has left a legacy across many health systems of defunded community-based care and prevention projects (Kalofonos, 2014; Kenworthy, 2017; Maes and Kalofonos, 2013), overworked and overburdened health systems (Pfeiffer and Chapman, 2015; Pfeiffer, et al., 2014), and increasingly fragmented and disjointed landscapes of care (Geissler, 2014; Moyer, 2015; Whyte, 2014). Of course, health systems, particularly in Africa, were already diminished by resource extraction, structural adjustment, and human resource depletion before HIV scale-up took place in earnest. But the fact that 'End of AIDS' discourses have promoted largely limited, vertical, biomedical interventions in the face of both older and newer health system depletions holds a particular irony that deserves more critical attention (Kenworthy, et al., 2018).

These trends are also evident in the US, where such scale-up has left many health systems defunded, overburdened, or simply gutted, particularly in the US South (Adimora, et al., 2014; Reif, et al., 2017; Sangaramoorthy, 2014). Funding mechanisms, and the creation of new surveillance systems targeting at-risk populations, serve to obscure the fact that increased HIV vulnerability within these communities arises, at least in part, from the degradation of local and regional health systems. As news reports in 2017 highlighted, extremely high HIV prevalence in these populations is threatened by resource shortages and threats to the Affordable Care Act – health system depletions that have led states such as Mississippi to charge for HIV testing (Kempner, 2017; Villarosa, 2017). Both in the US and abroad, clinicians and institutions are especially underprepared to face a population with HIV that is both aging and suffering from comorbid chronic conditions – syndemics that greatly complicate HIV care and treatment efforts (Mendenhall, et al., 2017).

In addition to these general and much-remarked upon trends, we wish to highlight three under-examined impacts. The first is the especially perverse effect of the biomedical turn on activism, whereby the far-reaching rights-based dialogues of previous decades become distilled into a narrow focus on the right to (biomedical) treatment, as access to rights-based prevention modalities, structural interventions, and broad-based socio-economic support fall by the wayside. A second, related impact is the institutionalisation of a two-tiered system of treatment access, where patients in poorer countries can only access the cheapest and most toxic drug cocktails, which threatens adherence (MSF, 2014; Zaidi, 2011). Limited access to second- and especially third-line treatments, along with inconsistent viral-load monitoring, is leading to increasing levels of HIV drug resistance (WHO, 2017). These trends point to the dual effects of an increasingly neutralised and side-lined AIDS activism combined with the power of the pharmaceutical industry, which has continued to wage battles around intellectual property, trade, and pricing schemes while fuelling 'End of AIDS' discourses (Aggleton and Parker, 2015; David, et al., 2015; Parker, 2011). Finally, an acute environment of fiscal austerity following the 2008 financial crisis, combined with the additional demands placed on health systems by uneven and overly biomedical methods of HIV programme scale-up, has produced a depleted, overworked, and increasingly disillusioned health workforce in many countries.

## The need for long-term commitment

It seems clear to many observers that the end of AIDS is not around the corner, and that a future *with* AIDS will be with us for some time to come. At the same time, the Trump administration in the US and nationalist movements across Europe make the future of global health funding increasingly uncertain. In the US, global health funding cuts are under review and there is talk of USAID being folded into the State Department, as well as a broader effort to link US funding for international development and global health to issues of US national security (Harris, et al., 2017).

The Trump administration has already proposed a reduction in funding for PEPFAR (Harris, 2017), and, more ominously, is reinstating and extending the so-called 'Global Gag Rule' (Redden, 2017), which blocks US aid to any organisations that provide services or information regarding abortion. Trump's executive order extends funding restrictions to include HIV-related programmes that had been exempted under the policy as implemented by the George W. Bush administration. As of now, the gag rule's blockade is limited to US global health assistance programmes, but exempts US funding to public–private partnerships such as The Global Fund to Fight AIDS, Tuberculosis and Malaria and GAVI, the Vaccine Alliance (Lieberman, 2017; Sampathkumar, 2017). Indeed, the Trump administration's broader assault on women's health and rights seems almost guaranteed to continue to spill over into HIV and AIDS funding which is a key part of current aid for reproductive and sexual health and rights more generally (Girard, 2017).

During his first year in office, Trump and his administration announced a series of changes to the US PEPFAR programme that involve not only a reduction in the overall level of funding (a 17 per cent reduction in the administration's proposed budget for 2018, from US$4.6 billion to US$3.8 billion), but a 'concentration' of resources in order to 'accelerate implementation in a subset of 13 high-burden countries that have the potential to achieve epidemic control by 2020' (US Department of State, 2017, n.p.). While PEPFAR will reportedly continue to provide some more limited support for HIV related work in as many as 50 countries, the concentration of resources is clearly predicated on an 'End of AIDS' logic, based on the prediction that these countries can effectively control the epidemic in only three years, by 2020, according to an unnamed State Department representative (Igoe, 2017). This plan is justified as the first step towards longer-term reductions of funding, which are nonetheless framed as providing sufficient support to fully control the global epidemic. It is a view which provides perhaps the ultimate vindication of enlightened US policy,

> This strategy will also reduce the future costs required to sustain the HIV and AIDS response, the report says: 'In less than two decades of commitment and funding since PEPFAR's launch by President George W. Bush in 2003, the pandemic will have progressed from tragedy to control.'
>
> *Igoe, 2017, n.p.*

Given the rise of populist politics not only in the US, but in many of the key donor countries in recent years, it seems clear that the 'End of AIDS' narrative can all too easily become a justification (or even a smoke screen) for what is in fact the scaling down of the global response to HIV – an agenda that is particularly clear in the US State Department strategy announcement mentioned previously. In such divisive times, we must underscore the importance of continued funding commitments to HIV and AIDS while at the same time advocating for more equitable, long-term, and socially responsive policies and programmes than what the global AIDS establishment has given us in the most recent phase of biomedicalised policy initiatives and social marketing slogans. While aspirational ideals are important, so too is pragmatic solidarity and a realistic assessment of the gaps and shortcomings in our response to HIV to date. Getting to a future without AIDS requires far more focus on the 'means' than the 'ends'.

## Acknowledgements

A more extended version of the analysis was published as an article in *Global Public Health* (see Kenworthy, et al., 2018). Readers interested in learning more about the development of the 'End of AIDS' discourse may wish to consult the longer argument included therein.

## References

Adams, V. (2016) *Metrics: What counts in global health*, Durham, NC: Duke University Press.

Adimora, A.A., Ramirez, C., Schoenbach, V., and Cohen, M. (2014) 'Policies and politics that promote HIV infection in the southern United States', *AIDS*, 28(10): 1393–7.

Aggleton, P. and Parker, R. (2015) 'Moving beyond biomedicalization in the HIV response: implications for community involvement and community leadership among men who have sex with men and transgender people', *American Journal of Public Health*, 105(8): 1552–8.

Amaya, A.B., Caceres, C.F., Spicer, N., and Balabanova, D. (2014) 'After the Global Fund: who can sustain the HIV/AIDS response in Peru and how?', *Global Public Health*, 9(1–2): 176–97.

amFAR. (2015) 'UNAIDS holds civil society meeting on fast-tracking the end of AIDS', available at www.amfar.org/UNAIDS-Holds-Civil-Society-Meeting/ (accessed on 28 May 2017).

Benton, A. (2015) *HIV Exceptionalism: Development through disease in Sierra Leone*, Minneapolis: University of Minnesota Press.

Berlin Declaration of G20 Health Ministers. (2017) 'Together today for a healthy tomorrow', available at www.bundesgesundheitsministerium.de/fileadmin/Dateien/3_Downloads/G/G20-Gesundheitsministertreffen/G20_Health_Ministers_Declaration_engl.pdf?utm_term=0_14504ce43d-7044d60fe7-298066201&utm_content=buffer324a0&utm_medium=social&utm_source=linkedin.com&utm_campaign=buffer (accessed on 29 May 2017).

Bhattacharya, S. (2003) '2003 worst ever year for HIV, says UN report', New Scientist.

Birn, A. (2014) 'Philanthrocapitalism, past and present: the Rockefeller Foundation, the Gates Foundation, and the setting(s) of the international/global health agenda', Hypothesis, 12(1): e8.

Clinton, H. (2011) 'U.S. Secretary of State Hillary Rodham Clinton to peak on global HIV/AIDS', available at https://videocast.nih.gov/Summary.asp?File=16952&bhcp=1 (accessed on 27 May 2017).

Coburn, B., Okano, J., and Blower, S. (2017) 'Using geospatial mapping to design HIV elimination strategies for sub-Saharan Africa', *Science Translational Medicine*, 9(383).

Cohen, J. (2010a) 'Anti-HIV pill protects against AIDS', *Science Magazine*.

Cohen, J. (2010b) 'A powerful and perplexing HIV prevention tool', *Science*, 330(6009): 1298–9.

David, P-M., Girard, G., and Nguyen, V-K. (2015) 'AIDS and biocapitalisation: the ambiguities of a "world without AIDS"', Books and Ideas, available at www.booksandideas.net/AIDS-Biocapitalisation.html (accessed on 24 March 2018).

Ellman, T. (2015) 'Demedicalizing AIDS prevention and treatment in Africa', *The New England Journal of Medicine*, 372(4): 303–5.

El-Sadr, W., Harripersaud, K., and Bayer, R. (2014) 'End of AIDS – hype versus hope', *Science*, 345(6193): 166.

Equal Eyes. (2015) 'Bangkok: UNAIDS holds civil society meeting on fast-tracking the end of AIDS' available at http://equal-eyes.org/database/2015/12/13/bangkok-unaids-holds-civil-society-meeting-on-fast-tracking-the-end-of-aids (accessed on 28 May 2017).

Esser, D.E. (2014) 'Elusive accountabilities in the HIV scale-up: "ownership" as a functional tautology', *Global Public Health*, 9(1–2): 43–56.

Fauci, A.S. and Marston, H.D. (2013) 'Achieving an AIDS-free world: science and implementation', *The Lancet*, 382(9903): 1461–2.

Furnish, D. (2015) 'We can make "Ending AIDS" more than just a slogan', The Independent, available at www.independent.co.uk/voices/we-can-make-ending-aids-more-just-than-a-slogan-10050840.html (accessed on 28 May 2018).

Geissler, W.P. (2014) 'The archipelago of public health: comments on the landscape of medical research in twenty-first-century Africa', In: R. Prince and R. Marsland (Eds.) *Making and Unmaking Public Health in Africa: Ethnographic and historical perspectives*, Athens: Ohio University Press, pp. 231–56.

Geng, E.H., Bwana, M.B., Kabakyenga, J., Muyindike, W., Emenyonu, N.I., et al. (2010) 'Diminishing availability of publicly funded slots for antiretroviral initiation among HIV-infected ART-eligible patients in Uganda', *PLOS ONE*, 5(11): e14098.

Girard, F. (2017) 'Implications of the Trump Administration for sexual and reproductive rights globally', *Reproductive Health Matters*, 25(49): 1301028.

Green, A. (2016) 'Obama dreams of an AIDS-free generation', Foreign Policy, available at http://foreignpolicy.com/2016/04/18/obama-wants-an-aids-free-generation-pepfar-africa/ (accessed on 27 May 2017).

Hafner, T. and Shiffman, J. (2013) 'The emergence of global attention to health systems strengthening', *Health Policy and Planning*, 28(1): 41–50.

Harris, B., Gramer, R., and Tamkin, E. (2017) 'The end of foreign aid as we know it', Foreign Policy, available at http://foreignpolicy.com/2017/04/24/u-s-agency-for-international-development-foreign-aid-state-department-trump-slash-foreign-funding/ (accessed on 27 May 2017).

Harris, G. (2017) 'Cuts to AIDS treatment programs could cost a million lives', The New York Times, available at www.nytimes.com/2017/05/23/world/africa/cuts-to-aids-treatment-programs-could-cost-a-million-lives.html?_r=0 (accessed on 28 May 2017).

Havlir, D. and Beyrer, C. (2012) 'The beginning of the end of AIDS?', *New England Journal of Medicine*, 367(8): 685–7.

Igoe, M. (2017) 'PEPFAR to "accelerate" implementation in 13 countries under new strategy', Devex, available at www.devex.com/news/pepfar-to-accelerate-implementation-in-13-countries-under-new-strategy-91064 (accessed on 13 October 2017).

Interagency Coalition on AIDS and Development. (2015) 'HIV, gender, sexual and reproductive health rights and the Post 2015 Development Agenda', available at www.icad-cisd.com/pdf/Publications/Post2015_EN-FINAL.pdf (accessed on 28 May 2017).

International AIDS Society Scientific Working Group on HIV Cure. (2011) 'Towards an HIV cure: a global scientific strategy', *Nature Reviews Immunology*, 12(8): 607–14.

International AIDS Society. (2017) 'Toward an AIDS cure', available at www.iasociety.org/HIV-Programmes/Towards-an-HIV-Cure/About-Towards-an-HIV-Cure (accessed on 28 May 2017).

Kaiser Family Foundation (KFF) and UNAIDS. (2017) *Financing the Response to AIDS in Low- and Middle-Income Countries: International assistance from donor governments in 2016*, Menlo Park, CA: KFF.

Kaiser, J. (2015) 'NIH drops special 10% set-aside for AIDS research', Science, available at www.sciencemag.org/news/2015/12/nih-drops-special-10-set-aside-aids-research (accessed on 29 July 2017).

Kalofonos, I. (2014) '"All they do is pray": community labour and the narrowing of "care" during Mozambique's HIV scale-up', *Global Public Health*, 9(1–2): 7–24.

Kates, J., Wexler, A., and Lief, E. (2016) *Financing the response to HIV in low- and middle-income countries: International assistance from donor governments in 2015*, Washington, DC: Kaiser Family Foundation and UNAIDS.

Kempner, M. (2017) 'Mississippi to start charging for HIV and STI testing', The Body, available at www.thebody.com/content/80019/mississippi-to-start-charging-for-hiv-and-sti-test.html (accessed on 26 June 2017).

Kenworthy, N. (2017) *Mistreated: The political consequences of the fight against AIDS in Lesotho*, Nashville: Vanderbilt University Press.

Kenworthy, N., Thomann, M., and Parker, R. (2018) 'From global crisis to the "end of AIDS": new epidemics of signification', *Global Public Health*, 13(8): 960–71.

Lieberman, A. (2017) 'Trump expands "global gag rule," targeting $8.8B in global health aid', Devex, available at www.devex.com/news/trump-expands-global-gag-rule-targeting-8-8b-in-global-health-aid-90291 (accessed on 28 May 2017).

Maes, K. and Kalofonos, I. (2013) 'Becoming and remaining community health workers: perspectives from Ethiopia and Mozambique', *Social Science & Medicine*, 87: 52–9.

Marchal, B., Cavalli, A., and Kegels, G. (2009) 'Global health actors claim to support health system strengthening – is this reality or rhetoric?', *PLOS Medicine*, 6(4): 1–5.

Mendenhall, E., et al. (2017) 'Non-communicable disease syndemics: poverty, depression, and diabetes among low-income populations', *The Lancet*, 389(10072): 951–63.

Moyer, E. (2015) 'The anthropology of life after AIDS: epistemological continuities in the age of antiretroviral treatment', *Annual Review of Anthropology*, 44: 259–75.

MSF. (2014) 'Untangling the web of antiretroviral price reductions, 17th edition July 2014', available at www.msfaccess.org/sites/default/files/MSF_UTW_17th_Edition_4_b.pdf (accessed on 29 July 2017).

Mugyenyi, P. (2009) 'Flat-line funding for PEPFAR: a recipe for chaos', *The Lancet*, 374(9686): 292.

Nattrass, N. and Gonsalves, G. (2009) 'Economics and the backlash against AIDS-specific funding', CSSR Working Paper No. 254, available at www.cssr.uct.ac.za/sites/cssr.uct.ac.za/files/pubs/WP254.pdf (accessed on 27 May 2017).

Packard, R. (2016) *A History of Global Health: Interventions into the lives of other peoples*, Baltimore, MD: Johns Hopkins University Press.

Parker, R. (2011) 'Grassroots activism, civil society mobilization, and the politics of the global HIV/AIDS epidemic', *Brown Journal of World Affairs*, 17(2): 21–37.

PEPFAR. (2012) *PEPFAR blueprint: Creating an AIDS-free generation*, Washington, DC: PEPFAR.

Pfeiffer, J. and Chapman, R. (2015) 'An anthropology of aid in Africa', *The Lancet*, 385(9983): 2144–5.

Pfeiffer, J., Robinson, J., Hagopian, A., Johnson, W., Fort, M., Gimbel-Sherr, K., Rowden, R., Friedman, E., Davis, P., Adedokun, L., and Gloyd, S. (2014) 'The end of AIDS and the NGO Code of Conduct', *The Lancet*, 384(9944): 639–40.

Piot, P. (2003) 'AIDS: the need for an exceptional response to an unprecedented crisis', *Presidential Fellows Lecture*, Washington, DC: UNAIDS.

Poku, N. K. (2016a) 'HIV prevention: the key to ending AIDS by 2030', *The Open AIDS Journal*, 10: 65–77.

Poku, N. (2016b) 'UN political declaration on HIV and AIDS: where to begin?', *The Lancet*, 388(10046): 743–4.

Porter, C. (2012) 'AIDS 2012: Clinton points way to AIDS-free generation', available at https://geneva.usmission.gov/2012/07/24/aids-2012-clinton-points-way-to-aids-free-generation/ (accessed on 27 May 2017).

Redden, M. (2017) '"Global Gag Rule" reinstated by Trump, curbing NGO abortion services abroad', *The Guardian*, available at www.theguardian.com/world/2017/jan/23/trump-abortion-gag-rule-international-ngo-funding (accessed on 19 July 2017).

Reif, S., Safley, D., McAllaster, C., Wilson, E., and Whetten, K. (2017) 'State of HIV in the US deep south', *Journal of Community Health*, available at https://link.springer.com/article/10.1007%2Fs10900-017-0325-8 (accessed on 9 November 2017).

Sampathkumar, M. (2017) 'Donald Trump "to give $9bn to health groups that refuse to provide abortions"', The Independent, available at www.independent.co.uk/news/world/americas/us-politics/trump-abortion-funding-mexico-city-rule-billions-global-gag-rule-health-services-a7736951.html (accessed on 28 May 2017).

Sangaramoorthy, T. (2014) *Treating AIDS: Politics of difference, paradox of prevention*, New Brunswick, NJ: Rutgers University Press.

Simbanda, A. (2000) 'A nation in pain: why the HIV/AIDS epidemic is out of control in Zimbabwe'. *International Journal of Health Services*, 30(4): 717–38.

Storeng, K. (2014) 'The GAVI Alliance and the "Gates approach" to health system strengthening', *Global Public Health*, 9(8): 865–79.

*The Economist*. (2014) 'Is an end in sight?: campaigners are now talking openly of beating the AIDS epidemic', available at www.economist.com/news/science-and-technology/21608568-campaigners-are-now-talking-openly-beating-aids-epidemic-end (accessed on 28 May 2017).

The Global Fund. (2014) 'Private & NGO partners: (RED)', available at www.theglobalfund.org/en/private-ngo-partners/red/ (accessed on 28 May 2017).

*The Guardian*. (2015) 'Elton John tells US Congress it has the power to end AIDS', The Guardian, available at www.theguardian.com/music/2015/may/07/elton-john-us-congress-senate-hearing-hiv-aids (accessed on 28 May 2017).

The Office of the U.S. Global AIDS Coordinator. (2014) 'PEPFAR 3.0: controlling the epidemic: delivering on the promise of an AIDS-free generation', available at www.pepfar.gov/documents/organization/234744.pdf (accessed on 29 May 2017).

UNAIDS. (2010) 'Getting to zero: 2011–2016 strategy', available at www.unaids.org/sites/default/files/sub_landing/files/JC2034_UNAIDS_Strategy_en.pdf (accessed on 27 May 2017).

UNAIDS. (2011) 'World AIDS Day report', available at www.unaids.org/sites/default/files/media_asset/JC2216_WorldAIDSday_report_2011_en_1.pdf (accessed on 26 July 2017).

UNAIDS. (2014a) 'Fast-track: ending the AIDS epidemic by 2030', available at www.unaids.org/sites/default/files/media_asset/JC2686_WAD2014report_en.pdf (accessed on 27 May 2017).

UNAIDS. (2014b) 'Press release: UNAIDS reports that reaching Fast-Track targets will avert nearly 28 million new HIV infections and end the AIDS epidemic as a global health threat by 2030', available at www.unaids.org/en/resources/presscentre/pressreleaseandstatementarchive/2014/november/20141118_PR_WAD2014report (accessed on 28 May 2017).

UNAIDS. (2017) 'Ending AIDS: progress towards the 90-90-90 targets', available at www.unaids.org/en/resources/documents/2017/20170720_Global_AIDS_update_2017 (accessed on 9 November 2017).

UNICEF. (2015) 'UNAIDS, UNICEF and partners launch All In campaign to end the AIDS epidemic among adolescents', available at www.unicef.org/ceecis/hiv_aids_27418.html (accessed on 28 May 2017).

UN General Assembly. (2011) 'Political declaration on HIV and AIDS: intensifying our efforts to eliminate HIV and AIDS', available at www.unaids.org/sites/default/files/sub_landing/files/20110610_UN_A-RES-65-277_en.pdf (accessed on 27 May 2017).

UN General Assembly. (2016) 'Political declaration on HIV and AIDS: on the fast-track to accelerate the fight against HIV and to end the AIDS epidemic by 2030', available at www.hlm2016aids.unaids.org/wp-content/uploads/2016/06/2016-political-declaration-HIV-AIDS_en.pdf (accessed on 27 May 2017).

UN News Centre. (2014) 'World AIDS Day: UN, urban leaders endorse "fast track" to ending epidemic by 2030', available at www.un.org/apps/news/story.asp?NewsID=49473#.WSrChsm1uK5 (accessed on 28 May 2017).

US Department of State. (2017) 'Secretary Tillerson launches strategy for accelerating HIV/AIDS epidemic control', available at www.state.gov/r/pa/prs/ps/2017/09/274242.htm (accessed on 13 October 2017).

Vella, S. (2015) 'End of AIDS on the horizon, but innovation needed to end HIV', *The Lancet HIV*, 2(3): e74–5.

Villarosa, L. (2017) 'America's hidden HIV epidemic', The New York Times, available at www.nytimes.com/2017/06/06/magazine/americas-hidden-hiv-epidemic.html?_r=0 (accessed on 26 June 2017).

WHO. (2017) 'HIV drug resistance report 2017', available at http://apps.who.int/iris/bitstream/10665/255896/1/9789241512831-eng.pdf?ua=1 (accessed on 29 July 2017).

Whyte, S. (2014) *Second chances: Surviving AIDS in Uganda*, Durham, NC: Duke University Press.

Zaidi, S. (2011) 'Differential treatment: differential access to newer antiretrovirals', *UNChronicle*, available at https://unchronicle.un.org/article/differential-treatment-restricted-access-newer-antiretrovirals (accessed on 29 July 2017).

Zaracostas, J. (2012) 'Funding crisis threatens global fight against HIV/AIDS', *The Lancet*, 12: 13–4.

# 26

# Enabling positive change

## Learning from progress and setback in HIV and sexual and reproductive health

*Purnima Mane and Peter Aggleton*

Despite significant progress throughout the 1990s and early 2000s, the field of sexual and reproductive health and rights (SRHR) has currently reached a challenging stage. The adverse political climate in many countries, funding cutbacks, and a backtracking in progressive policies make it difficult to advance the momentum made earlier in areas such as maternal mortality (WHO, UNICEF, UNFPA and the World Bank, 2010), HIV infection rates (UNAIDS, 2017), and contraceptive access (Department of Economic and Social Affairs, UN Population Division 2015). Admittedly making headway against conservative forces has always been difficult, but it will help boost confidence if those in the field feel that change is possible, even in the most adverse of conditions, and that many of the challenges that confront us now are those that have been dealt with successfully, in the past.

Against this background, and from an international perspective, this chapter reflects on some of these changes in countries the authors have witnessed, participated in, and celebrated. It identifies factors which collectively have shaped and promoted changes in three instances in the highly polarised, complex, and often frustrating field of HIV and SRHR. Through case studies developed from a review of existing literature and key informant interviews, we examine the early response to HIV and AIDS in India; changes in the penal code in Mozambique to make abortion more accessible to women; and the increase in the age at marriage and uptake of contraception among adolescents in some districts of Bihar State, in India. The three areas together cover a number of critical aspects of SRHR where change has proved to be challenging to secure, although successful and much needed.

## From considering banning sex with foreigners to an evidence-informed response: evolution in the Indian AIDS response

When AIDS was first identified in India in the late 1980s, it was estimated that the country would face a serious epidemic (Dube, 2000; Mane, 1996; Mane and Maitra, 1992; World Bank, 1993), similar to that in many African countries. Prevalent conditions such as poverty, population size, labour migration, and gender disparities, along with cultural taboos surrounding sex, limited programmes for vulnerable populations, and the stigmatisation of sexual minorities made it particularly challenging for India to respond to HIV with the programmes and resources the epidemic needed.

In the mid-1990s in India, health received less than 4 per cent of the GDP (World Bank, 2018), and national authorities saw diseases of the circulatory and respiratory system, and infectious and parasitic diseases as more important than HIV (Bhende and Kanitkar, 1997). In addition, the government had no experience nor stated priority for working with populations seen as being on the fringes of society such as sex workers, injecting drug users, and men who have sex with men. The initial reaction of the government was therefore not surprising – constituting a refusal to see AIDS as a problem for India. It was argued that HIV was limited to socially marginalised groups, resulted from issues alien to Indian culture, and that cultural norms would protect India from HIV, and could be dealt with by 'solutions' such as banning sex with foreigners (Dube, 2000; Ramachandran, 2005).

Fortunately, early in the epidemic, donors and multilateral organisations with a history of cordial and mutually respectful relations with the Indian government such as the World Bank, the World Health Organization, US and European bilateral funding agencies, and charitable foundations like the Ford Foundation, offered financial and technical assistance to aid understanding of the epidemic and examine evidence-informed, rights-based approaches for implementation. For a country seized with socio-economic development as a priority and with limited foreign exchange, the World Bank loan of US$84 million to fight AIDS, for instance, was a major incentive and fostered the establishment of the National AIDS Control Organization (NACO). Multiple phases of work have subsequently been funded by the World Bank (2013). The donors who funded the initial government response encouraged national and state-level authorities to work more closely with civil society and invest in building capacity. Health activists including affected community groups and legal stalwarts, and subsequently the media, also put pressure on the government to respond appropriately and justly.

The results were evident in the nature of the policies and programmes developed by NACO, which involved evidence-gathering on the extent and nature of the epidemic through scientific means; setting aside longstanding biases and cultural taboos in the development of effective programmes; and the involvement of eclectic groups led by the corporate media to develop information and communication strategies. Innovation and pace were encouraged, both of which were not hitherto characteristic of Indian government operations (Dube, 2000). The leadership consciously worked to develop a coordinated approach, tackling prevalent norms and taboos.

The Indian government engaged those impacted by the epidemic in all its advisory bodies and provided direct funding to them, taking a pragmatic and sound approach to the epidemic (UNAIDS, 2016). The engagement of civil society including the media and the legal community, and the direct funding of community groups became integral to the response since community groups had a better understanding of the most vulnerable populations in particular and how to engage with norms around sexual behaviour and stigma and discrimination. In these ways, and through the media and the legal community's extensive reach, the government and its partners boosted their capacity to act swiftly and boldly.

Not surprisingly, the statistics over the years proved the soundness of this approach. Although India still has the third largest population of people living with HIV and one of the largest epidemics, its prevalence rate today is 0.26 per cent (as compared to the estimate in 1990 of 5 per cent among vulnerable populations identified as sex workers, people who inject drugs, men who have sex with men, transgender populations, migrant labourers, and frequently traveling men including truck drivers), with an overall reduction of 66 per cent in estimated annual infections since 2000 (NACO, 2015; UNAIDS, 2016). UNAIDS has subsequently commended India for the comprehensive, multi-sectoral, evidence-informed, and rights-based approach which characterised the nation's response for many years, and which fostered this reduction. Of course, challenges persist in terms of the reduced legal and financial resources allocated to HIV in recent years and the dwindling attention given to HIV as in many other countries.

## Overcoming a colonial legacy: amending the penal code for access to abortion in Mozambique

Abortion continues to be the most elusive reproductive right for women to access, worldwide (Center for Reproductive Rights, 2017; Guttmacher Institute, 2016, 2017). Developing countries like Mozambique have inherited attitudes towards abortion from their colonisers and the influence of religious teachings which denounced abortion. With the exception of five countries, abortion remains restricted in all African states and is not legally permitted for any reason in 11 out of 54 countries (Guttmacher Institute, 2016). Despite this, one in five pregnancies ends in an induced abortion and results in a higher rate of unsafe abortion, the world over, endangering the lives of women; the African continent has the dubious distinction of having the highest rates of deaths related to unsafe abortion-related complications (Guttmacher Institute, 2016).

Mozambique inherited a penal code dating back to 1886 from its Catholic rulers, the Portuguese, when it gained independence in 1975. This code kept access to abortion extremely restricted. Post-independence, a more progressive government had the appetite to make changes in the law but kept the issue on the back burner mainly due to a civil war lasting 16 years after independence (Center for Reproductive Rights, 2017; Pathfinder International, 2016).

In addition, Mozambique had one of the highest rates of maternal mortality in the world, much of it fuelled by unsafe abortion. In 1990, the maternal mortality ratio was 1,390 for every 100,000 live births, much of it due to pregnancy or childbirth-related complications as a result of unsafe abortion; in 2015, though the drop was extensive, the number (489 per 100,000) was still too high (WHO, UNICEF, UNFPA, and the World Bank, 2010). These data and the political leadership's interest in improving national development indicators created strong foundations for the changes that followed.

### The Maputo Protocol as an instrument for change

The Protocol to the African Charter on Human and Peoples' Rights on the Rights of Women in Africa (the Maputo Protocol) was a watershed moment for Mozambique. In 2003, the Assembly of the African Union passed a ground-breaking resolution which upheld the right of women to 'control their fertility' through contraception, and sought to 'protect the reproductive rights of women by authorising medical abortion in cases of sexual assault, rape, incest, and where the continued pregnancy endangers the mental and physical health of the mother or the life of mother or the foetus' (African Union, 2003, p. 16). Significantly progressive as a document, as many as 46 out of the 54 member states of the African Union signed it, with 37 ratifying it by March 2015 according to a report by the Special Rapporteur to the 60th Meeting of the Commission on the Status of Women, in 2016 (Asuagbor, 2016).

With the push for the Millennium Development Goals (MDGs), Mozambique seized upon the protocol to improve its maternal mortality rates, and in 2013 signed and ratified the protocol, which included ensuring safe abortion (Center for Reproductive Rights, 2017; Pathfinder International, 2016). In December 2014, Mozambique became one of only five African countries to legalise abortion. One of the key steps to securing this goal involved revising its penal code, which was successfully achieved with civil society engagement and endorsement, and the involvement of the legal groups and the media, thereby removing a major barrier to women's access to safe abortion and sound health.

The leadership of Pascoal Mocumbi had a major impact in moving things along. Mocumbi had held key government positions from the 1980s including being Prime Minister for a decade until 2004. His prior involvement in the freedom movement and his key leadership roles, as well as his own medical background, contributed to his stature and made a major difference in accelerating the change process (Ramsay, 2003). The Mozambique government also involved civil society by creating inter-sectoral working groups working closely with an existing Coalition for the Defence of Sexual and Reproductive Rights which had made abortion reform its main focus from 2011 (Pathfinder International, 2016). A striking feature of the coalition was its inter-sectoral nature. It involved trusted international NGOs like Ipas and Pathfinder International who played a supportive and educational role and helped raise funds. It also included local NGOs and representatives of the health professions as well as legal professionals. These groups not only promoted a best practice approach but also worked with the media to create an enabling environment by building community awareness and educating parliamentarians who would vote on the reform.

## Increasing the age at marriage in rural Bihar

For many years in India's history, Bihar was considered as a major development challenge. The third most-populated Indian state, with almost 90 per cent of its population living in rural areas (Government of India, 2011), Bihar's total fertility rate (TFR) even today remains at 3.4 while that of India as a whole has dropped to 2.7 (Ministry of Health and Family Welfare, 2016). According to the 2015–16 National Family Health Survey, 40.9 per cent of rural women in Bihar who were between 20–24 years (as compared to 26.9 per cent in urban areas) were married before the age of 18 years, the legal age at marriage for girls; more disturbingly, 25 per cent of women between the ages of 15 to 19 years were already mothers (Ministry of Health and Family Welfare, 2016) and contraceptive prevalence remained low among women below 25 years even though it increased with older age groups (Daniel, et al., 2008).

Girls' age at marriage and conception matter significantly for their future including survival. Early conception is tied to death during pregnancy and childbirth – girls aged 15 years and under are five times more likely to die than women in their 20s – as well as to poor health and higher mortality of infants (UNFPA, 2012; UNICEF, 2014). Early marriage and motherhood also precipitate school drop-out and deny girls access to future social, economic, and political participation, depriving themselves, their families, and their countries by not contributing to national development.

In 2001, an ambitious project was taken on by Pathfinder International with the support of Packard Foundation in three Bihar districts working with the state government and NGOs to change social norms and behaviour around age at marriage and conception, and contraception and birth-spacing.[1] A multi-pronged programme, PRACHAR as it was called, ran in phases for more than ten years, with each phase learning from the previous one. The main components included working with adolescents, both unmarried young people and married couples, their parents, mothers-in-law, teachers, community health workers, community leaders, and local NGOs to build knowledge and shape norms around marriage and contraception, thereby influencing reproductive behaviour and age at marriage.

A focus on gender equity was integrated throughout the programme especially since son preference often featured as a reason for frequent pregnancies. The methodology included diverse avenues ranging from home visits, couple sessions, group training sessions to community meetings, and education through entertainment and programmes for the community. Working with boys and girls, married couples, and home visits proved to be the most effective strategies (Pathfinder International, 2013) but a formal evaluation concluded that it was the multi-pronged approach adopted by PRACHAR that was the major contributor to its success (Jejeebhoy, et al., 2015). What made the approach sustainable was the training of a cadre of male communicators in adolescent and youth sexual and reproductive health who worked with and through local NGOs, and the training of government community health workers or Accredited Social Health Activists (ASHAs) to work with couples, in-laws and parents, and with community leaders.

Evidence was gathered throughout the project and three-year and five-year data showed dramatic differences between intervention and comparison districts in knowledge and use of contraception, age at marriage (going up in intervention districts by 2.6 years vis-a-vis comparison districts), and age at first birth (1.5 years later than before) (Pathfinder International, 2013). The independent evaluation in 2012 went further by showing that these results lasted beyond the intervention phase and also influenced the behaviour of those more indirectly exposed to the project's work through cultural meetings on reproductive health in the PRACHAR districts (Jejeebhoy, et al., 2015).

The PRACHAR project continued until 2013 (with additional UNFPA support) and its approach was eventually integrated into the government health structure through a less intensive, pared-down model which continued to work with ASHAs and through NGOs. Government interest and support throughout had bolstered the success of the project as had civil society engagement, making diversity of partners a strong contributor to PRACHAR's success.

## Common factors collectively influencing change in the three case studies

A number of common factors coalesced to bring about change in the three examples presented, along with other contextual factors (c.f. Kippax, et al., 2013). Just one of these factors alone would not have made the difference. Success was the result of the combined force of evidence, civil society engagement, and political will or leadership with values, often enshrined in the existing laws of the country, acting as enablers.

In each of the three cases, *evidence* came from both local data as well as global data. The testimonies of those affected by HIV in India or other countries, or by those who were forced to marry and conceive early in Bihar, made an impact. An informed media spread the word far and wide. The opinions of health experts were also instrumental in having an impact along with the statistical data. When India began to take HIV seriously, the evidence from its own established bodies and from trusted international organisations about the problem – its existence and its potentially negative impact on multiple facets of life for the individual, family, and nation especially on its development trajectory – was undeniable. Evidence of the interconnectedness of AIDS with many other problems of the country helped increase commitment from the political leadership.

There was also data on how countries could benefit if they took early, evidence-informed action and what could happen to others who chose to ignore the warning signs. Clear scientific evidence that enhancing access to safe abortion would reduce maternal mortality appealed to the Mozambique government, which wished to reduce its high maternal mortality ratio, be responsive to the MDG commitments, and foster national development. In Bihar, worldwide data indicated that early age at marriage and conception were major barriers to development; the monitoring data collected and shared widely throughout the PRACHAR initiative also showed that multi-pronged, intensive efforts involving multiple stakeholders had a positive impact on changing both behaviour and entrenched community norms around these issues. Evidence therefore came in diverse forms, creating pressure to act based on what the data had shown to be effective.

While evidence is essential, however, it alone is often not enough to lead to action. In 2000, President Mbeki spent precious time and resources on an Advisory Panel on AIDS to look into what caused AIDS when HIV's role in causation had already been clearly established (McIntyre, et al., 2008; Sidley, 2000) and the epidemic spread rapidly in South Africa. For years, the US prioritised abstinence-only programmes when the evidence clearly showed that these had limited impact (Gorman, 2016; Kirby, et al., 2007; Santelli, et al., 2006).

In all three of the key examples discussed in this chapter, strong *political leadership* and *civil society involvement* were central to success, often through a partnership model with each element doing its bit. In Mozambique, Pascoal Mocumbi's leadership and the involvement of the interdisciplinary coalition were central to Mozambique's success in penal code reform and abortion access. In India, the prime minister chaired the AIDS National Council involving all ministries, thereby sending out the right message from the very top; NACO leadership was central in making the HIV response truly multisectoral – it consulted and engaged a range of players from media, communications, social work, and health and affected communities and funded them directly to expedite action (UNAIDS, 2016). HIV and AIDS were presented as needing the support of all sectors, and the education of the media as well as parliamentarians, the legal community, the corporate sector, and community groups was prioritised. Civil society in turn worked with the legal community and media, using constitutional rights and social justice as the basis to promote action around AIDS and change in discriminatory laws and policies to deal with stigma. A similar situation was observed in Bihar where both local NGOs and government systems like ASHA were central to PRACHAR's success, keeping government and communities engaged from the start.

## Additional lessons learned

Despite what has been learned, there is no formula for success in influencing change. Change has to harness context-specific factors such as was evidenced in the foreign exchange imperative in India related to the World Bank loan, or the timing of the Maputo Protocol in Mozambique's case. Other strategies like quiet diplomacy and working behind the scenes also play a role – for example, in Iran and India where needle exchange in prisons was implemented without a public hue and cry, or in China where change to the one child policy was achieved not always through vociferous advocacy but by multilateral organisations working with the government to pilot test loosening of the policy in some districts.

It is also important to recognise that change is not a linear process and is often slow, fluid, and fragile. Its outcomes cannot be entirely predicted and can prove short-lived. Change by its nature is susceptible to being reversed over time by political, social, and economic circumstances, or stalled especially when organised forces or events push it back. However, being prepared for the fact that priorities will (and do) change is imperative. Examples witnessed include governments seeing the availability of antiretroviral treatment as a 'quick-fix' solution to the HIV epidemic, thereby downplaying the importance of education and a fully social response to HIV (Aggleton and Parker, 2015); the growing attention given to non-communicable diseases and other conditions at the expense of SRHR (Islam, et al., 2014); and adverse economic and political climates causing a reduction in resources for health (Kirigia, et al., 2011) and decreasing support for socially just policies in countries such as the USA (Girard, 2017).

It is critical to recognise therefore that change-making involves a long-term commitment and there is still work to be done in each of the three cases – age at marriage and contraceptive acceptance among the younger population is still low in Bihar (Ministry of Health and Family Welfare, 2016); in India, HIV is no longer given the attention it received earlier on (Agooramoorthy, 2015); and the implementation of non-stigmatising access to abortion will need vigilant tracking in Mozambique.

## Celebrating change

Despite how tough change may be to bring about and retain, we need to celebrate the extent of improvement which has in fact happened in SRHR over the last two decades. Some examples of this can be seen in total fertility rate reductions; increased access to contraception; reduction in maternal and infant mortality; and improved HIV rates and ART access. Undoubtedly, there is a long way to go – for example, rates of HIV are rising among most-at-risk populations in many countries (Beyrer, et al., 2012; UNAIDS, 2017); 45 per cent of all abortions globally are still unsafe (Ganatra, et al., 2017; WHO and Guttmacher Institute, 2017); girls continue to be married early in many countries (UNICEF, 2014); and young women are still among those most vulnerable to HIV infection (UNAIDS, 2017). However, our conviction should be that positive change will and does happen even if there is more work ahead of us. The cost of not acknowledging and celebrating the change that has happened is too high. Without it, those engaged in the process will not benefit from the reassurance that staying the course is critical to bringing about results, and they will lose out on the imperative of learning and persevering while doing so.

## Note

1   Much of the detail in this section come from a technical brief prepared by Pathfinder International (2013), papers produced by Pathfinder International staff (e.g., Daniel, et al., 2008), and an evaluation conducted by the Population Council (Jejeebhoy, et al., 2015).

## References

African Union. (2003) 'Protocol to the African Charter on Human and Peoples' Rights on the rights of women in Africa', available at www.achpr.org/files/instruments/women-protocol/achpr_instr_proto_women_eng.pdf (accessed on 1 January 2017).

Aggleton, P. and Parker, R. (2015) 'Moving beyond biomedicalization in the HIV response: implications for community involvement and community leadership among men who have sex with men and transgender people', *American Journal of Public Health*, 105(8): 1552–8.

Agooramoorthy, G. (2015) 'India's budget reduction and AIDS initiatives', *The Lancet Infectious Diseases*, 15(6): 6636.

Asuagbor, L. (2016) 'Report to the 60th meeting of the Commission on the Status of Women', New York.

Bhende, A. and Kanitkar, T. (1997) *Principles of Population Studies*, 10th edn, Mumbai: Himalaya Publishing House.

Beyrer, C., Baral, S., van Griensven, F., Goodreau, S., Chariyalertsak, S., Wirtz, A., and Brookmeyer, R. (2012) 'Global epidemiology of HIV infection in men who have sex with men', *The Lancet*, 380(9839): 367–77.

Center for Reproductive Rights. (2017) *The World's Abortion Laws*, New York: Center for Reproductive Rights, available at www.worldabortionlaws.com/ (accessed on 1 January 2017).

Daniel, E., Masilamani, R., and Rahman, M. (2008) 'The effect of community-based reproductive health communication interventions on contraceptive use among young married couples in Bihar, India', *International Family Planning Perspectives*, 24(4): 189–97.

Department of Economic and Social Affairs, UN Population Division. (2015) *Trends in Contraceptive Use Worldwide*, New York: United Nations.

Dube, S. (2000) *Sex, Lies and Drugs*, New Delhi: Harper Collins India.

Ganatra, B., et al. (2017) 'Global, regional, and subregional classification of abortions by safety, 2010–14: estimates from a Bayesian hierarchical model', *The Lancet*, 390(10110): 2372–81.

Girard, F. (2017) 'Implications of the Trump administration for sexual and reproductive rights globally', *Reproductive Health Matters*, 25: 49.

Gorman, C. (2016) 'US anti-AIDS abstinence efforts in Africa fail to prevent HIV', Scientific American, available at www.scientificamerican.com/article/u-s-anti-aids-abstinence-efforts-in-africa-fail-to-prevent-hiv/ (accessed on 1 January 2017).

Government of India. (2011) *List of States with Population, Sex Ratio and Literacy, Census, 2011*, New Delhi: Government of India.

Guttmacher Institute. (2016) 'Fact sheet: abortion in Africa', available at www.guttmacher.org/fact-sheet/facts-abortion-africa (accessed on 1 March 2018).

Guttmacher Institute. (2017) 'Induced Abortion Worldwide, Fact Sheet May 2016', available at www.guttmacher.org/fact-sheet/induced-abortion-worldwide (accessed on 1 March 2018).

Islam, S., Purnat, T., Phuong, N., Mwingira, U., Schacht, K., and Froschl, G. (2014) 'Non- communicable diseases (NCDs) in developing countries: a symposium report', *Journal of Global Health*, 10(81):1–7.

Jejeebhoy, S., Prakash, R., Acharya, R., Singh, S., and Daniel, E. (2015) 'Meeting contraceptive needs: long term associations of the PRACHAR project with married women's awareness and behavior in Bihar', *International Perspectives on Sexual and Reproductive Health*, 41(3): 115–25.

Kippax, S., Stephenson, N., Parker, R., and Aggleton, P. (2013) 'Between individual agency and structure in HIV prevention: understanding the middle ground of social practice', *American Journal of Public Health*, 103(8): 1367–75.

Kirby, D., Laris, B., and Rolleri, L. (2007) 'Sex and HIV education programs: their impact on sexual behaviors of young people throughout the world', *Journal of Adolescent Health*, 40(3): 206–17.

Kirigia, J., Nganda, B., Mwikisa, C., and Cardoso, B. (2011) 'Effects of global financial crisis on funding for health development in nineteen countries of the WHO African Region', *BMC International Health and Human Rights*, 11(4).

McIntyre, J., Bruyn, G., and Grey, G. (2008) 'HIV/AIDS in Southern Africa', In: D. Celentano and C. Beyrer (Eds.) *Public Health Aspects of HIV/AIDS in Low and Middle Income Countries: Epidemiology, prevention and care*, New York: Springer Science and Business Media, pp. 290–329.

Mane, P. (1996) 'Evolving impact of HIV/AIDS on India', In: J. Mann and D. Tarantola (Eds.) *AIDS in the World: Global dimensions, social roots, and responses*, New York: Oxford University Press, pp. 124–7.

Mane, P. and Maitra, S. (1992) *AIDS Prevention: The socio-cultural context in India*, Mumbai: Tata Institute of Social Sciences.

Ministry of Health and Family Welfare. (2016) *NFHS-4, 2015–2016 State Fact Sheet Bihar*, Mumbai: IIPS and Macro International.

NACO. (2015) *India HIV Estimations 2015: Technical Report*, New Delhi: NACO and National Institute of Medical Statistics, ICMR, Ministry of Health and Family Welfare.

Pathfinder International. (2013) *PRACHAR, Technical Brief*, Watertown, MA: Pathfinder International.

Pathfinder International. (2016) *Strategies to Advance Abortion Rights and Access in Restrictive Settings: A cross-country analysis*, Watertown, MA: Pathfinder International.

Ramachandran, R. (2005) 'Remembering Paintal', Frontline, available at www.frontline.in/static/html/fl2220/stories/20051007002308900.htm (accessed on 1 January 2017).

Ramsay, S. (2003) 'Pascoal Mocumbi – international health advocate', *The Lancet*, 361(9355): 400–3.

Santelli, J., Ott, M., Lyon, M., Rogers, J., Summers, D., and Schieffer, R. (2006) 'Abstinence and abstinence-only education: a review of US policies and programs', *Journal of Adolescent Health*, 38(1): 72–81.

Sidley, P. (2000) 'Mbeki appoints team to look at cause of AIDS', *British Medical Journal*, 320(7245): 1291.

UNAIDS. (2016) *Governments Fund Communities: Six country experiences of financing community responses through governmental mechanisms*, Geneva: UNAIDS.

UNAIDS. (2017) *UNAIDS Data 2017*, Geneva: UNAIDS.

UNFPA. (2012) *Marrying Too Young: End child marriage*, New York: UNFPA.

UNICEF. (2014) *Ending Child Marriage: Progress and prospects*, New York: UNICEF.

WHO and Guttmacher Institute. (2017) 'Worldwide, an estimated 25 million unsafe abortions occur each year' Joint WHO and Guttmacher Institute press release, available at www.guttmacher.org/news-release/2017/worldwide-estimated -25-million-unsafe-abortions-occur-each-year (accessed on 1 January 2017).

WHO, UNICEF, UNFPA and the World Bank. (2010) *Trends in Maternal Mortality 1990–2008*, Geneva: WHO.

World Bank. (1993) *World Development Report 1993: Investing in health, world development indicators*, New York: Oxford University Press.

World Bank. (2013) 'India: World Bank approves $255 million for National AIDS control support project', World Bank press release, available at www.worldbank.org/en/news/press-release/2013/05/01/india-world-bank-approves-255-million-for-national-aids-control-support-project (accessed on 3 February 2018).

World Bank. (2018) 'Health expenditure, total', available at https://data.worldbank.org/indicator/SH.XPD.TOTL.ZS (accessed on 28 March 2018).

# 27

# The global politics of polio eradication

*William S. Schulz and Heidi J. Larson*

The Global Polio Eradication Initiative (GPEI) is widely recognized as an extraordinary humanitarian enterprise, made possible in part by its political neutrality. It is undoubtedly true that the GPEI's successes to date are due in large part to the efforts of many laudably idealistic members of the global health community, dedicated to the goal of eradicating polio from the entire world. But when the program has encountered actors who do not share this goal, progress has necessitated a negotiation of interests – that is, it has required engaging in politics. This chapter explores these processes as a window into the workings of global health generally, and as a guide to those who seek to pursue such idealistic goals in the future.

## Introduction: the political origins of polio eradication

In 1988, the World Health Assembly (WHA) resolved to eradicate polio globally by the year 2000. Health and humanitarian ideals aside, this resolution was a significant political milestone, since it required many countries – each with different national priorities – to collectively fight a single disease. In theory, the member countries of the World Health Organization (WHO) would deliberate carefully about which disease was most suitable for eradication, taking into account such factors as global burden of disease or case fatality rate. In reality, although the member countries' votes are necessary to move a resolution forward, the real genesis of polio eradication was a series of smaller events that built towards the global project, and which provide valuable insights into the politics of global health.

Rather than agreeing to eradicate polio in an international forum, the decision was mainly driven by a relatively small cadre of doctors and epidemiologists who believed that eradication was a global good, despite the prevailing preference for Primary Health Care over disease-specific vertical programmes. Following the successful eradication of smallpox, these 'true believers' organised a series of conferences with the objective of identifying the next disease they would eradicate. Remarkably, the speakers at these events offered little support for eradication – smallpox veteran D.A. Henderson himself came out strongly against it, believing smallpox had been eradicated largely by luck – yet in the sidelines eradication proponents encouraged each other, and gradually narrowed their list of target diseases, from which polio emerged as a frontrunner (Muraskin, 2012).

These advocates had a variety of motivations for supporting the principle of eradication. Albert Sabin, for example, believed passionately in the potential of his live-attenuated oral polio vaccine (OPV), and wanted to see it used as widely as possible. He advocated for mass vaccination campaigns that successfully eliminated polio in the Dominican Republic, Cuba, and Brazil (though he was expelled from the latter initiative for publicly criticising the Brazilian government, which had hoped polio elimination would improve its public image (Hampton, 2009)). The successes in these countries set the stage for Ciro de Quadros (a Brazilian epidemiologist) to convince the Pan American Health Organization (PAHO) to undertake a project of regional polio elimination throughout the Americas in 1985 (Brookes and Khan, 2007).

De Quadros saw polio as a 'banner disease' that could rally support for broader immunisation programmes (de Quadros, 2008, p. 61, cited by Muraskin, 2012), a view shared by the newly elected PAHO director (and fellow Brazilian) Carlyle Guerra de Macedo. They received financial support for their regional elimination project from Rotary International, which was hoping to unite its international membership in an idealistic cause (Muraskin, 2012).

For Rotary leadership, as for many other eradication advocates along the way, polio's appeal lay not only in its idealism, but also in its high level of public visibility. In the twentieth century, polio was a particularly high priority in the United States. President Franklin D. Roosevelt, who was disabled by polio, helped make the 'March of Dimes' the largest medical charity in history (Barrett, 2008), supporting research that ultimately produced both the inactivated polio vaccine (IPV) and the oral polio vaccine (OPV). These vaccines made eradication technically conceivable, and (as noted earlier) OPV developer Albert Sabin was instrumental in agitating for elimination programmes early on. Polio's notoriety also made it ideal as a 'banner disease' for people like de Quadros, who successfully used this argument to win over Jim Grant, then Executive Director of UNICEF (Closser, 2010, p. 37). Yet in many ways, polio remained an unlikely candidate for global eradication: it caused relatively few deaths worldwide, and many argued that the resources required for eradication would be better spent on less ambitious programmes to control more deadly diseases (Muraskin, 2012).

The notion of scaling-up from PAHO's regional elimination project to a global polio eradication programme was seeded, quite unexpectedly, in the midst of a busy meeting of the Task Force for Child Survival in Talloires, France in 1988. UNICEF's Jim Grant and smallpox eradication veteran Bill Foege handed around drafts of a so-called 'Declaration of Talloires', proposing to eradicate polio, neonatal tetanus, and measles. The Talloires meeting was only supposed to decide the Task Force's agenda for the 1990s, but it proved a highly effective venue for promoting the eradication idea: by Ciro de Quadros' reckoning, most of the world's population was represented by the Ministers of Health in attendance, along with the president of the World Bank and many other influential figures in global health. Yet the person whom Foege and Grant most needed to convince was D.A. Henderson, who, as the acting rapporteur, was the ultimate gatekeeper as to how the Declaration was portrayed in the meeting report (Muraskin, 2012; Brooks and Khan, 2007; The Task Force for Child Survival, 1988).

Henderson, already a noted eradication sceptic, found their proposal unrealistic. Meeting privately with Grant and Foege, he exhorted them 'not [to] make fools of ourselves' (Muraskin, 2012, p. 49) by publicly proposing to globally eradicate tetanus, whose spores could not be removed from the soil, and measles, which had never been interrupted even in the United States. Grant and Foege relented on both counts, but they would not be dissuaded from polio. Grudgingly, Henderson agreed to include this revised 'Declaration of Talloires' in the meeting report. This document was then strategically deployed to mobilise support for the official WHA resolution to eradicate polio, which passed with unanimous support just a few months after Talloires (Muraskin, 2012). In this way, a relatively small group of people managed to put polio on the global agenda.

In its final wording, the WHA resolution stated that '... eradication efforts should be pursued in ways which strengthen the development of the Expanded Programme on Immunization as a whole, fostering its contribution, in turn, to the development of the health infrastructure and of primary health care' (WHA, 1988, p. 1). This helped to justify the programme in poorer countries where basic health services were a higher priority than an idealistic enterprise like polio eradication: the resources rallied around the eradication goal would, along the way, help build up basic health services such as routine immunisation (RI). With this, the resolution passed, and the GPEI was created. But, despite an international agreement being forged, the process of convincing the world to eradicate polio had only just begun. As we shall see, executing a global goal still depends on the commitment of individual countries and, ultimately, that of their people.

## Latin America

Polio's earliest experiences in overcoming countries' internal divisions come from Latin America, where the first large-scale polio vaccination campaigns were conducted under the aegis of PAHO's regional polio elimination programme. Most challenging of all were those settings in which violent conflict threatened to interfere in vaccination activities.

In the 1980s Salvadorian Civil War, for example, there was a substantial risk of vaccination teams being caught in the crossfire between the government and guerrilla fighters. In El Salvador, PAHO collaborated with UNICEF, the Red Cross, and the Catholic Church to organise one-day truces, dubbed 'days of tranquillity', through a lengthy process of briefing guerrilla representatives in faraway Washington, DC on why collaboration was needed to be able to deliver the vaccines. The representatives then relayed the message to field commanders, who determined whether a truce was agreeable:

> During the actual immunisation days, around 20 000 people – health workers, volunteers, and members of guerrilla forces – gave the vaccinations. On one occasion, one of the PAHO epidemiologists who was leading a team of vaccinators was returning from the field at the end of the day and was stopped by a group of guerrilla fighters. Initially, he was terrified, but then he realised that the guerrilla fighters wanted the team to return to a village that was left without vaccination!
>
> Eventually, 3 days of tranquillity were held every year from 1985 to 1991 for vaccination of practically every child in El Salvador, until peace was achieved in the early 1990s. It is difficult to measure the contribution of polio eradication to the final achievement of peace in that region, but, undoubtedly, the collaboration among all those working in health helped to raise the level of trust among people.
>
> *de Quadros and Epstein, 2002, p. 26*

Processes like this were part of PAHO's 'Health as a Bridge for Peace' plan, which sought to capitalise on the universal value of good health, to negotiate Days of Tranquillity and successfully arrange for polio eradicators to operate despite conflicts in Sri Lanka, the Philippines, Afghanistan, Tajikistan, Sudan, and DR Congo (Mach, 1999).

PAHO faced a different situation in Peru, where *Sendero Luminoso* (Shining Path) guerrilla insurgents lacked the command structure that had facilitated negotiation in El Salvador:

> The only option was to try to inform everybody, through the mass media, that the [recently diagnosed] case in Junin could be the last case of polio in the western hemisphere and that only with the cooperation of every individual in the country could the outbreak represented by this boy be contained. This approach had a certain amount of risk, because the Shining Path could have used this opportunity to disrupt the operation as a show of power. Press conferences were held and appeals were made to every member of society to participate and cooperate with the mop-up vaccination campaign.
>
> *de Quadros and Epstein, 2002, p. 26*

No disruption occurred in the ensuing campaign. By saturating the public with messages emphasising the imminence of eradication, eradicators seemingly captured enough popular support that Sendero Luminoso could not benefit politically from interfering. Thus, humanitarian neutrality has, at times, allowed polio to forge some improbable partnerships.

## Nigeria

Eradicators faced a tougher challenge in July 2003 in Nigeria, where internal political divisions fuelled a boycott of polio vaccination by five Northern states. While other states only held short boycotts, Kano state persisted for 11 months, with Governor Ibrahim Shekarau apparently blocking the national eradication agenda as a show of defiance to President Obasanjo. Obasanjo was a Southern Christian who had recently won re-election, defeating a candidate who was close to Shekarau, and popular in Nigeria's predominantly Muslim North. In the wake of this defeat, Shekarau sought to consolidate his political base by appealing to his constituents' identity, and promoted a rumour that OPV was a Western conspiracy, abetted by the Christian president, to kill and sterilise Muslims (Ghinai, et al., 2013; Jegede, 2007; Obadare, 2005).

Several factors may have exacerbated this rumour. First, the free provision of OPV in Kano may have appeared suspicious to people with few health services and more serious diseases, and biomedicine's historical association with colonialism redoubled those suspicions. Moreover, the post-9/11 conflicts in Iraq and Afghanistan had heightened perceptions that the West was at war with Muslims, and the memory of recent deaths during Pfizer's Nigerian trials of its anti-meningitis drug, Trovan, heightened the plausibility of Western medicines killing children, even though the deaths were found to be unrelated to the trial (Ghinai, et al., 2013).

Through religious networks, the polio programme sought to dispel anti-vaccination rumours. The Organisation of the Islamic Conference approved a resolution in October 2003 urging member countries to hasten eradication, and also helped GPEI secure pro-vaccination *fatwas* from the Islamic Fiqh Academy (Kaufmann and Feldbaum, 2009). GPEI had been cultivating ties with these groups since before the boycott, following the recognition that its Western links could be a liability. Internationally, this rebranding took the form of international agreements. At the local level, it meant connecting health workers with local *imams* to relay health messages through their mosques – the idea being to dispel arguments that polio vaccination was contrary to Islam, so as to clear the path for a solution through diplomatic channels.

Ibrahim Gambari, the UN Secretary-General's senior advisor for African affairs, was the GPEI's chief diplomat in the efforts to end the persisting boycott in Kano State. As the child of a Northern Muslim father and a Southern mother, Gambari was a political bridge – in President Obasanjo's words, 'You get to where I find it difficult to get to' (Kaufmann and Feldbaum, 2009, p. 1094). Yet Gambari was unable to win the Governor over. 'You are going to condemn a whole people to this life of misery', Gambari said to the Governor, before he left Kano, 'at least consider you may be wrong' (Kaufmann and Feldbaum, 2009, p. 1094). Nonetheless, his work opened a dialogue with the North, conveying that the boycott would not only harm children's health, but also damage Nigeria's (and Kano's) international reputation.

The government of the United States (the chief GPEI donor at the time) incorporated the polio issue into official visits to Nigeria by the Health and Human Services secretary and deputy-secretary, raising it in Secretary of State Colin Powell's meeting with his Nigerian counterpart, and sending further emissaries through the African Union and regional diplomats (Kaufmann and Feldbaum, 2009). These routes of influence targeted the central government, which was unable to overrule Shekarau outright, but still had means to push him towards capitulation.

While applying these different forms of pressure and persuasion, the Programme and its partners simultaneously created ways for Shekarau to back out of his boycott while avoiding embarrassment. For example, UNICEF sourced new OPV stocks from Indonesia, allowing Shekarau to justify his capitulation by saying the vaccines could be trusted if manufactured in a Muslim country (despite the fact that the Indonesian vaccine had already been used in Nigeria before the boycott) (Kaufmann and Feldbaum, 2009). The Indonesian factory was opened for inspection by the Nigerian government, and, when the Kano authorities were still not satisfied, a second delegation was sent from the Kano state government.

Shekarau's capitulation was fumbled, according to WikiLeaks cables allegedly penned by US Ambassador John Campbell: the Governor planned to announce resumed polio activities on 14 June 2004 (Campbell, 2004b), but balked when his decision was prematurely revealed by Dere Awosika, the leader of the National Programme on Immunisation (NPI). Campbell allegedly proposed devolving the NPI to state governments, removing Awosika from the picture and allowing Shekarau to resume vaccination on his own authority, without appearing to give in to the federal government. At this stage, '… public pressure on either the

GON [Government of Nigeria] or the Kano state governor could prove counterproductive … the Nigerian aversion to public criticism and arm-twisting could be strengthened, delaying implementation even further' (Campbell, 2004a). Vaccination in Kano finally did resume in August 2004, but serious damage had been done: the boycott was estimated to have quintupled polio incidence in Nigeria between 2002–6, seeded polio outbreaks across three continents, and cost over US$500 million to contain (Ghinai, et al., 2013).

In the decade following the boycott, Nigeria gradually brought polio cases back to pre-boycott levels, and in September 2015 Nigeria was officially removed from the list of polio-endemic countries (National Primary Health Care Development Agency, 2015). Celebration of this milestone was short-lived, however, as in August 2016 two children were discovered paralysed by wild poliovirus in Borno state, indicating that the disease still lingered in the North, where population movements and violent conflict hinder vaccination and surveillance activities (WHO, 2016). By the end of 2016 four cases of wild polio virus were confirmed in Nigeria and it was returned to the list of endemic countries along with Pakistan and Afghanistan.

## Pakistan

Pakistan has seen some of the most extreme opposition to polio eradication, including outright violence. One Saturday in December 2013, two masked men stormed an immunisation office in Khyber, ordered women and children out of the building, then fatally shot polio campaign supervisor Ghilaf Khan and escaped on motorcycles, leaving behind a one-sentence note: 'Those who follow foreigners will meet the same fate' (Afridi, 2013, n.p.).

This conforms to the rhetoric of anti-state militants in Pakistan, who oppose any symbol of compliance with Western interests. As of September 2016, attacks like this had killed 41 people, and injured an additional 40, including polio workers as well as police assigned for their protection (Yusufzai, 2016). Facing violence and poor pay, health workers and teachers refused to work on polio campaigns in Khyber and Peshawar (AFP, 2014; *The Express Tribune*, 2014a; Dawn, 2014; *The Express Tribune*, 2014b).

Around the same time as the killing of Ghilaf Khan, polio cases started appearing in North Waziristan (Firdous, 2013; IMB, 2013), where militant leader Hafiz Gul Bahadur had banned polio vaccination the previous year:

> Dated: 15/06/2012
>
> In the name of Allah!
>
> Shura of Mujahideen's Administrator Hafiz Gul Bahadur has taken this decision in consultation with his shura that unless the series of drone attacks are stopped, there will be a ban on the administration of polio drops. Because what is the use of the well wishes of such a well-wisher who on one hand, spends billions on the administration of drops for the protection against polio disease, and polio happens to one in hundred thousand, on the other hand the same well-wisher (USA) with the help from his servant (Pakistan) is conducting relentless drone attacks […] Also in the polio campaigns there are strong chances of spying over the Mujahideen by the US and an example of which is Dr. Shakil Afridi…
>
> *RUSI, 2014, p. 1*

With vaccinators under fire, and Waziristan rapidly becoming a polio reservoir, the International Monitoring Board of the Global Polio Eradication Initiative (IMB) urged that 'all means be used to ensure that the polio programme in every country is known to be politically neutral' (IMB, 2013, pp. 58–9), adding, 'The goal of eradicating polio from the world should be an apolitical, humanitarian endeavor' (IMB, 2013, p. 43).

The CIA received considerable blame for politicising health programmes after it was revealed that the agency had employed Dr. Shakil Afridi to stage a fake hepatitis B vaccination campaign, in an attempt to locate Osama Bin Laden (Shah, 2011). The incident was denounced for undermining trust in polio vaccination teams and humanitarian workers worldwide (Roberts and VanRooyen, 2013; *The Lancet*, 2014; Buekens, et al., 2013).

However, it is an over-simplification to blame the CIA for the violence and bans against vaccinators in Pakistan. First, violence towards vaccinators preceded the CIA-Afridi incident. During the 2006–9 occupation of Swat, for example, Tehreek-e-Taliban Pakistan (TTP) leader Mullah Fazlullah prohibited polio vaccination and issued *fatwas* condemning lady health workers (LHWs) as prostitutes and servants of America, and exhorted Muslim men to kidnap, forcibly marry, or kill them if they came knocking (Ud Din, et al., 2012). As in Nigeria, Fazlullah saw polio vaccination as 'a conspiracy of the Jews and Christians to stunt the population growth of Muslims' by sterilising their children (Yusufzai, 2007, n.p.). The CIA incident may have reinforced these attitudes, but it did not create them (Roberts, 2013).

Second, militants in Pakistan should not be presumed to operate as a unified front. The fragmentary groups that fall under the umbrella of the TTP generally consider themselves to be at war with the Pakistani state, which they see as a puppet of the West. The groups in North Waziristan, in contrast, exist primarily as bases of operation for Taliban fighters in Afghanistan, and it is an open secret that they receive covert support from the Pakistani military (who consider these groups to be useful agents for influencing events across the border in Afghanistan).

Polio eradicators have therefore faced very different challenges with respect to the Waziristan ban and the targeted attacks by TTP groups. The attacks appear to be opportunistic strikes against the Pakistani government and the West – the groups behind them make no demands, claim no responsibility, and their only apparent goal is to undermine the government, leaving no basis for negotiation. The ban, by contrast, lays out clear demands, and bears the signature of the leader sponsoring it, who has a longstanding relationship with the Pakistani military (International Crisis Group, 2015). What the ban and the attacks have in common is that the gatekeepers do not value polio eradication, and are willing to compromise it to pursue other ends – mainly to express grievances to the government and to send a broader ideological message to the world at large.

This is in contrast with Afghanistan, where eradicators have successfully negotiated with the Taliban to get access for vaccinators. The organisational hierarchy of the Taliban allowed the polio programme to overrule local opposition through a high-level agreement with Taliban leader Mullah Omar, facilitated by the International Committee of the Red Cross. Omar signed a letter of protection, which vaccination teams used to gain access in areas under Taliban control (Crossley, 2013; Trofimov, 2010). So, the Afghan and Pakistani groups differ: '… whereas the Taliban in Pakistan is a militant group that is dependent upon a show of power to maintain their control over a small geographical area, the Taliban in Afghanistan is potentially the government-in-waiting' (Abimbola, et al., 2013, p. 1).

The Taliban have a sense of stewardship in Afghanistan, and a responsibility to provide public services to communities under their control. This illustrates how, in any given country, there are often multiple centres of power that operate in parallel to (or in opposition to) the traditional civilian government that is recognised by the international community. These informal authorities – beneficent civil society groups, freedom fighters, fragmentary armed mafias, and many others in between – can exert great influence in facilitating or disrupting a global initiative like polio eradication, despite lacking a seat at the WHA.

But all political powers, formal and informal alike, depend to some extent on the will of the people who live under their regime – leaders who fail to satisfy the public are at risk of being voted out of office, or being supplanted by a rival faction. This, in general, is a great advantage for global health programmes, which can offer something that is of great value to nearly every human being: a longer and healthier life. These benefits are so universally valuable at the grassroots level, that even the most indifferent leaders can sometimes be persuaded to acquiesce to a health programme's requests, especially when it costs these leaders little and they are still able to claim credit for the benefits given to their constituents.

Yet the polio programme has often struggled to gain grassroots support. Particularly in Pakistan and Nigeria (and in contrast to Latin America), as polio became far less visible it was seen as far less important than other local needs, especially in communities where basic public services are crumbling. Sometimes such communities have bargained for services or infrastructure (e.g., a borehole for drinking water) by strategically refusing polio vaccinators entry (Taylor, 2014; Closser, Jooma, et al., 2016; Closser, Rosenthal, et al., 2016).

The GPEI therefore adopted a strategy in Pakistan, used in India and Nigeria a decade earlier, of accompanying polio vaccination drives with other health services that addressed the felt needs of the community. For example, the *Sehat ka Insaf* (Justice for Health) model, in Peshawar, Pakistan, folded polio vaccination in amongst vitamin A drops, hygiene supplies, and vaccines for tuberculosis, diphtheria, pertussis, tetanus, hepatitis B, haemophilus influenza, pneumonia, and measles (Yusufzai, 2014). Particularly in Pakistan, with its security threats, de-centring polio from being a highly visible campaign may make it a less attractive target for attackers, since its symbolism of Western interests is defused by the fact it is providing services that many people value.

Pakistani expert Zulfiqar Bhutta has, moreover, proposed that 'Polio eradication hinges on child health in Pakistan', on the basis that providing basic health services is the most genuine and direct way to win community trust for polio eradication (Bhutta, 2014, p. 285). In a way, this turns the original promise of polio eradication on its head: basic health services, once supposed to follow on the GPEI's coat-tails, now appear crucial to achieving eradication itself.

## Polio eradication endgame and legacy

Another political challenge facing the GPEI is polio eradication's endgame and legacy. The endgame strategy requires sustained political commitment – even after the last case of polio is identified – in order to maintain polio surveillance and immunisation activities, and eventually to certify the success of global polio eradication.

At the core of this plan is the fundamental need to close the book on polio, which has become a symbolic flag-bearer for global health writ large. Its success or failure is expected to have implications for future disease eradication efforts, global health institutions, the people who work within them, and the ideals which motivate them. Success would be the ultimate show of strength, demonstrating the capacity of the partner organisations, validating the vast investments made, and giving a much-needed injection of confidence. Indeed, polio eradication is one of the most expensive global health projects in history, with 2016 costs totalling nearly US$1 billion – supplied by an array of donors led by the Bill & Melinda Gates Foundation, the US government, Rotary International, and many other country governments and private philanthropists (WHO, 2017). Failure could discourage future investment in such initiatives and undermine the very idea of eradication.

In addition to epidemiological, financial, managerial, and many other factors, maintaining political commitment to eradication at all levels is critical. As seen in the example of Nigeria, countries must be prepared to mount a strong and rapid response in the case of outbreaks, even after being certified polio-free. An unexpected resurgence of the disease after eradication is certified would undermine the credibility of the polio programme. It is therefore necessary to prepare politicians and the public to celebrate certification without letting surveillance and containment falter.

Each step towards global eradication raises the risk of the programme being held hostage by actors who seek to use the global commitment to eradication as an opportunity to leverage other local political ends. At the same time, successful eradication creates the possibility of polio bioterrorism – though it is not considered a likely bioterrorism agent (CDC, 2017), being neither as deadly or fearsome as other pathogens that might be used in this way. Nevertheless, the un-eradication of a disease would deal a serious blow to global health institutions and public and political confidence in them.

The legacy of polio eradication will also reflect upon the outcome of the promise, made in 1988, that polio eradication would contribute to health systems strengthening, and thereby benefit low-income countries which otherwise might not have considered polio eradication to be in their national interest. If this promise goes unfulfilled, it may undermine future efforts at disease eradication, as well as other public health endeavours requiring global commitment to a shared goal.

To some extent it is already possible to estimate the GPEI's impact on national health systems. It is widely agreed, for example, that the surveillance system set up for polio eradication greatly benefitted Nigeria's response to the 2014 Ebola outbreak (IMB, 2014), however, more systematic analyses are necessary for understanding how widespread and sustainable the polio programme's contribution is.

One large mixed-methods analysis (Closser, et al., 2014), focusing on Africa and South Asia, found little quantitative evidence that polio eradication activities were associated with improvements in routine immunisation (as measured through DTP3 coverage). Their qualitative analysis found that polio eradicators had made contributions to national health systems, but these were often built in parallel to routine health programmes, rather than within them. For example, countries had improved disease surveillance systems, but often these were reserved for polio while other diseases were monitored using older, weaker systems; polio vaccinators had created unprecedented maps of marginalised communities, but these were rarely used to deliver any services other than polio vaccination. Cold chain systems stood out as the only significant improvement that was consistently integrated into the wider health system. The greatest improvements, the authors noted, were found in countries which already had relatively strong health systems to begin with.

A more recent set of analyses, focused on seven African countries, found more encouraging evidence that polio surveillance systems were repurposed for priority diseases like measles, yellow fever, cholera, and anthrax (Mwengee, et al., 2016). They noted an increase in routine immunisation coverage in the years since polio activities began, but did not assess whether this was directly attributable to GPEI support, nor whether this was likely to be sustained after eradication. Likewise, they observed that GPEI-funded personnel and resources had been used to benefit other health services, but identified no plans for sustaining these once GPEI funding lapsed (Anya, et al., 2016; Gumede, et al., 2016).

It remains to be seen whether gains beyond polio will be sustained when GPEI funding ends and the networks of international advocacy for polio eradication are relaxed. A study in ten African and South Asian countries found that polio-funded staff were supporting surveillance and routine immunisation, and many expected routine immunisation coverage to suffer if this support disappeared, noting, 'The disparity in pay between polio workers and other health workers also indicates that there is not a clear path to transitioning human resources from the polio eradication effort to other responsibilities' (GPEI, 2015, p. 36). According to this view, the apparent strengthening of health systems is dependent on GPEI's financial support, or at least the equivalent sustained support beyond polio-specific efforts. Only when this support is withdrawn will we know how real and sustained the promised 'value-added' system strengthening of the polio eradication effort turns out to be.

## Conclusion

Polio eradication began with an agreement, made at the most elite levels of international health diplomacy. In this chapter, we tracked this commitment from the halls of power in which it was forged to the local pathways to implementation trod by volunteers and community leaders working to bring the commitment to fruition. We highlight three conclusions that can be drawn from this discussion.

First, the common saying, 'all politics is local', is just as applicable to global health as to any other sphere of politics. Even with an international coalition backing their effort, eradicators have frequently had no choice but to sit down at the negotiation table with the local gatekeepers – priests, politicians, militants, and revolutionaries – to engage their local support in order to achieve the global eradication goal. These negotiations succeeded in many instances because the gatekeepers themselves appreciated the value of health to their communities and followers, and realised that support for the programme could win them praise.

Second, eradication is a high-payoff, high-risk strategy of communicable disease control. In particular, it is a strategy vulnerable to being held hostage by local leaders or other stakeholders, when large sums of money have already been invested and high visibility attained for global goals, which are perceived as inconsistent with local priorities. Among the many considerations that must be taken into account if another disease is selected for eradication, the political contexts and feasibility will need to be assessed, particularly in priority endemic regions. Rather than leaving the most difficult settings for last, it will be important to make a concerted effort to address isolationist enclaves first, and monitor the ebb and flow of conflict situations to take advantage of any windows of opportunity to clear infection from those areas affected by violence and instability.

Finally, a global programme like eradication depends fundamentally on trust. The 'true believers' (Closser, 2010) of polio eradication believe fervently in the power of the international community to be a force for good in the world, but not everyone in the world shares this view. For many, the global order is a menace; a vestige of imperialism that imposes unwanted ideologies under a pretext of humanitarianism. The greater good of polio eradication is not self-evident; rather, each locality judges the GPEI by the amount of good it brings to their community in particular. This makes it a practical necessity, as well as a moral obligation, that eradicators earn their trust the hard way, listening to and answering the needs of the people, if they are to reach their goal.

# References

Abimbola, S., Malik, A.U., and Mansoor, G.F. (2013) 'The final push for polio eradication: addressing the challenge of violence in Afghanistan, Pakistan, and Nigeria', *PLoS Medicine*, 10(10): 1–4, available at https://dx.doi.org/10.1371%2Fjournal.pmed.1001529 (accessed on 15 January 2018).

AFP. (2014) 'Vaccinators refuse to join polio campaign in Jamrud', The Express Tribune, available at http://tribune.com.pk/story/657327/vaccinators-refuse-to-join-polio-campaign-in-jamrud/ (accessed on 2 April 2017).

Afridi, A. (2013) 'Warning shots: polio vaccinator shot dead in Khyber Agency', The Express Tribune, available at http://tribune.com.pk/story/648962/warning-shots-polio-vaccinator-shot-dead-in-khyber-agency/ (accessed on 2 April 2017).

Anya, B.M., Moturi, E., Aschalew, T., Tevi-Benissan, M.C., Akanmori, B.D., Poy, N.A., Mbulu, K.L., Okeibunor, J., Mihigo, R., and Zawaira, F. (2016) 'Contribution of polio eradication initiative to strengthening routine immunization: lessons learnt in the WHO African region', *Vaccine*, 34(43): 5187–92.

Barrett, W.P. (2008) 'March of Dimes' second act', Forbes, available at www.forbes.com/2008/11/19/march-dimes-revinvention-pf-charities08-cx_wb_1119dimes.html (accessed on 2 April 2017).

Bhutta, Z.A. (2014) 'Polio eradication hinges on child health in Pakistan', Nature, 511: 285–7, available at www.nature.com/news/infectious-disease-polio-eradication-hinges-on-child-health-in-pakistan-1.15540 (accessed on 15 January 2018).

Brookes, T. and Khan, O.A. (2007) *The End of Polio?*, Washington, DC: American Public Health Association Press.

Buekens, P.M., Curran, J.W., Finnegan, J.R., Frenk, J., Fried, L.P., Frumkin, H., Goldman, L.R., Heymann, J., Klag, M.J., Philbert, M., Rimer, B.K., and Shortell, S.M. (2013) 'Letter to President Obama', available at www.jhsph.edu/news/news-releases/2013/Klag letter to President Obama.pdf (accessed on 2 April 2017).

Campbell, J. (2004a) 'Nigeria: next steps: political action to restart the Polio Eradication Initiative (PEI)', available at http://wikileaks.org/plusd/cables/04ABUJA1186_a.html (accessed on 2 April 2017).

Campbell, J. (2004b) 'The state of play: Polio Eradication Initiative (PEI)', available at https://wikileaks.org/plusd/cables/04ABUJA1132_a.html (accessed 2 April 2017).

CDC. (2017) 'Bioterrorism agents/diseases', Emergency Preparedness and Response, available at https://emergency.cdc.gov/agent/agentlist.asp (accessed on 31 March 2017).

Closser, S. (2010) *Chasing Polio in Pakistan: Why the world's largest public health initiative may fail*, Nashville, Tennessee: Vanderbilt University Press.

Closser, S., Cox, K., Parris, T.M., Landis, R.M., Justice, J., Gopinath, R., Maes, K., Banteyerga Amaha, H., Mohammed, I.Z., Dukku, A.M., Omidian, P.A., Varley, E., Tedoff, P., Koon, A.D., Nyirazinyoye, L., Luck, M.A., Pont, W.F., Neergheen, V., Rosenthal, A., Nsubuga, P., Thacker, N., Jooma, R., and Nuttall, E. (2014) 'The impact of polio eradication on routine immunization and primary health care: a mixed-methods study.' *The Journal of Infectious Diseases*, 1–10, available at www.ncbi.nlm.nih.gov/pubmed/24690667 (accessed on 1 August 2014).

Closser, S., Jooma, R., Varley, E., Qayyum, N., Rodrigues, S., Sarwar, A., and Omidian, P. (2016) 'Polio eradication and health systems in Karachi: vaccine refusals in context', *Global Health Communication*, 1(1): 32–40.

Closser, S., Rosenthal, A., Maes, K., Justice, J., Cox, K., Omidian, P.A., Mohammed, I.Z., Dukku, A.M., Koon, A.D., and Nyirazinyoye, L. (2016) 'The global context of vaccine refusal: insights from a systematic comparative ethnography of the global polio eradication initiative', *Medical Anthropology Quarterly*. DOI: https://doi.org/10.1111/maq.12254

Crossley, A. (2013) Polio vaccination access in high risk areas of Afghanistan: policy options, masters thesis, London School of Hygiene & Tropical Medicine.

Dawn. (2014) 'Health workers threaten boycott of anti-polio drive in Kohat', Dawn, available at www.dawn.com/news/1112397/health-workers-threaten-boycott-of-anti-polio-drive-in-kohat (accessed on 2 April 2017).

de Quadros, C.A. (2008) 'The whole is greater: how polio was eradicated from the Western hemisphere', In: D, Perlan and A. Roy (Eds.) *From the Practice of International Health: A case orientation*, New York: Oxford University Press, pp. 54–69.

de Quadros, C.A. and Epstein, D. (2002) 'Health as a bridge for peace: PAHO's experience', *The Lancet*, 360(December): 25–6, available at www.thelancet.com/journals/lancet/article/PIIS0140-6736(02)11808-3/fulltext (accessed on 15 January 2018).

Firdous, I. (2013) 'Paralysing virus: 10 fresh polio cases detected in North Waziristan', The Express Tribune, available at http://tribune.com.pk/story/609024/paralysing-virus-10-fresh-polio-cases-detected-in-north-waziristan/ (accessed on 15 January 2018).

Ghinai, I., Willott, C., Dadari, I., and Larson, H.J. (2013) 'Listening to the rumours: what the northern Nigeria polio vaccine boycott can tell us ten years on', *Global Public Health*, 8(10): 1138–50.

GPEI. (2015) 'Polio eradication & endgame midterm review: July 2015', available at http://polioeradication.org/wp-content/uploads/2016/07/GPEI-MTR_July2015.pdf (accessed on 2 April 2017).

Gumede, N., Coulibaly, S.O., Yahaya, A.A., Ndihokubwayo, J., Nsubuga, P., Okeibunor, J., Dosseh, A., Salla, M., Mihigo, R., Mkanda, P., and Byabamazima, C. (2016) 'Polio Eradication Initiative (PEI) contribution in strengthening public health laboratories systems in the African region', *Vaccine*, 34(43): 5164–9.

Hampton, L. (2009) 'Albert Sabin and the Coalition to Eliminate Polio from the Americas', *American Journal of Public Health*, 1(99): 34–44.

IMB. (2013) '8th Report of the Independent Monitoring Board of the Global Polio Eradication Initiative: October 2013', available at www.polioeradication.org/Portals/0/Document/Aboutus/Governance/IMB/9IMBMeeting/9IMB_Report_EN.pdf (accessed on 30 January 2014).

IMB. (2014) '10th Report of the Independent Monitoring Board of the Global Polio Eradication Initiative: October 2014', available at http://polioeradication.org/wp-content/uploads/2016/07/03E.pdf (accessed on 2 April 2017).

International Crisis Group. (2015) 'Winning the War on Polio in Pakistan', Asia Report N°273. International Crisis Group, Avenue Louise 149, 1050 Brussels, Belgium, available at www.crisisgroup.org/file/475/download?token=CE53wMYY (accessed on 17 Oct 2017).

Jegede, A.S. (2007) 'What led to the Nigerian boycott of the polio vaccination campaign?', *PLoS Medicine*, 4(3): e73.

Kaufmann, J.R. and Feldbaum, H. (2009) 'Diplomacy and the polio immunization boycott in Northern Nigeria', *Health Affairs (Project Hope)*, 28(4): 1091–101.

Mach, A. (1999) 'Congo polio immunisation campaign gets go ahead', *BMJ*, 318(March), available at www.ncbi.nlm.nih.gov/pubmed/10082690 (accessed on 15 January 2018).

Muraskin, W. (2012) *Polio Eradication and Its Discontents: A historian's journey through an international public health (Un)Civil War*, Hyderabad: Orient BlackSwan Private Ltd.

Mwengee, W., Okeibunor, J., Poy, A., Shaba, K., Kinuani, L.M., Minkoulou, E., Yahaya, A., Gaturuku, P., Landoh, D.E., Nsubuga, P., Salla, M., Mihigo, R., and Mkanda, P. (2016) 'Polio Eradication Initiative: Contribution to improved communicable diseases surveillance in WHO African region'. *Vaccine*, 34(43): 5170–4, available at http://dx.doi.org/10.1016/j.vaccine.2016.05.060 (accessed on 15 January 2018).

National Primary Health Care Development Agency. (2015) '2016 Nigeria Polio Eradication Emergency Plan', available at http://polioeradication.org/wp-content/uploads/2016/08/3.2_14IMB.pdf (accessed on 15 January 2018).

Obadare, E. (2005) 'A crisis of trust: history, politics, religion and the polio controversy in Northern Nigeria', *Patterns of Prejudice*, 39(3): 265–84, available at www.tandfonline.com/doi/abs/10.1080/00313220500198185 (accessed on 30 January 2014).

Roberts, L. (2013) 'Killings force rethinking of Pakistan's anti-polio drive', *Science*, 339(January): 259–60, available at www.sciencemag.org/content/339/6117/259.short (accessed on 28 August 2014).

Roberts, L. and Van Rooyen, M. (2013) 'Ensuring public health neutrality', *New England Journal of Medicine*, 368: 1073–5, available at www.nejm.org/doi/full/10.1056/NEJMp1300197 (accessed on 28 August 2014).

RUSI. (2014) 'Royal United Services Institute discussion notes', Personal communication, Jennifer Cole.

Shah, S. (2011) 'CIA organised fake vaccination drive to get Osama bin Laden's family DNA', The Guardian, available at www.guardian.co.uk/world/2011/jul/11/cia-fake-vaccinations-osama-bin-ladens-dna/ (accessed on 15 January 2018).

Taylor, S.A.J. (2014) 'Culture and behaviour in mass health interventions: lessons from the global polio eradication initiative', *Critical Public Health*, (July): 1–13, available at www.tandfonline.com/doi/abs/10.1080/09581596.2014.895799 (accessed on 10 July 2014).

*The Express Tribune*. (2014a) 'Collective caution: teachers follow LHWs in polio drive boycott', *The Express Tribune*, available at: http://tribune.com.pk/story/663013/collective-caution-teachers-follow-lhws-in-polio-drive-boycott/ (accessed on 15 January 2018).

*The Express Tribune*. (2014b) 'Unrealised demands: LHWs boycott polio drive in Charsadda', *The Express Tribune*, available at http://tribune.com.pk/story/747332/unrealised-demands-lhws-boycott-polio-drive-in-charsadda/ (accessed on 2 April 2017).

*The Lancet*. (2014) 'Polio eradication: the CIA and their unintended victims', *The Lancet*, 383(9932): 1862, available at www.ncbi.nlm.nih.gov/pubmed/24881975 (accessed on 19 August 2014).

The Task Force for Child Survival. (1988) 'Declaration of Talloires', March, available at www.unicef.org/about/history/files/Talloires_declaration_1988.pdf (accessed on 2 April 2017).

Trofimov, Y. (2010) 'Risky ally in war on Polio: the Taliban', The Wall Street Journal, A1, available at www.wsj.com/articles/SB126298998237022117 (accessed on 15 January 2018).

Ud Din, I., Mumtaz, Z., and Ataullahjan, A. (2012) 'How the Taliban undermined community healthcare in Swat, Pakistan', *BMJ (Clinical research ed.)*, 2093(March): 10–13, available at www.ncbi.nlm.nih.gov/pubmed/22438368 (accessed on 30 January 2014).

WHA. (1988) 'WHA41.28 Global eradication of poliomyelitis by the year 2000', May, available at www.who.int/ihr/polioresolution4128en.pdf (accessed on 2 April 2017).

WHO. (2016) 'Government of Nigeria reports 2 wild polio cases, first since July 2014', Media Centre, available at www.who.int/mediacentre/news/releases/2016/nigeria-polio/en/ (accessed on 31 January 2017).

WHO. (2017) 'Global Polio Eradication Initiative Annual Report 2016', Annual Reports, available at http://polioeradication.org/wp-content/uploads/2017/08/AR2016_EN.pdf (accessed on 16 February 2018).

Yusufzai, A. (2007) 'Impotence fears hit polio drive', BBC, available at http://news.bbc.co.uk/1/hi/world/south_asia/6299325.stm (accessed on 2 April 2017).

Yusufzai, A. (2014) '"Sehat Ka Insaf" a complete health package for KP children', Dawn, available at www.dawn.com/news/1084354 (accessed on 2 April 2017).

Yusufzai, A. (2016) 'Militant attacks on polio workers haunt KP', Dawn, available at www.dawn.com/news/1284090 (accessed on 2 April 2017).

# Part VI
# Intellectual property rights, trade relations, and global health

# 28

# Politics of access to medicines and human rights

*Anand Grover*

Access to essential medicines is an integral component of the Right to Health, which has been explicitly enunciated in a number of international instruments. However, it has been most elaborated under article 12 of the International Covenant on Economic, Social and Cultural Rights (ICESCR). The right to health under article 12 is elaborated by the Committee on Economic, Social and Cultural Rights in General Comment No. 14 (United Nations, 2000). It provides for the right of everyone to the highest attainable standard of physical and mental health. States have an obligation to respect (not interfere with the right itself), protect (prevent interference by others), and fulfil (take all administrative measures) the right to health. It also provides that all health services, goods, and facilities, including medicines, are to be made available, accessible, acceptable, and of good quality. Furthermore, the provision of essential medicines to all persons in a non-discriminatory manner is a core obligation of the state, which would also include ensuring availability and access to quality affordable medicines.

The role of the law in saving lives is evident from the time HIV was wreaking havoc all over the world. Before the mid-1990s there was no treatment for HIV. The mid-1990s saw the advent of triple-combination antiretroviral therapy (ART), which became available in the West immediately, while millions of People Living with HIV (PLHIV) in the developing world could not access ART till much later. During this period, the drugs were priced about US$10,000 per patient annually, denying access to life-saving ART to PLHIV in most developing countries. It was only when developing countries like Brazil took initiative to provide better health care that the movement to make ART more accessible in developing countries began.

When at the turn of the century Indian generic companies announced that they would provide ART at US$350 per patient per annum, accessibility of ART became more possible in the developing countries (McNeil, 2001). The resulting increased competition in the generic market thereon led to a 99 per cent drop in the prices of ARV drugs from 2000–10, to about US$10,000 per patient per annum, providing affordable access to ARVs to millions of people across the world.

Indian generic companies were able to sell ARVs at low prices because the Indian patent law at the time did not recognise product patents on pharmaceutical products. Before 1972, the original Patents Act, 1911 in India, allowed patent protection for both products and processes, allowing the patent holder to exercise absolute monopoly rights and control on both the availability of the drug and its price. One of the main consequences of the 1911 Act was that drug prices in India were amongst the highest in the world. Realising the need to prioritise the public health agenda, after a lot of study, the Patent law in India was amended in 1970, but in a very simple manner. Patent only for process was protected but no patent for pharmaceutical products was allowed. This simple measure allowed generic companies to manufacture drugs through alternative processes. Competition amongst drug companies flourished, and by the 1990s, Indian generic industry was offering the lowest medicine prices in the world. Thus, by the late 1990s, 90 per cent of the ARVs in the developing world were provided by the Indian generics (Waning, et al., 2010). India became the pharmacy of the developing world.

In the early days of the fight for access to ART, Brazil had a major role to play. The 1996 policy of the Brazilian government to provide free ART to PLHIV was instrumental in improving health and providing access to medicines to thousands of Brazilians. This was possible, partly because of the expertise of the Brazil's domestic pharmaceutical industry, which allowed the country to produce generic versions of ARV drugs. Thus, Brazil provided a shining example to the rest of the developing world. Unfortunately, unlike in Brazil, in India the free ARV support for PLHIV was introduced only in 2004, almost ten years after its introduction in Brazil, despite the fact that India had the largest pool of generic companies in the developing world.

At the global level, the Brazilian policy of free access to ART was regularly used as an example to demonstrate that goal of access to medicine is achievable. The '3 by 5' initiative from the WHO, implemented in 2003, is one such instance. In fact, the Doha Declaration, which emphasised on TRIPS flexibility for better access to medicine, is often seen as an acknowledgement of Brazil's policy of free ART. Because of Brazil, the rest of the developing world started free ART thanks to the Global Fund on HIV, TB and Malaria, PEPFAR and UNAIDS.

While protection of pharmaceutical product patent could be excluded earlier, as in India, the TRIPS agreement of 1995 changed all that.[1] Under TRIPS, protection had to be provided to both product and process patents. India and the developing countries agreed to the TRIPS Agreement because of the flexibilities that could be used in their domestic IP Laws. The flexibilities in the TRIPS Agreement were fought for on the basis of public health interests. These flexibilities, amongst others issues, aided the objective of making medicines available at affordable prices. These include allowing members to define their own patentability criteria; the opportunities to challenge patent applications by pre- and post-grant oppositions; revocation; to provide for issuing of compulsory licensing; amongst others.

Exercising this facility provided under TRIPS, in 2005, India used all the flexibilities and amended its patent laws and, amongst other amendments, added a higher standard of patentability to address the evergreening of patents. India found that the experience in the US and EU showed that over 76 per cent of pharmaceutical patents were for new forms of known drugs without any additional therapeutic effect. Such evergreening also allowed for increasing the patent period for the originator companies. So, India amended its patent law and inserted Section 3(d) in the Patents Act. Section 3(d) does not allow patents on new forms of known drugs unless there is significantly more efficacy in the new form as compared to that of the known drug.

Section 3(d) was challenged by Novartis when its patent application on cancer drug 'Gleevec' was rejected by the Madras High Court on the ground of 3(d). Novartis claimed that Section 3(d) violated the TRIPS Agreement and the equality provision in the Indian Constitution. The Madras High Court (2007) rejected the contentions of Novartis and upheld Section 3(d). It held that Section 3(d) was to promote the fulfilment of the right to health obligations of the government. Section 3(d) is crucial for promoting generic competition and reducing the prices of costly drugs by not allowing patenting of new forms of known drugs.

Later, again in the *Novartis* case, the Supreme Court (2013) clarified the scope of Section 3(d) making it clear that it does not apply to physical properties but applied to other properties relating to therapeutic efficacy and the Patent Applicant would have to show in each case that the efficacy was significantly more than that of the known substance.

However, developed countries and powerful multinational corporation (MNC) blocs such as 'Big Pharma' are increasingly focusing on furthering their narrow industry agenda of super profits, forcing developing countries to do away with their laws, which would ensure access to affordable medicines. India, for example, had been facing immense pressure from the US to dilute Section 3(d) of the Patents Act. The pressure is also on countries not to introduce provisions, like Section 3(d). Though it would stand to reason that provisions like 3(d) should be introduced in developing countries, till date only the Philippines and Argentina have introduced provisions similar to Section 3(d) in their patent laws.

Today, access to affordable medicines is under threat from a variety of fronts. The primary danger, as always, is the pressure that the US, the EU, and Japan are exerting on developing countries to dilute their IPR (intellectual property rights) regime through threats of trade sanctions such as US 301, and the introduction of Free Trade Agreements (FTAs) like the North American Free Trade Agreement (NAFTA), the Trans Pacific Partnership Agreement (TPPA), the Regional Comprehensive Economic Partnership (RCEP), and so on. Though the US has withdrawn from negotiations in the TPPA, the deal is being pursued by other countries like Japan, Australia, and South Korea.

All the so-called FTAs have common provisions which seek to extend patent monopolies and restrict competition from generic companies that ultimately allow exorbitant profits to be reaped by the MNCs. These include patent for new or second use, patent term extensions, data exclusivity, limiting oppositions to grant of patents, limiting conditions for issuing compulsory licenses, data exclusivity, patent linkage, enhanced enforcement measures, all of which enhance monopolies and restrict introduction of generic competition in the market and thereby allow the reaping of exorbitant profits by the Patentees.

Most problematic in these FTAs is the inclusion of Investor State Dispute arbitration tribunals. This allows only the private corporations to sue states for doing any act, which would potentially adversely impact on the potential profits of the corporation. It is a one-way street. Pertinently states are not allowed to sue the private corporations. The tribunals are not accountable to any communities and are only a boon for lawyers, who appear for the states and private corporations on a regular basis. There are no appellate procedures. Proceedings, unlike domestic courts, are held in closed door hearings. There are a huge number of disputes pending in the private arbitral tribunals which are set up. These tribunals are totally outside the domestic legal system and are totally unaccountable to the members of the public. A number of awards have been rendered against states, mostly developing countries, awarding millions of dollars against them. Developing countries are now realising the negative impact of such tribunals. States need to review such arbitration agreements and refuse to enter into them.

The access to the new drugs like sofosbuvir for hepatitis C and bedaquiline and delamanid for TB are good examples with which the problems of access to medicines can be illustrated in the present-day scenario.

Sofosbuvir is an effective drug for hepatitis C. Apart from the fact that there is a dispute about the actual entity, which 'invented' sofosbuvir, in respect of which there is an ongoing dispute in the US, the drug does not deserve to be patented. It has been disallowed a patent in Egypt, in Ukraine, and host of other countries. Where it has been granted a patent, like Malaysia, the government rightly issued a compulsory license to make it available to the patients who need the drug. Unfortunately, in India, which boasts of the best patent law for access to medicines, it was patented, but no compulsory license has been issued. Instead Gilead, the patentee in India, has issued voluntary licenses to at least 11 generic companies, making the drug available at about US$900 for a 12-week treatment (Pillai, 2015). There is no genuine competition but controlled access through voluntary licensing.

Voluntary license granted to the generic players in India is the latest tool of the big pharma companies influencing accessibility and affordability of medicines. Because of this, the generic companies are not filing patent oppositions or demanding compulsory licenses. For example, in the case of sofosbuvir in India, the generic companies who filed patent oppositions withdrew them and did not even demand a compulsory license because of the voluntary license offered to them. Though the countries in Latin America and the Middle East and North Africa are most in need of drugs like sofosbuvir, they have not been included in the list of countries to which Indian generic companies having voluntary licenses can export the drug.

Voluntary licenses have passed on the initiative from the state to the private sector and have put the MNCs in the driver's seat to control the accessibility and affordability of medicines. Though this challenge has to be met internationally, unfortunately civil society organisations, which were united at the turn of the century, are now divided over voluntary licenses.

There is a worse story to tell with respect to Multi-Drug Resistant (MDR) TB. India also has the largest number of people living with TB, estimated at 2.7 million. It also has the largest number of people living with MDR TB, at 147,000 (Central TB Division, 2018). New drugs bedaquiline, with the combination of another drug, delamanid, has shown a lot of promise as a new and effective therapy for MDR TB. Bedaquiline and delamanid for adult formulations were added to the WHO Essential Medicines List (EML) for TB in 2015 while delamanid was added to the WHO EML for children in 2017. In India, bedaquiline and delamanid have been patented by Janssen (a division of Johnson and Johnson) and Otsuka respectively. Despite the patent having been granted for both the drugs, they are not available to People Living with MDR TB (PLDTB) in India who desperately need them. They are being given as donations to the Government of India through USAID who get it from Johnson and Johnson, and Otsuka. However, these drugs are made available to only about 1,000 PLDTB when according to independent estimates about 20,000 PLDTB are in need of those drugs in India.

Donations are likely to stop sometime next year. Then, if at all available in the market, the price for a six-month course of bedaquiline in India will be US$900 and an exorbitant US$1,700 for a six-month delamanid course, the price of which is not expected to decrease substantially.

What can the government do? It can issue a 'government use license' under Section 92 of the Indian Patents Act and then invite generic companies to manufacture them. With generic competition, drug prices will fall dramatically and become available to the PLDTB in India who need them at affordable prices. This will be in accord with the TRIPS Agreement, the DOHA Declaration, and the UN High Level Panel on Access to Medicines. However, because of the US government pressure, this is not seen as an option. This would be detrimental to the government's own programme to eliminate TB by 2025, five years ahead of the deadline under the Sustainable Development Goals.

## Conclusion

The framework on the right to health makes it clear that medicines must be available, accessible, acceptable, and of good quality, and reach ailing populations without discrimination throughout the world. Affordable access to medicines cannot be achieved sustainably without sufficient market competition. The need of the hour is for developing countries to utilise and preserve the flexibilities embodied in the TRIPS Agreement in their national laws and prioritise the right to health above all.

In the case of patenting of drugs, which makes the drugs unavailable, inaccessible, or affordable, compulsory licenses, in accordance with law, should be resorted to. This will also cut into the strategy of voluntary licenses which Big Pharma has adopted. For this, the civil society again needs to be united across continents, from Latin America to Europe, Africa and Asia, to challenge the agenda of MNCs of the voluntary license regime, FTAs, and bilateral agreements. This is required so that the state can be back in the driver's seat to make medicine accessible and affordable for its own people.

## Note

1   Though the TRIPS Agreement was entered into 1995, different countries were given different time lines for full compliance depending on their development, and they were categorised into developed (which had to comply with TRIPS one year after 1 January 1995), developing (which had to comply within ten years of 1 January 1995, that is 1 January 2005), and least developed (which had to comply initially in 2006, which was extended to 1 January 2016, and later to 2033).

# References

Central TB Division. (2018) 'India TB report 2018, revised National TB Control Programme, annual status report', Ministry of Health and Family Welfare, available at https://tbcindia.gov.in/showfile.php?lid=3314 (accessed on 3 April 2018).

Madras High Court. (2007) 'Novartis v. Union of India', *Madras Law Journal*, 4: 1153.

McNeil, D.G. (2001) 'Indian company offers to supply AIDS drugs at low costs in Africa', *The New York Times*, available at www.nytimes.com/2001/02/07/world/indian-company-offers-to-supply-aids-drugs-at-low-cost-in-africa.html (accessed on 3 April 2018).

Pillai, V. (2015) 'Natco Pharma gets nod to sell hepatitis C medicine in India', Livemint, available at www.livemint.com/Industry/JdXdj9kUOOmEHFftB1cYTO/Natco-Pharma-gets-nod-to-sell-Hepatitis-C-medicine-in-India.html (accessed on 3 April 2018).

Supreme Court. (2013) 'Novartis Ag v. Union of India, 2013, 6 SCC 1', available at www.supremecourtcases.com/index2.php?option=com_content&itemid=99999999&do_pdf=1&id=43380 (accessed on 3 April 2018).

United Nations. (2000) 'Substantive issues arising in the implementation of the international covenant on economic, social and cultural rights, general comment no. 14', available at http://docstore.ohchr.org/SelfServices/FilesHandler.ashx?enc=4slQ6QSmlBEDzFEovLCuW1AVC1NkPsgUedPlF1vfPMJ2c7ey6PAz2qaojTzDJmC0y%2B9t%2BsAtGDNzdEqA6SuP2r0w%2F6sVBGTpvTSCbiOr4XVFTqhQY65auTFbQRPWNDxL (accessed on 2 April 2018).

Waning, B., Diedrichsen, E., and Moon, S. (2010) 'A lifeline to treatment: the role of Indian generic manufacturers in supplying antiretroviral medicines to developing countries', *Journal of the International AIDS Society*, 13(1): 35.

# 29

# Trading away global health?

## Unravelling the intellectual property, trade, and investment nexus and the impact on the right to health

*Karen van Rompaey*

## Introduction

Paradoxically, in the era of accelerated progress in medical sciences and biotechnology, global health is undermined by inequality within and amongst countries. Universal access to health and medicines is far from being accomplished worldwide. To illustrate this, every year 100 million people are pushed below the poverty line because of health care expenditure (World Health Organization, 2015). An additional 400 million people lack access to health care, including access to medicines (UNSGHLP, 2016). In most developing countries, individuals – instead of health insurances – bear the costs of access to medicines (Velásquez, 2011).

Access to essential medicines is a constitutive element of the right to health (hereafter RTH). States have a legal obligation – as they have ratified several international human rights instruments – to protect, promote, and fulfil the right to the highest attainable standard of physical and mental health of their peoples on an equitable and non-discriminatory basis (UN, 2000). Equality ensures fairness involving that 'people's needs, rather than their social privileges, guide the distribution of opportunities for wellbeing' (World Health Organization, 2002, p. 22).

A human rights approach to access to medicines and health envisages that whilst states have primary responsibility for the progressive realisation of the RTH, individuals, communities, international organisations, nongovernmental organisations, health professional, and private business have responsibilities regarding this right, too (Hunt, 2004). Amongst them, pharmaceutical companies play a key role in the development and distribution of medicines and health technologies in the world (TNI, 2016). Their investment and pricing decisions have a significant impact on access to medicines worldwide. Hence, they need to act with due diligence, preventing and mitigating adverse impacts of their actions on human rights (Ruggie, 2009).

Moreover, access to medicines entails physical accessibility and affordability of drugs (Hunt, 2007). Currently, pharmaceutical research and development (R&D) initiatives are predominantly led by large private companies which are profit driven. Profits are, in turn, ensured by the global intellectual property (IP) regime[1] – which includes the IP related rules under trade and investment agreements – enabling pharmaceutical companies to recoup investments through the exploitation of a patent monopoly for 20 years or more.

On one hand, this market-driven scheme discourages R&D in so-called neglected diseases whose target markets are people living in poverty. This results in a lack of physical accessibility to medicines for the affected populations (t'Hoen, 2005). In 1990, a seminal report by the Commission on Health Research from Development revealed that 10 per cent of funding for R&D was devoted to 90 per cent of the global health issues – the so-called 90/10 gap – showing there is a market failure for diseases primarily affecting the developing world (Milstein and Kaddar, 2006).

On the other hand, where there is a profitable market, for instance in antiretroviral (ARV) drugs to treat HIV/AIDS, the system of patents and the relative inelasticity of demand render drugs highly priced, thus, unaffordable for large groups of the world's population (Hunt, 2004). At a price of US$4,000, ARV treatments are unaffordable for low-income countries (Velásquez, 2011). Another example is related to the treatment of hepatitis C, an epidemic that affects 71 million people worldwide (World Health Organization, 2017). At an estimated production cost for the whole treatment in the range of US$68 to US$136 (Sachs, 2015), the patent holder in the United States sells the treatment at US$84,000, and out of reach for a large number of people (Hill, et. al., 2014).

This work delves into the IP, trade, and investment nexus and the relationship to access to medicines through the prism of the RTH. In so doing, it argues that the RTH for large and vulnerable groups of the world's population is threatened by the current profit-driven IP regime embedded in trade and investment agreements. Underlying the access to medicines' global moral dilemma (Pakes, 2006) is a policy and accountability incoherence regarding the IP regime, human rights international law, and global/national public health goals that urges to be corrected.

This chapter is structured as follows: after the present introduction, the next two sections unravel the evolution and main characteristics of the IP regime and its impact on access to medicines and the RTH. The fourth section discusses the latest attempts at gaining policy coherence between global health and the IP regime to advance access to medicines and global health. The final section presents some concluding remarks.

## The IP regime, access to medicines, and the right to health

At the outset, it is crucial to unpack the relation between the level of economic development and IP protection. In the past, many of the current developed countries established a weak system of patent protection, which paved their way to technological development (Brenner-Beck, 1992; Reidl, 1990). The link between weak protection and industrialisation is given by the 'opportunities it allows for local producers to acquire foreign technology and accumulate production capabilities' (Eren-Vural, 2007, p. 111). In fact, as soon as a sector becomes competitive enough to innovate it starts demanding for stronger IP protection.

Until the 1970s, developing countries benefited from weak/non-patent regimes which were favourable to their industrialisation via import substitution efforts. This, in turn, led to the development of domestic pharmaceutical industries (Eren-Vural, 2007). Consequently, the generics industry flourished which, in turn, brought the prices of medicines down (World Health Organization, 2006) and helped to advance the affordability and accessibility of essential medicines and the progressive realisation of the RTH.

Since the 1980s, the major pharmaceutical companies started lobbying their host governments for stronger patent protection in response to the decline of profit margins. A parallel process of health privatisation took place provoking the fragmentation and multiplication of health actors which, in turn, rendered the articulation of health responses at the international level more difficult (Ingram, 2005). Meanwhile, the global pharma-sector increased its power during the 1990s with the spread of neoliberal globalisation, pushing developed countries to seek to strengthen IP rights through the world trade regime.

During the Uruguay round of multilateral trade negotiations, an agreement on Trade Related Aspects of Intellectual Property Rights (hereafter TRIPS) aimed at harmonising a minimum set of (high) patent protection standards amongst member parties was achieved in 1994. As Rangnekar (2013a) signals, most accounts of the process point to corporate lobby groups informally influencing the TRIPS Agreement, alongside the US dominating the agenda through the threat of trade sanctions. TRIPS became the 'main vehicle for the introduction of medical patents in developing countries' (Cullet, 2005, p. 183) under 'strong surveillance provisions' (Rangnekar, 2007, p. 3).

Although the TRIPS Agreement upgrades patent protection to comply with developed countries' standards, it allows for some flexibilities on public policy and developmental grounds. Flexibilities include the freedom to determine patentability criteria so as to ensure that patents are only awarded for genuine innovation (articles 27.3(a) and 30), as well as provisions for pre- and post-grant opposition and strict disclosure standards. Moreover, article 31 allows for the issuance of compulsory licences (CLs)[2] on public health grounds to ensure access to medicines for all (UNSGHLP, 2016).

As Forman and Kohler (2012) note, concerns about the impact of TRIPS on access to medicines came to the spotlight in the face of the AIDS pandemic, especially in sub-Saharan Africa, and the struggle of millions of people living with HIV to access costly ARV drugs protected under TRIPS' standards. In February 1998, the South African Amendment Act no. 90 was challenged by several multinational pharmaceutical companies. The amendment introduced generic substitution of off-patent medicines, transparent pricing, and the parallel importation of patented medicines in order to increase accessibility and affordability of medicines (t'Hoen, 2005). In 2001, the case was dropped due to increasingly strong opposition promoted by AIDS activists and human rights' campaigners worldwide, and a weak legal position on the part of the pharmaceutical companies (t'Hoen, 2005).

In 2001, the Doha Declaration on TRIPS and Public Health – an initiative of the coalition of developing countries as well as a triumph of NGO advocacy (Rangnekar, 2007) – was agreed upon in the recognition of the gravity of the public health problems afflicting developing countries, such as HIV/AIDS, tuberculosis, malaria, and other epidemics. Paragraph 4 constitutes the core of the Declaration as it clarifies that '(…) the Agreement can and should be interpreted and implemented in a manner supportive of WTO members' right to protect public health and, in particular, to promote access to medicines for all…' (Declaration on the TRIPS Agreement and Public Health, 2001, par. 4).

Paragraph 5 further clarifies that each member has the freedom to determine the grounds upon which CLs are granted and the right to determine what constitutes a national emergency. Since the wording of this article does not provide a closed list of diseases, non-communicable diseases (NCDs) such as heart disease, diabetes, cancer, or others may as well be subject to compulsory licenses (Correa and Matthews, 2011).

Whilst the Doha Declaration clarifies some of the uncertainty in the interpretation of the TRIPS Agreement, it does not address the prohibition of a third country to issue a CL for a developing country with no manufacturing capacity (Cullet, 2005). To address this matter, states negotiated the WTO-Decision 30.08.03, which allows developing and least developed members lacking pharmaceutical manufacturing capacity to grant a CL for the importation of generics on public health grounds. Yet to benefit from the waiver, the country must comply with several conditions. As a result, only a few countries have reformed their legislation to act as potential exporters and it has only been used in one case to supply an ARV from Canada to Rwanda (Correa and Matthews, 2011, p. 21). Despite criticism, WTO members transformed the decision 30.08.03 into a permanent amendment, when two-thirds of the membership accepted it in 2017.

Thus, the TRIPS Agreement poses several threats on access to medicines and the RTH. First, the introduction of patents on pharmaceuticals inexorably leads to higher drug prices, and developing countries cannot afford to pay monopoly prices attached to patents without compromising their level of access to medicines. Second, the shift of resources to the global pharmaceutical sector that followed the introduction of patents has not enabled the much-needed development of drugs on neglected diseases, which mostly affect people living in poverty (Commission on Intellectual Property Rights, 2002).

Third, the current IP regime encourages a process of 'evergreening' patents through artificial improvements which keeps prices high whilst few new treatments are developed. As Rangnekar (2013a, n.p.) puts it, '(p)articularly perverse in pharmaceuticals are patent thickets around a single molecule when minor modifications such as changes in size, colour, dosage, delivery mechanism and composition are either simultaneously or sequentially patented'. To illustrate this, only 15 per cent of drugs approved by the US Food and Drug Authority between 1989 and 2000 were considered 'highly innovative', and over 75 per cent of the patented drugs were modifications of known substances (Grover, 2013). Fourth, enforcement of TRIPS rules impacts negatively on local manufacturing capacity and affects 'generic, innovative, quality drugs on which developing countries depend' (Hestermeyer, 2007, p. 279). All things considered, the TRIPS Agreement represents a 'deliberately retrogressive step' on access to medicines, and, thus, on the realisation of the RTH and ultimately on the right to life (Cullet, 2005, p. 194).

## The political problem: IP rules under post-TRIPS trade agreements and bilateral investment treaties

Developing countries have been strengthening their bargaining positions through a process of social and institutional learning at the WTO (Hurrell and Narlikar, 2006). In so doing, they have gained flexibilities to meet their human rights and development duties. Partly as a result of this, multilateral trade negotiations came to a halt in the 2000s. Instead, a new wave of bilateral free trade agreements (FTAs) and bilateral investment treaties (BITs) were prompted by the US and increasingly the European Union (EU).

In recent years, mega-regional trade and investment agreements such as the Trans Pacific Partnership and the Transatlantic Trade and Investment Partnership, as well as Economic Partnership Agreements (EPAs) 'are largely overshadowing the deadlocked WTO negotiating process' (McNeill, et al., 2017, p. 760). All of these agreements enforce or aim to enforce stricter IP regulations between parties than those negotiated at the multilateral level.

According to Correa (2017), provisions contained in these FTAs can be categorised either as TRIPS*plus*, because they expand existing obligations under the TRIPS Agreement, or TRIPS*extra*, when they introduce issues not addressed by the TRIPS Agreement. Moreover, they do not always provide for the full range of flexibilities offered by the TRIPS Agreement with regard to CLs, revocation of patents or the option to exclude the patentability of plant and animal varieties (Liberti, 2010).

Additional obligations contained in these agreements include: extension of patent terms due to delays in the examination of a patent application or in the marketing approval for a drug; patent 'administrative linkage' that prevents the marketing approval of generics when patents of the original drug exist; patents for second indications of known pharmaceuticals; test data exclusivity periods; stricter enforcement provisions such as retention at the custom of medicines for import, export, or in transit on suspicion of infringement of a patent (Correa and Matthews, 2011).

Finally, several academic studies and UN documents have signalled the negative impact of FTAs in relation to access to medicines (Correa, 2017). All TRIPS*plus* and TRIPS*extra* provisions delay the production of generics and hinder access to affordable medicines, especially by the poor and in developing countries, thus undermining the progressive realisation of the RTH (Correa, 2017).

Less studied in the academic literature are the IP-related aspects of bilateral investment treaties (BITs) and investment chapters of FTAs and EPAs. BITs that define IP as a covered investment can also lead to strengthened IP protection 'through the unqualified operation of "Most-Favoured-Nation" and "National Treatment" obligations and expropriation provisions' contained in these agreements (Liberti, 2010, p. 8).

Through an IP rights lens, it could be argued that a CL granted for public health reasons for domestic use or for export needs to be compensated as it represents an investment expropriation. Following this reasoning, parallel imports of a generic drug could damage the value of the investment or diminish a patent holder's market share, which would also need compensation. To avoid this wrongful interpretation, some post-TRIPS FTAs have explicitly excluded from the expropriation provisions the issuance of CLs granted in relation to IP rights in accordance with the TRIPS Agreement (Liberti, 2010).

Hence, if a CL is to be invoked under BITs and post-TRIPS FTAs, investors could bring the developing country to international arbitration to dispute the quantum of compensation as well as the decision to grant the license itself. Because international 'arbitrators tend to defend private investor rights above public interest, revealing an inherent pro-corporate bias' (Eberhardt and Olivet, 2012, p. 8), this could lead to a ruling in favour of IP rights, thus, hindering access to medicines and the RTH of the people living in the sued country.

Finally, since trade and investment generate winners and losers in each country, it is of utmost importance to compensate the losing sectors/communities. This is unlikely to happen in developing countries which enter bilateral or regional agreements with developed countries, due to restricted domestic budgets. FTAs and BITs produce both positive and negative effects on the conditions in which people live, work, and die. In these types of agreements, the negative effects on the social determinants of health are significant, yet indirect and harder to measure (McNeill, et al., 2017).

Therefore, the signature of a FTA or BIT with TRIPS*plus* and TRIPS*extra* provisions that hinder access to medicines results in a violation of article 12 of the International Covenant on Economic, Social and Cultural Rights (ICESCR), which requires states to take positive measures towards the fulfilment of the RTH, including ensuring access to medicines for all. All of this suggests that despite articulated efforts of developing countries and civil society, post-TRIPS agreements are 'rewriting the rules that govern the global economy, promoting corporate interests at the expense of public health priorities' (McNeill, et al., 2017, p. 760).

## The political remedy: embedding the RTH and TRIPS flexibilities in national legislations

There is a growing recognition that access to medicines and the progressive realisation of the RTH are hindered by the existing policy incoherence between the IP regime, human rights international law, and (global) public health. Incoherence becomes apparent in divergent goals and different accountability mechanisms (UNSGHLP, 2016).

On one hand, the global IP regime has been erected to protect rights which are personal and corporate entitlements. Their goal is to protect material interests arising from an invention/creation which are granted for a fixed term, and can be subject to exploitation (Verma, 2007). This is so for all inventions, including medicines and medicine development processes, irrespective of the disease burden or level of development of countries (Forman and Kohler, 2012).

This leads to a tension between exclusive protection through monopolies, on one hand, and development goals through public-oriented dissemination and competition, on the other (Verma, 2007). In the case of patents for medicines, there is a further conflict between the expectations of the pharmaceutical industry to recover investments, and the need of the government to keep the cost of health under control (Cullet, 2005). Arguably, the pharmaceutical industry needs the incentives provided by a system of patent protection as it invests significantly in R&D whilst it is easy to copy a new drug (Cullet, 2005). However, FORBE's numbers show that with a profit margin of around 20 per cent, patent monopolies outstrip their original purpose, since the pharmaceutical industry is the world's most profitable industry (Anderson, 2014).

In turn, states have an obligation to protect the RTH of their people. Furthermore, in 2015 they committed themselves to achieve 17 Sustainable Development Goals by 2030. Through the third Sustainable Development Goal, states are committed to ensure healthy lives and promote well-being for all ages by 2030. To do so, they need to end the epidemics of AIDS, tuberculosis, malaria and neglected tropical diseases, and combat hepatitis, water-borne diseases, and other communicable diseases. Additionally, they are to reduce by one-third premature mortality from NCDs through prevention and treatment, and promote mental health and well-being, amongst other health targets (United Nations General Assembly, 2015). All of this will imply that states ensure access to affordable medicines for all.

However, the current profit-driven IP regime, which is disconnected from historical, social, political, and economic factors of countries (Rangnekar, 2013b, p. 39), is hampering the production of generics and, thus, hindering affordable medicines as well as investment in R&D in neglected diseases. The fact that waivers to pharmaceutical patents provided in TRIPS and the Doha Declaration are granted only under health emergencies, on a product-by-product, time-bound, and *ad-hoc* basis, is unsatisfactory from the perspective of the RTH. This is so 'in so far as the central concern of health is consistently framed as an exception to a property right' (Cullet, 2005, p. 193) and not as a fundamental right to be promoted, protected, and fulfilled over profit concerns.

On the other hand, trade and investment treaties are generally negotiated in secret, making it difficult for civil society, health authorities, and citizens to assess plausible impacts and hold negotiators to account. Moreover, their IP related accountability mechanisms are regulated by dispute settlement bodies whose rulings are binding for Member Parties. Furthermore, there is a lack of accurate and up-to-date information on existing and expired patents, which obscures governments' procurement decisions and delays generic manufacturing. In contrast, accountability mechanisms for both human rights and public health have 'limited degrees of precision, legal weight and enforceability' (UNSGHLP, 2016, p. 9).

There is an urgent need to achieve a humanitarian IP system (Rangnekar, 2013b). Although the Doha Declaration was a step forward in the right direction, 15 years after its launching, developing countries still lag behind in relation to access to essential medicines, and thus, the progressive realisation of the RTH of their peoples. The Declaration has not led to an increased use of TRIPS flexibilities. The explanation for this is manifold. First, many countries adjusted their IP legislations – without fully realising the impacts of TRIPS on access to medicines and the RTH – before the end of the transitional period for developing countries[3] and prior to the Doha Declaration (Correa and Matthews, 2011). Second, given the sensitivity of IP issues, states have been reluctant to review the adopted legislation to incorporate flexibilities not present in the existing legislation (Correa and Matthews, 2011). Third, some developing countries lacked technical assistance to embed the full range of TRIPS flexibilities in their national IP laws (Matthews, 2005).

In the light of this, both the Special Rapporteur on the RTH (Correa, 2017) and the United Nations' Secretary General's High Level Panel on Access to Medicines established in 2015 recommended that developing countries (re)adjust their laws and policies to make full use of the flexibilities allowed by the TRIPS Agreement. Moreover, national patent laws should be adjusted in the spirit and letter of the Doha Declaration to facilitate the issuance of CLs in an efficient, fair, predictable, and practical way on legitimate public health interests to ensure access to essential medicines (UNSGHLP, 2016).

Developing countries that did amend their national patent legislation accordingly have improved their stance on access to medicines. For instance, through the introduction of Section 3(d) of the Indian Patents Act of 2005 (third amendment), India found a way to avoid the evergreening of drugs. Section 3(d) states that the mere discovery of a new form of a known substance is not to be considered an invention. Moreover, in 2013 the Indian Supreme Court ruled against claims for a patent in India on the grounds of Section 3(d) (Rangnekar, 2013a). Similarly, China amended its patent law in 2010 introducing the standard of absolute novelty, the 'research or Bolar exception', and provisions on CLs to be produced and consumed in China or to export it to a developing country without manufacturing capacity (Correa and Matthews, 2011).

The UN High Level Panel further recommended that governments which engage in trade and investment negotiations need to conduct a global impact assessment to evaluate the costs and benefits as well as a public health impact assessment prior to signing the treaty. They moreover should refuse any provisions in the treaty that could interfere with their obligations to fulfil the RTH. To increase their level of accountability they should avoid conducting the negotiations in secret and disclose the results of the impact assessments (UNSGHLP, 2016).

To shield their obligations towards public health and human rights, states need to mainstream the RTH in all relevant national and international policy-making processes (Hunt, 2004). Once domestic constitutional and legal provisions on the RTH are in place, they shall elaborate a list of essential medicines to define their minimum needs which has to be updated in consultation with stakeholders (Hogerzeil, 2006). Essential medicines should be made available on an affordable and non-discriminatory basis to all. To do so, both the 'judicial' and the 'policy' approach to human rights need to be pursued. Whereby the judicial approach is a way for individuals to make governments honour their commitments on the RTH via the courts or *ombud* processes, the policy approach is an attempt at gaining policy space for development and international solidarity for the realisation of the RTH globally. It moreover provides (developing) countries with the moral and legal basis to enhance their physical accessibility and affordability of medicines much needed to improve global health (Hunt, 2004).

Finally, competition law is another way to enhance access to medicines. The legal and political umbrella for this is article 31(k) of the TRIPS Agreement which enables CL to be granted on grounds of remedying anti-competitive abuses, such as excessive pricing, refusals to license, or the denial of an essential facility. Moreover, claims could be triggered either by governments themselves, competitors, and eventually patients and civil society (Correa and Matthews, 2011).

## Conclusions

This chapter has sought to demonstrate that the current IP regime is undermining states' capacities – in particular of low- and middle-income countries – to maintain and increase their access to medicines, needed to fulfil the RTH of their peoples. Local production and export of generic drugs – which had flourished under the weak/no patent system until the 1980s – faced increasing obstacles as a result of the adoption of the TRIPS Agreement which enforced stricter IP protection standards globally.

Because most developing countries – with the exception of LDCs – reformed their patent laws to comply with TRIPS in the aftermath of the agreement and before realising its global impact on access to medicines, they did not incorporate the full range of flexibilities offered by the multilateral agreement.

In 2001, developing countries completed the negotiation of the Doha Declaration to clarify some of the flexibilities contained in the TRIPS Agreement regarding public health. Under the TRIPS Agreement, CLs are permitted on a case-by-case, time-bound, and local basis, provided that an adequate remuneration is given to the patent holder on the grounds of health emergencies. A cumbersome mechanism was later established for developing countries with no manufacturing capacity to import more affordable generic drugs.

Yet, with the halt of multilateral trade negotiations, further attempts at strengthening IP rules through the signing of FTAs and BITs and the negotiation of mega regional FTAs were advanced. These agreements produce more harmful direct and indirect effects over access to medicines and the realisation of the RTH.

Hence, the global IP regime which crystallised in TRIPS and beyond rendered medicines more expensive under patent monopolies. This profit-driven system is not succeeding in expanding the much-needed R&D of drugs for tropical diseases affecting the world's poor. Moreover, countries still suffer from external and internal political pressures if they try to issue compulsory licenses. All this hinders equal access to medicines and results in a violation of the RTH, and ultimately the right to life of large and vulnerable sectors of the world's population.

To conclude, there is a need to correct the policy and accountability incoherence between the IP regime, international human rights law, and global health. This can be achieved by embedding and making the most use of the full scope of TRIPS flexibilities into national IP laws. When negotiating FTAs or BITs, states should avoid secrecy as well as any IP clauses that deny the letter and spirit of the Doha Declaration. They ought to conduct and disclose health and global impact assessments prior to entering FTAs and make use of anti-competitive laws to avoid excessive pricing of medicines. Additionally, mainstreaming the RTH in all national constitutions will also grant governments – in particular of developing countries – with the moral and legal basis to enhance their physical accessibility and affordability of medicines much needed to improve global health.

## Notes

1 Regimes have been defined as social institutions around which actor expectations converge in a given area of international relations. They consist of principles, norms, rules, and procedures (Ruggie, 1982).
2 Compulsory licensing is the mechanism by which a state allows the production of a patented medicine or process without the consent of the patent holder but for an adequate compensation defined by the state itself. In the TRIPS Agreement, compulsory licensing is allowed only after negotiations with the patent holder proceeded, unless there is a situation of national emergency or the state wants to make public non-commercial use of the object of patent, on a case-by-case basis.
3 Developing countries were given a transition period until the year 2000 to adjust their national IP legislation to comply with TRIPS provisions. In recognition of their vulnerability, the TRIPS Council extended the transition period for least developed countries (LDCs) until 2016. In 2015, the Council decided to further extend the transition until January 2033 or when a country graduates from the least developed category.

## References

Anderson, R. (2014) 'Pharmaceutical industry gets high on fat profits', *BBC News*, available at www.bbc.com/news/business-28212223 (accessed on 6 October 2017).

Brenner-Beck, D. (1992) 'Do as I say, not as I do', UCLA Pacific Basin Law Journal, 11: 84–118.

Commission on Intellectual Property Rights. (2002) 'Integrating intellectual property rights and development policy', available at www.iprcommission.org/papers/pdfs/final_report/CIPRfullfinal.pdf (accessed on 6 January 2017).

Correa, C. (2017) 'Mitigating the regulatory constraints imposed by intellectual property rules under free trade agreements', research paper no. 74, South Centre.

Correa, C. and Matthews, D. (2011) 'The Doha Declaration ten years on and its impact on access to medicines and the right to health', discussion paper, available at www.undp.org/content/dam/undp/library/hivaids/Discussion_Paper_Doha_Declaration_Public_Health.pdf (accessed on 5 May 2017).

Cullet, P. (2005) 'Patents and medicines: the relationship between TRIPS and the human right to health', In: S. Grunskin, M. Grodin, G. Annas, and S. Marks (Eds.) *Perspectives on Health and Human Rights*, New York: Routledge, pp. 179–202.

Declaration on the TRIPS Agreement and Public Health (2001) WT/MIN(01)/DEC/2, 20, Ministerial Conference, fourth session, Doha, 9–14 November 2001.

Eberhardt, P. and Olivet, C. (2012) 'Profiting from injustice', available at www.tni.org/files/download/profiting frominjustice.pdf (accessed on 26 June 2017).

Eren-Vural, I. (2007) 'Domestic contours of global regulation: understanding the policy changes on pharmaceutical patents in India and Turkey', *Review of International Political Economy*, 14(1): 105–42.

Forman, L. and Kohler, J. (2012) 'Introduction: access to medicines as a human right – What does it mean for pharmaceutical industry responsibilities?', In: L. Forman and J.C. Kohler (Eds.) *Access to Medicines as a Human Right Implications for Pharmaceutical Industry Responsibility*, Toronto: University of Toronto Press, pp. 3–23.

Grover, A. (2013) 'Analysing the Supreme Court Judgment', *Economic & Political Weekly*, 48(32).

Hestermeyer, H. (2007) *Human Rights and the WTO: The case of patents and access to medicines*, Oxford: Oxford University Press.

Hill, A., et. al. (2014) 'Minimum costs for producing Hepatitis C direct acting antivirals, for use in large-scale treatment access programs in developing countries', *Clinical Infectious Diseases*, 58(7): 928–36.

Hogerzeil, H. (2006) 'Essential medicines and human rights: what can they learn from each other?', *Bulletin of the World Health Organisation*, 84(5): 371–5.

Hunt, P. (2004) 'The right of everyone to the enjoyment of the highest attainable standard of physical and mental health', available at www.who.int/medicines/areas/human_rights/E_CN_4_2004_49_Add_1.pdf (accessed on 30 May 2017).

Hunt, P. (2007) 'Neglected diseases: a human rights analysis', available at www.who.int/tdr/publications/publications/seb_topic6.htm (accessed on 12 April 2008).

Hurrell, A. and Narlikar, A. (2006) 'A new politics of confrontation? Brazil and India in multilateral trade negotiations', *Global Society*, 20(4): 415–33.

Ingram, A. (2005) 'Global leadership and global health: contending meta-narratives, divergent responses, fatal consequences', *International Relations*, 19(4): 381–402.

Liberti, L. (2010) 'Intellectual property rights in international investment agreements: an overview', available at www.oecd.org/daf/inv/investment-policy/WP-2010_1.pdf (accessed on 10 June 2017).

Matthews, D. (2005) 'TRIPS flexibilities and access to medicines in developing countries: the problem with technical assistance and free trade agreements', *European Intellectual Property Review*, 28(11): 420–27.

McNeill, D., Deere Birkbeck, C., Fukuda-Parr, S., Grover, A., Schrecker, T., and Stuckler, D. (2017) 'Political origins of health inequities: trade and investment agreements', *The Lancet*, 389: 760–2.

Milstein, J. and Kaddar, M. (2006) 'Managing the effect of TRIPS on availability of priority vaccines', *Bulletin of the World Health Organisation*, 84: 360–5.

Pakes, B. (2006) 'Public health ethics and intellectual property policy', *Bulletin of the World Health Organisation*, 84(5): 341.

Rangnekar, D. (2007) 'Context and ambiguity: a comment on amending India's Patent Act', CSGR working paper, available at www2.warwick.ac.uk/fac/soc/csgr/research/workingpapers/2007/wp2240 7.pdf (accessed on 3 May 2008).

Rangnekar, D. (2013a) 'Novartis firmly put in place' available at www.hardnewsmedia.com/2013/07/5983?page=show (accessed on 14 May 2017).

Rangnekar, D. (2013b) 'The Supreme Court judgment: "lawmaking" in the south', *Economic and Political Weekly*, 48(32), available at www.epw.in/journal/2013/32/glivec-precedent-special-issues/supreme-court-judgment.html (accessed on 20 March 2018).

Reidl, R. (1990) 'A brief history of the pharmaceutical industry in Basel', In: J. Liebenau, G.J. Higby, and E.C. Straud (Eds.) *Pill Peddlers: Essays on the history of the pharmaceutical industry*. Madison, WI: American Institute of the History of Pharmacy.

Ruggie, J. (1982) 'International regimes, transactions, and change: embedded liberalism in the postwar economic order', *International Organization*, 36(2): 379–415.

Ruggie, J. (2009) 'Business and human rights: towards operationalizing the "protect, respect and remedy" framework: report of the special representative of the Secretary-General on the issue of human rights and transnational corporations and other business enterprises', available at www.ivr.uzh.ch/institutsmitglieder/kaufmann/archives/HS09/vorlesungen/Text-13.pdf (accessed on 20 March 2018).

Sachs, J. (2015) 'The drug that is bankrupting America', available at www.huffingtonpost.com/jeffrey-sachs/the-drug-that-is-bankrupt_b_6692340.html (accessed on 15 June 2017).

t'Hoen, E. (2005) 'TRIPS, pharmaceutical patents, and access to essential medicines: a long way from Seattle to Doha', In: S. Gruskin, M.A. Grodin, G.J. Annas, and S.P. Marks (Eds.) *Perspectives on Health and Human Rights*, New York: Routledge, pp. 203–22.

TNI. (2016) 'Hold TNCs responsible for violating a human right if they block access to medicines', available at www.tni.org/en/publication/hold-tncs-responsible-for-violating-a-human-right-if-they-block-access-to-medicines (accessed on 15 May 2017).

United Nations General Assembly. (2015) 'Transforming our world: the 2030 agenda for sustainable development', available at www.un.org/ga/search/view_doc.asp?symbol=A/RES/70/1&Lang=E, (accessed on 16 June 2017).

UNSGHLP (United Nations Secretary General High-Level Panel on Access to Medicines). (2016) 'Promoting innovation and access to health technologies', available at https://static1.squarespace.com/static/562094dee4b0d00c1a3ef761/t/57d9c6ebf5e231b2f02cd3d4/1473890031320/UNSG+HLP+Report+FINAL+12+Sept+2016.pdf (accessed on 13 June 2017).

Velásquez, G. (2011) 'The right to health and medicines: the case of recent Negotiations on the Global Strategy on Public Health Innovation and Intellectual Property', research paper 35, available at http://apps.who.int/medicinedocs/documents/s21392en/s21392en.pdf (accessed on 3 June 2017).

Verma, S.K. (2007) 'Seminar on intellectual property rights, globalization and related issues', Department of Economics, University of Delhi.

World Bank. (2006) 'Vaccine-preventable diseases', available at http://files.dcp2.org/pdf/expressbooks/vaccine.pdf (accessed on 4 May 2008).

World Health Organization. (2002) '25 questions & answers on health and human rights', *Health & Human Rights Publication Series*.

World Health Organization. (2006) 'Essential medicines and health products', available at www.who.int/medicines/services/essmedicines_def/en/ (accessed on 17 June 2017).

World Health Organization. (2015) 'Health and human rights fact sheet', available at www.who.int/mediacentre/factsheets/fs323/en (accessed on 11 June 2017).

World Health Organization. (2017) 'Cancer factsheet', available at www.who.int/mediacentre/factsheets/fs297/en/ (accessed on 18 June 2017).

# 30

# Will the amendment to the TRIPS Agreement enhance access to medicines?

*Carlos Correa*

## Introduction

After the entry into force of the Agreement on Trade Related Aspects of Intellectual Property Rights ('TRIPS Agreement'), all members of the World Trade Organization (WTO) were obliged to grant patents on pharmaceutical products. As a result, generic producers that in some countries were formerly able to supply low-cost generic pharmaceuticals to local and foreign markets could not continue to reverse engineer and sell new, patented drugs. This new scenario affected not only the producing countries, but also those importing generic drugs that were left with the only option of purchasing them from the patent owner, often at unaffordable prices. While those countries could issue compulsory licenses, their grant would not provide a solution if there was no manufacturing capacity in the country and the needed pharmaceuticals could not be imported from low-cost producers. The TRIPS Agreement did not allow the granting of compulsory licenses for exports only, thereby preventing generic manufacturers from eventually exporting the required products to countries unable to produce them.

The problem created by the limitations imposed by the TRIPS Agreement was addressed, in the context of the WTO, through paragraph six of the Doha Declaration on the TRIPS Agreement and Public Health (hereinafter 'the Doha Declaration'), which instructed the Council for TRIPS 'to find an expeditious solution' to address this serious public health problem: if a medicine is patented in a country where there is insufficient or no manufacturing capacities in the pharmaceutical sector, and the medicine is unavailable (because of high prices or other reasons) granting a compulsory license (that is, authorising a third party to produce and sell the medicine against payment of a remuneration to the patent owner) becomes ineffective, since the medicine might not be produced anyway (Thapa, 2011). It could be exported from a country where such manufacturing exists, but paragraph (f) of article 31 of the TRIPS Agreement banned the grant of a compulsory license for export only.

Hence, the country in need of a medicine would be in a trap: it will be unable to ensure the supply of the needed medicine, even if the medicine were available and could actually be sold by the patent owner (or its licensees). Importantly, this situation may arise even in countries where a medicine is not protected by any patents, such as in the case of least developed countries (LDCs), which were temporarily exempted from complying with the TRIPS Agreement under article 66.2 of said agreement. The initial transitional period of ten years was subsequently extended; it will expire on 1 January 2033 for pharmaceuticals, unless renewed again.

In fact, many developing countries and LDCs cannot produce either active ingredients or formulations, due to lack of technological capacity, equipment, human resources, or simply because domestic production would not be economically viable, especially when the markets are small and economies of scale cannot be realised.

This is the problem the Council for TRIPS was instructed to deal with and solve. It took the WTO members more than one and a half years to strike an agreement: a decision was adopted by the WTO General Council on 30 August 2003 (hereinafter 'the WTO Decision').

Significantly, the problem addressed under Paragraph six of the Doha Declaration is not the unavailability of a particular medicine but the effects of the monopoly created by patents and the conduct of the patent owner. The system developed by the WTO Decision (hereinafter 'the system') is meant to apply in a scenario where the world supply of a patented product is controlled by the owner of one or more patents (often a large number of patents are obtained around a single active ingredient) and, therefore, no alternative supply of *generic* products is available (Correa, 2014). The use of that system becomes necessary because the patent owner refuses to supply a patented product in a country (with insufficient or no manufacturing capacity in pharmaceuticals) at an affordable price or under other conditions that the demanding country cannot meet.

Paragraph six addressed the described problem by adopting two 'waivers' in respect of the obligations set out in article 31 paragraph (f), regarding the ban to grant compulsory licenses exclusively to export, and paragraph (h), regarding the obligation to pay a remuneration to the patent owner in the country where the medicines are imported. A waiver under WTO rules can be granted 'in exceptional circumstances' and allows a member not to comply with certain obligations; it must be reviewed annually by the WTO Conference (article 9.4 of the Agreement Establishing the WTO). The WTO Decision that adopted these waivers provided for an annual reporting on the operation of the system set out, and stipulated that the waivers would be terminated on the date on which an amendment to the TRIPS Agreement replacing its provisions takes effect for a member.

An agreement to amend the TRIPS Agreement by incorporation (as article 31*bis*) of the text of the decision was reached in December 2005, subject to further approval by two-thirds of the WTO members, as requested by the WTO rules (article X(3) of the Agreement Establishing the WTO). The process of approval demanded ten years, an extremely long period as compared, for instance, to that required for the approval of the Trade Facilitation Agreement (TFA), which entered into force a little more than three years after its adoption.

## The compulsory license system

The process leading to the adoption of the Doha Declaration was highly controversial, particularly due to the initial opposition by the US government and pharmaceutical industry. Its adoption was a significant achievement for developing countries, as it recognised the 'gravity' of the public health problems afflicting many developing and LDCs, confirmed the 'flexibilities' allowed under the TRIPS Agreement (such as compulsory licenses and parallel imports), and, although it specifically referred to HIV/AIDS, tuberculosis and malaria, it covered all diseases, including non-communicable diseases (Correa and Matthews, 2011).

The negotiation and adoption of the WTO Decision (often called 'the paragraph six solution') was equally, or perhaps even more, controversial. In particular, the US rejection to a broad scope for the system to be established – covering all diseases and not just malaria, tuberculosis, and HIV/AIDS – significantly delayed the conclusion of an agreement. A final compromise was reached upon issuance by the chair of the WTO General Council of a 'statement' intended to further expand some of the conditions established to export a pharmaceutical product under the compulsory license system (Correa, 2004).

In order to use the system, a potential importing country must send a notification to the Council for TRIPS:

(i) specifying the names and expected quantities of the pharmaceutical product(s) needed;

(ii) confirming (unless the importing country is an LDC) that it has insufficient or no manufacturing capacities in the pharmaceutical sector for the product(s) in question; and

(iii) confirming that, where a pharmaceutical product is patented in its territory, it has granted or intends to grant a compulsory license in accordance with Article 31 of the TRIPS Agreement and the provisions of the WTO Decision. Complying with this condition would mean, *inter alia*, that a prior request of a voluntary license needs to be made to the patent owner (unless grounds of extreme urgency or anti-competitive practices were invoked or the non-commercial public use of the patent/s decided) and, only if refused or deemed to be refused, a compulsory license can be subsequently granted. (WTO, 2003, n.p.)

In addition, the potential supplier of the required product should seek a voluntary license from the patent owner on commercially reasonable terms to produce the required drug in the exporting country and, once refused or deemed to be refused, submit to the competent authorities an application for the grant of a compulsory license, which will be subject to a number of conditions:

(i) only the amount necessary to meet the needs of the eligible importing Member(s) may be manufactured under the license and the entirety of this production shall be exported to the Member(s) which has notified its needs to the Council for TRIPS;

(ii) the products manufactured under the license shall be clearly identified through specific labelling or marking. Suppliers should distinguish such products through special packaging and/or special colouring/shaping of the products themselves, 'provided that such distinction is feasible and does not have a significant impact on price'; and

(iii) before shipment begins, the licensee shall post on a website the following information:
  • the quantities being supplied to each destination; and
  • the distinguishing features of the products;

(iv) a remuneration must be paid to the patent owner in accordance with article 31(h) of the TRIPS Agreement. (WTO, 2003, n.p.)

These conditions must be fulfilled over and over even if the same importing country requests an additional quantity of the same product, since only the amount necessary to meet the needs initially notified by the importing country may be manufactured under the license.

Two additional notifications to the Council for TRIPS are needed. On one hand, prior to using the system as prescribed, an interested country (unless it is an LDC) must notify of its intention to use the system as an importer. Significantly, not a single notification for this purpose has been made so far in accordance with the WTO 'Dedicated page' on the WTO Decision.

On the other hand, if a compulsory license has been granted, the exporting country is bound to notify of the grant of the license and the conditions attached to it, including the name and address of the licensee, the product(s) for which the license has been granted, the quantity for which it has been granted, the country to which the product is to be supplied, the duration of the license, and the address of the website where the licensee will post the information required about the quantities and features of the products.

It is also to be noted that the implementation of the WTO Decision or article 31*bis* may require some changes in national patent laws if they only provide for the granting of compulsory licenses for the manufacture of patented subject matter, and not for importation. More importantly, since most countries introduced in their legislation the limitation imposed by article 31 (f) of the TRIPS Agreement (that is, compulsory licenses may be granted only to supply 'predominantly' the domestic market), they would not be able to grant compulsory licenses exclusively for export to countries without sufficient manufacturing capacity in pharmaceuticals, unless the national law is amended accordingly. So far only Canada, the

European Union, the Netherlands, Norway, India, China, Switzerland, and Australia seem to have amended their legislation accordingly. Out of these countries, only India and China would have the potential to supply pharmaceutical products, including active ingredients, at low cost under the established export/import system.

The required notifications and the nature of the information required – plus the obligation to adopt measures to avoid the 'diversion' of the products to other countries – would seem more suitable for the export of weapons or dangerous materials than for products to address public health needs. The adoption of the WTO Decision, and later of the amendment to the TRIPS Agreement, was described by the WTO as a proof that this organisation 'can handle humanitarian concerns' (WTO, 2003) and as 'an extremely important amendment … that helps the most vulnerable access the drugs that meet their needs, helping to deal with diseases such as HIV/AIDS, tuberculosis or malaria, as well as other epidemics' (WTO, 2017, n.p.).

However, the procedural burden imposed on governments and potential suppliers to deal with an essentially humanitarian issue has raised significant criticism from academics, non-governmental organisations (NGOs) and potential suppliers, and scepticism about the effectiveness of the adopted 'solution'.

The scholars' prevailing view has been summarised as follows:

> Among the scholars, it is a common view that the Decision will create more hurdles than solution to paragraph 6 problem of the Doha Declaration. It is saddled with many administrative pre-requisites, which will hamper the very purpose of the Para 6 System. A country in need of required drugs to meet the health emergency, and lacking manufacturing capacity will have to go through many layers of procedure … All these measures not only will delay the manufacture and supply but increase the cost of the drugs. Decision is termed to be a temporary solution which is difficult to operate. It is considered not faithful to Doha Declaration on TRIPS and Public Health.
>
> *Verma, 2006, pp. 90–1*

The practical hurdles that, in particular, a potential supplier would have to face under the system have been highlighted in some of the academic literature. For instance, Cohen-Kohler, et al. (2007) have noted the need to negotiate a voluntary license with potentially multiple patent holders (which is a lengthy, complex, and expensive process), that the quantity of the license is limited to that which was originally applied for by the country, and that there is heavy front-end investment and little incentive, particularly if a company would need to adjust and/or increase their manufacturing infrastructure for products which are not normally part of their product portfolio.

The view of many NGOs is exemplified by a statement of Doctors Without Borders (MSF) – a humanitarian organisation that was awarded the Nobel Prize in 1999. It noted that,

> The Decision flies in the face of the practical reality of managing a health programme, where flexibility and rapidity of response to ever-changing circumstances are vital. It also ignores the fact that economies of scale are needed to attract interest from producers: without the pull of a viable market for drugs, generic manufacturers will not seek to produce for export.
>
> *MSF Canada, 2006, p. 3*

The opinion of generic pharmaceutical companies – the potential suppliers under the system created by the WTO Decision – was equally sceptical. The Director General of the European Generic Medicine Association (EGA), for instance, declared that the 'WTO's 2003 August 30 Decision concerning compulsory licenses is complicated, unworkable and unable to deliver any significant improvement in access to medicines' (Rehman, 2011, n.p.).

The same scepticism was expressed by the main potential suppliers of generic medicines – the Indian firms who are major providers of medicines to developing countries. Thus, the representative of

CIPLA – one of the top global pharmaceuticals companies in India – observed that the paragraph 6 system is 'a cumbersome and ineffective process and that CIPLA will not use para 6 in its current state of writing' (Nightingale, 2016, n.p.).

Since, by hypothesis, when a particular pharmaceutical product is demanded for supply under the system created by the WTO Decision – and incorporated in article 31*bis* of the TRIPS Agreement – its global production and commercialisation is controlled by the patent owner, any alternative supplier would have to take several steps to be able to sell the (limited) quantity that may be supplied under such system.

First, research and development need to be conducted on the chemical composition of the needed product. This exercise, sometimes characterised as 'reverse engineering', has to be made without the technical cooperation of the patent owner. Patent specifications normally do not disclose the know-how necessary to develop a protected chemical compound; hence considerable experimentation may be needed to develop an efficient and reliable process to obtain the required product. Second, once this step is completed, an appropriate salt (if produced in solid form) and stable formulation (tablet, capsule, etc.) for the particular drug must be developed. In designing the formulation and its packaging, the producer would need to investigate the shape, colouring, labelling, and packaging of the patent-holder's product in the importing country in order to differentiate the product for export. Finally, the producer will also need to seek marketing approval and, eventually, demonstrate bioequivalence and bioavailability, when required by national law. In some cases, such approval would be needed both in the importing and exporting country.

While these activities may take several months or more than one year for a chemical compound, in the case of biologicals the investment and time necessary to develop a 'biosimilar' would be much longer – so long that the use of the export/import system would become illusory. Given the costs and risks involved in the development of biosimilars, the lack of automatic substitution and need to undertake (at least some) new clinical studies (Blackstone and Fuhr, 2013), it is practically unthinkable that a producer will consider a request under the article 31*bis* system for the supply of a small quantity of a biological product. In fact, the number of potential producers of biosimilars is several times less than generic producers (of chemically synthesised drugs) and the market is still largely controlled by a few large companies (Desai, 2016).

A potential supplier must, therefore, make a considerable investment and devote a significant amount of time to develop the limited quantity of the product demanded under the system. This is to be done, in addition, in a context of high risk: *at any time*, the patent owner may decide to lower the price or even donate the required medicines to the country in need, and thereby frustrate the whole process and deprive the investment made of any possible return.

Even worse, the patent owner may exploit the intricacies and complexities of the system, for instance, by delaying a response to a request of a voluntary license – as mentioned earlier, one of the conditions to put the system into operation – or exercising his rights under the relevant national laws to block the grant or execution of a compulsory license. For instance, this can be done through an appeal against a decision granting a compulsory license in the importing and/or exporting country. Although some national laws (e.g., Argentina) have stipulated that an appeal by the patent owner against the grant of a compulsory license does not suspend its immediate execution (e.g., article 49, Argentine Patent Law No. 24.481, as amended) this is not the case in many other countries. The patent owner may file for an injunction and thereby stop exports until a final administrative or judicial decision is taken, perhaps a few years later.

In countries where test data are protected under the so-called 'data exclusivity' regime, an additional hurdle may be created by the marketing approval of the product to be imported under a granted compulsory license. Unless the national law of the importing country specifies (such as in the case, for instance, of Chile) that data exclusivity may not be invoked when a compulsory license has been granted, the needed products may not be authorised for commercialisation, or the right-holder may request a court to prevent it. It is worth noting, however, that data exclusivity could not normally be invoked in the exporting country, since that form of protection only relates to the commercialisation of a product in the territory where the protection was not acquired, and not to exports (Correa, 2017).

As noted, the basic assumption for the application of the system is a situation where a product is available and could effectively be supplied to the country in need by the patent owner. In the last instance, the system legitimises the conduct of a patent owner who refuses to sell a product under his monopolistic control. By subjecting the use of the system to a large number of stringent conditions, it seems to be designed to protect the patent owner rather than facilitating access to pharmaceutical products where needed. Whatever humanitarian reasons may underpin a country's demand of a given drug, nothing in the adopted system compels the patent owner to supply the required drugs or to grant a voluntary license to a potential exporter. The patent owner may just passively watch how the country in need and a potential supplier strive to fulfil the conditions imposed by the WTO Decision (now article 31*bis*), while people remain without treatment.

The WTO Decision was apparently built upon the assumption that a patent owner is legitimised to prevent access to products under his control, even in the presence of compelling humanitarian reasons. This is inconsistent with the Doha Declaration (particularly paragraph 4) and with the states' commitments under the International Covenant on Economic, Social and Cultural Rights, especially its article 12 (recognising the human 'right of everyone to the enjoyment of the highest attainable standard of physical and mental health' and obliging states to take steps to fully realise this right, including 'those necessary for … the prevention, treatment and control of epidemic, endemic … and other diseases').[1]

## Use of the WTO Decision

The system set out by the WTO Decision was used only once for the export by a Canadian firm, Apotex, of a combination of antiretrovirals (Apo-TriAvir) to Rwanda. The active ingredients were protected by patents held by Boehringer Ingelheim (Canada) Ltd. and GlaxoSmithKline Inc. in Canada, to whom Apotex was bound to request voluntary licenses as the first step to comply with the WTO Decision and the national law. The case was instigated by Medicines Without Borders to test the viability of the system and the suitability of the Canadian legislation. The Canadian Access to Medicines Regime (CAMR) was adopted in 2004 as the first law in the world to implement the WTO Decision. The process took nearly four years, due to various factors (including the delay in finding a candidate importing country and the tender process). Apotex representatives have made the following statements in relation to their experience in this case:

> We've spent millions of dollars on the [research and development] we've spent lawyers' time at our cost, just because it's the right thing to do. It would be difficult to do again unless the legislation is made simpler … Imagine if … another country, like Malawi, comes forward asking for the drugs, we'd have to start this whole process again.
>
> *Gandhi, 2008, n.p.*

> Well, we might end up with a couple of orders, but at the end of the day we won't make any money out of it, and I'm going to get to a point where someone else comes along, like [NGO], and say 'we want this other compound', I'm not going to be able to develop it, because I'm in business to make money and I can only do so many products.
>
> *Cohen-Kohler, et al., 2007, n.p.*

It has been reported that if Rwanda had procured the required medicine from generic manufacturers, it would not have needed to use the WTO Decision at all, since the products were not patented in India. In accordance with one estimate, Apotex lost US$3–4 million by offering a lower price to win Rwanda's tender, as it could not compete with other low-cost producers (Nightingale, 2016). Another application for a compulsory license under the system was reportedly filed in September 2007 by a company with the Indian patent office to export an anti-cancer drug (erlotinib) to Nepal. However, Nepal's government never notified that it intended to carry out the importation from India of that drug and no compulsory license was issued (WHO, et al., 2012).

The way in which the system was used in the case of Canada, and the absence of other uses, certainly raises questions about its appropriateness and effectiveness to address the problem it was intended to solve. As noted by one commentator,

> [I]n the light of theoretical analysis and the two cases (Rwanda and India), it is hard to construe the Waiver Decision 2003 as a positive measure which can solve the problem of access to medicine. The decision is cumbersome and rigid and beyond its textual constraints, it also restricts the economic incentive which is essential to maintaining a manufacturing base.
>
> *Rehman, 2011, p. 13*

In addition, given the intricacies of the system as now incorporated into the TRIPS Agreement, it does not put any pressure on patent owners to lower their prices or to negotiate voluntary licenses.

## Amending the system

The numerous conditions imposed for the use of the system show how difficult it was for developing countries, notably the African Group, to get the agreement of developed countries, notably the US (Abbott, 2005; Abbott and Reichman, 2007). As discussed earlier, the system has failed to deliver the expected outcomes. No systematic study has been made so far to explain why the system has not been effectively used. A better understanding of the factors that determine its failure would be useful in order to consider, in particular, what further steps need to be given or what amendments need to be introduced. Different hypotheses can, however, be made regarding those factors.

The main hypothesis that may be advanced relates to the barriers that the system creates for potential suppliers to exploit economies of scale. Since the markets that may be supplied (in countries where there is insufficient or non-existent manufacturing capacity in pharmaceuticals) are small, generic producers are unlikely to be interested – as the evidence so far indicates in becoming involved in complex legal procedures when there are no chances for economies of scale to recoup the investment made and generate at least a reasonable profit. As suggested in one of the Apotex's comments quoted earlier, generic producers are not philanthropic but business organisations that respond to economic incentives.

The WTO Decision, in fact, recognised that the viability of the 'solution' largely depended on the existence of economies of scale. Paragraph 6 of the Decision allowed, 'with a view to harnessing economies of scale for the purposes of enhancing purchasing power for, and facilitating the local production of, pharmaceutical products' to export products manufactured upon request of a country to other developing or LDC parties who are part of a regional trade agreement, provided that at least half of its membership is made up of LDCs. However, this latter requirement means that this possibility will only be open in the case of regional trade agreements established by African countries, whose aggregated demand for particular medicines would still be insufficient to generate a sizeable market and realise economies of scale.

It has been argued that the lack of incentives resulting from the impossibility of realising economies of scale may be overcome by '[r]egional approaches to procurement and joint notifications by countries with similar needs for accessible medicines' (WHO, et al., 2012; Abbott and Reichman, 2007). In some cases, progress has been made in pooled procurement for certain medicines to obtain lower prices. The Strategic Fund of the Pan American Health Organization (PAHO), for instance, is a system for the pooled procurement of essential medicines that has allowed governments to obtain significant savings (PAHO, 2017). Another initiative that has led to better bargaining for prices is PAHO's revolving fund for vaccine procurement (PAHO, 2016). However, pooling for the purposes of using the system discussed here is not a realistic approach since it is too complicated to organise given differences in planning, legal procedures, and regulatory frameworks. A well-functioning system should allow individual countries to expeditiously address their health needs.

It has also been argued that generic medicines have been available so far from non-patented sources, thereby making it unnecessary to use the WTO Decision system, and that the problem of access to patent drugs has been alleviated by voluntary licenses, particularly as a result of the operation of the Medicines Patent Pool established in 2010 (WHO, et al., 2012). It has also been argued, as noted in the Report of the UN High Level Panel on Access to Medicines, that the availability of multilateral health financing for resource-constrained countries explains the lack of use of the system (UN High Level Panel on Access to Medicines, 2016).

In fact, the political and economic pressures felt by some countries not to use compulsory licenses – which are highlighted in the same report (UN High Level Panel on Access to Medicines, 2016) – may have played a role in discouraging the use of the system. Most probably, there has been a multiplicity of factors that determined the lack of interest in using it. They probably included 'burdensomeness and complexity, economic and political pressures, reluctance in implementation and its failure to recognize the need for economies of scale for exporting countries' (Thapa, 2011, p. 474).

In light of the failure of the WTO Decision, the High Level Panel on Access to Medicines established by the UN General Secretary in 2016 recommended that:

> WTO Members should revise the paragraph 6 decision in order to find a solution that enables a swift and expedient export of pharmaceutical products produced under compulsory license. WTO Members should, as necessary, adopt a waiver and permanent revision of the TRIPS Agreement to enable this reform.
>
> *UN High Level Panel on Access to Medicines, 2016, p. 27*

It will be worth pursuing this recommendation, as the problem of access to medicines may aggravate in the years to come. On one hand, probably due to new humanitarian demands (such as the refugee crises) and the fiscal austerity in many countries, recent years have seen a regression of donor funding, for instance, for the HIV response in low- and middle-income countries; it declined by almost 13 per cent between 2014 and 2015 (Avert, 2017). This trend may be further aggravated by the announced budgetary cuts in the US for foreign aid, including funding for the President's Emergency Plan for AIDS Relief (Aizenman, 2017).

On the other hand, while many countries have some manufacturing capacity (albeit in most cases for pharmaceutical formulations, not active ingredients) relating to drugs produced by chemical synthesis, the production of biologicals (such as the growth hormone, interferon, erithropoetin, monoclonal antibodies) is much more complex and only a few countries have manufacturing capacity in this field. Biologicals account for a growing share of the pharmaceutical market, which reflects their increasing importance in the arsenal of therapeutic tools available to treat diverse diseases (Blackstone and Fuhr, 2013; Desai, 2016). In fact, biologicals in some cases are the single option available to address some diseases (such as certain types of cancer), generally at a very high cost. Few countries have manufacturing capacity to produce biosimilars (that is generic versions of biologicals), and given the cost and time needed to develop them it seems unthinkable that the system, as currently designed, could contribute to facilitating access to those products.

An amendment to the system may be conceived in different ways. The most efficient one from the perspective of access to pharmaceutical products would be just to delete paragraph (f) of article 31 of the TRIPS Agreement that has created the problem addressed by the Doha Declaration.

Another possibility would be to clarify that the production for export of a patented product does not violate the patentee's exclusive rights as contemplated in article 28 of the TRIPS Agreement. An authoritative interpretation of this kind may be made by a three-fourths majority of the WTO members (article

IX(2) of the Agreement Establishing the WTO). However, individual members may adopt this interpret-ation, albeit with the risk of facing a complaint under the WTO Dispute Settlement Understanding that would clarify whether it is consistent or not with the TRIPS Agreement. In fact, there is considerable leeway for interpreting article 30 of said Agreement[2] which authorises exceptions to the patent owner's exclusive rights. Producing a protected product only for export does not affect the patent owners' *ius excluendi* in the territory where the patent has been granted. An exception that allows for such exports would be limited, would not unreasonably interfere with the normal exploitation of the patent (since patents are territorial and sales in the domestic market will not be affected), and would not unreasonably prejudice the legitimate interests of the patent owner (who may not claim interests based on rights he may have in other jurisdictions). In addition, such an exception would take into account the legitimate interests of third parties, in this case, patients in developing and LDCs.[3]

The referred two options were known to the negotiators of the WTO Decision, but discarded by developed countries. They had been discussed and proposed by the UK Commission on Intellectual Property Rights, which published its final report in 2002 (Commission on Intellectual Property Rights, 2002). Interestingly, on 3 October 2002, the European Parliament adopted Amendment 196 to the European Medicines Directive, which provided that,

> [M]anufacturing shall be allowed if the medicinal product is intended for export to a third country that has issued a compulsory licence for that product, or where a patent is not in force and if there is a request to that effect of the competent public health authorities of that third country.
>
> *Eur. PARL. Doc., AMEND. 196, 2002*

Less radical alternatives to the deletion of article 31(f) or the confirmation of an exception for exports would be to amend the system, as now incorporated into article 31*bis* of the TRIPS Agreement, to elim-inate some of its problematic conditions, such as the limitation of a compulsory license to the quantity of products initially demanded by the importing country, and the need to request the patent owner a volun-tary license prior to applying for and obtaining a compulsory license.

It is fair to recognise, however, that amending a provision that has just been approved by the WTO members, after ten years of its formal adoption, seems a very challenging objective. Ironically, perhaps, the most feasible approach might be to resort again to a waiver, which is easier to adopt than an amendment and may enter into force immediately. In any case, the process of reform should be initiated by a WTO member or a group of members, who would face the daunting task of reaching consensus (or the required majority under the WTO rules) to move forward. This would certainly need to recreate the sentiment of urgency that underpinned the debates on access to medicines at the time the Doha Declaration and the WTO Decision were adopted. In the meantime, article 31*bis* should be interpreted, in line with the Doha Declaration, in a manner that facilitates an increase in the supply of medicines to countries eligible to use the system.

## Conclusions

In order to be effective, a solution to the problem identified in Paragraph 6 of the Doha Declaration should provide the incentives necessary to attract the interest of potential suppliers of good quality pharmaceut-ical products at low cost. Pharmaceutical firms are unlikely to make the required investment and engage in complicated legal procedures if there is no expectation of a reasonable return, particularly through the realisation of economies of scale. This applies to drugs of chemical synthesis and, most importantly, to biosimilars that require significant investment and time to develop and get approved by regulatory authorities.

An amendment to the system has been suggested by the UN High Level Panel mentioned earlier. Such an amendment would be needed, indeed, to streamline the procedures and ensure access to pharmaceutical products in a timely manner. However, given the recent incorporation of the WTO Decision into the TRIPS Agreement, it would seem difficult to mobilise the needed support if the urgency to find a better solution is not fully acknowledged by the international community.

## Notes

1 See also the Resolution 32/L.23 of the Human Rights Council, adopted in its 32nd session (2016), which reaffirms the need for access to affordable, safe, efficacious, and quality medicines for all as a primary human right and underscores that improving such access could save millions of lives every year. The resolution also calls upon member states and other stakeholders to create favourable conditions at the national, regional, and international levels to ensure the full and effective enjoyment of the right of everyone to the highest attainable standard of physical and mental health.

2 See, e.g., the 'Declaration on Patent Protection. Regulatory Sovereignty under TRIPS' elaborated under the auspices of the Max Planck Institute for Innovation and Competition, available at www.mpg.de/8132986/Patent-Declaration.pdf (accessed 18 July 2017).

3 The EU Parliament 'Report on reindustrialising Europe to promote competitiveness and sustainability' (2013) recognised the feasibility of an exception for exports of medicines (including 'biosimilars') at least during the additional period of exclusivity granted to patent owners (under the supplementary protection certificate) in order 'to foster job creation in the EU, as well as to create a level playing field between European companies and their competitors in third countries' (EU Parliament, 2013, p. 19).

## References

Abbott, F.M. (2005) 'The WTO medicines decision: world pharmaceutical trade and the protection of public health', *American Journal of International Law*, 99(2): 317–58.

Abbott, F. and Reichman, J. (2007) 'The Doha round public health legacy: strategies for the production and diffusion of patented medicines under the amended TRIPS provisions', *Journal of International Economic Law*, 10(4): 921–87.

Aizenman, N. (2017) 'Trump's proposed budget would cut $2.2 billion from global health spending', available at www.npr.org/sections/goatsandsoda/2017/05/25/529873431/trumps-proposed-budget-would-cut-2-2-billion-from-global-health-spending (accessed on 18 July 2017).

Avert. (2017) 'Funding for HIV and AIDS', available at www.avert.org/professionals/hiv-around-world/global-response/funding (accessed on 20 November 2017).

Blackstone, E. and Fuhr, J. (2013) 'The economics of biosimilars', *American Health & Drug Benefits*, 6(8): 469–78.

Cohen-Kohler, J., Esmail, L., and Perez Cosio, A. (2007) 'Canada's implementation of the Paragraph 6 Decision: is it sustainable public policy?', *Global Health*, 3: 12.

Commission on Intellectual Property Rights. (2002) 'Integrating intellectual property rights and development policy', available at www.iprcommission.org/graphic/documents/final_report.htm (accessed on 20 July 2017).

Correa, C. (2004) 'Implementation of the WTO general council decision on paragraph 6 of the Doha Declaration on the TRIPS Agreement and public health', available at www.who.int/medicines/areas/policy/WTO_DOHA_DecisionPara6final.pdf (accessed on 20 July 2017).

Correa, C. (2014) 'Tackling the proliferation of patents: how to avoid undue limitations to competition and the public domain', research paper 52, available at www.southcentre.int/wp-content/uploads/2014/09/RP52_Tackling-the-Proliferation-of-Patents-rev_EN.pdf (accessed on 20 July 2017).

Correa, C. (2017) 'Mitigating the regulatory constraints imposed by intellectual property rules under free trade agreements', research paper 74, available at www.southcentre.int/wp-content/uploads/2017/02/RP74_Mitigating-the-Regulatory-Constraints-Imposed-by-Intellectual-Property-Rules-under-Free-Trade-Agreements_EN-1.pdf (accessed on 20 November 2017).

Correa, C. and Matthews, D. (2011) *The Doha Declaration Ten Years on and Its Impact on Access to Medicines and the Right to Health*, New York: UNDP.

Desai, P. (2016) 'The emergence of the biosimilars: a threat or an opportunity for biopharmaceutical innovation system?', *Asian Biotechnology and Development Review*, 18(2): 3–26.

EU Parliament. (2013) 'Report on reindustrialising Europe to promote competitiveness and sustainability', available at www.europarl.europa.eu/sides/getDoc.do?pubRef=-//EP//NONSGML+REPORT+A7-2013-0464+0+DOC+PDF+V0//EN (accessed on 20 July 2017).

Gandhi, U. (2008) 'Supplying generic AIDS drugs called pricey process', The Globe and Mail, available at www.theglobeandmail.com/news/national/supplying-generic-aids-drugs-called-pricey-process/article672157/ (accessed on 20 July 2017).

MSF Canada. (2006) 'Neither expeditious nor a solution: the WTO August 30th decision is unworkable', available at www.msfaccess.org/sites/default/files/MSF_assets/Access/Docs/ACCESS_briefing_NeitherExpeditiousNorSolution_WTO_ENG_2006.pdf (accessed on 20 July 2017).

Nightingale, A. (2016) 'WTO "Paragraph 6" system for affordable medicine: time for change?', Intellectual Property Watch, available at www.ip-watch.org/2016/11/14/wto-paragraph-6-system-affordable-medicines-time-change/ (accessed on 20 July 2017).

PAHO. (2016) 'PAHO's revolving fund for vaccine procurement' available at www.paho.org/immunization/toolkit/vaccine-procurement-fund.html (accessed on 18 July 2017).

PAHO. (2017) 'PAHO Strategic Fund', available at www.paho.org/hq/index.php?option=com_content&view=article&id=12163%3Apaho-strategic-fund&catid=8775%3Aabout&Itemid=42005&lang=en (accessed on 18 July 2017).

Rehman, H. (2011) 'WTO, compulsory export licences and Indian patent law', Nordic Journal of Commercial Law, available at http://njcl.dk/articles/2011-1/rehman_hafiz_aziz_ur.pdf (accessed on 20 July 2017).

Thapa, R. (2011) 'Waiver solution in public health and pharmaceutical domain under TRIPS Agreement', JWIP, 16: 470–6.

UN High Level Panel on Access to Medicines. (2016) 'Promoting innovation and access to health technologies', available at www.unsgaccessmeds.org/final-report/ (accessed on 20 July 2017).

Verma, S.K. (2006) 'TRIPS Agreement and access to medicines', available at www.kansai-u.ac.jp/ILS/publication/asset/nomos/29/nomos29-06.pdf (accessed on 20 July 2017).

WHO, WIPO, and WTO. (2012) 'Promoting access to medical technologies and innovation. Intersections between public health, intellectual property and trade', available at www.wipo.int/edocs/pubdocs/en/global_challenges/628/wipo_pub_628.pdf (accessed on 20 July 2017).

WTO. (2003) 'Decision removes final patent obstacle to cheap drug imports', available at www.wto.org/english/news_e/pres03_e/pr350_e.htm (accessed on 20 July 2017).

WTO. (2017) 'WTO IP rules amended to ease poor countries' access to affordable medicines', available at www.wto.org/english/news_e/news17_e/trip_23jan17_e.htm (accessed on 20 July 2017).

# 31

# Taking on the challenge of implementing public health safeguards on the ground

## The experience of Argentina and Brazil from a civil society perspective

*Marcela Fogaça Vieira and Lorena Di Giano*

### Introduction – health is separated from human rights and merged into the international trade agenda

The unsustainably high price of new medicines is increasingly becoming an issue of global concern. In developing countries, for the past two decades, it has been a central point of concern and action for governments and health activists. In high-income countries, austerity measures implemented after the 2008 economic crisis have shed new light and provided evidence of a persisting problem.

In responding to HIV and AIDS, the problem of unsustainable access to life-saving medicines due to high prices enforced by the protection of intellectual property rights reached global concerns, especially in developing countries. But the problem is by no means confined to HIV. Nor is it confined to developing countries. The more prominent debate currently involves access to expensive hepatitis C and cancer treatments, both in developing and developed countries. In fact, the problem of high prices, and its link with the monopoly created by exclusivity (private) rights, affects all diseases areas, and is one of the greatest challenges for the sustainability of public health policies and access to health technologies in the world.

The World Health Organization (WHO) estimates that the deaths of 18 million people, one-third of all deaths, are caused by treatable medical conditions (WHO, 2004). About 30 per cent of the world population has no access to necessary medical treatments and about 100 million people globally are pushed below the poverty line due to health care expenditures (WHO, 2015).

Even in the richest countries of the world, the issue is by no means new. For example, in the US, where HIV treatment has a price tag of US$20,000 per year, waiting lists exist for state HIV drug assistance. In 2012, 2,000 people remained on such lists. It is anticipated that once the patent term of HIV medications expires in the US, HIV treatment will become available for as little as US$200 per patient per year (Fojo and Grady, 2009; t'Hoen, 2014).

The newest available treatment for hepatitis C has a cure rate above 90 per cent, and was first put in the US market in 2013 at a price of US$1,000 per pill (Sovaldi ®, Gilead), leading to a treatment cost of

US$84,000 for a standard three-month period. The price is so high that treatment has been rationed and is available only for the sickest individuals, in the few countries that make it available at all. In the US, the release of this drug shocked the health care system (CBS News, 2014). In West Europe, France tried to challenge the high prices and faced the pressure of pharmaceutical companies (Le Figaro, 2014). Italy recently announced that the highest price it could pay for a three-month treatment was 4,000 euros, but Gilead refused to lower the price from the current 9,000 euros and the medicine was put in the list of non-reimbursable drugs by the national health system (Quotidiano Sanita, 2017). In countries in which generic versions of the drug are available, costs are as low as US$190 for the same treatment (HepCAsia, 2016), and cost of production has been estimated as US$178, including a profit margin of 50 per cent (Hill, et al., 2016a).

Another prominent debate is taking place around cancer drugs. Cancer drug prices have doubled in the US in the last decade from an average of US$5,000 per month to US$10,000 (Fojo and Grady, 2009; t'Hoen, 2014). In 2011, Roche stopped the supply of cancer drugs and other medicines to Greek state hospitals because of unpaid bills (t'Hoen, 2014). In the UK, the National Health Service has recently denied patients reimbursement to 25 cancer drugs, mostly due to high prices (*The Guardian*, 2015), including the drug lapatinib, which is used to treat breast cancer and is marketed by the company GlaxoSmithKline (GSK), a UK company that benefited from public resources for the development of the drug (Kanavos, et al., 2010).

## Why are drug prices so high?

The cost of production of a medicine can be very low. For example, a study by researchers at the University of Liverpool calculated the cost of production of some cancer drugs and concluded that generic production could achieve treatment prices in the range of US$128–4,020 per person-year (including a 50 per cent profit margin), versus current US prices of US$75,161–139,138 (Hill, et al., 2016b). The difference of the prices is impressive and it gives the pharmaceutical companies the largest margin of profit among all industries, including oil, gas, and banks (BBC News, 2014).

Pharmaceutical companies claim they need to recover the costs necessary to develop the drug, as well as costs related to research and development (R&D) of many other potential drugs that never became available and to reinvest in the development of new products. But how much does it cost to develop a new drug? The answer is unclear. The pharmaceutical industry claims that it costs US$2,870 million to develop a new medicine (in 2013 dollars) (DiMasi, et al., 2016). However, there are many criticisms about that figure, the main ones being the complete lack of transparency about R&D costs and the fact that about half of that figure corresponds to 'opportunity costs', that is, how much money could be made if the investment was made in something else. In 2011, *Health Policy* published a systematic review of drug R&D studies, with estimates ranging from US$161 million capitalised to US$1,800 million capitalised (in 2009 dollars). In 2006, the WHO's Commission on Intellectual Property Rights, Innovation and Public Health (CIPIH) published an estimation of the costs of developing a new drug between US$115 million and US$240 million (WHO/CIPIH, 2006).

Furthermore, it should be noted that a big part of the expenditures in health R&D is paid for with public resources. Different studies show that in most cases the discovery of new drugs is done by public institutions, which subsequent licensing to private companies (Avorn, 2015). In addition to the direct funding of R&D with public resources, many countries also provide fiscal incentives for private investments in health R&D, particularly for medicines, allowing for part of the investment to be recovered as a tax expenditure. Thus, public resources are behind most of the medicines, especially on those that are more innovative. However, these medicines are still priced very high, generally under monopolistic situations provided by patent protection, leading to even further private appropriation of the financial outcomes of drug R&D.

As concluded by Ellen t'Hoen,

> [t]he cost of drug development as an explanation for the high prices of new medicines is not convincing. A more likely explanation is that companies charge what the market can bear. And when it comes to healthcare and certainly in the case of potentially fatal diseases such as cancer, people are willing to bear a heavy burden even if the health benefits in reality turn out to be limited.
>
> *t'Hoen, 2014, p. 10*

But how is it possible to set the price so high? A significant part of the answer is because there is no competition. With only one producer, especially in cases of products that individuals don't really have a choice to buy or not (inelastic demand), it is possible for the producer to set the price as high as one can speculate people are willing to pay (Reichman, 2010). Exclusive rights, such as patents, is one form of allowing one producer to keep competition away for a period of time. The close relationship between the high price of a medicine and the fact that it is protected or not by patent is evidenced in several studies, which show there is a drastic reduction in the price of medicines due to competition from generic products as soon as patents expire. As an example, in the United States, a study conducted by the American government found that, on average, the price of generic drugs is equivalent to 43 per cent of the price of the reference medicine during the term of the patent (Reiffen and Ward, 2002).

Over the years too many people have assumed that the price of medicine is non-negotiable and that governments should provide them to people no matter what the cost. However, that assumption has already started to shift, and it needs to be completely removed from people's minds. The prices of medicines are way too high. Pharmaceutical companies are making huge profits out of people's lives and deaths and that can no longer be accepted.

## Health activists take on IP

The HIV epidemic and the millions of avoidable deaths that occurred after the development of life-saving treatment were the starting point of a global movement demanding greater access to medicines (Fire in the Blood, 2013). Questions about the reasons why there was no treatment available in developing countries started to be raised. One of the more important answers was because treatment was too expensive.

When in 1998 Nelson Mandela, then president of South Africa, changed the national IP law to allow for importation of cheaper versions of the treatment and was taken to court by multinational pharmaceutical companies accusing the government of violating their commercial rights, another element was added to the debate: the question of exclusivity rights. Exclusivity rights – usually granted to protect the 'intellectual property' over the product – allows a company to have control of the production, sales, and importation of a given medicine.

The protection of intellectual property had just been the object of an international treaty a few years previously, in December of 1994, with the constitution of the World Trade Organization (WTO). The WTO Agreement on Trade-Related Aspects of Intellectual Property Rights (TRIPS) set minimum but very strong common intellectual property protection standards to be adopted by the countries. They are called minimum standards because it is possible to adopt rules that give further protection to intellectual property (known as TRIPS-plus), but they represent the highest standard of IP protection granted by most countries at the time. Following TRIPS, WTO members had to recognise patents for all technological fields, including the pharmaceutical sector. Historically, many developing (and developed) countries did not grant patents on pharmaceuticals products. The TRIPS Agreement, therefore, placed medicines and other health-related technologies in the trade arena.

With the adoption of the WTO TRIPS Agreement, countries that were advocating for a stricter standard of protection for intellectual property worldwide got 95 per cent of what they wanted. But 95 per cent was never enough. They continued pressuring for the remaining 5 per cent (Sell, 2003). Governments of countries from the global North and their intellectual property rights holders' companies have continued to press for higher standards of IP protection mostly by direct negotiations with one or a small group of countries, outside of the framework of multilateral institutions. Free Trade Agreements negotiated mostly by the United States and the European Union consistently include protection and enforcement requirements that exceed those in the TRIPS Agreement (know as TRIPS-plus) given more rights to private companies and reducing the space for adoption of measures to promote the public interest (know as TRIPS flexibilities, or safeguards).

On the other hand, in developing countries such as Brazil and India, government officials, NGOs, communities, and health activists started to raise their concerns about access to medicines and the implications for the fulfilment of the human right to health, taking the debate to other international fora, especially at WHO and United Nations Human Rights bodies, but also back to the World Intellectual Property Organization (WIPO), with the 'Development Agenda' adopted in 2007. In 2001, even at WTO a more public health-based language was adopted with the 'Doha Declaration on TRIPS and Public Health' (WTO, 2001).

After more than 20 years, it has been shown that TRIPS generates great negative social impact, since high drug prices caused by patent monopolies exclude millions of people from access to health technologies in low-, middle-, and even high-income countries. The monopoly created by pharmaceutical patents increases the price of medicines because only one company can manufacture the medicine. It increases public and private spending on purchasing medicines and hinders the sustainability of the countries' health systems, at the same time as it works as a huge system of transferring public money to private companies due to over-excessive prices. On the other hand, it has not generated the expected positive outcomes. There is a lack of innovation oriented to meet the health needs of most of the world's population and an increasingly lower quality of the 'new' medicines being developed. This has been extensively shown in the literature.

While it is necessary to adopt an R&D system on health that does not have the innovation and access problems existing in the current IP system, there are also measures that can be adopted under the current system to reduce negative impacts of patents on access to medicines and innovation.

## Implementation of IP-related public health safeguards in global South countries

In order to minimise those negative effects of patents on health, TRIPS established that WTO members countries, 'shall be free to determine the appropriate method of implementing the provisions of this Agreement within their own legal system and practice' (article 1) and can 'adopt measures necessary to protect public health and nutrition, and to promote the public interest in sectors of vital importance to their socio-economic and technological development' (article 8) (TRIPS Agreement, 1994, articles 1 and 8), such as the health sector. Many measures can be adopted by countries under the TRIPS Agreement framework. It is important to say that the TRIPS Agreement does not bring an exhaustive list of measures, but merely some options, leaving room for countries to adopt other measures not listed in the Agreement, if such measures are consistent with the provisions of TRIPS (article 30). The main and most common safeguards are: parallel importation (exhaustion of rights) (article 6); interpretation of patentability requirements according to criteria established at national level (article 27); exceptions to patentability (article 27); Bolar exemption or early working (article 30); experimental use (article 30); public non-commercial use or government use (articles 30 and 31); compulsory license (article 31); third-party opposition to patent application (article 62.4); and a transition period for the implementation of some provisions (article 65).

International organisations have produced many reports, resolutions, and recommendations calling for a greater use of the measures within the TRIPS framework that can reduce the negative impact of IP on access to medicines, and have also called for the need for development of a new R&D system in health (WTO, et al., 2012). The UN Committee on Economic, Social and Cultural Rights has recognised that any intellectual property regime that makes it more difficult for a state party to comply with its core obligations in relation to health is inconsistent with the legally binding obligations of the state part (UN/CESCR, 2001, par. 12). Furthermore, the UN also recognised not only the right but also the duty of states to prevent high prices from hindering access to medicines, including using TRIPS safeguards to promote public health (UN/CESCR, 2006, par. 35). However, it is possible to say that after the initial challenges of including these measures in the text of the TRIPS Agreement, their actual use faces a triple challenge: first, the incorporation of the measures in the national laws (see example of 'fix the patent' law campaign in South Africa and Brazil); second, the political will to use them; and third, the threats and challenges posed by developed countries and pharmaceutical companies (UN/HLPA2M, 2016). In the following, we highlight some examples of implementation of TRIPS flexibilities by developing countries and some of the challenges faced.

## Compulsory license: the Brazilian experience

Compulsory licensing (CL), allowed under article 31 of TRIPS Agreement, can be issued for a number of reasons, among which cases of national emergency or public interest, the most relevant to health policies. A compulsory license allows the government to authorise third parties – public or private – to produce the patented product, without the authorisation of the patent holder subject to the payment of royalties. The TRIPS Agreement brings some conditions (article 31), but countries can determine its own bases for the issuance of compulsory license in their national law (article 5.b of the Doha Declaration on TRIPs and public health).

In Brazil, the response to the HIV epidemic in the 1990s was based on a public policy of providing free antiretroviral (ARV) treatment for all in need, which was possible especially through the local production of affordable generic drugs by national public laboratories. With the adoption of the new patent law in 1996 allowing for the granting of patents for pharmaceuticals, it was no longer possible to produce or import generic versions of the newer medicines. The constant increase in the price of ARV treatment has put the sustainability of the universal access to ARV policy in jeopardy, as alerted by the Ministry of Health in 2005.

From 2001 to 2007, the threat of issuing CLs was one of the main strategies used in price negotiations with pharmaceutical companies. Public-owned pharmaceutical laboratories could provide reference of cost of production and a credible threat of local production. At that time, pharmaceutical companies preferred to lower the price rather than have their IP rights licensed. However, since the Brazilian government had never actually issued a CL, this negotiating strategy grew increasingly less effective.

In 2005, during a round of negotiations with the pharmaceutical company Abbott (now Abbvie) to lower the price of lopinavir/ritonavir (Kaletra®, Abbott), the Brazilian government took a step towards a CL by declaring that the medicine was of public interest – the first step to issue a CL under Brazilian law. At the time, Brazil was paying US$1.17 per tablet, but estimates were putting the production cost at US$0.41 by public-owned laboratory Farmanguinhos. In the end, the Ministry of Health signed a contract with Abbott, which lowered the price to US$0.94 per pill, much higher than the estimate by the public laboratory and containing TRIPS-plus clauses.

The failure to issue a CL in this case prompted the Working Group on Intellectual Property of the Brazilian Network for the Integration of Peoples (GTPI/Rebrip) (see www.deolhonaspatentes.org) to file a civil public action to compel the government to issue a CL for lopinavir/r (Reis, et al., 2009). The case received a negative first decision, on the grounds that issuing a CL would trigger retaliation by developed countries, explicitly mentioning that Brazil could be included in the USTR Special 301 Watch list.[1] GTPI filed an appeal against this decision, which still awaits judgment by the Appeal Court. Although the price of US$1,380 per patient/year set by Abbott in the contract signed with the Brazilian government was initially supposed to be frozen for many years, the price lowered to US$1,000 just after a compulsory license for lopinavir/r was issued by Thailand in January 2007, leading Abbott to lower its price in several middle-income countries (AIDSMAP, 2007). This case shows that a CL issued in one country can also help to lower the prices in other countries as well.

A compulsory license was actually issued for the first – and only – time in Brazil in 2007, for the medicine efavirenz (Stocrin®, MSD), also used to treat HIV. Efavirenz was sold for US$1.59/pill or an annual cost of US$580 per patient/year. The Brazilian government attempted to negotiate a price reduction with MSD, mainly emphasising two points: (a) MSD was selling efavirenz at cheaper prices in countries at the same development level as Brazil, but with less people in need of treatment; and (b) Indian generic versions were much cheaper – as cheap as US$0.45/pill. MSD, however, did not present an acceptable proposal to the Brazilian government. The Brazilian government then issued a compulsory license in May 2007. The total savings in the purchase of generic efavirenz in a five-year period (2007–11) after the CL was issued was around US$104 million, allowing for the increase in the number of people on treatment with efavirenz from 70,000 in 2007 to 100,000 in 2011 (Viegas, et al., 2012).

Although the Brazilian government has indicated the possibility that it could make further use of compulsory licensing for other medicines, it has never happened, even if the issue of the CL in Brazil did not raise as many threats and acts of retaliation as faced by other countries. It is worth recalling that in Thailand the pharmaceutical company Abbott withdrew from the Thai market all medications awaiting registration and refused to register any new products in the country, as retaliation for the CL issued for lopinavir in 2007. We should also highlight the pressure currently being faced by the government of Colombia in the case of the cancer drug imatinib (Pharmalot, 2017). These pressures have led to an underuse of compulsory license. For example, in Latin America, only Brazil and Ecuador have used compulsory licenses for medicines.

Compulsory licensing is the most talked about IP health safeguard that can be used to lower the prices. However, countries face huge pressure from pharmaceutical companies and governments of developed countries when trying to use to it. Also, CL has a financial cost: the payment of royalties. Furthermore, CL is intended to be issued in cases in which a valid patent has been granted and it is usually more difficult to circumvent or remove a patent once it has been granted.

But there are also measures that can be used to prevent the grant of patents when they don't fulfil the legal requirements. Those measures used to be less costly in political terms, but have increasingly been the target of pharmaceutical companies and developed countries governments as well, as described later.

## Patent examination procedures

A key aspect of TRIPS implementation is how countries examine patent applications. Depending on how the examination guidelines are defined, more or less patents are granted or rejected. If more patents are granted, more monopolies are created, more technologies are taken away from the public domain, resulting in higher prices and lower access. If fewer patents are granted, more technologies are on the public domain, more producers can manufacture the technologies, prices drop, and access increases.

Filing multiple patents applications for the same medicine is standard practice in the pharmaceutical sector and several studies have suggested that pharmaceutical companies use this practice to block competition (European Commission DG, 2009). In addition to primary patents, companies commonly attempt to acquire secondary patents on alternative forms of molecules, different formulations, dosages, compositions, and new uses. These strategies used to extend periods of monopoly beyond the dates in which protection would otherwise lapse if the only protection came from the primary patent on the molecule are called 'life cycle management' by the pharmaceutical industry and 'evergreening' by international organisations, policymakers, and activists. Secondary patents are known to be of lower 'quality' than primary patents, in that they are less likely to be novel or manifest inventive step (non-obviousness). But they still can restrict competition and thus allow for supra-competitive prices, hindering access.

While the WTO TRIPS Agreement makes it mandatory to grant patents for pharmaceuticals, it is possible under the TRIPS framework to adopt measures to try to limit the grant of secondary patents and to increase the quality of patent examination in the pharmaceutical sector as a whole, to avoid the granting of unmerited patents. It is also possible to allow for the presentation of pre-grant or post-grant oppositions, a mechanism that has been increasingly used by civil society organisations (MSF, 2013). Pre-grant oppositions (including observations mechanisms) allow for any interested person to present arguments to the patent office to show that a particular patent application does not meet the criteria established by the national patent law, and therefore should not be awarded a patent. Post-grant opposition allows for any interested person to challenge the validity of a patent after it has been granted, either at administrative or judicial bodies. Some countries allow for one or the other type, and some for both. The TRIPS Agreement states that a country may have administrative procedures of patents annulment and/or opposition (article 62.4), leaving countries to decide which mechanisms will be provided. The TRIPS Agreement also states that any administrative decision may be challenged in the judiciary (article 62.5).

In 2001, Thai activists were among the first to successfully challenge a patent on HIV drug, didanosine. In India, oppositions started to be filed by civil society organisations and followed by generic producers, challenging patent applications for many medicines. In 2005, after the end of the transition period, India started to grant patents for pharmaceuticals. Civil society organisations and patients' groups have been engaged in litigation to use public health safeguards and also oppose attempts to introduce TRIPS-plus provisions in the Indian law (Lawyers Collective, 2017).

Civil society organisations in Brazil, drawing from the experience in India, also started in 2006 to question the patentability of essential medicines, by presenting arguments to the patent office against the granting of patent applications initially for HIV medicines and more recently also for hepatitis C medicines.[2] To date, there have been 12 patent oppositions filed by civil societies, challenging the patentability of seven medicines (five ARVs and two DAAs [direct-acting antiviral agents]). Four of the applications challenged were denied (related to tenofovir, lopinavir/r, and tenofovir/emtricitabine) and the others are still pending decision (GTPI, 2017). Public and private laboratories also filed oppositions for tenofovir, lopinavir/r, and sofosbuvir, increasing the challenge around the patentability of these medicines.

Today, tenofovir (TDF) is produced through a partnership between two Brazilian manufacturers and its price has been greatly reduced (MSF, 2012). The decision to deny the patent for tenofovir/emtricitabine was recently made in January 2017 and it is expected that it will influence the decision of the government to provide PrEP (Pre-exposure prophylaxis) for a greater number of people as the medicine will be able to be produced/imported at lower price than the one offered by Gilead.

In Argentina, civil society organisations have also taken on the challenge of presenting oppositions to avoid the granting of patents that do not fulfill the patentability criteria in the country. Argentina changed its patent law to become TRIPS compliant in 1995, but made use of part of the transition period and medicines were not patentable until 2000. During the transition period, Argentina developed its capacity to produce generic medicines, including first-line ARVs. The local production contributed to market competition, and the country's sovereignty to maintain a public policy of access to medicines. The grant of patents for pharmaceuticals changed this scenario and medicines under a monopoly situation where sold at very high prices.

Civil society organisations in Argentina decided to make use of one of the provisions under the patent law that allows for third-party participation in the process of analysis of patent applications.[3] They sent arguments to the patent office showing that the application did not fulfil the patentability requirements under Argentine law and therefore should not be granted. To this day, five pre-grant patent oppositions have been filed by civil society organisations in Argentina. Three of them on combinations of ARVs to treat HIV and two against patent applications on sofosbuvir, a DAA to cure hepatitis C. Three of the patent applications opposed are still pending of resolution. The patent application on lopinavir/r was rejected by the patent office in December 2016 since it does not meet legal patentability requirements. The one on TDF+FTC was withdrawn by the applicant, after the opposition was filed.

Other civil society groups have also challenged unmerited patent applications for medicines around the world, often in cooperation. An example is the case of sofosbuvir, used in the treatment of hepatitis C. Joint action to simultaneously file oppositions related to sofosbuvir was taken in Argentina, Brazil, China, Russia, and Ukraine (*The New York Times*, 2015). An opposition related to sofosbuvir was also filed at the European Patent Office (MdM, 2016).

Not by chance, pre-grant patent oppositions also started to be targeted by pharmaceutical companies and governments of countries in the global North. Free trade agreements (FTAs) have posed or intended to pose limitations on the use of safeguards against patent abuse, including the right of third parties to challenge patent applications (pre-grant opposition) (UN/HLPA2M, 2016, p. 25).

It is also possible to adopt stricter patentability criteria and examination procedures at the national level. One of the most important measures to protect health is the possibility that countries interpret the requirements for the grant of a patent according to the criteria set nationally. The TRIPS Agreement establishes that an invention is patentable if it is new, has an inventive step and industrial application (article 27.1). However, there are no standard criteria for the interpretation of these requirements, and each country has freedom to set them. TRIPS also says that countries shall be free to determine the appropriate method of implementing the provisions of the Agreement within their own legal system and practice (article 1.1).

International organisations have been recommending countries to adopt stricter patentability criteria and examination procedures to avoid the granting of low quality patents that hinder access and innovation. An example is the recommendation of the UN High Level Panel on Access to Medicines. The HLP report explicitly recommends countries to,

> [m]ake full use of the policy space available in Article 27 of the TRIPS Agreement by adopting and applying rigorous definitions of invention and patentability that are in the best interests of the public health of the country and its inhabitants. This includes amending laws to curtail the evergreening of patents and awarding patents only when genuine innovation has occurred.
>
> *UN/HLPA2M, 2016, p. 9*

The HLP report also recognises that 'many governments have not used the flexibilities available under the TRIPS Agreement for various reasons ranging from capacity constraints to undue political and economic pressure from states and corporations, both express and implied' (UN/HLPA2M, 2016, p. 8). However, there are countries that are trying to do that, not without facing political pressures. Three prominent examples of patent examination systems that try to reduce the number of undeserved patents are the cases of India, Brazil, and Argentina.

The Indian case is the one that has called most attention at the international level, especially with the Novartis case around the cancer drug imatinib (see Chapter 28 in this volume). Following extensive advocacy – both national and international India adopted some key public health safeguards when changing its patent law to become TRIPS-compliant in 2005. One such public health safeguard in the patent law is the establishment of stricter patentability criteria, introduced by the notorious session 3d of the patent law adopted by Indian Parliament excluding patenting of new forms of already known substances unless there is a significant enhancement in efficacy, in a bid to prevent evergreening of patents on medicines.

In the following we will develop on the cases of Argentina and Brazil and the pressures they are facing to keep implementing those measures.

## Patent examination guidelines in Argentina

In 2012, Argentina adopted new patentability examination guidelines for patent applications in the pharmaceutical sector. The guidelines were adopted as a joint resolution by the Ministry of Health, Ministry of Industry, and the National Institute of Industrial Property. As a motivation for adopting the new guidelines, it was said that low patentability criteria applied previously led to the granting of innumerous patents that do not meet the patentability requirements (novelty, inventive step, and industrial application). At the time, there was an estimation made that 90 per cent of all patent applications for pharmaceuticals would be rejected by the implementation of the new guidelines. A study conducted by FGEP (the Fundación Grupo Efecto Positivo, see http://fgep.org/en/about-us/) showed that 95 per cent of patent applications for ARVs have been rejected after 2012.

The Guidelines for the Examination of Pharmaceutical Patents Applications – also called 'Anti-Evergreening Resolution' – are a key tool to rationally establish an interpretation of patentability requirements stated in article 4 of Argentina's patent law (Law 24.481) in relation to 'novelty', 'inventive step', and 'industrial application'. These guidelines are considered an example worldwide in terms of public health perspective, since they guarantee an adequate administration of the pharmaceutical patents system and prevent abuses from the multinational pharmaceutical companies. However, they have been challenged by multinational pharmaceutical companies.

In 2015, the Argentine Chamber of Medicinal Specialties (CAEME in Spanish), an association that congregates mostly multinational pharmaceutical companies acting in Argentina, filed a court case against the examination guidelines. If they prevail, the guidelines would be annulled, removing a measure legitimately adopted by Argentina to prevent the grant of unmerited patents for medicines in the country. FGEP has filed a presentation at the court case as an interested third party in the defence of public health and access to medicines in Argentina. The aim is to support Argentina's right to defend public health against the abuse of multinational pharmaceutical companies that are attacking a set of high standards for patent applications' examination, therefore preventing unnecessary monopolies in the local medicine market that would result in a barrier for the access to treatment for HIV, hepatitis C, and many other diseases (FGEP, 2015).

Other pathways are also used to try to bypass the stricter examination guidelines adopted in 2012 in Argentina. In August 2016, following a change in administration of the patent office (INPI) under the new government, a new resolution was adopted (Res. 56/2016), which could dismantle the 2012 guidelines by establishing that Argentina could adhere to the search and examination conducted by foreign patent offices. There was strong mobilisation against this resolution from different sectors, including civil society and local manufacturers. As a response, INPI issued a new resolution (Res. 125/2016) asserting that the 2012 patentability guidelines are still in force. However, in March 2017 a new step was taken by INPI putting again in danger the applicability of the guidelines, by signing an agreement with the US patent office to share information related to patent examination (FGEP, 2017). The PPH (Patent Prosecution Highway) is considered by civil society organisations working on these issues as a danger for access to medicines, as it can undermine policies adopted at the local level to interpret the patentability criteria from a national perspective, adopting the standards used by developed countries that are usually much more lax.

### Anvisa's prior consent mechanism in Brazil

Since 2001, Brazil has adopted a double-step mechanism of examination of patent applications in the pharmaceutical sector. Anvisa (the Brazilian Health Regulatory Agency), a regulatory agency under the Ministry of Health, must give its 'consent' prior to the granting of a patent by the INPI – the Industrial Property National Institute, which is the patent office linked to the Ministry of Industry. The rationale behind this mechanism is to give as much accurate technical analyses as possible to patents filed in the pharmaceutical sector, by including the expertise and the interpretation of public health sector in the country. This way, the patent examination process reflects the understanding that patents are not just an industry and trade issue, but also have an impact on public health policies.

The 'prior consent' mechanism has been an important measure to avoid unmerited patent monopolies that could hinder the state's capacity to fulfil the human right to health and access to medicines in Brazil

(GTPI, 2016a). Anvisa has rejected over 400 patent applications. In addition, 40 per cent of the patent applications approved had to comply with demands such as to improve clarity or to reduce scope, before being granted, therefore increasing the quality of the patents that were granted.

Several international institutions have identified a close collaboration between health regulatory authorities and patent offices in the examination of pharmaceutical patent applications as a positive measure to enhance the examination of pharmaceutical patents from a public health perspective. WHO, for example, identified this as positive because it helps to prevent concession of unmerited patents (WHO/CIPIH, 2006, p. 134).

Anvisa's prior consent is repeatedly applauded around the world, but also has generated displeasure in some sectors, especially among transnational pharmaceutical companies that feel aggrieved, since they are not interested in rigorous analysis of patent applications. In some cases, pharmaceutical companies filed judicial actions over specific rejected patent requests that would question, additionally, the legitimacy of Anvisa's prior consent. In other cases, the companies filed judicial actions questioning directly Anvisa's participation in the patent granting process.

An important example of the second type of judicial case is the lawsuit filed by Associação da Indústria Farmacêutica de Pesquisa (Interfarma, see www.interfarma.org.br/), an association of 52 pharmaceutical companies, mostly transnational, responsible for most branded drugs sales in Brazil. In the case the lawsuit is judged in favour of Interfarma's request, it would be the end of Anvisa's prior consent and a great setback in the guarantee of the right to health in Brazil. Anvisa's prior consent mechanism has also been listed in the United States Trade Representative Special 301 list as a means to put pressure on Brazil to stop applying the mechanism. This is an illegitimate and illegal means of challenging Brazil's sovereignty rights, and duty to adopt TRIPS-compliant measures to fulfil the right to health.

## Drop the case campaign

To counter the attacks by pharmaceutical companies against the measures adopted in Argentina and Brazil to have a better patent examination in the pharmaceutical sector and avoid the granting of many undeserved patents that could hinder access to medicines, civil society organisations in both countries have launched a campaign asking pharmaceutical companies to drop their court cases. The campaign was launched in a side event held in the UN Human Rights Council in March 2016 (GTPI, 2016b). It has mainly two goals: (a) primary goal: abandonment of the court cases or rejection of the claims; (b) secondary goal: promote at the international level the understanding that companies must be held accountable and sanctioned for human rights violations.

Rigorous patent examination in the pharmaceutical sector is urgent to protect people's rights and to protect health systems from endless monopolies over essential drugs. Argentina and Brazil have adopted public health safeguards in their national laws to reduce the negative impacts of intellectual property rules on access to medicines. The attacks of the pharmaceutical companies against these measures are a violation of the human right to health and disrespect to the sovereignty of countries to adopt measures to protect the public health. As such, the international community should, in addition to writing reports and recommendations, join forces to demand companies and governments to respect the right of countries to adopt measures to protect people's rights (FGEP, et al., 2016).

## Final remarks

Over the last decades, the protection of intellectual property has been the main mechanism adopted to promote research and development. However, the IP system has been inefficient to promote R&D to address the main health problems of world's population. When products are developed, the IP system has created barriers to access to life-saving health technologies. Barriers to access include high prices that are

341

set by patent-holders during a period of time in which they have the exclusivity to explore the technology, allegedly as a mean to recoup their R&D investments. After two decades of the WTO TRIPS Agreement, there is plenty of evidence showing that this exclusivity leads to the increase of medicines' prices and the reduction of access to them, causing unnecessary suffering and death for millions of people around the world that cannot have access to the medicines they need. This is a systematic gross-violation of human rights, deliberately set in place by pharmaceutical companies and states defending their financial interests and deeply rooted in the international IP system.

While it is necessary to adopt an R&D system on health that will not have the innovation and access problems existing in the IP system, there are also measures that can be adopted under the current system to reduce negative impacts of patents on access to medicines. The negative impacts of patents in access to medicines is certain to remain a global challenge over the next years. Therefore, it is necessary to increase the use of health protective measures already existing in the IP system, in order to increase as soon as possible access to needed medicines. However, the use of TRIPS flexibilities, the promise of the Doha Declaration, has been broken through trade pressure like the US Special 301, excessive litigation by corporations and FTAs. This must stop.

The authors of this chapter have submitted a contribution (RedLAM, 2016) to the UN HLP on Access to Medicines on behalf of RedLAM – the Latin American Network for Access to Medicines (see www.redlam.org/) – highlighting the problems of the patent system for access to medicines and innovation and making some recommendations. In the following list we highlight some of the main recommendations:

- Adoption of alternative R&D systems and mechanisms for health.
- Abolition of the IP protection for health technologies, products, and processes in all countries, including those of TRIPS, FTAs, and national and regional legislation.
- Adoption of a system of automatic compulsory licenses for already granted patents for medicines and waivers of data exclusivity.
- For patent applications that are still pending analysis, a stricter and faster mechanism of analysing the fulfilment of the patent criteria should be implemented. And the adoption of measures necessary to produce or import generic versions when there is no patent in force (including when there are patent applications pending).
- Non-adoption of any measures that go beyond the obligations of the TRIPS Agreement (i.e., TRIPS-plus) and immediate exclusion of any such measures already adopted.
- Annulment of voluntary licenses that restrict the production/supply of active pharmaceutical ingredients (API) or finished products to a limited number of countries or undermine TRIPS flexibilities.
- Adoption of mechanisms of transparency of R&D costs and pricing of all medicines.

As this list makes clear, there is a need for a profound reform on the way that medicines and health technologies are developed and made available to the public. By no means can they continue to be treated as merchandise, commercialised by private companies that respond most of all to profits and the wills of their investors. Medicines and all health technologies should be developed and made available as public goods (WHO/CEWG, 2012), and should be treated as such by the legal and health systems of the world. It is not about trade, it is about human suffering, it is about people's ability to live healthier lives, and it is literally about people's life and death.

## Notes

1   The United States Trad Representative (USTR) 'Special 301' list is an outcome of an annual review of the global state of intellectual property rights (IPR) protection and enforcement, per US standards. Countries that do not

meet these US standards face commercial retaliation. The Special 301 list has been denounced for violating international human rights obligations. See: PIJIP, 2010.

2   It should be noted that Brazilian patent law (article 31, Law 9279/96) has adopted a mechanism called 'subsidies to the examination', which is weaker than an opposition system. The 'patent law reform' currently ongoing at the National Congress has a bill proposing to adopt a stronger opposition system, among many other changes to the law. For more information about the patent law reform in Brazil, please refer to: http://deolhonaspatentes.org/acoes/defesa-interesse-publico/legislativo/lista-pls-2/.

3   Argentine Patent Law (Law 24481, article 28) allows any party to file 'observations' and evidence related to a patent application. Although there are limitations on the period during which the observations can be submitted, the law states that they must be submitted within 60 days after the application has been published. This period is insufficient and the patent office by administrative practice receives observations and evidence under the modality of 'calls for attention'.

# References

AIDSMAP. (2007) 'Abbott announces Kaletra price cut for lower middle-income countries, makes new offer to Thailand', available at =www.aidsmap.com/Abbott-announces-iKaletrai-price-cut-for-lower-middle-income-countries-makes-new-offer-to-Thailand/page/1426966/ (accessed on 15 March 2017).

Avorn, J. (2015) 'The $2.6 Billion Pill – Methodologic and Policy Considerations', *New England Journal of Medicine*, 372: 1877–9.

BBC News. (2014) 'Pharmaceutical industry gets high on fat profits', available at www.bbc.com/news/business-28212223 (accessed on 16 March 2017).

CBS News. (2014) '$1,000-a-day miracle drug shocks U.S. health care system', available at www.cbsnews.com/news/1000-a-day-miracle-drug-shocks-us-health-care-system/ (accessed on 1 March 2017).

DiMasi J., et al. (2016) 'Innovation in the pharmaceutical industry: new estimates of r&d costs', *Journal of Health Economics*, 47: 20–33.

European Commission DG. (2009) 'Pharmaceutical Sector Inquiry: preliminary report', available at: http://ec.europa.eu/competition/sectors/pharmaceuticals/inquiry/communication_en.pdf (accessed on 17 March 2017).

Fire in the Blood. (2013) available at http://fireintheblood.com/ (accessed on 15 March 2018).

FGEP (2015) 'FGEP continues defense of public health in Argentina against the abuse of the patent system by multinational pharmaceutical companies', available at http://fgep.org/en/fgep-continues-defense-of-public-health-in-argentina-against-the-abuse-of-the-patent-system-by-multinational-pharmaceutical-companies/ (accessed on 16 March 2017).

FGEP (2017) 'Grave: políticas que afectan el derecho a la salud y conflictos de interés son la norma en el INPI de Dámaso Pardo', available at http://fgep.org/es/grave-politicas-afectan-derecho-salud-conflictos-interes-inpi-damaso-pardo/ (accessed on 16 March 2017).

FGEP, ABIA, GTPI. (2016) 'Big pharma's court cases in Brazil & Argentina threaten national laws considered important public health safeguards in the UN HLP report', available at http://fgep.org/en/big-pharmas-cases-brazil-argentina-threaten-national-laws-public-health-safeguards-hlp-report/ (accessed on 16 March 2017).

Fojo, T. and Grady, C. (2009) 'How much is life worth: cetuximab, non-small cell lung cancer, and the $440 billion question', *Journal of the National Cancer Instititute*, 101(15): 1044–8.

GTPI (2016a) 'Marcela Vieira, working group on Intellectual Property of the Brazilian Network for the Integration of the People_A', available at www.unsgaccessmeds.org/inbox/2016/2/28/marcela-vieira?rq=gtpi (accessed on 16 March 2017).

GTPI (2016b) 'GTPI anuncia campanha em evento no Conselho de Direitos Humanos da ONU', available at http://deolhonaspatentes.org/gtpi-anuncia-campanha-em-evento-no-conselho-de-direitos-humanos-da-onu/ (accessed on 16 March 2017).

GTPI (2017) 'Contestação de patentes', available at http://deolhonaspatentes.org/acoes/contestacao-patentes-2/ (accessed on 15 March 2018).

*The Guardian* (2015) 'UK NHS cancer patients denied drugs due to inflated prices', available at www.theguardian.com/business/2015/sep/23/uk-cancer-patients-being-denied-drugs-due-to-inflated-prices-say-experts (accessed on 17 March 2017).

HepCAsia. (2016) 'Generic DAAs pricing', available at http://hepcasia.com/wp-content/uploads/2016/03/Indian-generic-DAC-summary_7-March-16.pdf (accessed on 14 March 2017).

Hill, A., et al. (2016a) 'Rapid reductions in prices for generic sofosbuvir and daclatasvir to treat hepatitis C', available at www.ncbi.nlm.nih.gov/pmc/articles/PMC4946692/#jve5-bib-0008 (accessed on 14 March 2017).

Hill A., et al. (2016b) 'Target prices for mass production of tyrosine kinase inhibitors for global cancer treatment', Publishing on the Internet, available at http://bmjopen.bmj.com/content/6/1/e009586 (accessed on 17 March 2017).

Kanavos P., et al. (2010) 'The role of funding and policies on innovation in cancer drug development', *Ecancer Medical Science*, 4: 164.

Lawyers Collective. (2017) 'Access to medicines, background', available at www.lawyerscollective.org/our-initiatives/access-to-medicines (accessed on 15 March 2018).

Le Figaro. (2014) 'Hépatite C: "une solution d'urgence" pour Touraine', available at www.lefigaro.fr/flash-actu/2014/10/08/97001-20141008FILWWW00387-hepatite-c-une-solution-d-urgence-pour-touraine.php (accessed on 19 March 2017).

MdM – Medecines du Monde (2016) 'L'opposition au brevet sur le sofosbuvir', available at www.medecinsdumonde.org/fr/actualites/publications/2016/11/21/lopposition-au-brevet-sur-le-sofosbuvir (accessed on 19 March 2017).

MSF (2012) 'Patent opposition database, success story: the case ff Tdf in Brazil', available at www.patentoppositions.org/en/case_studies/4f106d0504a7f92f5b000003 (accessed on 15 March 2017).

MSF (2013) 'Patent Opposition Database', available at www.msf.org/en/article/patent-opposition-database (accessed on 15 March 2017).

Pharmalot. (2017) 'Pharma trade group urges US trade rep to take action against Colombia', available at www.statnews.com/pharmalot/2017/02/16/trade-rep-colombia/ (accessed on 15 March 2017).

PIJIP [Program on Information Justice and Intellectual Property of the American University]. (2010) Human Rights Groups to Challenge Special 301, available at www.wcl.american.edu/pijip/go/blog-post/human-rights-groups-to-challenge-special-301 (accessed on 19 March 2017).

Quotidiano Sanita. (2017) 'Le reazioni all'ultimatum di Aifa, sì dalla politica, dai medici e dai pazienti', available at www.quotidianosanita.it/scienza-e-farmaci/articolo.php?approfondimento_id=8929 (accessed on 19 March 2017).

RedLAM [Red Latinoamericana por el Acceso a Medicamentos] (2016) 'Maria Lorena Di Giano and Marcela Fogaça Vieira, RedLAM, contribution to the UN HLP on access to medicines', available at www.unsgaccessmeds.org/inbox/2016/3/1/maria-lorena-di-giano-and-marcela-fogaa-vieira?rq=redlam (accessed on 19 March 2017).

Reichman, J.H. (2010) 'Compulsory licensing of patented pharmaceutical inventions: evaluating the options', In: C. Correa (Ed.), *Research Handbook on the Protection of Intellectual Property under WTO Rules: Intellectual property in the WTO*, volume I, Cheltenham, UK; Massachusetts, USA: Edward Elgar Publishing Limited, pp. 589–622.

Reiffen, D. and Ward, M. (2002) 'Generic drug industry dynamics', US Federal Trade Commission Working Paper 248, available at www.ftc.gov/be/workpapers/industrydynamicsreiffenwp.pdf (accessed on 1 March 2017).

Reis, R., Viera, M., and Chaves, G. (2009) 'Access to medicines and intellectual property in Brazil: a civil society experience', available at www.abiaids.org.br/_img/media/Intellectual_Property_internet.pdf (accessed on 15 March 2018).

Sell, S. (2003) *Private Power, Public Law: The globalization of intellectual property rights*, Cambridge: Cambridge University Press.

t'Hoen, E. (2014) 'Access to cancer treatment: a study of medicine pricing issues with recommendations for improving access to cancer medication', OXFAM, available at: http://apps.who.int/medicinedocs/documents/s21758en/s21758en.pdf (accessed on 1 March 2017).

*The New York Times*. (2015) 'High cost of sovaldi hepatitis c drug prompts a call to void its patents', available at www.nytimes.com/2015/05/20/business/high-cost-of-hepatitis-c-drug-prompts-a-call-to-void-its-patents.html?_r=0 (accessed on 19 March 2017).

UN/CESCR (2001) 'Human rights and intellectual property. Statement by the Committee on Economic, Social and Cultural Rights (CESCR), E/C.12/2001/15', available at: www2.ohchr.org/english/bodies/cescr/docs/statements/E.C.12.2001.15HRIntel-property.pdf (accessed on 1 March 2017).

UN/CESCR (2006) 'General comment No. 17: the right of everyone to benefit from the protection of the moral and material interests resulting from any scientific, literary or artistic production of which he or she is the author (Art. 15, Para. 1 (c) of the Covenant)', Committee on Economic, Social and Cultural Rights (CESCR), E/C.12/GC/17, available at www.refworld.org/docid/441543594.html (accessed 1 March 2017).

UN/HLPA2M (2016) 'Report of the United Nations Secretary-General's High Level Panel on Access to Medicines: promoting innovation and access to health technologies', available at www.unsgaccessmeds.org/final-report/ (accessed on 15 March 2017).

Viegas, F., Hallal, R., and Guimarães, A. (2012) 'Compulsory license and access to medicines: economic savings of efavirenz in Brazil', presentation at the International AIDS Conference, available at http://pag.aids2012.org/session.aspx?s=228#2 (accessed on 15 March 2017).

WHO. (2004) 'The world health report', available at www.who.int/whr/2004/en/ (accessed on 16 March 2018).

WHO. (2015) 'Health and human rights, fact sheet 323', available at www.who.int/mediacentre/factsheets/fs323/en/ (accessed on 15 March 2017).

WHO/CEWG. (2012) 'Research and development to meet health needs in developing countries: strengthening global financing and coordination', available at www.who.int/phi/cewg_report/en/ (accessed on 14 March 2017).

WHO/CIPIH. (2006) 'Public health: innovation and intellectual property rights', Report of the Commission on Intellectual Property Rights, Innovation and Public Health, available at www.who.int/intellectualproperty/documents/thereport/ENPublicHealthReport.pdf (accessed on 15 December 2016).

WTO. (2001) 'Declaration on the TRIPS Agreement and public health', available at www.wto.org/english/thewto_e/minist_e/min01_e/mindecl_trips_e.htm (accessed on 14 March 2017).

WTO, WHO, WIPO. (2012) 'Promoting access to medical technologies and innovation: intersections between public health, intellectual property and trade', available at www.wipo.int/edocs/pubdocs/en/global_challenges/628/wipo_pub_628.pdf (accessed on 14 March 2017).

# 32

# The politics of malnutrition

## Achieving policy coherence in a globalised world

*Anne Marie Thow and Biraj Patnaik*

### Action on nutrition will be critical for achieving global health goals

Poor nutrition hampers development at a personal, household, community, and societal level. The imperative for action on all forms of malnutrition and food security is explicit in Sustainable Development Goal 2, 'End hunger, achieve food security and improved nutrition, and promote sustainable agriculture'. Achieving the Sustainable Development Goals (SDGs), signed off in 2015, will require sustained improvements in nutrition – not only for Goal 2 but also for broader goals related to poverty, education, employment, female empowerment, and inequality (IFPRI, 2016).

In 2016, the United Nations (UN) declared a decade of action on nutrition. This reflects rising political attention for nutrition since the mid-2000s (Nisbett, et al., 2015). A growing number of countries have recognised access to food as a fundamental human right, supported by grassroots activism against hunger and food insecurity.

However, countries around the world are struggling to end hunger and persistent undernutrition. Economic growth over the past three decades has been associated with reductions in hunger, but translating economic growth into improved nutritional outcomes has proved challenging (FAO, 2015). Despite declines in hunger and undernutrition globally in the past two decades, 795 million people remain undernourished (FAO, 2015). Hunger continues to exact a devastating human toll, hampering personal, societal, and economic development (Ziegler, et al., 2011). Undernutrition is estimated to contribute to 45 per cent of child deaths (Bhutta, et al., 2013).

At the same time, diet-related non-communicable diseases (NCDs) are a major cause of death and disability globally, and the prevalence of these diseases continues to rise (WHO, 2013a). The number of adults with diabetes, worldwide, has quadrupled since 1980 (NCD, 2016). Cardiovascular disease is the largest contributor to global mortality (Sacco, et al., 2016). Obesity prevalence doubled between 1980 and 2008, with half of this rise occurring between 2000–8 (Stevens, et al., 2012). In 2012, there were 14 million new cases of cancer per year – more than 60 per cent occurring in the developing world – and this number is expected to more than double over the next two decades (Stewart and Wild, 2015). In 2010, dietary risk factors (particularly diets low in fruits and vegetables and those high in sodium, but also including diets high in fats and sugars) were the largest contributors to the global disease burden (Lim, et al., 2013).

In addition to the human and social costs described, the economic consequences of malnutrition represent losses of 11 per cent of gross domestic product (GDP) every year in Africa and Asia (IFPRI,

2016). Almost every country is facing escalating health care costs and lost productivity; the World Economic Forum has estimated that the economic cost of NCDs over the following 20 years could amount to US$47 trillion – more than US$2 trillion per year (Bloom, et al., 2011). In contrast, preventing malnutrition delivers $16 in returns on investment for every one dollar spent (IFPRI, 2016).

This double burden of malnutrition is proving intractable, and the world is off track to meet global nutrition targets (IFPRI, 2016). It is widely acknowledged that a 'broken' food system underlies these persistent nutritional problems (World Economic Forum, 2017). Current food systems are not sustainable, and biodiversity is at risk. Lengthening supply chains are compromising food safety (Alders, et al., 2016). In modern food systems, distancing – separation between production and consumption decisions in the food system – constrains feedback of information, and contributes to the externalising of environmental, health, and social costs (Clapp, 2014).

## What needs to be done?

Overall, we largely know what to do to improve nutrition. Addressing undernutrition will require delivery of direct nutrition interventions, particularly in the first 1,000 days of life and in emergency situations (Morris, et al., 2008; Bryce, et al., 2008). These interventions are well established, and include promotion of appropriate breastfeeding and complementary feeding practices, provision of food and micronutrient supplements, community-based supportive strategies to improve nutrition, and reduction of disease burden through interventions promoting behaviours such as handwashing (Bhutta, et al., 2013).

However, nutrition represents a complex and long-term outcome of personal, household, community, and policy decisions (Black, et al., 2013). At a personal and household level, preferences, economic capacity, food skills, and culture can consciously or unconsciously influence food choice. The food environments in which these choices are made also have a significant influence, and in some ways underpin these decisions. The food environment can either exploit or limit people's 'biological, psychological, social, and economic vulnerabilities', through shaping their access to – and the relative attractiveness of – healthy and unhealthy foods (Roberto, et al., 2015; De Vet, et al., 2013). As a result, policy decisions in sectors as diverse as agriculture, commerce, water and sanitation, and social protection have direct impacts on nutritional status.

Therefore, for maximum effect, these direct nutrition interventions must be situated within a larger context of supportive and 'nutrition-sensitive' policy (Pinstrup-Andersen, 2013). This includes agricultural policies that support access to affordable, diverse healthy food, and social policies that promote sustained poverty reduction, livelihoods, and women's empowerment (Ruel and Alderman, 2013). Similarly, strong social policies are essential for achieving food and nutrition security – particularly in rural areas, where the majority of those who are hungry and food insecure live (Pritchard, 2016; Ziegler, et al., 2011).

Recommendations to prevent diet-related NCDs are similarly multi-sectoral. Direct behavioural interventions to improve diets and nutrition must be accompanied by agricultural, commerce, procurement, and other policies that support a food environment in which healthy foods are accessible and affordable (WHO, 2013a). Nutrition is thus an issue of political economy, and progress on implementation of global recommendations reflects this. In this chapter, we present a policy-focussed analysis of the global politics of malnutrition, considering political priorities, actors and institutions, and the frames and narratives that surround the challenge that nutrition presents.

## The politics of malnutrition

The inclusion of a specific SDG on hunger and malnutrition, and the commencement of the UN Decade of Action on Nutrition, are evidence of the significant rise in political attention for undernutrition over the past decade (Nisbett, et al., 2014). Since the first *Lancet* series on maternal and child undernutrition in 2008, recognition of the need for consideration of politics and policy action has resulted in strategic and coordinated policy advocacy (Gillespie, et al., 2013; WHO, 2013b). However, policy action on undernutrition faces challenges – in particular, sustained commitment, investment, and action from sectors outside of health (Pelletier, et al., 2016). The 2008 global food crisis highlighted the vulnerability of the preceding 'wins' in malnutrition, as rising prices of staple foods rendered many people food insecure (Clapp, 2014).

Analyses of the political economy of undernutrition find that continuing undernutrition is 'rooted in wider structural causes of poverty and unequal access to resources' (Nisbett, et al., 2014, p. 422). In line with this, social movements and campaigns that focus on the right to food take a structural and rights-based approach to access to food and food security. These efforts have also gained momentum over the past decade. In 2004, the Food and Agriculture Organization of the United Nations (FAO) published the *Voluntary Guidelines to Support the Progressive Realization of the Right to Adequate Food in the Context of National Food Security* (also known as the Right to Food Guidelines), which provide guidance on strengthening legal and accountability frameworks, for countries seeking to implement the right to food (which is enshrined in the International Covenant on Economic, Social and Cultural Rights) (Vidar, et al., 2014). Thirty countries now have an explicit recognition of the right to adequate food in their national constitution (FAO, 2017). However, an analysis of the SDGs shows a disconnect between the stated aims related to ending poverty, illiteracy, and hunger, with commitments to universal access to education, health care, and social protection, but no mention of the right to food. The authors conclude that 'human rights commitments are pitched against economic interests', undermining coherence in food policy (Vivero Pol and Schuftan, 2016, p. 2).

As the double burden of malnutrition has emerged, the need to reorient food systems to support access to affordable healthy food for NCD prevention – highlighted by SDGs 2 and 3 – has also faced challenges from economic interests (Hawkes and Popkin, 2015). The majority of World Health Organization (WHO) recommendations for healthy diets are focused on creating positive incentives for the production and consumption of healthy foods (WHO, 2013a). However, implementation of recommendations to date has focused on interventions to promote individual behaviour change – much of this due to prevailing policy frames that locate the cause of NCDs at the individual – rather than environmental level (Roberto, et al., 2015).

Threaded through these nutrition issues is the challenge of an environmentally sustainable food system. There are many synergies between the nutritional and environmental demands for food system reform (De Schutter, 2014; Monteiro, et al., 2015); for example, rising consumption of meat, associated with deforestation and environmental degradation, diversion of cereals from human consumption (hunger), and the NCD risk associated with overconsumption (De Schutter, 2014). In addition, climate change is threatening productivity and increasing demand for biofuels is contributing to volatility in staple food prices.

## The political challenge of action to improve nutrition

Achieving nutrition goals will require structural, policy-led change to the global food system. Policy theory tells us that such decisions are fundamentally political (Shiffman and Smith, 2007; Kingdon, 2003). Power, paradigms, and political contexts shape decisions as much as – if not more than – evidence for best practice. Understanding this can help to explain the limited action on even the 'straightforward' policy recommendations for direct nutrition intervention, as well as on the complex multisectoral recommendations for nutrition-sensitive policy, food security, and NCD prevention. Where significant progress has been seen in reducing malnutrition – for example, in Brazil, Ghana, Peru, and the Indian state of Maharashtra – this was supported by overt political commitments, and structural, policy-led, food system change (IFPRI, 2016).

In the following section, we examine the politics, actor interests and power differentials, and policy frames that underlie the evident incoherence in food system policy making.

## Global nutrition actors

Margulis describes a 'regime complex' governing food security, at the intersection between agriculture and food, international trade, and human rights (Margulis, 2013). This situation becomes even more complex when also considering undernutrition and NCD prevention.

Historically, nutrition as a health issue at the global level has been the purview of WHO and UNICEF, as institutions with a specific health mandate. In the post war era, these institutions led action on maternal and child nutrition, with a particular focus on breastfeeding and vertical interventions (Brown, et al., 2006). The United Nations World Food Program (WFP) was created in the 1960s as a multilateral food aid programme, focused on providing access to food during emergencies, initially with a limited nutrition mandate. At the same time, FAO was advocating a (marginalised) human rights and sociopolitical based approach to food policy (Pritchard, 2016). Historically, the role of the FAO had been coordinating surplus food distribution, and it had a major focus on increasing food production (Margulis, 2013). However, during the 1980s and 1990s its mandate and definition of food security expanded from a narrow focus on food availability to food access (Pritchard, 2016).

During the late 1980s and early 1990s, the World Bank rose to be arguably the most powerful actor in health, nutrition, and development. The 1993 World Development Report on investing in health was a milestone in framing nutrition as an economic and development issue, with a major focus on economic cost-effectiveness analysis (World Bank, 1993). The implication of this was a focus on targeted, 'vertical', cost-effective interventions that would support attainment of good nutrition as the underpinning of a healthy and productive workforce (Sridhar, 2007). However, World Bank spending on nutrition peaked in the period 1990–3, and then declined again to less than 5 per cent of health, nutrition, and population spending (Sridhar, et al., 2017). This was in part a result of a shift in priorities to health systems funding, and was also influenced by the difficulty in showing outcomes within relatively short periods of time (as is possible with, for example, immunisation) and the multiplicity of factors that influence nutritional status (Sridhar, 2007). More recently, the Scaling Up Nutrition (SUN) Movement, initiated by the World Bank in 2010 in collaboration with the WHO and the Global Alliance for Improved Nutrition (GAIN), acts as a focal point for implementation of best-practice direct interventions to address undernutrition in the first 1,000 days of life (Gillespie, et al., 2013).

Coordination of such diverse actors with a nutrition mandate at the global level has continued to present challenges. The Committee on World Food Security (CFS) was established by the United Nations in 1974, to coordinate action on food security and nutrition. In 2009, the CFS was reformed to increase stakeholder engagement through a Civil Society Mechanism and Private Sector Mechanism (Claeys, 2015). The CFS has emerged as a leading UN agency for governance of food and nutrition (increasingly addressing the double burden of malnutrition, in addition to food security), and the Civil Society Mechanism has offered a formal mechanism for input by global food movements, such as the Via Campesina and Peoples' Health Movement. These movements offer opportunities for marginalised voices – regarding, for example, producer rights and public health – to be heard (Mann, 2014). However, the nutrition agenda is still in many cases sidelined by economic agendas (discussed in detail in the next section). The inclusion of a stakeholder platform for the private sector, and the growing role of private philanthropic foundations in financing nutrition interventions, means that rights-based and pro-poor strategies are often marginalised (Mann, 2015).

The growing prevalence of diet-related NCDs in low- and middle-income countries (LMIC) and emergence of the double burden of malnutrition during the last two decades of the twentieth century has led to a shift in focus in the key global nutrition agencies. Mandates for 'nutrition' have expanded to include food security, undernutrition, and diet-related NCD prevention in the WHO, FAO, World Bank, UNICEF, and CFS. Even the WFP has identified, in its 2016 nutrition policy update, its role in addressing the double burden of malnutrition in its emergency response. One key implication of this expanded mandate has been increased attention to the fact that the global food system is not delivering affordable healthy foods. The Second International Conference on Nutrition, a member-state meeting jointly hosted by the WHO and FAO in 2014, described the global food system as 'broken'.

## Food as a politico-economic issue

The food system is subject to widely divergent policy objectives. From a policy perspective, the food system contributes not only to nutrition, food security, and health, but also to economic growth and development, livelihoods, rural development, environmental sustainability, and biodiversity. At the global level, food is thus governed by economic, health, and agricultural institutions.

Food is one of the most highly traded commodities globally, and contributes significantly to measures of economic growth and productivity in all countries (Singh and Gupta, 2016). Although international trade presents opportunities to grow agricultural markets, expand productivity (also contributing to rural development and poverty reduction), in practice trade liberalisation has also been associated with rising inequality, fluctuations in global staple food prices, and increasing trade in low quality, unhealthy food (Murphy, 2016; Friel, et al., 2013; Thow and Hawkes, 2009). Increased global trade over the past 40 years has not supported improved nutrition. Dependence on trade for food security has not delivered a quality, diverse food supply (Murphy, 2015). Developing countries are dependent on trade for staple crops, compared to high-income countries, which import 'luxury' foods. As a result, fluctuations in global staple food prices are more likely to hurt the poor (Otero, et al., 2013).

Because food is one of the most highly traded commodities globally, policy space in which governments can take action on nutrition and food security is constrained by global trade and investment agreements. Recently, interpretive nutrition labelling – an intervention recommended for NCD prevention – has been the subject of specific trade concerns in the Technical Barriers to Trade Committee (Thow, et al., 2017). Under the World Trade Organization (WTO) Agreement on Agriculture, India has been called to defend its public stockholding programme that supports its constitutional implementation of the Right to Food (Patnaik, 2017). The main concern raised by such challenges is a restriction of innovation at a time when food and nutrition policy needs new approaches (Singh and Gupta, 2016).

The politics of food and nutrition is also closely tied to the politics of agriculture and production. Agriculture has become increasingly financialised over the past several decades, in part arising from the colonial structure of commodity trade (Gertel and Sippel, 2016). Now, four agribusiness firms control over 70 per cent of global grain production (Clapp, 2015). A key limitation of existing agricultural systems is the focus on a few staple grains – these systems are not set up for production of a diversity of nutrient-dense foods (Jones and Ejeta, 2015). Financial actors have gained significant power in food production decision-making, as a result of the 'distancing' between production and consumption decisions, and contribute to the ongoing volatility of commodified food markets (Clapp, 2014). The financialisation of food was a significant contributor to the global food crisis of 2007–9, in which shocks such as speculative behaviour in food commodity markets and the diversion of food crops to fuel production led to sudden increases in the prices of staple foods (De Schutter, 2009). It was estimated that the number of outstanding contracts in maize futures increased from 500,000 in 2003 to almost 2.5 million in 2008, and that commodity index fund holdings increased from US$13 billion in 2003 to US$317 billion by 2008 (De Schutter, 2010).

## Conflicts of interests and power differentials

The multiple goals for food system policy across economic, social, health, environmental, and other sectors give rise to policy incoherence and conflicts of interest. The current food system is not delivering optimal health, environmental, or economic outcomes. This raises the question of whose interests are served by the status quo, since governments seek legitimacy in balancing interests of different food system actors (Murphy, 2016).

The food industry (across the entire supply chain) is a major contributor to GDP in most countries, which acts as a significant source of influence in policy decisions (Nestle, 2013; Monteiro, et al., 2013). There are two major implications of the influential position of the food industry in shaping global food policy priorities. The first is that economic, rather than health or human, concerns are the major consideration. The second is that economically profitable (technical) solutions are preferred to structural, food system-oriented reforms; for example, the development of 'functional' foods, or 'therapeutic' foods to address malnutrition. In both of these instances, the food industry is positioned as a critical part of the 'solution' to malnutrition (Yach, et al., 2010). Much of the scepticism regarding the potential role of industry in nutrition stems from unethical behaviour by the food industry in the past (Balarajan and Reich, 2016); in particular, the inappropriate and aggressive marketing of breast milk substitutes, that led to child malnutrition and death and eventually the creation of the International Code of Marketing of Breast Milk Substitutes (WHO, 1981).

Balancing public health needs with commercial interests and managing conflicts of interest requires transparent systems and mechanisms, as well as clear limits on the influence of vested interests on nutrition policy making (Kraak, et al., 2011). The WHO and the United Nations Standing Committee on Nutrition have both identified the need to monitor and regulate the activity of the private sector with respect to nutrition interventions and policy (Balarajan and Reich, 2016; WHO, 2016). The WHO Framework for Engagement with Non-State Actors (FENSA) outlines broad principles for engagement and associated risks and benefits, but has been critiqued as implicitly acting as a mechanism for increased access by private sector interests to global policy dialogues (Labonté, 2016). If anything, the FENSA negotiations at the WHO revealed that the conflicts of interest may be deepening at the institution, rather than vice versa. Several global non-government organisations have raised concerns publicly about the investments of the Bill & Melinda Gates Foundation Trust endowment – the source of revenue for the Foundation – in many of the food, alcohol, and physical inactivity related consumer products that contribute to NCDs, including Coca-Cola and Walmart (PHM-SA, 2017). Such conflicts of interest weaken the capacity of WHO to make strong recommendations and potentially develop international treaties that support the regulation of such industries.

The inclusion of 'transparency' and 'regulatory coherence' provisions in recent trade and investment agreements are likely to also undermine efforts to protect nutrition policy from the influence of vested interests at the national level. For example, provisions such as that in the Korea–United States Free Trade Agreement requiring governments to allow 'persons [a national or an enterprise] of the other party to participate in the development of standards, technical regulations, and conformity assessment procedures' (Thow, et al., 2015, p. 91; Labonté, 2016).

This imbalance of power between economic and nutrition actors in food supply policy making is also enshrined through significant power differentials in multilateral forums. On the one hand are non-binding recommendations ('soft law') for nutrition and 'guidelines' for implementing the right to food. On the other are binding international trade and investment agreements ('hard law') and conditionalities attached to loans from international financial institutions. Economic institutions dominate decision-making – and 'forum shopping' by industry groups is evident, particularly with the rise of regional and bilateral trade and investment agreements (Labonté, 2016). The food industry presents clear arguments in such forums for its pivotal role in contributing to economic growth, resulting in reluctance among governments to implement strong regulation for nutrition that challenges the status quo (Friel, et al., 2016).

## Powerful, persistent frames

Nutrition is thus a contested and political space. One manifestation of this is a range of diverse frames for 'the problem' by different actors, which have led to widely different solutions. The term 'frame' refers to 'ideas, packaged as values, social problems, metaphors or arguments', and can range from general ideological orientations to specific policy positions (Koon, et al., 2016, p. 801).

A powerful framing of nutrition, resonant with economic simplification, is the equating of undernutrition with insufficient calories (Jones and Ejeta, 2015; Headey, et al., 2012). For example, as global attention to hunger and food insecurity has led to increasing cooperation across the UN system, the Bretton Woods institutions, the WTO, and the Group of 20 (G20) leaders, malnutrition has been progressively reduced to issues of poverty and an adequate (aggregate) supply of food (Margulis, 2013; Margulis, 2014). This frame is particularly unhelpful in the context of the double burden of malnutrition, as the corollary to undernutrition as insufficient calories is the framing of overweight/obesity and NCDs as 'overconsumption': a problem of 'too many' calories (Thow, et al., 2016). This framing thus avoids the issues of food quality, dietary diversity, and access to healthy, nourishing food that are central to addressing food security and nutrition.

The food industry also presents clear frames for nutrition. Relevant to obesity and NCDs, the food industry frames nutrition as primarily an individual responsibility, and the role of the food industry as the provision of technical solutions to support individuals in making healthier choices (Roberto, et al., 2015; Brownell, et al., 2010; Scott, et al., 2017); for example, through reformulating processed foods to reduce the content of unhealthy nutrients (rather than addressing issues of access to healthy foods). Similarly, with respect to undernutrition and food security, technological solutions that increase production – vis-à-vis the Green Revolution – are portrayed as essential (Jones and Ejeta, 2015). A result of these frames is a strong perception that the transnational food industry is a critical contributor to the solution. This reflects broader philanthrocapitalist approaches to development, with a focus on markets and technological solutions, an approach that minimises the role of food distribution in determining access (Brooks, 2013; Holt Giménez and Shattuck, 2011). This framing is in direct contrast to Amartya Sen's framing of hunger as an issue of entitlements and a product of social and political arrangements that shape access to food, and to a human rights approach to ensuring the right to adequate food (Pritchard, 2016; Margulis, 2013; Sen, 1983).

## Issue characteristics

The nature of the nutrition challenge itself also creates political challenges to policy action. The technical and social complexity of nutrition means that it is hard to demonstrate effectiveness of policy change to reduce malnutrition, which is not conducive to political cycles (Balarajan and Reich, 2016). For example, the difficulty in attributing (and quantifying) changes in nutritional status to intervention was one of the reasons for the decline of nutrition on the World Bank's agenda during the 1990s (Sridhar, 2007).

Another challenge is the fact that nutrition requires multisectoral action. Nutrition is often seen as a health sector issue, as it is the health sector that monitors, and is tasked to address, the human outcomes of poor nutrition. However, as described earlier, addressing the determinants of nutrition requires policy action across sectors. At both the global and national level it has proved difficult to get nutrition on other sectors' agendas – and in particular, to work across sectors to identify specific actions that will promote nutrition through addressing its determinants in a coherent approach (Mwadime, 2012).

A third characteristic of nutrition that has led to challenges in attaining political priority and the coordinated implementation of global policy recommendations is the fragmentation of the nutrition community (Morris, et al., 2008; Balarajan and Reich, 2016). This has resulted in multiple policy narratives, and no clear prioritisation of actions (Balarajan and Reich, 2016). For example, despite being brought together under Sustainable Development Goal 2, global nutrition and health recommendations demonstrate significant diversity in priorities and frames. Existing frames and recommendations for priority action include the need to protect and promote maternal and child health through direct interventions (undernutrition), limit access to unhealthy foods (NCD prevention), and implement public stockholding (food security and the right to food). These divergent narratives and demands regarding appropriate policy responses do not lend themselves to a cogent vision for global food system change.

## Towards policy coherence

Addressing the double burden of malnutrition will require food security and nutrition advocates and researchers to engage with global economic institutions and politics. Although there is strong evidence for best-practice nutrition interventions and the policies needed to reorient food systems to ensure access to affordable healthy food, the implementation of food systems change runs into very real politico-economic challenges (Alders, et al., 2016; Gillespie, et al., 2015).

In order to increase capacity among nutrition and food security advocates to engage with such agendas, four practical strategies can be identified. First, learning from local innovation in practice and policy – particularly in low- and middle-income countries – can provide evidence of not just impact but also the political dimensions of policy design and implementation, as well as the management of competing agendas. For example, urban farms in Cuba and Thailand that are micro-examples of sustainable, economically productive, healthy food systems (Alders, et al., 2016). A robust global food movement will play a critical role in identifying and sharing lessons from such initiatives (Holt Giménez and Shattuck, 2011).

Second, fostering critical analysis of existing food governance and dominant frames in order to support renegotiation of governance structures for better outcomes for those who are food insecure. This can begin with small-scale reframing and redefinition of nutrition and food security from 'calories' – which often reinforces global macro-productionist perspectives on hunger and nutrition – to a more meaningful frame that focuses on access to healthy, quality, and diverse diets (Murphy, 2015). It can also begin with strategic support for nutrition leadership – both in global institutions and nationally, to coordinate and inspire action on nutrition (Balarajan and Reich, 2016).

Third, reshaping the global architecture of governance for food and nutrition security issues must be taken up as an urgent priority. The ascendance of the Private Sector Mechanism (PSM) in the CFS, representing food corporations and agribusiness, has for instance increasingly been at the cost of the Civil Society Mechanism (CSM). The private sector's engagement is no longer just through the PSM but also through organisations representing their interests who register charitable organisations and seek to become part of the CSM. The impact that the private sector has in these global governance bodies is multiplied many-fold, with the emerging power of philanthrocapitalism. Philanthropic institutions like the Gates Foundation are steeped in conflicts of interest vis-à-vis the private sector, especially in the food industry.

Last, policy coherence cannot be achieved for the progressive realisation of the right to adequate food unless trade policies reflect the interests of the hundreds of millions of small and marginalised farmers in developing countries and not those of a handful of developed countries. This would need a fundamental change in the global trade rules on agriculture, especially at the WTO and a re-drafting of the Agreement on Agriculture (AoA). The unfinished agenda of the Doha Development Round, which saw a quiet burial at the Nairobi ministerial of the WTO, needs to resurrected and resolved in favour of those who are food insecure rather than corporations.

## References

Alders, R., Nunn, M., Bagnol, B., Cribb, J., Kock, R., and Rushton, J. (2016) 'Approaches to fixing broken food systems', In: M. Eggersdorfer, K. Kraemer, J. Cordaro, et al. (Eds.) *Good Nutrition: Perspectives for the 21st century*, Basel: Karger, pp. 132–44.

Balarajan, Y. and Reich, M.R. (2016) 'Political economy challenges in nutrition', *Globalization and Health*, 12(1): 70.

Bhutta, Z.A., Das, J.K., Rizvi, A., et al. (2013) 'Evidence-based interventions for improvement of maternal and child nutrition: what can be done and at what cost?' *The Lancet*, 382(9890): 452–77.

Black, R.E., Victora, C.G., Walker, S.P., Bhutta, Z.A., Christian, P., and Onis, M. (2013) 'Maternal and child undernutrition and overweight in low-income and middle-income countries', *The Lancet*, 382(9890): 427–51.

Bloom, D.E., Cafiero, E.T., Jané-Llopis, E., et al. (2011) *'The global economic burden of noncommunicable diseases'*, Geneva: World Economic Forum.

Brooks, S. (2013) 'Investing in food security? Philanthrocapitalism, biotechnology and development', University of Sussex, available at www.opendemocracy.net/sally-brooks/investing-in-food-security-on-philanthrocapitalism-biotechnology-and-development (accessed on 20 September 2017).

Brown, T.M., Cueto, M., and Fee, E. (2006) 'The World Health Organization and the transition from "international" to "global" public health', *American Journal of Public Health*, 96(1): 62–72.

Brownell, K.D., Kersh, R., Ludwig, D.S., et al. (2010) 'Personal responsibility and obesity: a constructive approach to a controversial issue', *Health Affairs*, 29(3): 379–87.

Bryce, J., Coitinho, D., Darnton-Hill, I., Pelletier, D., and Pinstrup-Andersen, P. (2008) 'Maternal and child undernutrition: effective action at national level', *The Lancet*, 371(9611): 510–26.

Claeys, P. (2015) 'The right to food: many developments, more challenges', *Canadian Food Studies/La Revue Canadienne des Études sur L'alimentation*, 2(2): 60–7.

Clapp, J. (2014) 'Financialization, distance and global food politics', *The Journal of Peasant Studies*, 41(5): 797–814.

Clapp, J. (2015) 'ABCD and beyond: from grain merchants to agricultural value chain managers', *Canadian Food Studies*, 2(2): 126–35.

De Schutter, O. (2009) 'The right to food: fighting for adequate food in a global crisis', *Harvard International Review*, 31(2): 38.

De Schutter, O. (2010) 'Food commodities speculation and food price crises', Rome: United Nations Special Rapporteur on the Right to Food.

De Schutter, O. (2014) 'The transformative potential of the right to food', report submitted to the United Nations Human Rights Council, New York: United Nations.

De Vet, E., de Wit, J.B.F., Luszczynska, A., et al. (2013) 'Access to excess: how do adolescents deal with unhealthy foods in their environment?', *The European Journal of Public Health*, 23(5): 752–6.

FAO. (2015) 'The state of food insecurity in the world', Rome: UN Food and Agriculture Organization, International Fund for Agricultural Development, and World Food Programme.

FAO. (2017) 'The human right to adequate food', available at www.fao.org/righttofood/right-to-food-home/en/ (accessed on 20 September 2017).

Friel, S., Hattersley, L., Snowdon, W., et al. (2013) 'Monitoring the impacts of trade agreements on food environments', *Obesity Reviews*, 14: 120–34.

Friel, S., Ponnamperuma, S., Schram, A., et al. (2016) 'Shaping the discourse: what has the food industry been lobbying for in the Trans Pacific Partnership trade agreement and what are the implications for dietary health?', *Critical Public Health*, 1–12.

Gertel, J. and Sippel, S.R. (2016) 'The financialisation of agriculture and food', In: M. Shucksmith and D.L. Brown (Eds.) *Routledge International Handbook of Rural Studies*, London: Routledge, pp. 215–26.

Gillespie, S., Haddad, L., Mannar, V., Menon, P., and Nisbett, N. (2013) 'The politics of reducing malnutrition: building commitment and accelerating progress', *The Lancet*, 382(9891): 552–69.

Gillespie, S., Menon, P., and Kennedy, A.L. (2015) 'Scaling up impact on nutrition: what will it take?', *Advances in Nutrition: An International Review Journal*, 6(4): 440–51.

Hawkes, C. and Popkin, B.M. (2015) 'Can the sustainable development goals reduce the burden of nutrition-related non-communicable diseases without truly addressing major food system reforms?', *BMC Medicine*, 13(1): 1–3.

Headey, D., Chiu, A., and Kadiyala, S. (2012) 'Agriculture's role in the Indian enigma: help or hindrance to the crisis of undernutrition?', *Food Security*, 4(1): 87–102.

Holt Giménez, E. and Shattuck, A. (2011) 'Food crises, food regimes and food movements: rumblings of reform or tides of transformation?', *The Journal of Peasant Studies*, 38(1): 109–44.

IFPRI (2016) 'Global nutrition report 2016: from promise to impact, ending malnutrition by 2030', Washington, DC: International Food Policy Research Institute.

Jones, A.D. and Ejeta, G. (2015) 'A new global agenda for nutrition and health: the importance of agriculture and food systems', *Bulletin of the World Health Organization*, 94: 228–9.

Kingdon, J.W. (2003) *Agendas, Alternatives and Public Policies*, New York: Longman.

Koon, A.D., Hawkins, B., and Mayhew, S.H. (2016) 'Framing and the health policy process: a scoping review', *Health Policy and Planning*, 31(6): 801–16.

Kraak, V.I., Swinburn, B., Lawrence, M., and Harrison, P. (2011) 'The accountability of public-private partnerships with food, beverage and quick-serve restaurant companies to address global hunger and the double burden of malnutrition', *SCN News*, 39: 11–25.

Labonté, R. (2016) 'Health promotion in an age of normative equity and rampant inequality', International Journal of Health Policy and Management, 5(12): 675–82.

Lim, S.S., Vos, T., Flaxman, A.D., et al. (2013) 'A comparative risk assessment of burden of disease and injury attributable to 67 risk factors and risk factor clusters in 21 regions, 1990–2010: a systematic analysis for the Global Burden of Disease Study 2010', *The Lancet*, 380(9859): 2224–60.

Mann, A. (2014) *Global Activism in Food Politics: Power shift*, New York: Palgrave MacMillan.

Mann, A. (2015) 'Food sovereignty: alternatives to failed food and hunger policie', *Contemporanea*, 18(3): 445–68.

Margulis, M.E. (2013) 'The regime complex for food security: implications for the global hunger challenge', *Global Governance: A Review of Multilateralism and International Organizations*, 19(1): 53–67.

Margulis, M.E. (2014) 'Trading out of the global food crisis? The World Trade Organization and the geopolitics of food security', *Geopolitics*, 19(2): 322–50.

Monteiro, C.A., Moubarac, J.C., Cannon, G., Ng, S.W., and Popkin, B. (2013) 'Ultra-processed products are becoming dominant in the global food system', *Obesity Reviews*, 14: 21–8.

Monteiro, C.A., Cannon, G., Moubarac, J-C., et al. (2015) 'Dietary guidelines to nourish humanity and the planet in the twenty-first century. A blueprint from Brazil', *Public Health Nutrition*, 18(13): 2311–22.

Morris, S.S., Cogill, B., and Uauy, R. (2008) 'Effective international action against undernutrition: why has it proven so difficult and what can be done to accelerate progress?', *The Lancet*, 371(9612): 608–21.

Murphy, S. (2015) 'Food security and international trade: risk, trust and rules', *Canadian Food Studies/La Revue canadienne des études sur l'alimentation*, 2(2): 88–96.

Murphy, S. (2016) 'International trade, food security and nutrition', In: B. Pritchard, R. Ortiz, and M. Shekar (Eds.) *Routledge Handbook of Food and Nutrition Security*, London: Routledge, pp. 268–82.

Mwadime, R.K.N. (2012) 'Accelerating national policymaking across sectors to enhance nutrition', In: S. Fan, and R. Pandya-Lorch (Eds.) *Reshaping Agriculture for Nutrition and Health*, Washington, DC: International Food Policy Research Institute.

NCD. (2016) 'Worldwide trends in diabetes since 1980: a pooled analysis of 751 population-based studies with 4.4 million participants', *The Lancet*, 387(10027): 1513–30.

Nestle, M. (2013) *Food Politics: How the food industry influences nutrition and health*, Berkeley: University of California Press.

Nisbett, N., Gillespie, S., Haddad, L., and Harris, J. (2014) 'Why worry about the politics of childhood undernutrition?', *World Development*, 64: 420–33.

Nisbett, N., Wach, E., Haddad, L., and El Arifeen, S. (2015) 'What drives and constrains effective leadership in tackling child undernutrition? Findings from Bangladesh, Ethiopia, India and Kenya', *Food Policy*, 53: 33–45.

Otero, G., Pechlaner, G., and Gürcan, E.C. (2013) 'The political economy of "food security" and trade: uneven and combined dependency', *Rural Sociology*, 78(3): 263–89.

Patnaik, B. (2017) *Unpacking Trade and Investment 2: The WTO Chessboard: Queens vs Peasants*, Brussels: Rosa Luxemburg Stiftung.

Pelletier, D., Gervais, S., Hafeez-ur-Rehman, H., Sanou, D. and Tumwine, J. (2016) 'Multisectoral nutrition: feasible or fantasy?', *The FASEB Journal*, 30(1 Supplement): 669.9.

PHM-SA (People's Health Movement-South Africa). (2017) 'Open letter to the executive board of the World Health Organization. Re: Conflict of interest safeguards far too weak to protect WHO from influence of regulated industries (the case of the Bill and Melinda Gates Foundation)', available at http://phm-sa.org/open-letter-to-the-%E2%80%A8executive-board-of-the-%E2%80%A8world-health-organization/ (accessed on 20 September 2017).

Pinstrup-Andersen, P. (2013) 'Nutrition-sensitive food systems: from rhetoric to action', *The Lancet*, 382(9890): 375–6.

Pritchard, B. (2016) 'Food and nutrition security', In: B. Pritchard, R. Ortiz, and M. Shekar (Eds.) *Routledge Handbook of Food and Nutrition Security*, Abingdon: Routledge, pp. 1–24.

Roberto, C.A., Swinburn, B., Hawkes, C., et al. (2015) 'Patchy progress on obesity prevention: emerging examples, entrenched barriers, and new thinking', *The Lancet*, 385(9985): 2400–9.

Ruel, M.T. and Alderman, H. (2013) 'Nutrition-sensitive interventions and programmes: how can they help to accelerate progress in improving maternal and child nutrition?', *The Lancet*, 382(9891): 536–51.

Sacco, R.L., Roth, G.A., Reddy, K.S., et al. (2016) 'The Heart of 25 by 25: achieving the goal of reducing global and regional premature deaths from cardiovascular diseases and stroke: a modeling study from the American Heart Association and World Heart Federation', *Global Heart*, 11(2): 251–64.

Scott, C., Hawkins, B., and Knai, C. (2017) 'Food and beverage product reformulation as a corporate political strategy', *Social Science & Medicine*, 172: 37–45.

Sen. A. (1983) 'Development: which way now?' *The Economic Journal*, 93(372): 745–62.

Shiffman, J. and Smith, S. (2007) 'Generation of political priority for global health initiatives: a framework and case study of maternal mortality', *The Lancet*, 370(9595): 1370–9.

Singh, J.P. and Gupta, S. (2016) 'Agriculture and its discontents: coalitional politics at the WTO with special reference to India's food security interests', *International Negotiation*, 21(2): 295–326.

Sridhar, D. (2007) 'Economic ideology and politics in the World Bank: defining hunger', *New Political Economy*, 12(4): 499–516.

Sridhar, D., Winters, J., and Strong, E. (2017) 'World Bank's financing, priorities, and lending structures for global health', *BMJ*, 358: j3339.

Stevens, G.A., Singh, G.M., Lu, Y., et al. (2012) 'National, regional, and global trends in adult overweight and obesity prevalences', *Population Health Metrics*, 10(1): 22.

Stewart, B. and Wild, C. (2015) *World Cancer Report 2014*, Lyon, France: International Agency for Research on Cancer, World Health Organization.

Thow, A.M. and Hawkes, C. (2009) 'The implications of trade liberalization for diet and health: a case study from Central America', *Globalization and Health*, 5(5).

Thow, A.M., Snowdon, W., Labonté, R., et al. (2015) 'Will the next generation of preferential trade and investment agreements undermine implementation of the Global Action Plan for Prevention and Control of Noncommunicable Diseases? A prospective policy analysis of the Trans Pacific Partnership Agreement', *Health Policy*, 119: 88–96.

Thow, A.M., Kadiyala, S., Khandelwal, S., Menon, P., Downs, S. and Reddy, K.S. (2016) 'Towards food policy for the dual burden of malnutrition: an exploratory policy space analysis in India', *Food and Nutrition Bulletin*, 37: 261–74.

Thow, A.M., Jones, A., Hawkes, C., Ali, I., and Labonte, R. (2017) 'Nutrition labelling is a tradepPolicy issue: lessons from an analysis of specific trade concerns at the World Trade Organization', *Health Promotion International*, 10.1093/heapro/daw109.

Vidar, M., Kim, Y., and Cruz, L. (2014) 'Legal developments in the progressive realization of the right to adequate food: thematic study', Rome: Food and Agriculture Organisation of the United Nations Legal Office.

Vivero Pol, J.L. and Schuftan, C. (2016) 'No right to food and nutrition in the SDGs: mistake or success?', *BMJ Global Health*, 1(1).

WHO. (1981) 'International code of marketing of breastmilk substitutes', Geneva: World Health Organization.

WHO. (2013a) 'Follow-up to the political declaration of the high-level meeting of the general assembly on the prevention and control of non-communicable diseases', Geneva: World Health Organization.

WHO. (2013b) 'Global nutrition policy review: what does it take to scale up nutrition action?', Geneva: World Health Organization.

WHO. (2016) 'Addressing and managing conflicts of interest in the planning and delivery of nutrition programmes at country level', technical report, Geneva: World Health Organization.

World Bank. (1993) *World Development Report 1993: Investing in health*. New York: Oxford University Press.

World Economic Forum. (2017) 'Shaping the future of global food systems: a scenarios analysis', Davos: World Economic Forum System Initiative on Shaping the Future of Food Security and Agriculture and Deloitte Consulting LLP.

Yach, D., Feldman, Z.A., Bradley, D.G., and Khan, M. (2010) 'Can the food industry help tackle the growing global burden of undernutrition?' *American Journal of Public Health*, 100(6): 974–80.

Ziegler, J., Golay, C., Mahon, C., and Way, S-A. (2011) *The Fight for the Right to Food: Lessons learned*, London: Palgrave Macmillan UK.

# Part VII

# Humanitarian emergencies and global health politics

# 33

# Forced migration and health

## Problems and responses

*Eduardo Faerstein and Anete Trajman*

In 2016, the images of overcrowded, small boats crossing the Mediterranean Sea, often sinking tragically off the coast of Europe, raised worldwide concern about the magnitude and risks of contemporary forced migration. In fact, the most recent wave of migration from Syria, Iraq, and Afghanistan to European and North American countries became a leitmotif of current global politics, dividing public opinion and strongly influencing general elections in several countries, such as the US, the UK, the Netherlands, Austria, and France.

Forced migrations, however, are not new to humankind. About two million years ago, our *Homo* ancestors moved out of Africa. Even if this occurred out of curiosity in specific situations, it is widely acknowledged that the genus *Homo* evolved as it did due to the climatic vicissitudes of the Pleistocene (Finlayson, 2005). Since then, forced migration has been an inherent part of humankind's history, including massive dispersions of religious and ethnic groups, such as the African, Jewish, Armenian, Palestinian, Irish, and Chinese diasporas (Cohen, 2008).

In this chapter, we review concepts of interest and describe the origins and magnitude of the contemporary phenomenon, and we note the convergence of academic disciplines into the relatively new field of forced migration studies. We then present selected data on the main health issues related to forced migration, as well as on current institutional responses to those issues. We conclude by outlining a potential agenda for health-related global policies with respect to forced migrants.

According to the International Organization for Migration,

> Forced migration is a migratory movement in which an element of coercion exists, including threats to life and livelihood, whether arising from natural or man-made causes e.g. movements of refugees and internally displaced persons as well as people displaced by natural or environmental disasters, chemical or nuclear disasters, famine, or development projects.
>
> *IOM, 2015, n.p.*

## Convergence of disciplines in forced migration studies

Women and men have migrated over long distances since ancient times, but during the twentieth century forced migrations were intensified by many armed conflicts, including the two World Wars, colonial wars, conflicts in the Balkans, Africa, the Caucasus, Afghanistan and Iraq, state partitions and territorial claims in

South Asia and the Middle East, and also by human rights violations under authoritarian regimes. People were displaced across international borders, traveling into neighbouring states or roaming over continents in search of international protection; others were displaced across borders as stateless or environmentally displaced people. An even greater number of people were forced to leave their homes but remained within their country of origin as internally displaced persons (IDP).

Although the migrant crisis that began in 2015 has many features common to migrations across other historical periods, it became an exceptionally severe and large-scale phenomenon. In 2015, 24 new individuals were displaced every minute, compared to six per minute in 2005. Of the 250 million international migrants worldwide in 2016, 65 million were forced migrants, of whom 21.3 million were refugees (World Bank Group, 2016) and 37.5 million were internally displaced persons (UNHCR, 2016). During 2015, over one million individuals fled to Europe by sea, of whom 84 per cent left typical refugee-producing countries, such as Syria (49 per cent), Afghanistan (21 per cent), and Iraq (9 per cent) (Médecins Sans Frontières, 2016). However, even if the recent influx of refugees in Europe has caught the world's attention, South–South migration, i.e., migration among developing countries, remains larger than South–North migration, and is estimated at 38 per cent of all international migrants. Latin America, India, and South Africa are frequent destinations of international migrants (KNOMAD, 2016; World Bank Group, 2016).

Defining whether migration is voluntary or forced can be difficult, since most combine elements of both coercion and volition along a continuum of situations. These can vary from a natural search for better opportunities to a dramatic escape from death due to persecution or civil war. At this extreme are refugees and persons living in refugee-like conditions.

The United Nations High Commissioner for Refugees (UNHCR) has defined five categories of persons of concern: (1) refugees, (2) asylum seekers, (3) internally displaced persons, (4) returnees, and (5) stateless persons. According to the 1951 United Nations (UN) Refugee Convention, a refugee is a person who:

> Owing to a well-founded fear of persecution for reasons of race, religion, nationality, membership of a particular social group or political opinions, is outside the country of his nationality and is unable or, owing to such fear, is unwilling to avail himself of the protection of that country.
>
> *UNHCR, 2010, n.p.*

Later statements, from the Organization of African Unity (1969) and the 1984 Cartagena Declaration, did not change the basic definition of refugee in the 1951 UN Convention (UNHCR, 2010).

Refugees and other UNHCR persons of concern are the only groups protected under international law. However, contemporary forced migration is increasingly driven by situations such as hunger, economic crises, and unemployment. In addition, catastrophes such as floods, hurricanes, earthquakes, and tsunamis may also force people to migrate, without the short-term possibility of return. Populations from poor countries tend to suffer more from these catastrophes; for example, about 22 per cent of Haitians live outside their country (Abrams, 2010), mainly as 'environmental refugees'.

As happened to our early ancestors, climate change – man-made this time – will most likely be associated with growing population movements in coming decades. Myers (2002) estimated that climate change would create up to 200 million additional environmental refugees by 2050, motivated by the perception or expectation of an increased frequency of extreme weather events and the resulting food and water shortages. The Darfur crisis of the past decade exemplifies an explosive combination of environmental, political, and economic factors (Flint and Waal, 2008). The 2010 Cancun Climate Adaptation Framework Agreement called for 'measures to enhance understanding, coordination and cooperation with regard to climate change-induced displacement, migration and planned relocation, where appropriate, at national, regional and international levels' (UNFCCC, 2010, n.p.).

Finally, an under-studied subcategory of forced migration worth mentioning is associated with infrastructure interventions, such as dams, railway development, and building complexes – the so-called 'development refugees' (McMichael, et al., 2012). Although extremely vulnerable and prone to massive internal or international migration, environmental and development refugees do not qualify for refugee status or any international mechanisms of protection.

## Health consequences of forced migration

Despite the scale of the global forced migration phenomenon, little attention has been given to the health needs of the migrants themselves. For example, at the Global Knowledge Partnership on Migration and Development (KNOMAD) website, migrants' health is nowhere mentioned (KNOMAD, 2016). United Nations documents (OCHA, 2004; UNHCR, 2010) highlight education, freedom, and protection against violence as rights of internally dislocated persons and refugees, but health is surprisingly omitted from the list of their rights, despite being designated as a priority issue by the UNHCR (UNHCR, 2014).

Meanwhile, the academic discipline of forced migration studies has drawn predominantly on the social sciences, analysing the causes and consequences of human displacement from the migrants' perspective, and has arguably neglected a 'top-down' analysis that might be essential to understand the macro-level structures that influence states' responses to forced migration (Betts, 2012). Within the public health research field, migrant populations have traditionally been investigated (mainly by epidemiologists) as a 'natural experiment', with the focused aim of disentangling genetic (stable) from environmental (dynamic) determinants of specific diseases across generations (Susser, et al., 1985). In spite of growing interest and scientific output, research about the health of forced migrants still lacks more solid connections with forced migration studies, a challenge that should be taken up by global health academics and activists alike.

Studies investigating relations between and among migration, health status, and health-seeking behaviour are conceptually and methodologically challenging. One such challenge is the 'healthy migrant effect' (for example, the so-called 'Latino health paradox') (Abraído-Lanza, et al., 1999), namely the fact that those who choose and are able to migrate tend to be healthier than their compatriots. However, the increasing heterogeneity of contemporary migrant populations and their circumstances presents a more mixed picture. For example, an 'unhealthy re-migration effect' (Razum, et al., 1998, p. 302), also described as the 'salmon bias' phenomenon (Abraído-Lanza, et al., 1999, p. 1543), was observed in Germany, where socially successful migrants with a lower mortality risk tended to stay in the host country, but those less successful tended to return home before or after a disease episode. While a study of migrants to Mexico found weak evidence for the healthy migrant effect (Rubalcava, et al., 2008), a study of migrants to Spain found that the longer they stayed, the worse their overall health status became (Gimeno-Feliu, et al., 2015). A meta-analysis of global literature on schizophrenia and migration disclosed no difference between first- and second-generation migrants, with both groups showing a threefold increased risk of developing the disorder (Cantor-Graae and Selten, 2005).

As for the healthy migrant effect among individuals forced to migrate, the picture is as mixed as with migrants in general. For example, the effect was observed among migrants originating from the former Yugoslavia, a group that included many conflict refugees (Janevic, et al., 2011). In contrast, in Ontario, Canada, the risk of severe neonatal morbidity was less among refugees compared to non-refugee immigrants (Wanigaratne, et al., 2016).

For the most part, forced migrants are at higher risk of poor health, depending on the stage of migration (Toole and Waldman, 1997), but because both health status and behaviour are influenced by the diversity of characteristics of the origin and host environments, as well as the cause and time of migration, findings on migrants' health in host countries are conflicting.

Health issues common among migrants before their journeys begin include chronic infectious diseases such as hepatitis and tuberculosis, non-communicable diseases, and post-traumatic stress syndrome. Food insecurity is also worrisome. Transmission of malaria during the transit phase of international migration, and the development of anti-malarial resistance during transit, have been described as a potent threat of a treatment-resistant malaria pandemic (Lynch and Roper, 2011).

Mental health is a special concern at all stages of migration. Individuals forced to flee their home countries have often endured war, persecution, and long travel in adverse conditions. A particular threat to forced migrants' mental and physical health is gender-based violence, which in addition to physical wounds and maternal health problems, notably those accompanying unwanted pregnancy as a result of rape (Stark and Ager, 2011), has associated depression, anxiety, post-traumatic stress syndrome, and other manifestations. More than half of migrants who arrived in Germany in the last few years show signs of mental disorder, and a quarter of them have PTSD, anxiety, or depression (Abbott, 2016). Muslims, in particular, face the long-term effects of Western nations' responses to the attacks of 11 September 2001 (Gould and Klor, 2016). Hate crimes against Muslims have been on the rise since then.

Due to the high prevalence of psychological trauma among forced migrants, the so-called 'treatment gap' for mental conditions is wider for these migrants than for other migrants. One must consider, however, the ongoing controversy between proponents of global mental health (GMH), which espouses the global upscaling of evidence-based treatment as practiced in the world's most developed medical cultures, and a number of transcultural psychiatrists and anthropologists who see mental health treatment as locally contingent (Bemme and D'souza, 2014). While GMH puts forward a humanitarian moral argument for global action based on shared biology and the universality of human rights, some criticism of GMH and its biomedical model has appeared in the literature, echoing critiques of other 'global' projects – capitalism, colonialism, imperialism – and their associated imagery of harmful expansion, hegemony, exploitation of indigenous people, and extraction of natural resources without local benefit.

Another view of mental health in the global context is that economic, social, and political processes leading to stigma, stereotyping, prejudice, and discrimination against forced migrants can be classified as dimensions of structural violence (Parker, 2012). More recently, attention has been drawn to discrimination and marginalisation that sexual and gender non-conforming (SGN) refugees suffer (Türk, 2013). In some countries such as Mexico, South Africa, and Uganda, SGN refugees encounter extra barriers when applying for refugee protection (ORAM, 2013, p. 4). Many LGBTI, including adolescents, flee their country because of persecution motivated by their sexual orientation and find themselves in a particularly vulnerable situation, subject to violence, rape, and even murder. Because they fear further harm from officials, they will eventually not seek protection. UNHCR's Code of Conduct sets out clear norms and requires managers to take action when inappropriate behaviour is identified but recognise that staff sensitisation and training will often be necessary (UNHCR, 2011).

There is evidence that migrants face greater health risks in refugee camps than in their countries of origin. Overcrowding poses the danger of transmission of infectious diseases: hepatitis, infectious diarrhoea, tuberculosis, and other oral-faecal and respiratory infection outbreaks have been consistently reported. Communicable diseases prompt over 91 per cent of all refugee medical consultations, and respiratory infections have now surpassed malaria as the leading cause of death among this population (UNHCR, 2014). Potable water supply and sanitation, adequate nutrition, prevention of malaria, psychosocial support, vaccination, and child-maternal care are the main health priorities in refugee camps (UNHCR, 2014). To this list should be added all the pre-existing chronic conditions that need attention.

Various studies have highlighted the specific health needs of women and adolescents in refugee camps (Norwegian Refugee Council, 2015). Menstrual problems have often been cited; other reported health issues in the camps are skin diseases, nutritional deficiencies, kidney disease, and asthma (Samaddar, 2003). As host countries begin to limit or foreclose entry to immigrants in general, and asylum seekers in particular, refugee camp stays may be prolonged and these health needs may intensify.

Other complex health needs emerge once refugees arrive in their host countries. Some pre-departure health problems will continue to affect these individuals for the long term, and in addition various new health issues can supervene post-arrival. Assimilation in urban settings and acculturation in Western countries result in increased risk of chronic non-communicable diseases. Tooth decay and missing teeth are also more prevalent among migrant children, especially refugees, than in host countries' general populations (Hoover, et al., 2016).

Forced migrant workers often have undesirable, low-skill jobs, with consequent insecure and precarious employment, long working hours, and low income. Undocumented migrants (asylum seekers whose refugee visas are denied) are especially vulnerable to exploitation, since they fear job loss, incarceration, and deportation if they complain of working conditions. Thus, urgent health issues for this population include occupational safety, injury prevention, and work-related illnesses (Benach, et al., 2011).

## Agenda for global policies

Evidence is scarce about the public health component of interventions during humanitarian crises (Blanchet, et al., 2017). Policies to protect forced migrants' health will possibly be most effective if they address the multiple phases of the migratory process, including pre-departure, travel, destination, interception, settlement, and return. Health intervention opportunities exist at each stage (Zimmerman, et al., 2011), and policymakers should take care that their decisions on these issues are evidence-based. Often, this is not the case, as discussed in the following.

Several countries implement outdated screening programmes for migrants. Screening for tuberculosis, for example, is widely conducted by immigration services, although treatment of latent infection detected through screening may require coercive and ethically questionable measures to maximise impact and cost-effectiveness (Mandalakas and Menzies, 2011; Dasgupta and Menzies, 2005). Similarly, absence of other communicable conditions and good mental health status are often included in the conditional health requirements for an entry visa.

For social, economic, environmental, and health reasons, the consequences of placing refugees in camps are often negative, not only for the refugees themselves but also frequently for the national populations and governments of receiving states. Historical and political reasons explain the long-term survival of some refugee camps. Currently there is a clear trend among refugees to go to cities rather than camps, but some refugee camps (e.g., in Gaza, Palestine) have turned into urbanised agglomerations.

The course of the recent Ebola epidemic in Guinea, Liberia, and Sierra Leone illustrates the dramatic consequences of restrictions on travel to and from affected countries. Despite the statement of the World Health Organization (WHO) opposing Ebola-related travel restrictions, some airlines cancelled some of their flights, and immigration authorities in several other countries restricted the entry of any person coming from these countries, regardless of their health status. These policies made international help difficult to deliver to these countries. During the same epidemic, the closure of the borders of neighbouring countries resulted in further dislocations, for example, the trapping of thousands of Ivorian refugees in Liberia who were prevented from returning to Ivory Coast (Adele, 2015).

Health aid to forced migrants in refugee camps is often provided by humanitarian non-governmental organisations such as the International Red Cross and Médecins Sans Frontières, usually coordinated by the United Nations agencies – mainly UNHCR – that also train physicians and nurses for psychosocial support (UNHCR, 2016). These organisations plan the logistics of mass vaccinations, protective bed nets against vectors, mental health support, and paediatric and obstetric facilities in refugee and displaced person camps (WFPHA, 2015). Médecins Sans Frontières (2017) reported over eight million outpatient consultations in 2015.

Contemporary forced migrants mostly settle in cities, and in many cases, contribute to the growing population of the 'urban poor' in the global South, who experience an 'urban health penalty' due to their exposure to unhealthy physical and social conditions (Freudenberg, et al., 2005, pp. 2–3). Forced migrants should not be added to a 'surplus humanity' (Davis, 2007, p. 175) that should not exist in the first place. It is therefore of utmost importance to monitor the implementation of the United Nations *Habitat III* report, which explicitly recognised 'the need to give particular attention to addressing multiple forms of discrimination faced by, inter alia, … refugees, returnees, internally displaced persons and migrants, regardless of their migration status', and to:

> support [these individuals'] host cities in the spirit of international cooperation, taking into account national circumstances and recognizing that, although the movement of large populations into towns and cities poses a variety of challenges, it can also bring significant social, economic and cultural contributions to urban life.
>
> *United Nations, 2016, n.p.*

Once refugees and asylum seekers are settled, their safety and well-being are the responsibility of their host countries, which should prepare them for such challenges. UNHCR advocates that, at a minimum, emergency and primary health care should be provided free of charge to refugees during an emergency. UNHCR also recommends that essential services such as prenatal and delivery care, vaccination and management of communicable diseases should be available free of charge in post-emergency situations and should be of the same quality as services provided to the local population. Thus, UNHCR encourages the use, wherever possible, of governmental health services. In other words, countries with universal, free-of-charge health systems are ideal hosts and should make efforts to increase their response to the current humanitarian crisis. Developing countries should expand their role as host countries in this scenario.

An invaluable example is the decades-long health system experience of the United Nations Relief and Works Agency for Palestine Refugees in the Near East (UNRWA), which has now adopted the Family Health Team approach (UNRWA, 2017), on principles of person-centredness, comprehensiveness, and continuity of care. By 2020, all 137 UNRWA health centres should have implemented this approach. Other innovative policies and interventions, including migrant-focused health plans, such as the 'Migrant-Friendly Hospitals' project in Europe (Koskinen and Vimpeli, 2011), should be encouraged. To provide adequate health care to migrants, specific cultural norms should be considered (such as the need for same-gender professionals), as well as linguistic barriers indicating the need for comprehensive translation services.

Multilateral political solutions are needed to resolve the conundrum of forced migrants' frequent inability to meet the strict legal definitions of refugees and other UNHCR 'persons of concern'. An especially important recent instance of the problem is the massive migration of Haitians to other countries after the earthquake of 2010 and the floods of 2016. Many Haitians who arrived in Brazil were denied refugee visas because their circumstances did not fit the 1951 Geneva Convention definition of 'refugee'. Formal definitions notwithstanding, the Brazilian government eventually granted 'humanitarian' visas to these forced migrants (Annoni, et al., 2016; Godoy, 2011; Pacifico, et al., 2015); but the health of populations forced to flee natural disasters or other tragedies should not have to depend on one-time dispensations from a host government.

International research funding agencies and universities need to agree on an agenda for research strategies and data collection systems about population movements and migrant health indicators and needs. Innovative methods are needed, since displaced populations can be difficult to reach as people move within and across geographic borders and through formal and informal systems and regimes.

In times where border walls and legal barriers are being built to restrict immigration, it should be remembered that refugees and other forced migrants are mostly young adults who will work, pay taxes, and contribute to social security funds, raising badly needed revenue in countries with aging populations where retirement health funding has become a challenge. A 2016 study in the US (National Academies of Sciences, Engineering, and Medicine, 2017) estimated that immigration would have few if any longer-term negative effects on the overall wages or employment rates of native-born workers. Moreover, immigration brings with it cultural diversity and the 'brain gain' of well-trained professionals into host countries.

In 2015, 193 United Nations member states adopted the 2030 Agenda for Sustainable Development. Among the Agenda's stated goals is to 'facilitate orderly, safe, regular and responsible migration and mobility of people, including through the implementation of planned and well-managed migration policies' (United Nations, 2015, n.p.).

To achieve these goals requires global governance based on a thorough debate among governments and international institutions (Betts, 2012). The international political climate, particularly the growing politicisation of migration, precludes optimistic predictions about forced migration and the fate of forced migrants in the near future. During the second half of the 2010s, rising xenophobia and racism paralleled the growth of populist isolationism, exemplified by sociopolitical phenomena such as the UK Brexit, Trump's election in the US, and the strengthening of right-wing political parties in several European countries.

Globally, however, both population health and societal welfare will benefit if forced migrants are welcomed and integrated into host nations, even if the causes of forced migration cannot be eliminated from human experience.

# References

Abbott, A. (2016) 'The mental-health crisis among migrants', *Nature*, 538(7624): 158–60.

Abraído-Lanza, A.F., et al. (1999) 'The Latino mortality paradox: a test of the "salmon bias" and healthy migrant hypotheses', *American Journal of Public Health*, 89(10):1543–48.

Abrams, E. (2010) 'What Haiti needs: a Haitian diaspora', Council on Foreign Relations, available at www.cfr.org/haiti/haiti-needs-haitian-diaspora/p21270 (accessed on 10 February 2017).

Adele, A. (2015) 'A long wait for home – how Ebola kept refugees stuck in Liberia', IRIN, available at www.irinnews.org/analysis/2015/03/18-0 (accessed on 5 December 2016).

Annoni, D., Manzi, L., Júlia, M., Annoni, D., Manzi, L., and Júlia, M. (2016) 'Brazilian migration policy and its consequences for the states of UNASUR: a study from the treatment given by Brazil to the Haitian case', *Bol. Mex. Derecho Comp.*, 49: 61–83.

Bemme, D., and D'souza, N.A. (2014) 'Global mental health and its discontents: an inquiry into the making of global and local scale', *Transcult. Psychiatry*, 51: 850–74.

Benach, J., et al. (2011) 'Migration and "low-skilled" workers in destination countries', *PLOS Medicine*, 8(6): e1001043.

Betts, A. (2012) *Global Migration Governance*, Oxford: Oxford University Press.

Blanchet, K., Ramesh, A., Frison, S., Warren, E., Hossain, M., Smith, J., Knight, A., Post, N., Lewis, C., Woodward, A., Dahab, M., Ruby, A., Sistenich, V., Pantuliano, S., and Roberts, B. (2017) 'Evidence on public health interventions in humanitarian crises', *The Lancet*, 390: 2287–96.

Cantor-Graae, E. and Selten, J.P. (2005) 'Schizophrenia and migration: a meta-analysis and review', *The American Journal of Psychiatry*, 162(1): 12–24.

Cohen, R. (2008) *Global Diasporas: An introduction*, London: Routledge.

Dasgupta, K. and Menzies, D. (2005) 'Cost-effectiveness of tuberculosis control strategies among immigrants and refugees', *European Respiratory Journal*, 25(6): 1107–16.

Davis, M. (2007) *Planet of Slums*, London, New York: Verso.

Finlayson, C. (2005) 'Biogeography and evolution of the genus Homo', *Trends in Ecology & Evolution*, 20(8): 457–63.

Flint, J. and Waal, A. (2008) *Darfur: A new history of a long war*, London, New York: Zed Books.

Freudenberg, N., Galea, S., and Vlahov, D. (2005) 'Beyond urban penalty and urban sprawl: back to living conditions as the focus of urban health', *Journal of Community Health*, 30(1): 1–11.

Gimeno-Feliu, L.A., et al. (2015) 'The healthy migrant effect in primary care', *Gaceta Sanitaria*, 29(1): 15–20.

Godoy, G.G. de (2011) 'O caso dos haitianos no Brasil e a via da proteção humanitária complementar', In: F.H. Ramos, A. de Carvalho, G. Rodrigues, and G. de Almeida (Eds.). *60 Anos de ACNUR: Perspectivas de futuro*. São Paulo: CLA Cultural Editora, pp. 45–68.

Gould, E.D. and Klor, E.F. (2016) 'The long-run effect of 9/11: terrorism, backlash, and the assimilation of Muslim immigrants in the West', *The Economic Journal*, 126(597): 2064–114.

Hoover, J., Vatanparast, H., and Uswak, G. (2016) 'Risk determinants of dental caries and oral hygiene status in 3-15-year-old recent immigrant and refugee children in Saskatchewan, Canada: a pilot study', *Journal of Immigrant and Minority Health*, 27: 1–7.

IOM. (2015) 'Key migration terms', International Organization for Migration, available at www.iom.int/key-migration-terms (accessed on 10 February 2017).

Janevic, T., Savitz, D.A., and Janevic, M. (2011) 'Maternal education and adverse birth outcomes among immigrant women to the United States from Eastern Europe: a test of the healthy migrant hypothesis', *Social Science & Medicine*, 73(3): 429–35.

KNOMAD. (2016) 'Global knowledge partnership on migration and development (KNOMAD)', available at www.knomad.org/ (accessed on 10 February 2017).

Koskinen, N. and Vimpeli, R. (2011) *Migrant Friendly Hospital: A literature review*, VDM Verlag Dr. Müller.

Lynch, C. and Roper, C. (2011) 'The transit phase of migration: circulation of malaria and its multidrug-resistant forms in Africa', *PLoS Medicine*, 8(5): e1001040.

Mandalakas, A.M. and Menzies, D. (2011) 'Is screening immigrants for latent tuberculosis cost-effective?' *The Lancet: Infectious Diseases*, 11(6): 418–19.

McMichael, C., Barnett, J., and McMichael, A.J. (2012) 'An ill wind? Climate change, migration, and health', *Environmental Health Perspectives*, 120(5): 646–54.

Médecins Sans Frontières. (2016) 'Obstacle course to Europe: a policy-made humanitarian crisis at EU borders', available at www.doctorswithoutborders.org/sites/usa/files/2016_01_msf_obstacle_course_to_europe_-_final_-_low_res.pdf (accessed 10 February 2017).

Médecins Sans Frontières. (2017) 'Overview – Médecins Sans Frontières (MSF)', available at www.msf-me.org/en/article/about-us/overview.html (accessed on 10 February 2017).

Myers, N. (2002) 'Environmental refugees: a growing phenomenon of the 21st century', *Philosophical Transactions of the Royal Society B: Biological Sciences*, 357(1420): 609–13.

National Academies of Sciences, Engineering, and Medicine. (2017) *The Economic and Fiscal Consequences of Immigration*, Washington, DC: The National Academies Press.

Norwegian Refugee Council. (2015) 'Listening to women and girls displaced to urban Afghanistan', available at www.flyktninghjelpen.no/globalassets/pdf/reports/listening-to-women-and-girls-displaced-to-urban-afghanistan.pdf (accessed on 10 February 2017).

OCHA. (2004) 'Guiding principles on internal displacement', available at www.unhcr.org/43ce1cff2.pdf (accessed on 10 February 2017).

ORAM. (2013) 'Blind Alleys Part I, guidance for NGOs, governments, UNHCR & program funders', available at http://oramrefugee.org/wp-content/uploads/2016/03/oram_recommendeng_final_lr.pdf (accessed on 12 June 2017).

Pacifico, A.P., Ramos, E.P., Abreu Bastista Claro, C. de, and Cavalcante de Farias, N.B. (2015) 'The migration of Haitians within Latin America: significance for Brazilian law and policy on asylum and migration', In: D. Cantor, L.F. Freier, and J.-P. Gauci (Eds.), *A Liberal Tide? Immigration and asylum law and policy in Latin America*, London: School of Advanced Study, University of London, pp. 139–52.

Parker, R. (2012) 'Stigma, prejudice and discrimination in global public health', *Cadernos De Saude Publica*, 28(1): 164–9.

Razum, O., et al. (1998) 'Low overall mortality of Turkish residents in Germany persists and extends into a second generation: merely a healthy migrant effect?' *Tropical medicine & International Health*, 3(4): 297–303.

Rubalcava, L.N., et al. (2008) 'The healthy migrant effect: new findings from the Mexican Family Life Survey', *American Journal of Public Health*, 98(1): 78–84.

Samaddar, R. (2003) *Refugees and the State: Practices of asylum and care in India, 1947–2000*, New Delhi, Thousand Oaks, CA: Sage Publications Pvt. Ltd.

Stark, L. and Ager, A. (2011) 'A systematic review of prevalence studies of gender-based violence in complex emergencies', *Trauma, Violence & Abuse*, 12(3): 127–34.

Susser, M.W., Hopper, K., and Watson, W. (1985) *Sociology in Medicine*, New York: Oxford University Press.

Toole, M.J. and Waldman, R.J. (1997) 'The public health aspects of complex emergencies and refugee situations', *Annual Review of Public Health*, 18: 283–312.

Türk, V. (2013) 'Ensuring protection for LGBTI persons of concern', *Forced Migration Review*, 42: 5–9.

UNFCCC. (2010) 'Outcome of the work of the ad doc working group on long-term cooperative action under the convention', available at http://unfccc.int/files/meetings/cop_16/application/pdf/cop16_lca.pdf#page=3 (accessed on 10 February 2017).

UNHCR. (2010) 'Convention and protocol relating to the status of refugees, Geneva, Switzerland', available at www.unhcr.org/3b66c2aa10.pdf (accessed on 10 February 2017).

UNHCR. (2011) 'Working with lesbian, gay, bisexual, transgender & intersex persons in forced displacement', available at www.refworld.org/pdfid/4e6073972.pdf (accessed on 12 June 2017).

UNHCR. (2014) 'Global strategy for public health – HIV and reproductive health – food security and nutrition water, sanitation and hygiene (WASH), Geneva, Switzerland', available at www.unhcr.org/530f12d26.pdf (accessed on 10 February 2017).

UNHCR. (2016) 'Global trends: forced displacement in 2016', available at www.unhcr.org/globaltrends2016 (accessed on 10 February 2017).

United Nations. (2015) 'Sustainable development goals: 17 goals to transform our world', United Nations Sustainable Development, available at www.un.org/sustainabledevelopment/ (accessed on 10 February 2017).

United Nations. (2016) 'The new urban agenda. Habitat III', available at https://habitat3.org/the-new-urban-agenda/ (accessed on 10 February 2017).

UNRWA. (2017) 'Family health teams, UNRWA', available at www.unrwa.org/what-we-do/family-health-teams (accessed on 10 February 2017).

Wanigaratne, S., et al. (2016) 'Severe neonatal morbidity among births to refugee women', *Maternal and Child Health Journal*, 20(10): 2189–98.

WFPHA. (2015) 'WFPHA newsletter November 2015', available at www.wfpha.org/component/acymailing/mailid-44.html?tmpl=component (accessed on 5 December 2016).

World Bank Group. (2016) 'Migration and development: a role for the World Bank Group', available at http://pubdocs.worldbank.org/en/468881473870347506/Migration-and-Development-Report-Sept2016.pdf (accessed on 10 February 2017).

Zimmerman, C., Kiss, L., and Hossain, M. (2011) 'Migration and health: a framework for 21st century policy-making', *PLoS Medicine*, 8(5): e1001034.

# 34

# Geopolitics, political violence, and global health

## Ethical obligations for professionals acting within wars and conflict settings

*Cindy Sousa*

## Introduction

Political violence contributes to death, injury, and an increase in mental disorders like PTSD and depression of hundreds of millions of civilians (Krug, 2002). Political violence also undermines entire societies as it compromises citizens' investment and confidence in essential aspects of social and political life (Sousa, 2013).

To make matters worse, poor and unstable countries that already have vulnerable infrastructure, including legal and health care systems, are at a higher risk for political violence, which then worsens the already existing problems of poverty, inequality, and dependence (Baingana, et al., 2005; de Jong, 2010). As political violence weakens the welfare apparatus of states that already were suffering, health scholars charge that the neoliberal agenda fits exceedingly well within inter- and intra-state conflicts (Giacaman, et al., 2003; Hamid and Everett, 2007). While it might be unwitting, global health efforts may be complicit with taking advantage of the destabilised state to further dependence and the insertion of the private sector, a process Naomi Klein (2007) refers to as 'disaster capitalism'.

Enter into these already debilitated states models of public health recovery that rest on privatisation and the reification of health imperialism (Levich, 2015; Piachaud, 2008; Waitzkin and Jasso-Aguilar, 2015) and the neoliberal project of war recovery is solidified. Political violence and the neoliberal agenda work in tandem to impact public health in two key, interconnected ways: first, through the practice of privatisation and second, by increasing the reliance on outside assistance, including imported, 'expert' elites.

## Political violence, health, and neoliberalism: privatisation and parachuting health experts

A key component of the neoliberal model is moving essential functions from the public sphere (health care, education, resource management) over to private sectors. The role of nation-states in caring for the welfare of its citizens becomes less central; instead individuals and non-state actors, such as foundations and non-governmental organisations (NGOs) are impelled to take on more responsibility (Levich, 2015;

Ramon, 2008). Privatisation runs in direct opposition to theories of the welfare state, which posit that states must provide a sort of safety net for the inevitable failings of the economic system (Esping-Andersen, 1990). Further, some theorists and policy researchers hold strongly to the idea that responsibility for things essential for dignified lives and healthy societies (i.e., health care, education, delivery of essential services like water and electricity) should rest squarely with the public sector because the profit motive could so thoroughly corrupt its just provision (Katz, 2001).

Consistent with the neoliberal model, within political violence and its aftermath, the functions of the state with regards to health and welfare are increasingly privatised, and recovery efforts are pushed off to civil society (Carney, 2008; Lavalette and Ferguson, 2007). In this context, international agencies who move in to help are actually complicit with the misery, particularly as they approach collective health problems through a lens wherein normal responses to massive tragedy are treated with highly individualised and medicalised approaches (Kleinman, 1999; Sousa and Marshall, 2015).

Within the neoliberal process, citizens with rights are transformed into consumers endowed with choices and responsibilities (Horton, 2007). This is in sharp contrast to notions of social citizenship, wherein the welfare state provides universal benefits that establish and guarantee conditions to ensure achievement of full citizenship (Marshall, 1997). Under neoliberalism, as citizens become consumers, social rights, like that for health (including mental health), become mere aspects of the market. Health scholars maintain that the trend of tying health to markets or development goals (i.e., the United Nations Millennium Development Goals [MDGs]) pits health against economic development, thereby undermining the notion of health as a universal right in and of itself (Waitzkin and Jasso-Aguilar, 2015). This move towards market-ising health through intimately tying mental health recovery to the recovery of economic markets is a common theme in discourse about global conflict recovery (Baingana, et al., 2005; Bhavsar and Bhugra, 2008).

Efforts at privatisation with post-conflict recovery have resulted in an exorbitant growth of NGOs, particularly related to health (Lavalette and Ferguson, 2007; Pfeiffer, et al., 2008). One striking example of this is the deliberately increased relationship between NGOs and both the World Bank and the United Nations Development Program during the 1980s and 1990s; during this time, NGO inclusion in World Bank projects rose from 6 per cent in 1973–88 to 50 per cent by the late 1990s (Reimann, 2006). The ways that NGOs further the goals of privatisation have become so apparent that NGOs are often now termed the 'fourth sector', and critiques are mounting against their use to undermine the strategic relationships between the state, citizens, and the non-profit sector that are necessary for accountability and justice (Alessandrini, 2002; Incite! Women of Color Against Violence, 2007). Privatisation often rests on neoliberal rhetoric of 'civil society', and the long legacy of interference in sovereign nations 'for their own good' that is an integral part of the legacy of colonialism and imperialism (Lavalette and Ferguson, 2007; Waitzkin and Jasso-Aguilar, 2015). Horton notes that 'the entire project of neo-liberalism nationally and internationally is connected to a larger process of exporting the blame from the decisions of the dominant groups onto the state, and onto poor people' (Horton, 2007, p. 3). This blame usually is issued with rhetoric of corruption and inefficiency. As Klein asserts, '[the] theft of Iraq's reconstruction funds from Iraqis, justified by unquestioned, racist assumptions about U.S. superiority and Iraqi inferiority-and not merely the generic demons of "corruption" and "inefficiency" … doomed the project from the start' (Klein, 2007, p. 439).

The case of mental health in post-conflict Iraq is a good example of health imperialism. Iraq had been a country with deep investment in the public health system prior to the invasion. During the reconstruction period in 2007, a new mental health plan was generated by/with professionals who were from, in the most part, the United States and the United Kingdom (including SAMHSA and WHO). While this plan included a vast array of objectives and recommendations, the health system was highly dependent on outside aid and there was virtually no ability for the Iraqi government itself to control the system (Hamid and Everett, 2007, p. 1357).

As in the classic example of post-conflict 'recovery' in Iraq mentioned earlier, mental health treatment is often delivered and/or orchestrated by and through non-governmental institutions, effectively furthering the diminishing of states' role in recovery. The role these trans-governmental aid and development bodies play in the 'recovery' process is essential to understanding the destabilisation of the public health sector that often occurs in conflict settings. For example, Giacaman et al. (2003, p. 65) maintains that, with regards to the health sector in Palestine, the 'primary function of international aid is to sell the fragile and flawed peace process to the Palestinian people, by showing tangible results in their daily lives' at the cost of a commitment to long-term, authentic development. While expecting aid to solve political problems would be unfair, it has been charged that aid is used in political conflicts to substitute for actual political action. In other words, rather than dealing with the conflict itself, aid agencies, and the Western governments that support them, simply attempt to manage the worst symptoms of war (Shearer, 2000).

Furthermore, the attitude towards aid has fundamentally shifted in recent years; whereas it used to be quite limited so as to not undermine sovereignty, we now see a considerable 'humanitarian expansion', wherein aid agencies feel a right to intervene, and work around governments if they deem this approach necessary (Shearer, 2000, p. 197). Decisions about social services therefore are progressively made outside of the control of the state, with smaller non-state actors increasingly competing for funding. In this way, rather than actually empowering democratic rule and process and strengthening sovereignty, post-conflict aid is given or withheld to either reward or to punish political decisions (Brynen, 2000). Services are often deliberately defunded and organisations are hijacked (Brynen, 2000).

In line with the neoliberal model, assistance in post-conflict settings is done with rhetoric about community organising and civil society. As Swartz (2008, p. 306) points out, in South Africa, the state 'in its failure to provide adequate social care to all its vulnerable citizens, uses the language of community empowerment to justify non-delivery of services.' Civil society, though, is a contested concept, and does not 'necessarily mean more democracy' (Lavalette and Ferguson, 2007, p. 452). Paramount to the controversy is the fact that 'multinationals, vast corporation and smaller local enterprises all inhabit civil society' (Lavalette and Ferguson, 2007, p. 452). While essential for many functions (including keeping the government accountable to its citizens), civil society 'should not be compelled to take responsibility for the failure of the welfare state through neglect' (Alessandrini, 2002, p. 16). Rather than a substitute for a functioning government, actions by civil society operate best in relation to a responsive government that 'guarantee[s] a comprehensive set of rights' (Marmot, et al., 2008, p. 1667).

As the role of the state in ensuring the basic means for individual, family, and societies' well-being deteriorates and 'civil society', or the private sector, takes on increasing importance, control becomes increasingly concentrated in the hands of 'global elite networks' (Scholte, 2005, p. 24). Sklair (2002) refers to this network of elites as the Transnational Capitalist Class, noting that it is not comprised only of those who control means of production. While it does include individuals who operate for the good of transnational corporations, it also includes individuals who function within three other important spheres of society: state, technology, and culture. This includes transnational governance and development agencies who are highly present in post-conflict situations (i.e., US Agency for International Development, or USAID) as well as NGOs, however unwilling individual NGOs or workers may be to collude with neoliberalism (Lavalette and Ferguson, 2007; Sklair, 2002).

The rise in NGOs works alongside the problem of brain drain, or the flight of professionals that tends to be particularly acute within countries experiencing conflict, and which further undermines sovereignty within post-war recovery (Pfeiffer, et al., 2008). Among other problems, the parachuting in of outside 'experts' tends to create a situation where treatment and interventions are neither culturally appropriate nor sustainable (Summerfield, 1999; Weiss, et al., 2003).

What, then, is the responsibility of public health within these complex contexts? I end this chapter with some suggestions that may help us move forward as a field as we engage more deeply in geopolitical analyses of public health crises around the world, particularly focused on understanding the colonial and neoliberal legacies of suffering that are related to both violence and recovery efforts. I also present examples that might guide us in establishing viable agendas for global public health practice that counter neoliberal tendencies through emphasising advocacy, self-determination, and social justice.

First, we must gather energy from the theoretical direction put forth by the World Health Organization's Commission on Social Determinants of Health, who maintains the 'unequal distribution of health-damaging experiences is … the result of a toxic combination of poor social policies and programmes, unfair economic arrangements, and bad politics' (Marmot, et al., 2008, p. 1661). According to the Commission, global differentials in power and economic configurations are key to understanding global disparities in health.

Second, given the dilemmas laid out in this chapter, what global public health goals might be sound within conflict recovery, particularly with regards to the role of nongovernmental bodies? NGOs may indeed have something to offer, especially when they turn their attention to interrupting facets of neoliberalism (such as de-regulation of private industries and roll back of public provision of services) that we know exasperate inequality and mental health (Marmot, et al., 2008). Countries also may indeed lack workforce (Kabeera and Sewpaul, 2008). Also, atrocities of the political violence may be so severe and entrenched that international presence is crucial (Ludwin, 2003). However, the issue is how we, as public health workers, researchers, and advocates approach the intersection of health and political violence. Respectful work done in true partnership with those who suffer should not come to a standstill. Rather, a critique of the increasing presence of neoliberal frameworks should inspire the global public health community to (1) establish real and thoughtful partnerships, which includes deep reflection on where we go wrong, (2) connect the work to larger frameworks and imperatives for action, and (3) learn and promote understanding of the unique deep political and historical contexts of political conflicts.

Working with thoughtfulness regarding partnership may be found in the movement for codes of ethics that counter neoliberalism, which is an energising example of globalisation for liberation. For example, the NGO Code of Conduct for Health Systems Strengthening, launched in 2008, provides a formidable and clear challenge to the de-stabilisation of the public sector under neoliberalism (Health Alliance International, 2008). This is part of a larger movement addressing ethical conduct in globalised projects. The Global Development Research Center has amassed an array of conduct codes, including those specific to work in disaster zones, authored by the International Red Cross/Crescent (Global Development Research Center, n.d.). As evident in recent critiques of the Red Cross' work during Hurricane Katrina, codes of conduct are helpful only to the degree that they are upheld (Salmon, 2006).

The field of global public health absolutely can engage in emancipatory processes as we respond to the ways political violence undermines health. Global public health is well positioned to approach political violence from a perspective that honors our historic emphases on prevention and the political dimensions of health through frameworks that prioritise questions about the antecedents of global conflict, as well as questions about power, accountability, and agency (de Jong, 2010; Krieger, 2001). We must see our work within conflict and post-conflict settings as intimately tied to our imperatives towards social justice, dignity, and self-determination (American Public Health Association, 2009; Farmer, 2005; Hagopian, et al., 2009). Our ability to do so rests in our commitment to social justice, political education, and individual and professional self-reflection as we work towards a thoughtful and holistic solidarity with those most affected by political violence.

## References

Alessandrini, M. (2002) 'A fourth sector: the impact of neo-liberalism on non-profit organisations', paper presented at the Jubilee Conference of the Australasian Political Studies Association at Australian National University, Canberra.

American Public Health Association (APHA). (2009) 'The role of public health practitioners, academics and advocates in relation to armed conflict and war', available at www.apha.org/policies-and-advocacy/public-health-policy-statements/policy-database/2014/07/22/13/29/the-role-of-public-health-practitioners-academics-and-advocates-in-relation-to-armed-conflict (accessed on 20 November 2017).

Baingana, F., Bannon, I., and Thomas, R. (2005) 'Mental health and conflicts: conceptual framework and approaches', working paper, available at http://documents.worldbank.org/curated/en/829381468320662693/Mental-health-and-conflicts-conceptual-framework-and-approaches (accessed on 20 November 2017).

Bhavsar, V. and Bhugra, D. (2008) 'Globalization: mental health and social economic factors', *Global Social Policy*, 8(3): 378–96.

Brynen, R. (2000) *A Very Political Economy: Peacebuilding and foreign aid in the West Bank and Gaza*, Washington, DC: United States Institute of Peace Press.

Carney, T. (2008) 'The mental health service crisis of neoliberalism – an antipodean perspective', *International Journal of Law and Psychiatry*, 31(2): 101.

de Jong, J.T. (2010) 'A public health framework to translate risk factors related to political violence and war into multi-level preventive interventions', *Social Science and Medicine*, 70(1): 71–9.

Esping-Andersen, G.S. (1990) *The Three Worlds of Welfare Capitalism*, Princeton, NJ: Princeton University Press.

Farmer, P. (2005) *Pathologies of Power: Health, human rights and the new war on the poor*, Berkeley, CA: University of California Press.

Giacaman, R., Abdul-Rahim, H.F., and Wick, L. (2003) 'Health sector reform in the Occupied Palestinian Territories (OPT): targeting the forest or the trees?', *Health Policy and Planning*, 18(1): 59–67.

Global Development Research Center (GDRC). (n.d.) 'NGO Codes of Conduct', available at www.gdrc.org/ngo/codes-conduct.html (accessed on 20 November 2017).

Hagopian, A., Ratevosian, J., and deRiel, E. (2009) 'Gathering in groups: peace advocacy in health professional associations', *Academic Medicine: Journal of the Association of American Medical Colleges*, 84(11): 1485.

Hamid, H.I. and Everett, A. (2007) 'Developing Iraq's mental health policy', *Psychiatric Services*, 58(10): 1355–7.

Health Alliance International. (2008) 'NGO code of conduct for health systems strengthening', available at http://ngocodeofconduct.org/ (accessed on 20 November 2017).

Horton, E. (2007) 'Neoliberalism and the Australian healthcare system (factory)', paper presented at the Philosophy of Education Society of Australasia.

Incite! Women of Color Against Violence. (2007) *The Revolution Will Not be Funded: Beyond the non-profit industrial complex*, Cambridge, MA: South End Press.

Kabeera, B. and Sewpaul, V. (2008) 'Genocide and its aftermath: the case of Rwanda', *International Social Work*, 51(3): 324–36.

Katz, M.B. (2001) *The Price of Citizenship: Redefining the American welfare state*, New York: Metropolitan Press.

Klein, N. (2007) *The Shock Doctrine: The rise of disaster capitalism*, New York: Metropolitan Books/Henry Holt.

Kleinman, A. (1999) 'Commentaries – social violence: research questions on local experiences and global responses', *Archives of General Psychiatry*, 56(11): 978.

Krieger, N. (2001) 'Theories for social epidemiology in the 21st century: an ecosocial perspective', *International Journal of Epidemiology*, 30: 668–77.

Krug, E.G. (2002) *World Report on Violence and Health*, Geneva: World Health Organization.

Lavalette, M. and Ferguson, I. (2007) 'Democratic language and neo-liberal practice: the problem with civil society', *International Social Work*, 50(4): 447–60.

Levich, J. (2015) 'The Gates Foundation, ebola, and global health imperialism', *American Journal of Economics and Sociology*, 74(4): 704–42.

Ludwin, E.B. (2003) 'Trials and truth commissions in Argentina and El Salvador', In: J.E. Stromseth (Ed.) *Accountability for Atrocities: National and International Responses*, Ardsley, NY: Transnational Publishers, pp. 273–317.

Marmot, M., Friel, S., Bell, R., Houweling, T., and Taylor, S. (2008) 'Closing the gap in a generation: health equity through action on the social determinants of health', *The Lancet*, available at www.thelancet.com/journals/lancet/article/PIIS0140-6736(08)61690–6/fulltext (accessed on 20 November 2017).

Marshall, T.H. (1997) 'Citizenship and social class', In: R.E. Goodin and P. Pettit (Eds.) *Contemporary Political Philosophy: An anthology*, Oxford: Blackwell Publishers, pp. 291–320.

Pfeiffer, J., Johnson, W., Fort, M., Shakow, A., Hagopian, A., Gloyd, S., and Gimbel-Sherr, K. (2008) 'Strengthening health systems in poor countries: a code of conduct for nongovernmental organizations', *American Journal of Public Health*, 98(12): 2134–40.

Piachaud, J. (2008) 'Globalization, conflict and mental health', *Global Social Policy*, 8(3): 315–34.

Ramon, S. (2008) 'Neoliberalism and its implications for mental health in the UK', *International Journal of Law and Psychiatry*, 31(2): 116.

Reimann, K.D. (2006) 'A view from the top: international politics, norms and the worldwide growth of NGOs', *International Studies Quarterly*, 50(1): 45–68.

Salmon, J. (2006) 'Counterparts excoriate Red Cross Katrina effort', Washington Post, A14.

Scholte, J. (2005) 'The sources of neoliberal globalization', available at www.unrisd.org/80256B3C005BCCF9/search/9E1C54CEEB19A314C12570B4004D0881 (accessed on 20 November 2017).

Shearer, D. (2000) 'Aiding or abetting? Humanitarian aid and its economic role in civil war', In: M.R. Berdal and D. Malone (Eds.) *Greed & Grievance: Economic agendas in civil wars*, Boulder, CO: Lynne Rienner Publishers, pp. 189–204.

Sklair, L. (2002) *Globalization: Capitalism and its alternatives*, Oxford; New York: Oxford University Press.

Sousa, C. (2013) 'Political violence, collective functioning and health: a review of the literature', *Medicine, Conflict and Survival*, 29(3): 169–97.

Sousa, C. and Marshall, D.J. (2015) 'Political violence and mental health: effects of neoliberalism and the role of international social work practice', *International Social Work*, 60(4): 787–99.

Summerfield, D. (1999) 'A critique of seven assumptions behind psychological trauma programmes in war-affected areas', *Social Science and Medicine*, 48(10): 1449–62.

Swartz, L. (2008) 'Globalization and mental health: changing views of culture and society', *Global Social Policy*, 8(3): 304–8.

Waitzkin, H. and Jasso-Aguilar, R. (2015) 'Imperialism's health component', *Monthly Review*, 67(3).

Weiss, M.G., Saraceno, B., Saxena, S., and van Ommeren, M. (2003) 'Mental health in the aftermath of disasters: consensus and controversy', *The Journal of Nervous and Mental Disease*, 191(9): 611–15.

# 35

# Sovereignty, development, and health

## Humanitarianism and health care provision in the Gaza Strip

*Ron Smith*

## Introduction

The health systems in Gaza are in a constant state of near collapse, and access to health care is steadily worsening in the strip. The state of the health system is so dire, that on numerous occasions the public hospitals periodically threaten closure due to lack of funds and lack of electricity and fuel (WHO, 2017; WHO and Halimah, 2017; Al-Mughrabi, 2018). This state of collapse is a direct consequence of Israeli attacks on the Gaza Strip, and an ongoing siege of the strip, enacted by Israel and Egypt, and supported by the international community since 2007. The state of the health system represents a failure of health care provision, with deep impacts on public health, but more precisely, is indicative of the necessity of an understanding of the political context within which health services are provided.

Hamas, or the Islamic Resistance Movement, is an Islamist political party that gained control over the Gaza Strip after winning the popular election in 2006. The collapse of the health systems in Gaza is a direct result of the Israeli occupation and siege of Gaza, which targets the health and well-being of civilian populations ostensibly as a means of achieving a political goal – the removal of the Hamas-led government from power in Gaza. While the international community seems willing to support a status quo on Gaza, numerous critics have alleged that the siege represents a form of collective punishment (Charbonneau, 2008; Falk, et al., 2014), and therefore is illegal under international law. The siege in Gaza is a mode of punishment that is far from unique (Wintour, 2017; Arnove, 2000; Gordon, 1999; Graham, 2006); the most salient contemporary examples of siege include the almost 20-year sanctions regime imposed on Iraq starting in 1991, and the siege imposed by the Gulf Cooperation Council (GCC) on Yemen.

This chapter considers the role of humanitarian aid in situations of siege. In the context of siege, what role does humanitarian aid play in alleviating the suffering of the targeted population, and in what ways does it abet and maintain the overall structures of violence that are imposed against these same populations? In what ways is humanitarian aid being proposed as a surrogate for sovereignty, and what are the consequences of this substitution?

## Development and health

Modernisation theorists understand development as a linear process, one where countries that follow prescriptions for development (usually imposed by the West either militarily, or through economic coercion) will inevitably progress and develop stronger economies, and improve the quality of life for their citizens. Numerous critics, many from the global South, have long critiqued this notion, instead putting forth a notion of under-development (Slater, 1973; Rodney, 1981; Marable, 1983; Stock, 1986; Wallerstein, 2004), wherein a society's progress is distorted, often enriching more powerful nations while maintaining high levels of poverty, large gaps between rich and poor, and negative health outcomes.

Under-development is a mode of development resulting from a lack of sovereignty, particularly in states that emerged from the horrors of colonialism and imperial violence (Galeano, 1981). In response to under-development, and the threat of continued violations of sovereignty by powerful countries, numerous countries in the global South joined together in an organisation designed to protect their self-determination, called the non-aligned movement (NAM) (Prashad, 2007). While the NAM has proven ineffective at countering the large-scale deleterious effects of neo-colonialism, including war and economic manipulation, it represented an attempt to curb the unchecked power of the former colonial states through collective organisation. The effects of colonialism on the health of subject populations is well documented (Krieger and Birn, 1998; Coovadia, et al., 2009), as are the impacts of policies like structural adjustment programmes imposed by the IMF and the World Bank, and austerity (Navarro, 2008).

This chapter considers a further mode of dispossession and immiseration, that of de-development. De-development is distinct from under-development in that it removes even the possibility of independent development of the targeted population (Roy, 1995). It can be understood as 'turning back the clock' on a society, dismantling progress made towards the development of economic autonomy. De-development is a denial of sovereignty and local control within a society, usually imposed by an occupying power. De-development is a process undertaken as an act of war, often enacted through debilitating comprehensive sanctions regimes coupled with military invasions and attacks on civilians and popular infrastructure (Graham, 2006), markers of modern military warfare, or 'war amongst the people' (Smith, 2005).

The process of de-development is deeply imbricated in debates centred around the relative benefits and consequences of harsh sanctions regimes imposed to create popular pressure for social change. Sanctions are considered alternately as alternatives to war (Lopez, 1999; Lopez and Cortright, 2004) or as collective punishment, and war by other means (Smith, 2016; Gordon, 1999; Gordon, 2010; Arnove, 2000; Garfield, 2001).

Sovereignty is violated whenever sanctions regimes are put into place, ministries of health are targeted, and humanitarian organisations attempt to provide health services without proper coordination. These scenarios are well documented in sites of crisis, from Haiti to Indonesia (Weiss, 1997; Gibbons and Garfield, 1999; Farmer, 2004). Ministries of health and other governmental health providers are subject to the vagaries of under-development throughout the 'third world', their inefficacy correlated directly to policies of austerity, structural adjustment, and neoliberalism (Navarro, 2008). Siege is unique because the greatest pressure on public health agencies is the result of explicit policy designed to destabilise the regime and immiserate the population to achieve a political result.

Israel's Ministry of Foreign affairs consistently denies the existence of a comprehensive siege on Gaza (Israel MFA, 2014), but the UN and other foreign observers make the siege visible and irrefutable (Hass, 2002; Gregory, 2004; Al Mezan Center for Human Rights, 2010; UN OCHA, 2017). It should be noted that Israel refuses to characterise its relationship with the 1967 occupied Palestinian territories as occupation, even though there is an international consensus on that characterisation. Israel refuses the moniker of 'occupier' because that term implies obligations under the Geneva conventions (International Committee of the Red Cross (ICRC), 1949). Israel has consistently denied the applicability of the Geneva conventions to its occupation of the West Bank, Gaza, and the Golan Heights. All of these territories were captured in the 1967 war, and all are the subject of UN Resolution 242 (UN Security Council, 1967), demanding Israel withdraw to the pre-1967 borders.

The siege operates through a complete detachment of the Gaza Strip from the region and the global economy through absolute control of all border crossings and the entry and exit of people and goods from the strip. All modes of entry – sea, land, and air – are controlled by Israel and its ally, the Egyptian government, in the case of the Gaza's sole entry outside of Israel's purview: Rafah Terminal in the South. Through international agreements, goods are banned from entry through Rafah, so trucks carrying goods from Egypt must pass to an Israeli checkpoint, notably Karm Abu Salam (Kerem Shalom) crossing, the only crossing in operation for goods into and out of the strip. People are limited to traveling through Rafah on the few days when it is open, and Erez Crossing, requiring an intense vetting procedure. Exit and entry are prohibited by sea, and Israeli warships patrol the unilaterally imposed maritime borders, and shoot and ram boats on sight. It is important to note that the siege is explained as a means of effecting regime change in Gaza, to remove Hamas from power, and replace them with a government that is satisfactory to Israel and other powerful political actors. What is worrying about this assumption is that since Israel denies any characterisation of its regime in Gaza as siege, there is no guarantee whatsoever that even if Hamas was removed from power that the siege regime would be removed.

The siege on Gaza is somewhat distinct from other contemporary models of siege, such as those imposed on Yemen by the GCC. This distinction is derived from the overall context of occupation, wherein Israel was established on the land inhabited by Palestinians, and is a process of dispossession, accompanied by practices of displacement aimed at changing the ethnic makeup of the population. The US and its allies in Iraq apparently had no such intentions, the claims of various military personnel notwithstanding (Peters, 2006). Likewise, Saudi Arabia and the GCC's siege on Yemen does not appear to be designed to alter the ethnic makeup of Yemen, but seeks to effect political change through the starvation of the population, and the precipitating of one of the worst medical crises in the twenty-first century so far (Almosawa, et al., 2017). Although the larger political context is distinct, the immediate goals of siege are the same: regime change brought about through the de-development of a society.

## Effects of siege as de-development on health systems

Failures within the health system of de-developed states are not coincidental; rather they are part and parcel of the programme of de-development (Garfield, et al., 1995). Programmes like the international sanctions regime on Iraq, the siege of Gaza, and the ongoing blockade of Yemen are often discussed in the literature as programmes seeking regime change. The Iraqi example is perhaps the most obvious case wherein it becomes clear that the sanctions were not simply about regime change, but a 'war against the Iraqi people' (Ismael and Ismael, 2015). This analysis suggests that the collapse of public health systems is a goal of siege, a means of applying further pressure to the targeted populations to achieve the stated geopolitical goals.

It needs to be stated that sanctions are useful as a potential tool that can provide pressure against regimes in contravention of international law and human rights. For this reason, it is vital to distinguish sanctions regimes such as those imposed by sovereign belligerents as an act of war from sanctions regimes brought about through popular organising and calls from the targeted population themselves, as in the case of South Africa during apartheid. The difference in efficacy of these two distinct classes of sanctions regimes is not coincidental: one is designed to punish a society through pressure on infrastructure including health systems until popular will buckles and topples a regime regardless of its democratic legitimacy, the other is a call for the international community to recognise injustices committed against a population by a regime. Thus, with the support of the targeted population, sanctions regimes can be crafted to protect the population and negative impacts of the sanctions will be seen as sacrifice for a greater good. Siege represents the former, and the support or opposition of the targeted population to the policies enacted through siege are irrelevant for the belligerents.

## Political violence and the health of the public

There exists an established literature on the deleterious effects of political violence on public health, including service provision and the overall health of the affected society (Sousa, 2013). Many researchers have considered these problems as unforeseen side effects of global policy, but in the case of Gaza as well as Yemen and Iraq in the timeframes laid out earlier, there is an intentionality of harm that is often ignored. This intentionality is made evident through documents such as those by Gisha, an Israeli NGO that published documents indicating that the siege was designed to manipulate nutrition in Gaza in such a way that food stores could be measured in days until starvation occurred (Gisha, 2010; Weizman, 2011). These policies are ostensibly designed to create political change by directly attacking the health of the public, not least through direct attacks on hospitals and caregivers (MSF, 2017a; MSF, 2017b; MSF, 2016; WHO, 2017; Mohyeldin, 2014; Fitzgerald, 2002; Craven, 2002; Lektzian, 2003).

While there have often been calls for a so-called 'smart-sanctions' (Fitzgerald, 2002; Craven, 2002; Lektzian, 2003) regime in response to claims of collective suffering by targeted populations, these modifications to sanctions regimes show little to no effectiveness. Even in the case when medical supplies are explicitly exempt from sanctions, the general impacts of sanctions on the larger economy often make the purchase of medical supplies difficult or even impossible (Borger and Dehghan, 2013).

Siege and sanctions regimes should be understood as war by other means, and the impact of siege should be understood in the context of deliberate military attacks on health care infrastructure, as in Yemen. Siege regimes directly impact the ability of health services providers to deliver quality, coordinated care to populations, as in Serbia and Montenegro (Black, 1993), Iraq (Akunjee and Ali, 2002), Iran, and Syria (Moret, 2015). Sanctions directly affect drug supplies and parts for medical equipment, but also affect the ability of targeted states to provide clean water, electricity, and transportation. Sanctions and siege regimes make health care delivery less effective and create additional strain on health systems already stretched beyond their ability to cope with health crises.

Perhaps most telling is the ongoing public debate being pursued at the medical NGO Médecins Sans Frontières (Doctors Without Borders, or MSF). MSF withdrew their operations from Misurata in Libya in 2012 because they saw themselves as supporting the ongoing torture in militia-run prisons: patching up victims who would then arrive again at the MSF clinic showing scars from continued torture. A similar conversation took place around MSF in Gaza, and their continued presence in the besieged strip (Whittall and Neuman, 2014).

In a very real sense, medical NGOs are patching up victims of Israel's siege, but in most cases providing nothing to solve the underlying problems of occupation, siege, and denial of self-determination. NGOs and medical practitioners have a unique ability and responsibility to address those concerns primarily relating to Israel's responsibility under the Geneva Conventions to provide for the health and well-being of Gazan civilians under occupation.

At the Lancet Palestinian Health Association conference in 2017, Professor Abu Al Noor described an aspect of the collapse of the health sector when he claimed that his nursing students, while working in post-op in Gaza's largest public hospital, had access to five pairs of gloves for each day on the floor (Abu El-Noor, 2017). He then presented a graph showing an alarming uptick of communicable diseases that can easily be attributed to the use of non-sterile gloves on multiple patients in the ward. While his presentation was met with fury by a representative of the Fatah Ministry of Health, it is emblematic of the siege overall, where quality medical talent is available, but hindered by lack of funding and a crushing lack of materials necessary for health care provision. Similar stories abound from medical staff operating during the sanctions period in Iraq, and from Yemen under the Saudi-imposed siege (UN OCHA Yemen, 2017; MSF, 2017a).

## Gaza as exception

Beyond the general context of Israel's occupation of Palestine, Gaza represents an exception to cases of siege and models of effective aid coordination. The case of Gaza is unique in the sense that Gaza has no fully functional public health sector, as the Ministry of Health (MOH) is an organisation whose existence is allowed by Israel primarily as a means of deflecting legal concerns due to Israel's unwillingness to live up to its role as occupier, outlined in the Geneva Conventions (Erakat, 2011; Giacaman, et al., 2003; Smith, 2015). As the MOH is part of the Palestinian Authority, an institution that is completely dependent on Israel, the Ministry of Health operates with no real sovereignty in Gaza.

Circumscribed by the siege, by Israel's limitations on imports and travel, and by the West Bank authority which has remained hostile to the governing power in Gaza – Hamas – the MOH is unable to fulfil its goals of health provision in the Gaza Strip. While the MOH represents the most important public-sector health care provider in Gaza, it is adjunct to Israel's responsibility to provide health care for the population of Gaza. Further support of the MOH, while absolutely essential, provides further evidence for Israel that it need not provide for health care for Palestinians, since they have their own institutions, but without independence or the structure of a sovereign state. In effect, humanitarian aid to the health sector in Gaza subsidises the siege (Smith, 2015), outsourcing the cost of health care from Israel to foreign aid donors, thus freeing Israel to operate as a belligerent, and to target health care facilities and strangle imports as it sees fit. This scenario presents a conundrum where humanitarian aid further erodes sovereignty, with no central health administration with the authority to claim sovereignty for the population.

While Gaza is exceptional in this regard, the effects of siege, and the ongoing collapse of the health sector in Gaza is mirrored in Yemen, as it was in Iraq, and elsewhere due to the targeting of civilians through the practice of siege (Arnove, 2000; Gordon, 1999). These sites suffer from the denial of sovereignty for targeted populations, and the destruction of the health sector by denial of necessary goods and the bombing of health care facilities. The violence depicted herein against the health sector is then justified as a means of developing popular pressure against the local regime, a practice with limited effectiveness historically.

## Conclusion

Health policy in Iraq, Yemen, and Gaza are exemplars of complete failures to provide for the needs of the populations. This failure does not reflect the will or intent of health care practitioners, rather it reflects political realities that no amount of humanitarian aid can provide succour to populations deprived of their basic human rights by belligerents and the apathy or complicity of the international community. Health care provision is deeply political, and the improvement of public health in targeted societies is contingent upon the willingness of medical staff as witnesses to speak out against the larger policies that precipitate massive health crises of the type addressed in this chapter (Redfield, 2006).

Material, sustainable improvements in public health demands that the political demands of sovereignty (Becker, et al., 2009) and independence be met. Continued humanitarian public health interventions represent a necessary, but insufficient means of bolstering health outcomes. In cases such as that of Gaza, humanitarian intervention even serves to hinder the larger goals of independence, and abets the occupying power in their abdication of the obligations to public health under international law (Erakat, 2011).

Medical service providers are an essential facet of humanitarian aid, and provide vital services to populations suffering from war and other forms of political violence. With that in mind, it becomes tempting to believe that in any given conflict, the geopolitical status quo can remain unchallenged by the international community. Particularly in cases of colonial violence and attacks that primarily affect civilians, humanitarian aid becomes a surrogate for policies that address the root of human rights and humanitarian crises. After more than 50 years of occupation and 10 years of siege, in the case of Gaza, the lingering aftereffects of sanctions on Iraq, and the ongoing humanitarian crises of famine and cholera in Yemen, humanitarian aid cannot be allowed to whitewash anti-civilian regimes or extend the intolerable status quo. Humanitarian aid staff and the agencies for whom they work must be vocal in their condemnations of human rights violations and their support of real sovereignty for the dispossessed. The harm caused by the humanitarian fig leaf is palpable, and tarnishes the very real and honest work done for humanity by medical relief staff.

## References

Abu El-Noor, N. (2017) 'Increase in communicable diseases in Al Shifa post operative ward', In: *Lancet Palestinian Health Association Conference*, Bir Zeit, Palestine.

Akunjee, M. and Ali, A. (2002) 'Healthcare under sanctions in Iraq: an elective experience', *Medicine, Conflict and Survival*, 18: 249–57.

Al Mezan Center for Human Rights. (2010) 'Israel reduces wheat supply to the Gaza Strip: food security at greater risk as siege continues', available at www.mezan.org/en/details.php?id=11120&ddname=Crossings&id_dept=9&id2=9&p=center (accessed on 1 August 2017).

Almosawa, S., Hubbard, B., and Griggs, T. (2017) '"It's a slow death": the world's worst humanitarian crisis', The New York Times, available at www.nytimes.com/interactive/2017/08/23/world/middleeast/yemen-cholera-humanitarian-crisis.html (accessed on 23 August 2017).

Al-Mughrabi, N. (2018) 'Gaza health facilities face closure due to fuel shortage: UN. Reuters February 6th 2018', available at www.reuters.com/article/us-palestinians-un-health/gaza-health-facilities-face-closure-due-to-fuel-shortage-u-n-idUSKBN1FQ25R?il=0 (accessed on 6 February 2018).

Arnove, A. (2000) *Iraq Under Siege: The deadly impact of sanctions and war*, Cambridge, MA: South End Press.

Becker, A., Al Ju'beh, K., and Watt, G. (2009) 'Keys to health: justice, sovereignty, and self-determination', *The Lancet*, 373: 985–7.

Black, M.E. (1993) 'Collapsing health care in Serbia and Montenegro', *BMJ*, 307: 1135–7.

Borger, J. and Dehghan, S.K. (2013) 'Iran unable to get life-saving drugs due to international sanctions', The Guardian, available at www.guardian.co.uk/world/2013/jan/13/iran-lifesaving-drugs-international-sanctions (accessed on 12 November 2017).

Charbonneau, L. (2008) 'Collective punishment for Gaza is wrong: U.N.', Reuters, available at www.reuters.com/article/us-palestinians-israel-un/collective-punishment-for-gaza-is-wrong-u-n-idUSN1832560020080118 (accessed on 13 November 2017).

Coovadia, H., Jewkes, R., Barron, P., Sanders, D., and McIntyre, D. (2009) 'The health and health system of South Africa: historical roots of current public health challenges', *The Lancet*, 374: 817–34.

Craven, M. (2002) 'Humanitarianism and the quest for smarter sanctions', *European Journal of International Law*, 13: 43–61.

Erakat, N. (2011) 'It's not wrong, it's illegal: situating the Gaza blockade between international law and the UN response', *Journal of Islamic and Near Eastern Law*, 11: 37–85.

Falk, R., et al. (2014) 'The international community must end Israel's collective punishment of the civilian population in the Gaza Strip', available at https://richardfalk.wordpress.com/2014/07/28/joint-declaration-by-international-law-experts-on-israels-gaza-offensive/ (accessed on 13 November 2017).

Farmer, P. (2004) 'Political violence and public health in Haiti', *The New England Journal of Medicine*, 350: 1483–6.

Fitzgerald, P.L. (2002) 'Managing smart sanctions against terrorism wisely', *New England Law Review*, 36: 957.

Galeano, E.H. (1981) *Las Venas Abiertas de America Latina*, Mexico, Madrid: Siglo Veintiuno Editores.

Garfield, R. (2001) 'Health and well-being in Iraq: sanctions and the impact of the oil-for-food program', *Transnat'l L. & Contemp. Probs.*, 11: 277.

Garfield, R., Devin, J., and Fausey, J. (1995) 'The health impact of economic sanctions', *Bulletin of the New York Academy of Medicine*, 72: 454.

Giacaman, R., Abdul-Rahim, H.F., and Wick, L. (2003) 'Health sector reform in the Occupied Palestinian Territories (OPT): targeting the forest or the trees?', *Health Policy and Planning*, 18: 59–67.

Gibbons, E. and Garfield, R. (1999) 'The impact of economic sanctions on health and human rights in Haiti, 1991–1994', *American Journal of Public Health*, 89: 1499–504.

Gisha. (2010) 'Press release: due to Gisha's petition: Israel reveals documents related to the Gaza closure policy', available at www.gisha.org/index.php?intLanguage=2&intItemId=1904&intSiteSN=113 (accessed on 21 October 2010).

Gordon, J. (1999) 'Sanctions as siege warfare', *The Nation*, 268.

Gordon, J. (2010) *Invisible War: The United States and the Iraq sanctions*, Cambridge, MA: Harvard University Press.

Graham, S. (2006) 'Cities and the War on Terror', *International Journal of Urban and Regional Research*, 30: 255–76.

Gregory, D. (2004) 'Palestine under siege', *Antipode*, 36: 601–6.

Hass, A. (2002) 'Israel's closure policy: an ineffective strategy of containment and repression', *Journal of Palestine Studies*, 31: 5–20.

International Committee of the Red Cross (ICRC). (1949) 'Convention (IV) relative to the protection of civilian persons in time of war. Geneva, 12 August 1949', available at https://ihl-databases.icrc.org/ihl/385ec082b509e76c412 56739003e636d/6756482d86146898c125641e004aa3c5 (accessed on 13 November 2017).

Ismael, T.Y. and Ismael, J.S. (2015) *Iraq in the Twenty-First Century: Regime change and the making of a failed state*, UK: Routledge.

Israel MFA. (2014) 'Behind the headlines: the myth of an Israeli siege on Gaza', available at http://mfa.gov.il/MFA/ForeignPolicy/Issues/Pages/The-myth-of-an-Israeli-siege-on-Gaza-17-Aug-2014.aspx (accessed on 13 November 2017).

Krieger, N. and Birn, A.E. (1998) 'A vision of social justice as the foundation of public health: commemorating 150 years of the spirit of 1848', *American Journal of Public Health*, 88: 1603–6.

Lektzian, D. (2003) 'Making sanctions smarter', PRIO, available at www.prio.org/Publications/Publication/?x=506 (accessed on 13 November 2017).

Lopez, G.A. (1999) 'More ethical than not: sanctions as surgical tools: response to "a peaceful, silent, deadly remedy"', *Ethics & International Affairs*, 13: 143–8.

Lopez, G. and Cortright, D. (2004) 'Containing Iraq: sanctions worked', *Foreign Affair*, 90–103.

Marable, M. (1983) *How Capitalism Underdeveloped Black America: Problems in race, political economy, and society*, Boston, MA: South End Press.

Mohyeldin, A. (2014) 'Another Gaza hospital hit by Israeli strike; four dead, 40 hurt', NBCNews, available at www.nbcnews.com/slideshow/palestinian-santas-clash-israeli-soldiers-n482596 (accessed on 13 November 2017).

Moret, E.S. (2015) 'Humanitarian impacts of economic sanctions on Iran and Syria', *European Security*, 24: 120–40.

MSF. (2016) 'MSF evacuates staff from six hospitals in Northern Yemen', available at www.doctorswithoutborders.org/article/msf-evacuates-staff-six-hospitals-northern-yemen (accessed on 13 November 2017).

MSF. (2017a) 'Yemen: crisis update – January 2017', available at www.msf.org/en/article/yemen-crisis-update-january-2017 (accessed on 13 November 2017).

MSF. (2017b) 'Yemen: MSF withdrawing from Ibb Al-Thawra hospital', available at www.msf.org/en/article/yemen-msf-withdrawing-ibb-al-thawra-hospital (accessed on 13 November 2017).

Navarro, V. (2008) 'Neoliberalism and its consequences: the world health situation since Alma Ata', *Global Social Policy*, 8: 152–5.

Peters, R. (2006) 'Blood borders: how a better Middle East would look', *Armed Forces Journal*, 6: 6.

Prashad, V. (2007) *The Darker Nations: A people's history of the third world*, New York, NY: The New Press.

Redfield, P. (2006) 'Humanitarianism, mediation, and intervention – a less modest witness: collective advocacy and motivated truth in a medical humanitarian movement', *American Ethnologist*, 33: 3.

Rodney, W. (1981) *How Europe Underdeveloped Africa*, Washington, DC: Howard University Press.

Roy, S. (1995) *The Gaza Strip: The political economy of de-development*, Washington, DC: Institute for Palestine Studies.

Slater, D. (1973) 'Geography and underdevelopment–1', *Antipode*, 5(3): 21–32.

Smith, R. (2005) *The Utility of Force: The art of war in the modern world*, London: Allen Lane.

Smith, R.J. (2015) 'Healthcare under siege: geopolitics of medical service provision in the Gaza Strip', *Social Science & Medicine*, 146: 332–40.

Smith, R.J. (2016) 'Isolation through humanitarianism: subaltern geopolitics of the siege on Gaza', *Antipode*, 48(3): 750–69.

Sousa, C.A. (2013) 'Political violence, collective functioning and health: a review of the literature', *Medicine, Conflict and Survival*, 29: 169–97.

Stock, R. (1986) '"Disease and development" or "the underdevelopment of health": a critical review of geographical perspectives on African health problems', *Social Science & Medicine*, 23: 689–700.

UN OCHA. (2017) 'Humanitarian bulletin – occupied Palestinian territory', Monthly Humanitarian Bulletin, available at https://reliefweb.int/report/occupied-palestinian-territory/humanitarian-bulletin-occupied-palestinian-territory-august-1 (accessed on 13 November 2017).

UN OCHA Yemen. (2017) 'Yemen's dialysis patients fear for their lives amid medical shortages', *Medium*.

UN Security Council. (1967) 'Resolution 242' available at https://unispal.un.org/DPA/DPR/unispal.nsf/0/7D35E1 F729DF491C85256EE700686136 (accessed on 13 November 2017).

Wallerstein, I.M. (2004) *World-Systems Analysis: An introduction*, Durham, NC: Duke University Press.

Weiss, T. (1997) *Political Gain and Civilian Pain: Humanitarian impacts of economic sanctions*, Lanham, MD: Rowman & Littlefield Publishers.

Weizman, E. (2011) *The Least of All Possible Evils: Humanitarian violence from Arendt to Gaza*, London: Verso.

Whittall, J. and Neuman, M. (2014) 'Opinion and debate: the limits of humanitarianism in Gaza', available at www.msf. org.uk/article/opinion-and-debate-limits-humanitarianism-gaza (accessed on 13 November 2017).

WHO. (2017) 'Thousands of lives at risk as Gaza public hospitals face fuel and electricity crisis', available at http:// reliefweb.int/report/occupied-palestinian-territory/thousands-lives-risk-gaza-public-hospitals-face-fuel-and (accessed on 13 November 2017).

WHO and Halimah, S. (2017) 'WHO steps up emergency response in the Gaza Strip, June 2017', available at www. emro.who.int/pse/palestine-news/who-steps-up-emergency-response-in-the-gaza-strip.html (accessed on 13 November 2017).

Wintour, P. (2017) 'Saudi Arabia still barring aid to Yemen despite pledge to lift siege', The Guardian, available at www. theguardian.com/world/2017/nov/24/saudi-arabia-continues-to-block-humanitarian-aid-to-yemen. (accessed on 24 November 2017).

# 36

# Drone operators, terrorists, and the biopolitics of public health in the War on Terror

*Neil Krishan Aggarwal*

National security support roles for physicians have been decried as 'a dramatic departure from conventional medical ethics, which are anchored in the "do no harm" principle' (Kimball and Soldz, 2014, p. g2947). However, physician involvement in national security dates at least to the sixteenth century (Maio, 2010), revealing contradictions in physician self-perceptions. What is the relationship of national security to mental health? Is physician involvement in national security truly a departure from medical ethics? Instead, what do we learn by viewing such physician involvement as normative throughout history?

A growing body of evidence has shown that the War on Terror has transformed psychiatry and psychology. Government psychiatrists and psychologists in treatment capacities have participated in what authorities call 'enhanced interrogations' that constitute torture according to the Geneva Conventions (Xenakis, 2014). Attorney interviews and policy analyses reveal that government standards have liberalised for diagnosing Posttraumatic Stress Disorder (PTSD) in soldiers but tightened for enemy combatants experiencing torture in detention facilities such as Guantanamo Bay (Aggarwal, 2009, 2015). In the guise of science, mental health scholarship has attributed violence and suicide bombing as pathologies inherent to Arabs and Muslims (Aggarwal, 2010), replicating popular stereotypes that cause fear and alienation within Muslim communities (Rousseau and Jamil, 2010). Not all have cooperated in national security: the American Psychiatric Association opposed the involvement of psychiatrists in detainee interrogations by invoking medical ethics to do no harm, but the American Psychological Association approved of psychologists' involvement until 2014 by invoking national security protections (Summergrad and Sharfstein, 2015).

This chapter presents a critical discourse analysis of mental health scholarship in the War on Terror that constructs drone operators and terrorists as new targets of public health intervention. The disciplinary boundary between politics and public health dissolves when governments regard public health as a security issue managed through institutions of governance, sparking new paradigms to critique this relationship (Davies, et al., 2014). To answer the questions earlier, this chapter unfolds in four sections. The first reviews work from the critical theorists Allison Howell and Michel Foucault on the public health–national security relationship, focusing on mental health. The second and third sections apply these theories to mental health scholarship that identifies drone operators and terrorists, now commonly known as 'violent extremists', as new foci of public health intervention. Even though drone operators kill violent extremists in the Middle East by piloting unstaffed, weaponised aircraft from the United States, mental health scholarship represents them as victims and extremists as victimisers. In the final section, I posit that this inversion of victim and victimiser emerges from the same logic whereby the pathology requiring treatment is each figure's capacity for violence vis-à-vis the state: drone operators require treatment for killing inefficiently whereas extremists challenge the state's monopoly on violence against citizens.

## Critical perspectives on global health and national security

We can investigate the national security–mental health relationship by viewing health as an instrument of politics rather than as a human right. Allison Howell (2014, p. 963) contends that modern warfare and medicine have evolved 'symbiotically' and 'homologously'; by 'symbiotic', she means 'warfare has produced medicine and medicine has produced warfare in their historical relation' and by 'homologous', she means 'both have been developed as strategic sciences for doing things to and with populations'. She defines medicine beyond only clinical interactions as 'a broad disciplinary and scientific set of practices directed at the management and health of the body and the population' (Howell, 2014, p. 963), a definition adopted here. Challenging the view that violent practices through medicine are anomalous, she names medical knowledge and practices that have maintained human resources during military drafts such as the rise of bacteriology to reduce casualties during the Russo-Japanese War and the Allies' hoarding of penicillin from the Nazis during World War II. Drawing upon Foucault's (2003) *Society Must Be Defended* lectures, Howell (2014, p. 974) asserts that medicine adopted non-therapeutic roles as warfare modernised in the nineteenth century; these roles include 'defending society from enemies without and degenerates within, and of shoring up "manpower" in both military and colonial spaces'. As contemporary examples of military–medical symbiosis, she points to the use of triage in assessing populations at risk for insurgency in American counterintelligence manuals; the false door-to-door immunisation campaign to find Osama bin Laden in Pakistan; and the US Department of Defence's research into helping soldiers tolerate sleep deprivation.

Foucault's (2003, pp. 243–6) lectures emphasise state racism in public health. He identifies public health as an objective of biopolitics: 'The birth rate, the mortality rate, longevity, and so on – together with a whole series of related economic and political problems ... in the second half of the eighteenth century, become biopolitics' first objects of knowledge' (Foucault, 2003, p. 243). The state's economy depends on public health since illnesses 'shortened the working week, wasted energy, and cost money' (p. 244). The rise of public health in Europe is tied to colonialism since public health functions in 'separating out the groups that exist within a population' (p. 255). State racism connects biopolitics with war through mutual exclusion: 'If you want to live, the other must die' (p. 255). Biology underlies warfare between two populations whose differences are constructed racially: 'The enemies who have to be done away with are not adversaries in the political sense of the term; they are threats, either external or internal, to the population and for the population' (p. 256).

In *Discipline and Punish*, Foucault (1995) castigates psychiatrists and psychologists for creating the knowledge through which the state justifies national security. Foucault (1995) criticises the psychiatrist for being:

> an adviser in punishment; it is up to him to say whether the subject is "dangerous," in what way one should be protected from him, how one should intervene to alter him, whether it would be better to try to force him or to treat him.
>
> *p. 22*

Mental health professionals supply knowledge and practices that the state adopts as standards of normality: 'The supervision of normality was firmly encased in a medicine or a psychiatry that provided it with a sort of "scientificity"; it was supported by a judicial apparatus which, directly or indirectly, gave it legal justification' (Foucault, 1995, p. 296). Foucault (1995) regards psychiatrists and psychologists as 'subsidiary authorities' to state power: 'A whole army of technicians took over from the executioner, the immediate anatomist of pain: warders, doctors, chaplains, psychiatrists, psychologists, educationalists; by their very presence near the prisoner, they sing the praises that the law needs' (p. 11).

These texts help to situate drone operators and terrorists as new objects of public health intervention. Howell and Foucault treat scientific publications as discourses that are subject to cultural analysis without subscribing to their truth claims, an assumption I also share. In the next two sections, I show that these themes pervade medical discourse: (1) warfare produces medicine and medicine produces warfare, (2) psychiatric knowledge and practices define 'normality' scientifically which the state supports through laws and institutions, and (3) public health acts as a means of biopolitics for population surveillance. I utilise Foucault's (1991) approach to discourse analysis, the close readings of texts, to show how boundaries of knowledge are defined and ideas circulate in society. My goal is not to review all possible texts, but those with clear impacts on the practice of medicine and politics.

## Drone operators and the new normal of PTSD

A forthcoming systematic review on the health of drone operators concluded that most military studies appear in technical reports, not in peer-reviewed journals (Armour and Ross, 2016). Because peer-review is the standard by which innovations in knowledge and practice disseminate within the medical community (Aggarwal, 2015), I reviewed the only peer-reviewed studies in the systematic review. These studies exemplify the production of knowledge and practices through institutional support from the state since the lead authors all work in American Department of Defence facilities.

The first paper, led by Wayne Chappelle (2014a) at the Air Force School of Aerospace Medicine, examines the incidence of PTSD through a web-based screening questionnaire known as the PTSD Checklist-Military Version (PCL-M) among 1,049 drone operators across 17 US bases. The paper declares that drone operators must be kept healthy for population surveillance:

> Bases are tasked to provide 24-hour support 7 days a week to military missions on the other side of the globe. The increased requirement for mission support has created a rapidly expanding need for Predator/Reaper operators (pilots, sensor operators, and mission intelligence coordinators) to keep pace with the surge in drone operations.
>
> *Chappelle, et al., 2014a, p. 63*

The phrase 'other side of the globe' draws attention to external security threats. Chappelle, et al. (2014a, p. 63) rationalise PTSD screening:

> Although such drone operators are not 'deployed' in hand-to-hand combat and are usually protected from direct threat, they are often involved in operations where they witness and make decisions that lead to the destruction of enemy combatants and assets. They can still become attached to people they track, experience grief from the loss of allied members on the ground, and experience grief/remorse when missions create collateral damage.
>
> *Chappelle, et al., 2014a, p. 63*

Drone operators are represented as experiencing novel pressures compared to battlefield warriors: 'There is also limited research in assessing if continuously balancing warfighter roles with domestic/personal lives and intermittent (and virtual) exposure to combat elevates their risk for clinical distress and post-traumatic stress disorder' (Chappelle, et al., 2014a, p. 63).

Referencing psychometric studies on the PCL-M's validity to identify PTSD, the authors use a PCL-M cut-off score of 50, finding that 1.57 per cent of the sample qualifies for PTSD. Correlating each respondent's demographic variables and PCL-M scores, they conclude that 'those working 50 hours a week were approximately four times more likely' to report scores at or above 50 (Chappelle, et al., 2014a, p. 67). The authors state that 'the repeated finding of operational stressors, as opposed to combat stressors, as the most problematic self-reported sources of stress is helpful for line commanders and medical personnel in developing interventions for mitigating stress' (Chappelle, et al., 2014a, p. 67). The original justification for PTSD screening due to witnessing digit combat becomes irrelevant; drone operators experience PTSD from occupational conditions within the military structure itself. This recalls Foucault's (2003) critique of the state's use of public health to ensure economic productivity. Here mental health is called upon to enable warfare, not to treat PTSD related to workplace conditions.

The second paper, also led by Wayne Chappelle, stratifies PCL-M scores among the same respondents. Writing in a different journal, the authors first justify that drone operators must 'keep pace with the national and international demand for drone operations' (Chappelle, et al., 2014b, p. 480). Again, they presuppose that 'defining combat of trauma exposure for this population is complex' since drone operators 'provide around-the-clock, real-time support to ongoing military operations worldwide, requiring sustained situational awareness and hypervigilance to threat' (Chappelle, et al., 2014b, p. 481).

However, Chappelle et al. establish different PCL-M cut-off scores to define PTSD. As with their previous article, they refer to 'previous research that used a score of 50 or more as the cut-off for high risk of PTSD', but then they add: 'When selecting for participants that met the DSM-IV criteria, a frequency distribution of PCL-M was run. The cut-off for the moderate risk category was chosen based on the minimum PCL-M score (37) for participants that met the DSM-IV criteria' (Chappelle, et al., 2014b, p. 481). We see circular logic: first they use the PCL-M to screen for PTSD risk with a cut-off score of 50, but then claim that scores less than 50 could also meet DSM-IV criteria. By broadening the cut-off score and defining a new standard of normality, they demonstrate that 2.7 per cent of the sample has a PCL-M total score between 37 and 49 and 1.6 per cent has a score above 50.

Despite the greater population that would meet criteria for PTSD, they still cannot identify combat-related stressors:

> Those working 25 months or more on station, and those working 51 or more hours per week were more likely to meet PTSD DSM-IV symptom criteria than their counterparts working less time on station and working less hours per week.
>
> *Chappelle, et al., 2014b, p. 483*

As before, stressors are occupational, and the authors conclude that 'military mental health providers and military leadership share the responsibility of maintaining and supporting a "fit to fight" and optimally ready military force' (Chappelle, et al., 2014b, p. 486).

Citing these studies, researchers at Wright-Patterson Air Force Base reviewed the implications of PTSD's revised definition in the fifth edition of the *Diagnostic and Statistical Manual of Mental Disorders* (DSM-5), published in 2013. They note that DSM-5 allows trauma to include 'exposure through electronic media, television, movies' so long as it is work-related and that 'the military's rapidly increasing use of remotely piloted aircraft (RPA) – commonly known as "drones" – may expose SMs [service members] to trauma' (Guina, et al., 2016, p. 43). The article then cites a statistic that subverts the entire rationale for PTSD screening among drone operators due to unique combat conditions:

> As of January 2016, the ACS [United States Air Force Aeromedical Consultation Service] has only diagnosed PTSD from video exposure on one occasion. This case involved an RPA pilot who was

involved in a 'friendly fire' incident which killed two American troops in the 'fog of war.' Following successful treatment, he received a waiver to return to full flying duties.

*Guina, et al., 2016, p. 43*

No paper states the locations where drone operators act, but Iraq, Afghanistan, and Syria are the three theatres of drone operations that the US has acknowledged (Office of the Director of National Intelligence, 2016). Some have pointed out that the US has inherited the British legacy of aerial counterinsurgency in colonial Afghanistan and Iraq that began in the 1920s, but spun a new human rights argument: drone operations are a virtuous form of war for their supposed precision and minimal civilian casualties (Gregory, 2011). The rationale for PTSD screening among drone operators ironically classifies the aggressors as victims of suffering while obscuring the actual suffering of those who are killed and their families (Pinchevski, 2016). Upon discharge from active duty, veterans have consistently protested against the military's focus on mission readiness over soldier well-being (Chua, 2018). Like the Army's positive psychology training to support a 'fit to fight' workforce (Howell, 2015), drone operator PTSD screening does not simply respond to conflict but constitutes a means to wage endless war.

## The public health of violent extremism

Compared to drone operators, the impetus to identify terrorists as targets of public health intervention originates not from psychiatrists in state institutions, but from those critiquing extant law enforcement strategies – though we shall see how such ideas become co-opted in government institutions. For example, Kamaldeep Bhui and colleagues propose a public health approach to violent radicalisation, defined as 'a social and psychological process, often facilitated by recruitment and training, by which an individual becomes increasingly committed to politically motivated violence, especially against civilians' (Bhui, et al., 2012, p. 1). Recognising that 'the term "violent radicalization" has been applied mostly to extreme Islamist groups as they have claimed responsibility for the majority of recent terrorist attacks across the world,' Bhui and colleagues also emphasise that 'the majority of the victims globally are in fact Muslim civilians' (Bhui, et al., 2012, p. 1). Law enforcement has too often treated Muslims as an internal threat requiring surveillance: 'Counter-terrorism initiatives by the British government stigmatized and alienated Muslim communities in the UK by treating them as a conspicuous religious group that was under suspicion rather than as allies in a preventive strategy' (Bhui, et al., 2012, p. 3). In contrast, Bhui and colleagues cite the work of terrorism researchers to advance a science of public health:

> We propose that a public health approach needs to be applied at the population level to engage a larger proportion of the population at risk of violent radicalization. This recognizes that very few people proceed all the way to committing a terrorist act and that many influences that make this more likely are potentially modifiable.

*Bhui, et al., 2012, p. 5*

Here, the priorities of warfare animate priorities in medicine. The language of 'risk' raises the possibility of internal security threats that require surveillance. A new science could emerge 'if public health research investigates promising new variables from the social and behavioural sciences such as social inclusion, exclusion, cultural identity and acculturation, stigma, discrimination, and political engagement' (Bhui, et al., 2012, p. 6). New interventions would focus on the factors that predispose individuals to violence, articulated in the idiom of primary prevention: 'Preventive interventions should focus on how negotiations of personal identity, social exclusion and marginalization can generate grievances that are not processed through political engagement, nor through democratic non-violent negotiations' (Bhui, et al., 2012, p. 6).

Similarly, Stevan Weine and colleagues situate 'violent extremism' within public health. They also discuss problematic law enforcement strategies:

> A frequently heard comment in our research interviews from community members impacted by violent extremism and law enforcement-driven responses is that there is hardly anything filling the space between a person at risk of crossing the line into terrorist activity and being investigated by the Federal Bureau of Investigation.

*Weine, et al. 2017, p. 209*

Weine, et al. (2017, p. 210) also criticise discrimination against Muslims: 'A key unintended consequence of the first wave of CVE [countering violent extremism] activities that emerged in both the US and UK was the stigmatization of Muslim community'. A paragraph then elaborates a science of public health in significant detail:

> Prevention activities of CVE refer to programs, policies, and interventions that promote inclusion of individuals and communities at risk and engage them to diminish exposure to the causes and promoters of violence as well as reduce the progression to violence. Additionally, these strategies increase their access to support and resources promoting individual and community well-being. From the perspective of public health, this can be thought of as primary prevention, which aims to prevent disease or injury before it ever occurs. Intervention activities of CVE refer to programs, policies, and interventions that serve youth and adult who are believed to be at risk of committing a violent act but are still in the pre-criminal space. This can be thought of as either or [*sic*] secondary prevention, which aims to reduce the impact of a disease or injury that has already occurred, or tertiary prevention which aims to soften the impact of an ongoing illness or injury that has lasting effects.

*Weine, et al., 2017, p. 210*

Both publications invoke the term 'risk' to argue for public health interventions. However, risk assessment in public health has come to signify that a population may be at danger without necessarily supplying a robust evidence base that specifies a relationship between an exposure and effect (Douglas and Wildavsky, 1982). In the articles previously mentioned, certain candidate variables are offered as putting populations at risk, but no clear relationship has been drawn between exposure and terrorist acts. Risk also distinguishes 'those at risk' for a health problem from 'those posing a risk', which has often stigmatised minority communities in multicultural societies (Lupton, 1993). Bhui, et al. (2012) observe that 'those posing a risk' may suffer from stigma, discrimination, and social exclusion, but a public health approach *risks* medicalising societal problems. Similarly, Weine, et al. (2017) define a 'pre-criminal' space for CVE activities in between licit and illicit activities, but this also *risks* medicalising societal problems that could be addressed through social work and criminology. It is not clear why public mental health should fill this pre-criminal space in the absence of psychopathology.

An agenda that targets terrorism through public health has found receptive government audiences. The US Department of Homeland Security has announced a funding mechanism titled the 'Countering Violent Extremism (CVE) Grant Program' that states: 'New grants will provide state, local and tribal partners and community groups – religious groups, mental health and social service providers, educators and other NGOs – with the ability to build prevention programs that address the root causes of violent extremism' (US Department of Homeland Security, 2016). Public health now becomes mobilised for domestic population surveillance. The US State Department has sponsored CVE summits since 2015 that are also attempts at international population surveillance, with a US Deputy Secretary and Italian Minister of Interior issuing this joint statement: 'To be effective, a strategy should be developed with input from a wide range of national government actors, including law enforcement, social services, education, health, and religious affairs' (Global Center on Cooperative Security, 2015, p. 2). In the UK, the National Health Service has mandated since 2011 that health professionals must screen all patients for signs of terrorism and report suspicious individuals to the police, with the result that the entire domestic population is under surveillance rather than only Muslim communities (Heath-Kelly, 2017). The burden of security now falls on physicians who become mandated reporters rather than state law enforcement and national security agencies, reinforcing the mental health–national security relationship. American and British policies thus construct terrorism as an internal and external security threat to domestic populations.

## Discussion

How can we understand the logic behind treating drone operators <u>and</u> terrorists as new at-risk populations for public health intervention? Foucault's (1995) critique of the state–psychiatrist relationship helps us reason through this. As I have shown throughout this chapter, psychiatrists have contributed to the 'scientificity' of new types of knowledge and practice that specify normal and abnormal behaviour in the War on Terror. Foucault's (1995) term 'subsidiary authority' underscores the psychiatrist's subservient position to state interests. It would be an overstatement to suggest like Foucault that psychiatrists are singing the praises the law needs in the examples previously mentioned – psychiatrists have clearly criticised extant law enforcement. Nonetheless, they have made recommendations to accommodate existing laws rather than to challenge them. They have colluded with the state to recommend PTSD screening among drone operators due to poor occupational conditions rather than interrogate the conditions themselves. They have recommended medicalising terrorism as a public health problem rather than scrutinise whether psychiatrists should address societal problems that are not psychiatric in their very nature.

What we see instead is the state's anxiety around losing the monopoly over life and death among its citizenry. A core assumption of classical political science advanced since the work of Max Weber (1864–1920) has been that states, not individual citizens, possess the power to put people to death, and individuals who challenge this power by transgressing laws against interpersonal violence are deemed irrational (Asad, 2007; Crenshaw, 2000). From this frame, the faulty relationship that requires repair is each population's capacity for violence in relation to the state. Drone operators threaten the efficiency of state violence and must be treated so that the state can wield violence against its enemies in optimal fashion, in the discourse of economic productivity. Terrorists transgress laws when individuals commit violence outside of state legal mechanisms to threaten social peace and security. In both instances, psychiatrists have recommended screening populations that endanger state interests in the absence of clear psychopathology. While the nature of psychiatric involvement in public health interventions that facilitate the War on Terror can and should be debated, what is beyond debate, as these examples show, is that war and medicine have influenced each other, psychiatric knowledge and practices construct new forms of normal and abnormal behaviour through the discourse of science, and that public health acts as a technology of biopolitical population surveillance. In this light, national security support roles for physicians in the War on Terror have not been a dramatic departure from conventional medical ethics but further proof that politics and public health remain intertwined.

## References

Aggarwal, N.K. (2009) 'Allowing independent forensic evaluations for Guantánamo detainees', *Journal of the American Academy of Psychiatry and the Law*, 37: 533–7.

Aggarwal, N.K. (2010) 'How are suicide bombers analysed in mental health discourse? A critical anthropological reading', *Asian Journal of Social Science*, 38: 379–93.

Aggarwal, N.K. (2015) *Mental Health in the War on Terror: Culture, science, and statecraft*, New York: Columbia University Press.

Armour, C. and Ross, J. (2016) 'The health and well-being of military drone operators and intelligence analysts: a systematic review', *Military Psychology*, 29: 83–98.

Asad, T. (2007) *On Suicide Bombing*, New York: Columbia University Press.

Bhui, K.S., Hicks, M.H., Lashley, M., and Jones, E. (2012) 'A public health approach to understanding and preventing violent radicalization', *BMC Medicine*, 10: 16.

Chappelle, W.L., McDonald, K.D., Prince, L., Goodman, T., Ray-Sannerud, B.N., and Thompson, W. (2014a) 'Symptoms of psychological distress and post-traumatic stress disorder in United States Air Force "drone" operators', *Military Medicine*, 179: 63–70.

Chappelle, W.L., Goodman, T., Reardon, L., and Thompson, W. (2014b) 'An analysis of post-traumatic stress symptoms in United States Air Force drone operators', *Journal of Anxiety Disorders*, 28: 480–7.

Chua, J.L. (2018) 'Fog of war: psychopharmaceutical "side effects" and the United States military', *Medical Anthropology: Cross-Cultural Studies in Health and Illness*, 1: 17–31.

Crenshaw, M. (2000) 'The psychology of terrorism: an agenda for the 21st century', *Political Psychology*, 21: 405–20.

Davies, S.E., Elbe, S., Howell, A., and McInnes, C. (2014) 'Global health in international relations: editors' introduction', *Review of International Studies*, 40: 825–34.

Douglas, M. and Wildavsky, A. (1982) *Risk and Culture*, Oxford: Basil Blackwood.

Foucault, M. (1991) 'Politics and the study of discourse', In: G. Burchell, C. Gordon, and P. Miller (Eds.) *The Foucault Effect: Studies in governmentality*, Chicago: University of Chicago Press, pp. 53–72.

Foucault, M. (1995) *Discipline and Punish*. A. Sheridan (tr.). New York: Vintage Books.

Foucault, M. (2003) *Society Must Be Defended: Lectures at the Collège de France, 1975–1976*, M. Bertani and A. Fontana (Eds.). New York: Picador.

Global Center on Cooperative Security. (2015) 'CVE summit process senior officials' check-in meeting: co-chairs' statement', available at https://drive.google.com/file/d/0BztW5QS-DfQjTlJlZzFfMW9oMEk/view (accessed on 1 February 2017).

Gregory, D. (2011) 'From a view to a kill: drones and late modern war', *Theory, Culture & Society*, 28: 188–215.

Guina, J., Welton, R.S., Broderick, P.J., Correll, T.L., and Peirson, R.P. (2016) 'DSM-5 criteria and its implications for diagnosing PTSD in military service members and veterans', *Current Psychiatry Reports*, 18: 43.

Heath-Kelly, C. (2017) 'Algorithmic autoimmunity in the NHS: radicalisation and the clinic', *Security Dialogue*, 48(1): 29–45.

Howell, A. (2014) 'The global politics of medicine: Beyond global health, against securitisation theory', *Review of International Studies*, 40: 961–87.

Howell, A. (2015) 'Resilience, war, and austerity: the ethics of military human enhancement and the politics of data', *Security Dialogue*, 46: 15–31.

Kimball, S.L. and Soldz, S. (2014) 'Medical professionalism and abuse of detainees in the war on terror: time for doctors to stand up our professional ethics', *British Medical Journal*, 348: g2947.

Lupton, D. (1993) 'Risk as moral danger: the social and political functions of risk discourse in public health', *International Journal of Health Services*, 23: 425–35.

Maio, G. (2010) 'History of medical involvement in torture – then and now', *The Lancet*, 357: 1609–11.

Office of the Director of National Intelligence. (2016) 'Summary of information regarding U.S. counterterrorism strikes outside areas of active hostilities', available at www.dni.gov/index.php/newsroom/reports-and-publications/214-reports-publications-2016/1392-summary-of-information-regarding-u-s-counterterrorism-strikes-outside-areas-of-active-hostilities (accessed on 27 January 2017).

Pinchevski, A. (2016) 'Screen trauma: visual media and post-traumatic stress disorder', *Theory, Culture & Society*, 33: 51–75.

Rousseau, C. and Jamil, U. (2010) 'Muslim families' understanding of, and reaction to, "the war on terror"', *American Journal of Orthopsychiatry*, 80: 601–9.

Summergrad, P. and Sharfstein, S.S. (2015) 'Ethics, interrogation, and the American Psychiatric Association', *American Journal of Psychiatry*, 172: 706–7.

US Department of Homeland Security. (2016) 'FY 2016 countering violent extremism (CVE) grant program', available at www.dhs.gov/cvegrants (accessed on 1 February 2017).

Weine, S., Eisenman, D.P., Kinsler, J., Glik D.C., and Polutnik, C. (2017) 'Addressing violent extremism as public health policy and practice', *Behavioral Sciences of Terrorism and Political Aggression*, 3: 208–21.

Xenakis, S.N. (2014) 'The role and responsibilities of psychiatry in 21st century warfare', *Journal of the American Academy of Psychiatry and the Law*, 42: 504–8.

# Part VIII

# Human rights, social justice, and global health

# 37

# The invisible reality of 'chintar rog' (a life of chronic worry)

## The illness of poverty in Dhaka's urban slum settlements

*Sabina Faiz Rashid*

## Introduction

Between 1989 and 1998, 20 slum settlement evictions and demolitions were carried out in various locations, displacing over 100,000 human lives in Dhaka, Bangladesh. Often, unexplained and 'accidental' fires led also to the destruction of slums and displacement of its residents. These are widely perceived to be ploys to evict the residents, in which a network of actors such as political leaders, police, and sometimes some of the residents (who are perhaps manipulated) themselves share complicity (Farid, 2017), and the eviction of informal settlements continues till now.

Compared to rural areas, residents in slum settlements live in crowded congested spaces and struggle to access basic services of housing, water, electricity, and sanitation. Crime and insecurity are pervasive. Endemic poverty is a part of daily life and with little to no education, most of them are engaged in low paid jobs (Baker, 2008). Insecure tenure is a way of life for millions of slum residents, as most settlements are prone to demolition by the government or landowners. There is yet to be a national urban poverty policy in Bangladesh (Banks, et al., 2011) which has implications for the distribution and quality of services provided. The life of the most impoverished living in slum settlements is one of unpredictability, managing one crisis after another, with chronic stressors faced daily. Do these deprivations place them at greater risk of vulnerabilities? Does it impact on how their health is understood and experienced?

Urban poverty is a global phenomenon persistently challenging sustainable public health. Most of the world's population increase is taking place in urban areas in developing countries. By 2050, it is projected that around ten billion people, two-thirds of the world's population, will live in cities, with rapid urbanisation mainly in Africa and South Asia (Satterthwaite and Mitlin, 2013). In Bangladesh, in 2009, 61.9 per cent of urbanites lived in slum areas (UN HABITAT, 2012), and a census by Bangladesh Bureau of Statistics (2015) shows a 77 per cent rise in the number of urban slum households between 1997–2014. Dhaka, the capital city, contains nearly 40 per cent of the total urban population (RAJUK, 2016), and Chittagong, a port city, has the second largest urban slum population (Islam, et al., 2009).

This chapter will draw on anthropological research narratives conducted in two slums (2001–2; and drawn from another slum in 2016 in Dhaka city) to reveal how urban slum residents endure and navigate through the maze of persistent insecurities and uncertainties of life. The narratives illustrate the complexities and underlying processes of poverty that are deeply interconnected to health and illness experiences for individuals living in slum settlements. The aim of this chapter is to reconsider how poverty is experienced and understood as a public health phenomenon through its intrinsic interconnectedness to all aspects of human health and well-being.

Why is it so important to reconceptualise our understandings of health? In many parts of the world, health continues to be embedded deeply in the personal, social, moral, economic, and political worlds people inhabit, challenging the widely accepted biomedical model of health and disease causation. As Farmer, et al. (2013) mentioned, illness and disease for the most vulnerable are often rooted in a complex array of emotional, mental, and physical factors coupled with macro social, economic, and political factors that subject them to destructive health realities (Farmer, et al., 2013). The newly laid out SDGs emphasise several goals, which includes paying increasing attention to those who are left behind economically and socially, and remain excluded from achieving progress. As urban populations increase globally, health indicators worsen, disparities increase, and their social exclusion persists creating urban vulnerable geographies. To address some of the issues raised, we first need to unpack what health means and how it is experienced by individuals living in slum settlements. Research conducted in 2001–2 and subsequently in 2015 and 2016, although 15 years apart, finds parallel health deprivations, vulnerabilities, and systemic chronic ill-health embedded in impoverished communities living in slum settlements.

## 2001–2: Slum Ajah

It is 2001, and Ajah slum (housing over 3,500 households) has been evicted, overnight in the span of one afternoon. Monsura is a small, malnourished girl, about 17 years of age. She has been married for four years to Sayed and has a baby boy, who is 11-months-old. Monsura and her Sayed were temporarily renting space at Sayed's uncle's home, in another slum, located near to what was previously Ajah (but now empty and vacant). Costs of other rentals at nearby slums sky-rocketed in prices when landlords heard about the eviction of Ajah. They were able to find immediate but temporary accommodation from his uncle. Three days after the eviction, I visited Monsura and found her sitting on the bed. She gave me a tired smile. Like most homes in Balurmat, this one roomed home was no bigger than 30 square feet, tiny, damp and dark. There was a torn sheet on the bed and her baby boy sat on the edge of the bed crying. Monsura informs me that she is three months pregnant. She whispers her news to me. She is anxious and tense because she does not know what to do. She is very worried about her husband Sayed (28-year-old) because he does not have a job. The World Bank together with Bangladesh government implemented a policy in September 2002 to reduce air pollution in Dhaka and banned thousands of diesel-run baby-taxis [local three wheelers transport] from the streets and introduced Carbon friendly three wheelers.

This was done with the intention to protect environmental pollution which was worsening in Dhaka city, however, political inefficiencies and poor governance led to the poorest being the most affected when the programme unfolded. In reality, climate change usually affects the most vulnerable, displacing many due to rising sea levels, natural disasters, and other adverse impacts.

Sayed used to rent a diesel run three-wheeler but with the new ban, and to get a 'legitimate' license to rent the new environment friendly three wheelers, required more money in bribes and navigating a host of brokers. Monsura's husband, like many hundreds of poor urban men, became unemployed. He was drinking heavily again and fights were common in the household. Monsura's uncle was threatening to evict them because they have not been able to pay any advance rent for moving in to this home.

Monsura claims Sayed's uncle is a heroin addict and wants the money to support his habit. Monsura and Sayed discuss her pregnancy and he admits that although they are both keen to have another baby, this was not the best time. He looks embarrassed and said, 'we can't keep the baby. Apa [sister] you know our situation now. You see how we are living. If I am lucky I can do some odd jobs and earn up to Taka/BDT 40 or 50 [A$1.00] a day but when I don't have work, which is often, we go without food for days. We already have one child and we cannot manage with another. We will also have to move soon.' Monsura remains quiet. She points to the corner of the room and tells us how she found a big dead rat drowned in her large bottle of cooking oil. She and her husband laugh. There were two cockroaches roaming around her tiny, muddy, uneven floor. I see one egg carefully set-aside on a plate on the floor. She is saving it to cook it for dinner. For a very poor household to purchase an egg is a luxury.

A few weeks later Monsura informs us that she had a crude abortion and was bleeding profusely. They rushed to the pharmacy and bought some medicines to control her fever and bleeding. Monsura is lying on her bed on a torn, stained sheet, looking tiny, pale and very ill. She says, 'I am very scared. I don't know what is happening to me. I feel very weak and I cannot get out of bed. I am terrified.' She decided to have an (illegal) abortion because it cost her very little money, whereas a termination from a clinic will cost about Taka/BDT400 [A$6], money that they did not have, and if they did, they could not afford to spend. The network of health providers that Monsura knew in the old Balurmat slum were no longer there for advice since the eviction. They needed money to meet their basic needs, food and rent.

Two months later, Monsura and Sayeed moved to another slum. Sayeed found some temporary work as a labourer. He was looking at jobs in garment factories, but after 9/11 2001 attacks in the USA, there was also a global recession, and garment factories were shutting down and many workers were left without work. Daily labour was available and he had found some temporary work. Monsura seems to prefer this new slum. While we chat, her baby plays on the muddy floor, half-naked playing with small stones and dirt. She proudly displays a sari her husband bought her with his income. A week later, her baby is sick with fever and severe diarrhoea, vomiting and they rush him to a nearby hospital for treatment. Monsura borrows Taka/BDT 2000 [A$30] from her elder brother for the treatment. Her husband would have to work for more than two months to repay that loan.

Monsura shares, 'apa the poor, we have chintar rog (worry illness) … my chest hurts from worrying so much. From the chest pains, my back hurts. Everyone says this is gastric pain.' When asked who is everyone, Monsura replies, 'doctors, pharmacies and others, but I know why my body is ill. I know what sort of pain this is. Whenever I worry too much I have this pain. This is the illness of poverty and tension and there is no cure … I worry about my husband. My child and I worry about our future. How will we manage? Everything is so uncertain …'

## 2016: Slum Dhakinath

An early morning walk in the informal settlements of Dhakinath, observation finds houses (rooms no bigger than 45 square feet) lined in rows, almost leaning into each other, crowded, leaving little room for privacy or space, with many having no windows for ventilation. Dark, dank and crowded. Next to one of the main lanes, one can see a line of men and women waiting to use the few latrines. There are two latrines, one built in with a broken door and the second latrine was an overhanging one, over a polluted pond, built on sticks and bamboos. Putrid stench fills the air and one can see the overflow of sewage, excretion and puddles of dirt flooding the narrow lanes leading up to this space. Farida, a 40-year-old woman, explained, 'in the hot summer months, there is usually an infestation of cockroaches, rats and mosquitoes, which one is constantly swatting or avoiding', as she uses an electronic racket (now widely available to kill the mosquitoes). She is sitting in a small space in the corner of one of the sections of this slum, selling snacks from a wooden small box.

She shares her story, 'I moved here two years ago, when the slum I lived in (in the periphery of Dhaka) was demolished. The private landowner decided to build a block of flats and after paying rising rents every few years, we had to finally leave. The shift took an enormous toll on us.' For Farida, it meant selling some of their hard-earned assets, including a television to collect more money to move their family to this new slum. They didn't know anyone except for another family that moved with them to this place. Rent on average was Taka/BDT 2,500 (A$42) per month and they were shocked by the size of the houses and the congestion. She shared, 'where we lived before was much less congested and crowded and we had some greenery nearby. In this space, there are hundreds of people jam-packed.' The unfamiliarity of the space and the lack of networks was difficult at first. Farida was used to borrowing money on credit from her neighbour in her previous slum settlement. She was used to regularly buying groceries for the family on credit as she was well known to the local neighbourhood and market sellers. This new move, meant building new relationships and having cash available at all times, as not a single person was willing to give them anything on credit initially. Her husband, Bashar also struggled to understand the local networks and politics of the new slum, but after two years they felt more settled in this new place.

After moving here, her son, Rahim, 15 years old, started hanging around with the wrong crowd. He had initially set up a small shop on the streets of Dhaka but there was a legal drive to get rid of hawkers from the streets of Dhaka in 2015. Farida's husband and son had to shut the small shop down. She worries about her son, Rahim is getting involved in gang politics, and with crime, heroin dealing and drug intake rife, he would hurt himself. Farida's neighbour, Shama, a young woman was married to a local gang leader. He was badly injured in a gang fight, a year ago. He was disabled and unable to work, and Shama worked in a garments factory to support the family.

Farida worries her son was friendly with the neighbour's husband and was getting influenced by him, 'I worry that so many of these boys don't listen to parents anymore. Gum candy (drugs) is common here. Even my son who was a good boy, is never home. My daughter [who is 10 years old] goes to school now, but I worry about the crime and insecurity in this place. One hears stories of harassment and rape. When I first moved here, I used to lock her inside the house (one room) when we went searching for work in the city. Then no one would know she is in there by herself. This was to keep her safe.

When we first moved here, money was tight, from chinta (worries) you can't eat. There were days we ate less, and when you have less food in your stomach, it aches in hunger … then slowly you lose your appetite and you won't be able to sleep. The chinta will invade into your blood and meat and bones, everywhere in your body. Then how will your health be okay? You tell me. Then your health will not be good. Then you will say, from worrying and worrying I don't feel good anymore. But will you let your worries go?'

Farida shares that although she is more settled in Dhakinath, she dreams of moving to a better place. Farida had managed to set up a small corner informal shop, where she sells local pita (sweet bread) and other snacks, which contributes to the household income (informal discussions with others revealed that one needs to pay an amount to the local leaders such as Mokbul (see following narrative) to maintain one's business without disruptions). Her husband, Bashar pulls a rickshaw, is often sick and complains of fever, body aches and pains and works erratically.

…

Mokbul, a 60-year-old and a local leader, who is more powerful than incoming temporary resident, owns a food shop and is a member of local committee of the slum. He discusses that to have a peaceful mind one should have all their basic needs met. He shared how slum life with its uncertainties and insecurities leads to too much mental stress, and then the person becomes a victim of 'chintar rog'. He shared how recently, there was an injury near the make shift latrine, as one child slipped and fell into the pond and was badly injured. The neighbours complained that the local NGO had promised to build a structured latrine, but the project had wrapped up and they had to use the locally made makeshift unsafe and unhygienic latrine. He said, 'the government doesn't care, no one cares about us!'

He shared how most urban poor residents lived in a cycle of poverty, with uncertain jobs, never knowing when an eviction may happen, worrying about food, and health expenses, paying more electricity and gas and water bills than other residents of Dhaka city. 'Poverty is huge problem. When someone has taken a loan and is unable to repay it, the pressure he receives from the other party (local extortionists) will automatically create 'chinta' (worry) for him'. He shared how his next-door neighbour now had a brain tumour, and this is because 'he was always suffering from 'chinta' (worries) from mental and emotional stress … now we have loss of faith, there is no iman in this city. Everything is going wrong as we are suffering from loss of faith … the people, government and everyone…'

What do these life stories tell us? These narratives are typical for many of the impoverished residents who live in slum settlements. It reveals an environment where individuals manage in conditions of continued deprivation and make ends meet, with temporary work and low wages, illnesses, and face constant economic instability. Many are juggling finances and supporting family members, and live in fear, hope, resignation, and frustration. One of the challenges is that the existing measurements of the poverty line for the urban poor of US$1.90 per day, as defined by World Bank (2013) and other agencies, are defined at a national level, and misrepresent levels of poverty. Those who are most vulnerable are not necessarily representative of the national average. The definitions do not take into consideration the temporal nature of slum residents' daily existence, with sudden evictions, unstable jobs, and health expenditures that are part of their lived realities. Crime and paying extorted higher fees to access basic water, electricity, and gas services add further to the cycle of debts. As studies report, in the absence of formal governance in slum settlements, groups of local leaders (*mastaans*) manage and control access to services, and residents pay inflated prices for poor quality basic utilities (Baker, 2008; Rashid, 2007). For Monsura, Farida, and their families, maintaining key relationships to individuals who belong to a hierarchy of powerful brokers was key to one's survival, and led to negotiating arrangements, where one could pay for services later, ask for credit and waiver of loans and other kinds of support. Evictions and sudden disruptions lead to the end of these carefully built up relationships over time and cause greater insecurity.

The emphasis on outcome measures of poverty tends to take away focus from the processes that cause poverty (Mitlin & Satterthwaite, 2013; Moser, 1995), and the fragility of existence, which can leave individuals who were managing or even graduating out of poverty suddenly at the bottom of the heap. For both Monsura and Farida and their families, eviction from the slum led to greater uncertainty and further deprivations. Assets were sold, and familiar networks and social capital were lost in this transition. Previously familiar networks who provided financial and social support are usually neighbours, community members who may lend money or loan some cash for emergencies, and often the local grocery shop and pharmacists provide goods on credit. In new spaces, these social networks and support cease to exist and temporary jobs that were previously nearby become too far to commute to daily because of transportation expenses in the city. The global recession in 2001 shut down many garment factories and led to unemployment of many, and the World Bank environmental policy to change the model of the three-wheeler vehicles in Dhaka city created corruption and a hike in the costs of buying a legitimate license, and the national drive to remove street hawkers resulted in a loss of income, overnight, for many urban poor families (Rashid, 2007). Occupations such as rickshaw pulling, which Farida's husband engaged in, make the urban poor susceptible to systematic health risks. Urban labour markets in Bangladesh remain intensely competitive. A majority of these jobs are informal, insecure, low waged, and often hazardous, including petty retail trade, transport, manufacturing, construction, and domestic services (Banks, 2016; Rashid, 2007). Rickshaw pulling, a predominant occupation for urban poor males, is an unsustainable livelihood, as one is physically unable to maintain working in this sector longer term with its labour intensive, hazardous working conditions (Begum and Sen, 2005). Worsening health, combined with mounting unpaid bills and debts, can impose a huge burden, pulling down the pace of upward mobility during their lifetime. It is critical for health and development practitioners and policymakers to understand how fragile and dependent the urban poor are on the forces of global and local market economies and politics and remain excluded.

The narratives reveal that despite the instability faced by Monsura and Farida and their families, they remained resilient and constantly looked for solutions to manage, but over time, the efforts put in and constant deprivations resulted in a debilitating effect on their minds and bodies, leading to much anguish and despair. The biomedical 'disease' model that dominates much of public health theory and practice is missing this important connection people make between their bodies and their everyday life worlds. *Chintar rog*[1] (an inadequate translation into English is 'worry illness') humanises the medical domain and processes by paying attention to people, not just disease-specific worlds to which human beings peripherally belong. *Chintar rog* reveals the hidden epidemic of uncertainty, the slum contexts of insecurity and deprivation, which is a part of daily life. For the poor, the illness is experienced and embodied in the social, economic, political, emotional, mental, physical, and spiritual.

The exhausting and relentless uncertainty of *chintar rog* becomes an explanatory model of everyday life, of time forcibly lived moment-to-moment, the past, present, and the future. *Chintar rog* is not an illness borne per say, but to them akin to a 'way of life' illness, it is their core being which embodies this everyday pain, worry and suffering and the body then becomes a form of truth telling, and the medicalisation of this illness speaks of the unspeakable of their existence. We need to understand not only the subjective experiences of illnesses and how they are personally and socially understood and experienced in different societies but also the root causes of illness and disease, to meaningfully address and improve health for the most disadvantaged. Continued neglect of ever-expanding urban slum populations in the world could inevitably lead to greater expenditures and worsening health for such populations. There is a pressing need to rethink and reframe how we write about, represent, and comprehend health as experienced in the most impoverished communities and how one understands the underlying causes of vulnerability which adversely impact personal, social, and public health of individuals and communities. The share of the world population who live in cities has increased steadily for decades, with 55 per cent of the world's population (~4.1 billion people) now living in cities, compared to 30 per cent in 1950 (UNDESA, 2014). In cities, health and other inequalities tend to be greater within slum settlements, where millions of people are affected with poor living conditions and health, and have limited health care (Ezeh, et al., 2017; Udofia, et al., 2014).

## Conclusions

Social, physical, and emotional suffering weave a complicated story between everyday lives and their health and personal well-being. There is a clear articulation of their position at the bottom of the hierarchy with little money, security, and support, and no services and an absence of basic needs being met. What does it mean for the global landscape of public health? How do we redefine health as these narratives clearly show how conditions are not divorced from poverty and their local idioms are expressed and lived in the body? The increasing marginalisation of these urban poorest parallels the global shift to capitalism where health is a commodity which further stigmatises them, decontextualises their social, economic, and political environment, and blames 'the poor' for being 'non-compliant' of health services. As Farmer, et al., (2013) argue, the challenge remains as to how the 'problem' is viewed, be it biological, environmental, or economic, which shape proposed interventions (solutions) and their ultimate effect. How does critical medical anthropology inform public health? Currently certain disciplines, epidemiology, and biostatistics predominantly inform public health agendas. A part of the problem is that most often critical medical anthropology doesn't inform public health, and public health goes on to create 'interventions' that don't make sense in terms of the realities of people's lived experience. It is apparent that many health challenges are syndemic with poverty (Singer, 2000); diseases are interactive and lived in every cell of the bodies of those who are suffering. *Chintar rog* speaks of precarious conditions, perpetual adversity, and impossible choices of the residents, as well as forcing us to think about the ontological insecurities present in the deprivations and how this is embodied in the meanings and experiences of health and illness.

Where is public health in all of this? How effective will public health be if we don't immediately reorient our approaches to how we understand health? Housing, water, food security, and social policies should be integrated into how we understand and approach public health interventions. The dominant disease inside the body model remains the primary way of managing health. Selective 'cost effective' vertical interventions based on the 'physical model' leave little room for focusing on achieving a comprehensive state of good health (World Bank, 1993). Health is viewed as a biomedical-commodity to be purchased, making the economically disadvantaged struggle perilous just to survive. Where are the other dimensions, the emotional, mental, spiritual, that impact on the individual and speak of the unliveable conditions of life? *Chintar rog* clearly highlights the limits of medicine as most people who live in slums are situated between hope, fear, anxiety, and chronic deprivations, and that is the 'normal' for them. By giving a name to it, they speak of their hard lives while also trying to normalise or articulate the uncertainty as many deal with chronic crisis situations and health adversities that plague them.

The history of public health and its agenda has usually been dominated by developed country public health leaders, UN and international agencies, and now private philanthropists (Farmer, et al., 2013). To add to this complex scenario, we live in a world where a market-based approach to health and development, as advocated by the World Bank and international bodies, and the private sector is the norm. There needs to be radical shift in the frameworks of health as currently conceptualised. This is critical to moving the public health of the most disadvantaged forward. We need to recognise that health is as much mental, emotional, and spiritual as it is physical, and directly impacted by the social, economic, and political conditions that people inhabit. Millions of individuals in slum settlements remain under perennial silent tyranny, managing one crisis after another, with comprehensive support from the development sector, donor community, and the state missing. Unless we own up to this fundamental reality of the illness of poverty and how it interacts and impacts on health, we will continue to produce short-term band-aid solutions, and the health, well-being, and lives of the most vulnerable will continue to remain deplorable.

## Acknowledgements

I would like to thank my colleague Mikhail Islam for his critical insights and feedback which greatly strengthened the quality of this chapter. Thank you to Richard Parker and Jonathan García for their edits and initial comments on the first draft.

## Note

1   A colleague and a friend came across this term while doing fieldwork in a rural village in Savar in 2006 and argued at the time that it was some form of mental anxiety. I recently came across a book by a medical doctor in Punjab, Dr. Marwah, who in the 1960s shared from a biomedical perspective the phenomenon of chintar rog, as an anxiety disorder of the poor.

## References

Baker, J. (2008) 'Urban poverty: a global view', (No. UP-5). World Bank Urban Papers, World Bank, Washington, DC available at http://documents.worldbank.org/curated/en/954511468315832363/Urban-poverty-a-global-view (accessed on 1 January 2018).

Bangladesh Bureau of Statistics. (2015) 'Preliminary report on census of slum areas and floating population 2014', Statistics and Information Division (SID), Ministry of Planning, Government of Bangladesh, May.

Banks, N. (2016) 'Livelihoods limitations: the political economy of urban poverty in Dhaka, Bangladesh', *Development and Change*, 47(2): 266–92.

Banks, N., Roy, M., and Hulme, D. (2011) 'Neglecting the urban poor in Bangladesh: research, policy and action in the context of climate change', *Environment and Urbanization*, 23(2): 487–502.

Begum, S. and Sen, B. (2005) 'Pulling rickshaws in the city of Dhaka: a way out of poverty?', *Environment and Urbanization*, 17(2): 11–25.

Ezeh, A., Oyebode, O., Satterthwaite, D., Chen, Y., Ndugwa, R., Sartori, J., Mberu, B., Melendez-Torres, G., Haregu, T., Watson, S., Caiaffa, W., Capon, A., and Lilford, R. (2017) 'The history, geography, and sociology of slums and the health problems of people who live in slums', *The Lancet*, 389(10068): 547–58.

Farid, C. (2017) 'A tale of two cities: the past in the present', University of Wisconsin Law School. Unpublished report.

Farmer, P., Kim, J.Y., Kleinman, A., and Basilico, M. (2013) *Reimagining Global Health: An introduction*, California: University of California Press.

Islam, N., Mahbub, A., and Nazem, N. (2009) 'Urban slums of Bangladesh', The Daily Star, 20 June, available at www.thedailystar.net/news-detail-93293 (accessed on 1 January 2018).

Mitlin, D. and Satterthwaite, D. (2013) *Urban Poverty in the Global South: Scale and nature*, London: Routledge.

Moser, C. (1995) 'Urban social policy and poverty reduction', *Environment and Urbanization*, 7(1): 159–72.

RAJUK. (2016) 'Dhaka: past and present, chapter 2, Dhaka structure plan 2016–2035', RAJUK Long Term Planning Policy Framework, available at www.rajukdhaka.gov.bd/rajuk/image/slideshow/5.Chapter%2002.pdf (accessed on 19 February 2018).

Rashid, S. (2007) 'Accessing married adolescent women: the realities of ethnographic research in an urban slum environment in Dhaka, Bangladesh', *Field Methods*, 19(4): 369–83.

Satterthwaite, D. and Mitlin, D. (2013) *Reducing Urban Poverty in the Global South*. London: Routledge.

Singer, M. (2000) 'A dose of drugs, a touch of violence, a case of aids: conceptualizing the SAVA syndemic', *Free Inquiry – Special Issue: Gangs, Drugs & Violence*, 28(1): 13.

Udofia, E., Yawson, A., Aduful, K., and Bwambale, F. (2014) 'Residential characteristics as correlates of occupants' health in the greater Accra region, Ghana', *BMC Public Health*, 14: 244.

UN HABITAT. (2012) 'State of the world's cities 2012/2013: prosperity of cities', World Urban Forum Edition, United Nations Human Settlements Programme.

UNDESA (United Nations Department of Economic and Social Affairs, Population Division) (2014) *World Urbanization Prospects: The 2014 revision, highlights (ST/ESA?SER.A/352)*, New York: Population Division of the Department of Economic and Social Affairs of the United Nations Secretariat.

World Bank. (1993) *World Development Report 1993: Investing in health*. Oxford: Oxford University Press.

World Bank. (2013) 'Understanding poverty, the World Bank', available at www.worldbank.org/en/topic/poverty/overview (accessed on 1 January 2018).

# 38

# Salmon, fire, and the environmental and political contexts of tribal health

*Kari Marie Norgaard and Ron Reed*

There is much emphasis within the global health field on epidemic disease in the global South. Yet even in the wealthiest regions of the United States, communities face dire poverty and extensive health challenges. This case study highlights how the politics of global health manifest in the contestation of unequal power dynamics that take place throughout the world, not just in the global South. Rather, our case highlihts the extreme marginalisation that also exists in the so-called global North – a marginsliation obscured by simple global North–South dichotomies. In 2004, the Karuk Tribe filed a report with the Federal Energy Regulatory Commission (FERC) describing the relationships between Klamath River dams, denied access to salmon, and elevated rate of diabetes and other diet-related diseases for Karuk people. This research was innovative in the policy world for the links it established between environmental and human health – no other Tribe had made such a claim that dams were giving them an artificially high rate of diabetes in a federal process. Since that time the Karuk Tribe has successfully influenced the California state water quality standards for the Klamath river to include Native American Cultural and Subsistence Beneficial Uses (Stoll, 2016), and made visible the role of human health in forest policies regarding fire suppression and climate change (Karuk Tribe, 2016; Norgaard, 2014).

We use a case study of long-term collaborations between academics and the Karuk Tribe to show how both policy debates and academic understanding can be meaningfully enhanced by including the broader environmental and social dimensions of human health. Whereas dominant health frameworks tend to de-contextualise social and political context of illness or disease (Krieger, 2011), from indigenous perspectives, social, political, cultural, and especially environmental dimensions of human health are key (Joe and Young, 1994; Ferreria and Lang, 2005; Kuhnlein, et al., 2009). In the absence of such context, work on tribal health in particular has negatively stigmatised and implicitly blamed Native communities for the health challenges they experience. In contrast, we describe the ways that the Karuk Department of Natural Resources has built on academic collaborations to situate health outcomes, from diabetes and obesity to mental anguish, as outcomes of failed federal forest and riverine policies. Our work builds on the environmental justice tradition in which affected groups collaborate with academics to conduct community-based science (Brown and Mikkelsen, 1997; Brown, 2013; Cordner, et al., 2012; Lynn, 2000; Pellow and Brulle, 2005). While there is an established literature on the benefits of collaborative community-based science for environmental health research, few of these collaborations are with indigenous communities, and even less has been written about the benefits of drawing upon indigenous cosmologies and knowledge frameworks for reshaping either research frameworks or policy debates. In this chapter, we describe the research and policy negotiation processes, as well as the ways that this type of policy driven work enriches existing theory (Brown, 2013; Krieger, 1994, 2011).

## Natural resource policy and the alteration of diet

The Karuk are the second largest American Indian Tribe in California with over 4,000 members and descendants. Their traditional territory and homelands is in the far northern part of the state along the Klamath River. Karuk people have used ceremony, fire, and sophisticated harvest techniques to sustainably manage salmon runs in coordination with neighbouring tribes for tens of thousands of years (Anderson and Lake, 2016; Lake, et al., 2010; Most, 2006). The Karuk are a fishing people: fish consumption prior to European contact is estimated at the enormous figure of 450 pounds per person per year (Hewes, 1973). Early anthropologists marvelled at the immense abundance of natural resources of the people living on the Klamath River. Indeed, the Karuk, together with their neighbouring tribes the Yurok and Hoopa, are considered to have been the wealthiest of all Indian people in the region now called California. This wealth was a direct result of the Klamath River's year-round abundance of food resources, particularly the multiple runs of salmon. However, salmon populations have been dramatically damaged by overfishing and habitat degradation since the arrival of non-Indians in the 1850s, and especially in the past generation.

The history of the Klamath Basin since contact between Europeans and indigenous tribes is a classic example of environmental injustice. The arrival of miners, the military, and settlers into Karuk territory in 1850 was accompanied by direct genocide in which many people and much knowledge of traditional culture, foods, social and political structure was lost (Madley, 2016; Norton, 1979). Whereas longstanding cultural traditions existed for regulating and sharing fish and other resources both within the Karuk Tribe and between neighbouring tribes, the entry of non-indigenous groups into the region led to conflict and dramatic resource depletion (McEvoy, 1986; Most, 2006). Over the past 150 years, state and federal natural resource management actions from dam building and irrigation diversions, to fire suppression and destructive mining and timber practices, have resulted in the degradation of the basin. At the same time, Karuk cultural management practices developed to care for the land, from burning the forest to fishing according to Karuk custom, have been criminalised (Norton, 1979; Norgaard, 2014). The Karuk did not have their Federal recognition reconfirmed until 1979. Karuk people still have no reservation and their fishing rights have yet to be acknowledged by the federal government outside the right to fish at one specific site for ceremonial purposes. Non-indigenous fishing regulations like those developed and enforced through California Department of Fish and Wildlife fail to account for the Karuk as original inhabitants, their inalienable right to subsistence harvesting, and the sustainable nature of Karuk harvests. As a result, they have attempted to balance the subsistence needs of Karuk people with recreational desires of non-indigenous peoples from outside the area.

In the face of these disruptions, populations of salmon, lamprey, sturgeon, and other aquatic food species have plummeted. Interestingly, despite 100 years of environmentally damaging practices, salmon continued to provide a significant food supply to Karuk people until the mid 1980s – about ten years after the lowermost dam blocked access to 90 per cent of the spawning habitat of the most important salmon run. Thus, while many Karuk people continued to consume salmon several times per day (during salmon season) up into the 1980s, in recent years consumption averages less than five pounds per person per year – giving Karuk people the ambiguous standing of having one of the most dramatic and recent diet shifts of any tribe in North America (Reed, et al., 2010; Norgaard, 2005).

## Research and policy process

Power companies are granted licenses to operate dams in the public interest by the Federal Energy Regulatory Commission. In 2006, the license application for the dams on the Klamath River expired. The relicensing process involves years of scientific investigation, input, and discussion from the impacted communities. Beginning in 2001, Ron Reed served as the Karuk tribal representative in this process, attending meetings for one week of every month for four years. During that time, his mother and several of his aunts passed on, all of them in their seventies or younger. Ron became convinced that the lack of healthy food, specifically the loss of salmon, was directly impacting the health of his people, leading to high rates of diabetes, heart disease, and a decreased life expectancy. He spoke passionately about this problem in the meetings. In February of 2004, PacifiCorp filed their final license application. Despite years of meeting with the Karuk and other tribes, commercial fishermen, scientists, and environmental groups who gave extensive testimony as to the ecological and cultural impacts of the dams, the power company claimed that there were no impacts from their operation below the dams. In the words of co-author Ron Reed, 'the document was five feet tall and contained no mention of our needs.'

It was at this time that we, the authors, began working together. Our research design and approach combined community perspectives and understanding with traditional ecological knowledge and Western science. Together we conducted a study and produced a report that made visible the relationship between ecological and human health. In October of 2004 the preliminary study, 'The effects of altered diet on the health of the Karuk people', was filed with the FERC and released. Our report, the preliminary draft of which was written in a few short months, became the first example of a tribe articulating how denied access to traditional foods led to artificially high rates of diabetes due to the presence of a dam. The full report containing survey data and additional interviews and analyses was filed and released one year later.

The central finding of these reports is that Karuk people face significant and costly health consequences as a result of denied access to many of their traditional foods, especially salmon (Norgaard 2004, 2005). Not only does a traditional diet prevent the onset of conditions such as obesity, diabetes, heart disease, kidney trouble, and hypertension, a traditional diet of salmon and other foods is one of the best treatments for such conditions. Lack of traditional food impacts tribal members not only in terms of the decreased nutritional content of specific foods, but also in an overall absence of food, leaving Karuk people with basic issues of food security. This report and the media attention it received generated significant public attention and became a key piece in the move towards dam removal (Gosnell and Kelly, 2010; Leimbach, 2009). Since developing this cultural resource and environmental justice angle, the Karuk Tribe has continued to use a combination of traditional and Western science to emphasise the environmental context of human health in policy struggles related to water quality, fire suppression, and climate change (Giles, 2017; Karuk Tribe, 2016; Kann, et al., 2010; Norgaard, et al., 2013; Stoll, 2016).

## Methods: integrating environmental and political context

We began our research by contacting everyone who could be a potential resource including diabetes researchers, medical practitioners, and traditional food experts and advocates. These people shared important research perspectives, medical data, and reports that formed the basis of our research design. We also began a series of interviews. We spoke to tribal elders and gathered testimony in oral interviews, including interviews with elders whose heart conditions had improved after eating salmon. In-depth interviews were used to gather detailed information from tribal members regarding health, diet, food access and consumption, and economic conditions. Information was also gathered on family history and health conditions over time. In-depth interviews were conducted with a total of 18 individuals. These individuals served as 'key informants' regarding a range of cultural and fisheries topics. Interviewees were selected to represent both women and men, a range of ages (30 to mid-70s), and various other aspects of the community (members of Tribal Council and Staff, as well as people who had no relationship to the tribal organisation). Karuk people are traditionally organised by family. Families are associated with regions of the river, and had particular rights and responsibilities within the community such as fishing and conducting specific ceremonies (Willette, et al., 2016). As this organisation persists today, interviewees were drawn from multiple families throughout ancestral territory to capture variation in these forms of experience and knowledge.

Simultaneously, we made connections with health practitioners within the Karuk Tribe and across California. The fact that the doctor heading the tribal clinic took a personal interest in the research was a major asset. In order to evaluate the prevalence of diet-related diseases, medical data on current rates of diabetes, heart conditions, high blood pressure, and obesity were obtained from the Happy Camp Tribal Office. Later, key medical staff provided major assistance in the distribution of the survey.

While medical data provided quantitative figures on disease rates and interviews provided the opportunity for in-depth information, we also conducted a survey to provide a wider view of community experience and to supplement medical data. The survey allowed for the collection of valuable quantitative data regarding economic patterns, health conditions, and fish consumption that had been long absent in the broader discussion of tribal impacts of riverine health. The 2005 Karuk Health and Fish Consumption Survey contained 61 questions designed to evaluate the range of economic, health, and cultural impacts for tribal members from the decline in quality of the Klamath River system. We developed open and closed ended questions on the consumption and harvesting of traditional foods based upon what people told us in the interviews. Questions about personal and family history, and information on medical conditions were included, as well as information on age of death of family members. Disease rates from medical and self-report survey data generally corresponded, suggesting accuracy in findings. The survey was distributed to all adult tribal members within the ancestral territory whom we could reach.[1]

Both the interview questions and survey design thus drew upon indigenous understanding and perspectives concerning the many social and cultural dimensions of food, health, and the forces creating denied access. Some of the most useful questions in our survey were about when various food sources ceased to be a significant portion of people's diets, and when various diet-related diseases first appeared in Karuk families. We would ideally like to have historical population data on food species, as well as historical data on diabetes rates. However, these did not exist. The tribe has only recently begun assembling good data on health conditions, so data from the 1980s was not available. And although agencies such as the US Fish and Wildlife Service collected data on salmon populations, they did not collect data on any of the many other important food sources for Karuks, such as lamprey 'eels' or freshwater mussels. Thus, asking people from memory filled important gaps. As we will discuss later, it was through the comparison of the answers on these questions that we were able to see that, just as Ron suspected, there was a direct relationship between the disappearance of the Spring Chinook salmon and the emergence of diet-related diseases.

## Findings

### Present and historical diet

Salmon are estimated to have made up close to 50 per cent of the energy and total protein in the pre-contact diet of Karuk people (Hewes, 1973). Deer elk, and tan oak acorns have also been of primary importance. According to both Karuk observations and scientific literature, a number of factors either deny or limit the access of people to their traditional foods. While earlier generations ate from the land, limited access to traditional food forces the present Karuk population to buy most of their food in stores and/or rely on government commodities. These changes represent a major dietary shift. Through our survey we learned that despite the reduced availability of salmon and other fish, a high percentage of Karuk families report that someone in their household still fishes or hunts for food, as indicated in Figure 38.1.

In the 2004–5 season, fishing for eels (Pacific Lamprey and other Lamprey species), Spring and Fall Chinook Salmon, Coho, and Sturgeon all reached record lows. Over 80 per cent of surveyed households indicated that they were unable to gather adequate amounts of eel, salmon, or sturgeon to

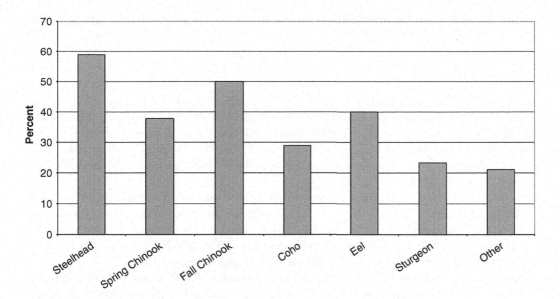

*Figure 38.1*  Percent of Karuk households who fish for various species, 2005

fulfil their family needs. For example, most households that caught salmon, steelhead, eels, and sturgeon report catching ten or fewer, and no households report catching more than 50 eels, Fall, or Spring Chinook salmon total for the season. Furthermore, 40 per cent of tribal members report that there are species of fish that their family gathered which they no longer harvest at all. For most of these species the decline is quite recent. For example, over half of respondents report that Spring Chinook became an insignificant source of food during the 1960s and 1970s, within a decade of the completion of Iron Gate dam, although some families continued to gather significant amounts of these foods into the 1980s and 1990s.

## Why have diets altered?

Genocide and forced assimilation over the past 150 years have led to a loss of traditional knowledge of relationships with the land (including the preparation and acquisition of traditional foods), and to a lesser extent, changes in the tastes and desires of people. Yet despite these dramatic earlier events, the testimony of elders about foods they ate until recently indicate that considerable changes have also occurred within the last generation. These most recent changes are largely due to denied access to traditional foods due to plummeting salmon populations, over-harvesting of mushrooms by competing commercial interests, and dropping acorn yields in the absence of proper fire management.

Spring Chinook have been a critically important food source for Karuk people and the salmon species whose decline is most visibly linked to the construction of the dams. But many species are affected. Until quite recently, the abundance of riverine and upslope forest food resources to which Karuk people had access provided a safety net of foods should one species fail to produce a significant harvest in a given year. Thus, while salmon were centrally important, other food resources were consumed fresh and preserved to provide throughout the year. Yet, as of 2017, every riverine food species consumed by Karuk tribal members is in a state of decline. Now so few fish exist that even ceremonial salmon consumption is limited. There are at least 25 species of plants, animals, and fungi that form part of the traditional Karuk diet to which Karuk people are currently denied or have only limited access. Furthermore, salmon and tan oak acorns, foods that were most central in the Karuk diet and provided the bulk of energy and protein, are amongst the missing elements.

## Diet-related diseases

The loss of traditional food sources is now recognised as directly responsible for a host of diet-related illnesses among Native Americans including diabetes, obesity, heart disease, tuberculosis, hypertension, kidney troubles, and strokes (Joe and Young, 1994). Indeed, diabetes is one of the most significant health problems facing Native peoples today (Olson, 2001; Fretts, et al., 2014). Diabetes is described as a new disease among this population and is the consequence of drastic lifestyle and cultural changes that have occurred since World War II (Joe and Young, 1994).

Survey and medical data indicate that as the presence of healthy traditional foods declined in the Karuk diet, a series of new health problems has emerged for Karuk people. Identified health consequences of the altered diet for the Karuk people include high rates of Type II diabetes, heart disease, and hypertension. The estimated diabetes rate for the Karuk Tribe is 21 per cent, nearly four times the US average. The estimated rate of heart disease for the Karuk Tribe is 39.6 per cent, three times the national average.

Despite their epidemic levels, diabetes has only recently appeared in the Karuk community. Self-report data from the Health and Fish Consumption Survey indicate that diabetes first appeared in most families (over 60 per cent) since the 1970s. Interestingly, it is the loss of Spring Chinook salmon that appears to correspond most closely with the rise in diet-related diseases. It was during the 1960s and 1970s that Spring Chinook dropped out of the diets of most Karuk tribal members, and shortly following this event, diabetes is reported in high numbers. Diabetes begins to appear in about 30 per cent of Karuk families roughly ten years following the loss of Spring Chinook salmon as a significant food source.

The relationship between the loss of large amounts of salmon in the Karuk diet and the emergence of diabetes is a correlation that may or may not be causal. The drop in gathering of Spring Chinook and the rise in diabetes rate could be happening by chance, or due to some other outside force (such as people moving away from the river, or some dramatic event). Causality cannot be determined from the statistical analysis itself, but can be inferred from induction. The fact that Native people around the world experience skyrocketing rates of diabetes with the shift from a traditional to a Western diet, coupled with the fact that salmon would be prescribed by a doctor as the ideal food as both preventative and cure for diabetes, together with the close temporal association between the two events, makes a very compelling case for a causal relationship. Based on this context we surmised that these health consequences stem from changes in the specific nutrient content of traditional foods such as salmon and acorns, as compared with the present-day diet, as well as a decrease in the physical benefits of exercise associated with their gathering.

Finally, the fact that Karuk tribal members are denied access to the healthy foods that supported them since time immemorial also costs society. When an entire tribe faces epidemic rates of expensive conditions such as diabetes, sizable state, county, and tribal medical resources will be used to address this problem. The American Diabetes Association reports that diabetes patients have an average annual per capita cost of health care at US$13,243 per person per year in the United States. Given the 148 diabetic tribal members within the ancestral territory in 2004, our report included a calculation of the annual cost for Karuk tribal members at over US$1.9 million. The report also noted that these increased medical care costs, paid by society as a whole, were not reflected in PacifiCorp's dam operation expenditures, nor were they withdrawn from the profits PacifiCorps receives from the production of electricity in a manner which damages the health of the Klamath riverine system. Instead the higher health care costs of increased diabetes in the Karuk population are born by society as a whole. PacifiCorps does not reimburse the Karuk Tribe, nor Siskiyou nor Humboldt Counties for the increased cost of health care that comes from the destruction of an abundant source of healthy food in the Klamath River. We contended that any cost-benefit analysis of the dams should include the 1.9 million annually that provides medical services for the artificially high incidence of diabetes in the Karuk Tribe.

When this information was compiled it was submitted to the Federal Energy Regulatory Commission docket. We also released the report publicly. Our work received coverage in the form of a front page of the *Washington Post*, a story on National Public Radio, and another *Associated Press* story that was widely reprinted, as well as dozens of additional news stories and coverage by local and regional radio stations. This helped keep the pressure on the power company.

Since the release of the report and the political pressure it brought to bear, the Karuk Tribe went on to be a part of the successful negotiation of a settlement agreement for dam removal. A decade later the report was again an important piece in the environmental impact statement for the dam removal. The Department of Natural Resources continues to conduct cutting edge research in the areas of fisheries, fire, food security, climate change, and water quality, and the environmental dimensions of human health remains a key framework for the tribe's work (Giles, 2017; Karuk Tribe, 2016; Lake, et al., 2010).

## What counts as knowledge? Re-framing policy debates

In his 2013 Reeder lecture Phil Brown reflected that,

> Combining medical sociology and environmental sociology have brought me ways to address pressing spheres of personal, professional, institutional and global importance. The linkage is more obvious each day that we discover additional connections that must be addressed together as with potential connections between obesity, diabetes, neighborhood walkability, and community gardens.
>
> *Brown, 2013, p. 160*

When Ron Reed first approached Kari Norgaard about documenting the heightened rates of diabetes and heart disease he was seeing in the Karuk community, the relationship he hypothesised between the loss of salmon and increased disease came from his direct experience. Salmon is a healthy food source, high in protein, iron, zinc, Omega 3 fatty acids, and lower in saturated fats and sugar. Yet until we combined this direct experience with medical and social science research it was dismissed as 'anecdotal evidence'. Without this three-part combination of direct community experience, indigenous epistemologies of interconnection, and Western science, our research could never have made such a substantial contribution.

Making visible the interconnections between environmental policy and human health required a number of innovations. When we began our work, Kari Norgaard was familiar with a number of tribal environmental justice cases involving traditional foods. She assumed that other tribes were making links between environmental decline, the loss of salmon, and increase in diet-related diseases, and figured that with a little investigation into the work of others she would be able to use the research methods of other tribes as a template to design the Karuk project. Much to her surprise, however, this was not the case. While there were many examples of tribes struggling with the health effects of the loss of their traditional foods, especially in Canada, this work was in response not to declining availability of the foods, but to environmental contaminants such as mercury. This literature, which had more of a justice framework, was not well linked with another body of literature from the medical community on the high rates of diabetes in among First Nations. In this second case, tribes such as the Navajo had well developed diabetes research programmes. However, these were not linking either the change in diet or the increase in diabetes with degradation of the environment.

The focus of our work, while building upon all these sources of material, was different. Karuk people described their situation as a case of 'denied access' to traditional foods; that is, diet change, rather than being inevitable, was tied to ecosystem decline due to the improper management of the rivers and forests. By bringing these three well established literatures together, we were able to illustrate how the inability of Karuk people to continue to eat their traditional foods – and hence the corresponding rise in diet-related diseases – was not coincidental or the fault of Karuk people. They had not become mysteriously poorly educated with respect to healthy foods, but instead the state had failed to protect tribal trust resources, despite its mandate to do so.

### Reframing academic conversations: context contributes to theory

Sociological approaches to epidemiology have contributed important insights to understanding the patterns of health inequalities – specifically regarding the importance of social structure and racism on health (Williams and Sternthal, 2010). These emphases on social context have been important additions to the dominant biomedical framework on health and disease that emphasises individual biology and behaviour. The inclusion of how the natural environmental and colonialism shape a community's health circumstances – as well as the interactions between them – provide further valuable context. There is an extensive literature on the benefits of community-based science in the context of environmental health research (Brown and Mikkelsen, 1997; Brown, 2013), but little of this work occurs in Native communities or employs indigenous cosmologies. By contrast, ecologists are beginning to describe in detail the scientific and applied benefits of indigenous–Western science collaborations in fields from restoration ecology (Charnley, et al., 2007; Hummel and Lake, 2015) to forestry (Kimmerer and Lake, 2001; Lake, et al., 2017) and fisheries management (Marin, et al., 2017).

Krieger (2011) argues that the act of engaging eco-social context of disease enables the greatest theoretical advancement for the field of epidemiology. Indigenous perspectives and understandings of the world include social, political, cultural, and environmental dimensions of human health that are enormously beneficial for advancing policies to promote human health (Colomeda and Wenzel, 2000). This case study not only illustrates the importance of community–academic collaboration in the politics of the production of knowledge, but it also draws attention to global health dynamics that result from power imbalances within global North settings. We encourage scholars in the field of global health to consider the many benefits of collaborations with indigenous communities as a means not only of improving community health, but advancing theoretical scholarship.

### Note

1   The survey had a response rate of 38 per cent, a total of 90 questionnaires. This is a relatively high response rate for such a remote and impoverished community; still we are unable to know the views of those who did not respond. Given the community demographics, we speculate that many of those who did not respond were more traditional, and had less income than those who did respond.

### References

Anderson, M.K. and Lake, F.K. (2016) 'Beauty, bounty, and biodiversity: the story of California Indian's relationship with edible native geophytes', *Fremontia,* 44(3): 44–51.
Brown, P. (2013) 'Integrating medical and environmental sociology with environmental health crossing boundaries and building connections through advocacy', *Journal of Health and Social Behavior,* 54(2): 145–64.
Brown, P. and Mikkelsen, E.J. (1997) *No Safe Place: Toxic waste, leukemia, and community action,* Berkeley, CA: University of California Press.
Charnley, S., Fischer, A.P., and Jones, E.T. (2007) 'Integrating traditional and local ecological knowledge into forest biodiversity conservation in the Pacific Northwest', *Forest Ecology and Management,* 246(1): 14–28.
Colomeda, L.A. and Wenzel, E.R. (2000) 'Medicine keepers: issues in indigenous health', *Critical Public Health,* 10(2): 243–56.

Cordner, A., Ciplet, D., Brown, P., and Morello-Frosch, R. (2012) 'Reflexive research ethics for environmental health and justice: academics and movement building', *Social Movement Studies*, 11(2): 161–76.

Ferreira, M.L. and Lang, G.C. (2005) *Indigenous Peoples and Diabetes*, Durham, NC: Carolina Academic Press.

Fretts, A.M., Howard, B.V., McKnight, B., Duncan, G.E., Beresford, S.A., Mete, M., Zhang, Y., and Siscovick, D.S. (2014) 'Life's simple 7 and incidence of diabetes among American Indians: the strong heart family study', *Diabetes Care*, 37(8): 2240–5.

Giles, N. (2017) 'Wildfires are essential: the forest service embraces a tribal tradition', available at www.yesmagazine. org/issues/science/wildfires-are-essential-the-forest-service-embraces-a-tribal-tradition-20170403 (accessed on 7 November 2017).

Gosnell, H. and Kelly, E.C. (2010) 'Peace on the river? Social-ecological restoration and large dam removal in the Klamath basin, USA', *Water Alternatives*, 3(2): 362.

Hewes, G.W. (1973) 'Indian fisheries productivity in pre-contact times in the Pacific Salmon Area', *Northwest Anthropological Research Notes*, 7(3): 133–55.

Hummel, S. and Lake, F.K. (2015) 'Forest site classification for cultural plant harvest by tribal weavers can inform management', *Journal of Forestry*, 113(1): 30–9.

Joe, J.R. and Young, R.S. (Eds.). (1994) *Diabetes as a Disease of Civilization: The impact of culture change on indigenous peoples*, vol. 50, Berlin: Walter de Gruyter.

Kann, J., Corum, S., and Fetcho, K. (2010) 'Microcystin bioaccumulation in Klamath River freshwater mussel tissue: 2009 results', technical memorandum.

Karuk Tribe. (2016) 'Karuk climate vulnerability assessment: assessing vulnerabilities from the increased frequency of high severity fire', Karuk Tribe Department of Natural Resources, available at https://karuktribeclimatechangeprojects.files.wordpress.com/2016/11/final-karuk-climate-assessment1.pdf (accessed on 7 November 2017).

Kimmerer, R.W. and Lake, F.K. (2001) 'The role of indigenous burning in land management', *Journal of Forestry*, 99(11): 36–41.

Krieger, N. (1994) 'Epidemiology and the web of causation: has anyone seen the spider?', *Social Science & Medicine*, 39(7): 887–903.

Krieger, N. (2011) *Epidemiology and the People's Health: Theory and context*, Oxford: Oxford University Press.

Kuhnlein, H.V., Erasmus, B., and Spigelski, D. (2009) *Indigenous Peoples' Food Systems: The many dimensions of culture, diversity and environment for nutrition and health*, Rome: Food and Agriculture Organization of the United Nations (FAO).

Lake, F.K., Tripp, W., and Reed, R. (2010) 'The Karuk Tribe, planetary stewardship, and world renewal on the middle Klamath River, California', *Bulletin of the Ecological Society of America*, 91: 147–9.

Lake, F.K., Wright, V., Morgan, P., McFadzen, M., McWethy, D., and Stevens-Rumann, C. (2017) 'Returning fire to the land – celebrating traditional knowledge and fire', *Journal of Forestry*, 115(5): 343–53.

Leimbach, J. (2009) *Preparation for FERC Hydropower Relicensing: An activist's guide for the six months to two years before a relicensing*, Washington, DC: Hydropower Reform Network.

Lynn, F.M. (2000) 'Community-scientist collaboration in environmental research', *American Behavioral Scientist*, 44(4): 649–63.

Madley, B. (2016) *An American Genocide: The United States and the California Indian Catastrophe, 1846–1873*, New Haven, CT: Yale University Press.

Marin, K., Coon, A., and Fraser, D. (2017) 'Traditional ecological knowledge reveals the extent of sympatric lake trout diversity and habitat preferences', *Ecology and Society*, 22(2): 20.

McEvoy, A.E. (1986) The Fisherman's Problem: Ecology and law in the California fisheries 1850–1980, Cambridge University Press.

Most, S. (2006) *River of Renewal: Myth and history in the Klamath basin*, Portland OR: Oregon Historical Society Press.

Norgaard, K.M. (2004) 'The effects of altered diet on the health of the Karuk people: A preliminary report', Karuk Tribe filed with the Federal Energy Regulatory Commission Docket P-2082, available at http://citeseerx.ist.psu.edu/viewdoc/download?doi=10.1.1.531.1540&rep=rep1&type=pdf (accessed on 7 November 2017).

Norgaard, K.M. (2005) 'The effects of altered diet on the health of the Karuk people', Karuk Tribe filed with the Federal Energy Regulatory Commission Docket P-2082, available at http://pages.uoregon.edu/norgaard/pdf/Effects-Altered-Diet-Karuk-Norgaard-2005.pdf (accessed on 7 November 2017).

Norgaard, K.M. (2014) 'The politics of fire and the social impacts of fire exclusion on the Klamath', *Humboldt Journal of Social Relations*, 36(1): 73–97.

Norgaard, K.M., Meeks, S., Crayne, B., and Dunnivant, F. (2013) 'Trace metal analysis of Karuk traditional foods in the Klamath River', *Journal of Environmental Management*, 4: 319–28.

Norton, J. (1979) *When Our Worlds Cried: Genocide in Northwestern California*, San Francisco, CA: The Indian Historian Press.

Olson, B. (2001) 'Meeting the challenges of American Indian diabetes: anthropological perspectives on treatment and prevention', In: C.E. Trafzer and D. Weiner (Eds.) *Medicine Ways: Disease, health and survival among Native Americans*, Walnut Creek, CA: Altamira Press, pp. 163–84.

Pellow, D.N. and Brulle, R.J. (2005) *Power, Justice, and the Environment: A critical appraisal of the environmental justice movement*, Cambridge, MA: MIT Press.

Reed, R. and Norgaard, K. (2010) 'Salmon feeds our people: challenging dams on the Klamath River', In: K. Painemilla, A.B. Rylands, A. Woofter, and C. Hughes (Eds.) *Indigenous People and Conservation: From rights to resource management*, Arlington County, VA: Conservation International, pp. 7–17.

Stoll, S. (2016) 'Transforming regulatory processes: Karuk participation in the Klamath River total maximum daily load (TMDL) process', unpublished thesis, University of Oregon.

Willette, M., Norgaard, K., and Reed, R. (2016) 'You got to have fish: families, environmental decline and cultural reproduction', *Families, Relationships and Societies*, 5(3): 375–92.

Williams, D.R. and Sternthal, M. (2010) 'Understanding racial-ethnic disparities in health sociological contributions', *Journal of Health and Social Behavior*, 51(1): S15–27.

# 39

# Research and sex work

## How neo-colonialism and biomedicalisation impact struggles for sex workers' rights

*Laura Murray, Elsa Oliveira, and Debolina Dutta*

During the 2014 *International AIDS Conference* in Melbourne, Australia, *The Lancet* launched their special issue on HIV and sex work. The series – comprised of seven papers that investigate the complex issues faced by sex workers worldwide – calls for the decriminalisation of sex work, citing law reform as the most effective measure in tackling the HIV epidemic (Das and Horton, 2014). Sex worker activists at the conference celebrated *The Lancet* conclusions; yet there was a stark contrast between the special issue conclusions and the biomedical direction where the broader field of HIV prevention appeared to be heading. The pre-conference statement by sex worker activists highlighted such disconnects, not only denouncing the pervasive biomedical focus of HIV prevention in their country contexts, but also calling for more sex worker community-led research and work stating: 'we have outreach data and want to share this evidence, but we need money for training and to analyse our data' (ScarletAlliance, 2014, p. 72).

Tensions between research, policy, and activist demands have also emerged in South Africa. Despite a lack of substantiated proof, South Africa was placed on the US Department of State's Tier-2 trafficking watch list from 2005–9. Pressure from the US for South Africa to address its so-called 'trafficking problem' gained momentum during the build-up to the FIFA World Cup, which was hosted in South Africa in 2010. Increasing popular anxiety about the connection between the mega-sporting event and trafficking coupled with the fact that South Africa is a signatory of the Palermo Protocol led to the development of the Trafficking in Persons (TiP) bill in 2010. Despite outcries from some sectors (including sex workers) that the bill conflated sex work with trafficking and was based on faulty evidence (Nyangairi and Palmary, 2015), it was eventually passed into law in 2013 at an unprecedented speed (Walker and Oliveira, 2015).

These two examples reveal some of the ways in which global structures impact and drive debates and policies surrounding issues of sexual commerce. Across global landscapes, activists and researchers have improved responses to HIV prevention, bringing critical attention to the inherent harms of conflating sex work with sex trafficking. Indeed, sex workers' voices in these debates is the result of decades of sex worker activists asserting the need for a protagonist role in the information produced about them (Delacoste and Alexander, 1998; Pheterson, 1989) and successfully shifting political, academic, and biomedical discourses about the sex industry (Chateauvert, 2013; Gira-Grant, 2014; Mancioti and Geymonat, 2016). Yet despite these advancements, the (re)medicalisation of the response to AIDS and continued conflation of trafficking with sex work also reveal gaps between what sex worker rights networks are demanding, what research is finding, and the types of policies regulating prostitution.

The regulation of prostitution under the auspices of 'public health' campaigns has roots in colonial governance structures that are reflected in global health governance structures today. The passage of the *Contagious Diseases Acts* in 1866 in England and the heated debates that followed between women's movements seeking to abolish prostitution and medical establishment that defended the regulatory approach as a way to control venereal diseases influenced prostitution laws across South America, South Asia, and Africa (Carrara, 1996; Guy, 1991; Walkowitz, 1992). During this time period, prostitution was the subject of medical surveillance and research. It is only with the emergence of the HIV epidemic in the late 1980s and early 1990s, however, that prostitution became a focus of large epidemiological studies as part of the HIV research industry (Csete, 2013). The goals of this early research were largely to identify risk factors, establish prevalence rates, and test interventions; sex workers' rights, or even their meaningful inclusion in this research, were not a central concern (de Zalduondo, 1991; Pheterson, 1990).

The HIV epidemic changed the course of sex work research and activism. As Joane Csete (2013) notes, 'For good or ill, sex work has a different place in the global health world and in the world of human rights than would have been the case without HIV/AIDS' (p. 45). Sex worker organising pre-dated the HIV epidemic, yet as Csete and many others have noted, funding for HIV prevention changed the shape, scope, and breadth of sex work activism and research on a global scale. In the 1990s and 2000s, activists fought for a place at the policy decision-making tables with international agencies of global health governance such as the World Health Organization, UNAIDS, and the World Bank. UN agencies and sex worker rights networks collaborated on a series of guidelines and reports on sex work and HIV that culminated in the early 2010s in a series of reports that endorse a rights-based and community mobilisation approach to the epidemic (WHO, 2012; UNAIDS, 2011; Kerrigan, et al., 2012). These guidelines, taken together with countless activist reports, statements, and policy documents, highlight connections between the criminalisation of sex work and vulnerability to HIV, explicitly endorsing decriminalisation. Yet as the examples at the beginning of our text demonstrate, not all voices and information are treated with equal authority when it comes to sex work.

In this chapter, we map global and regional trends in research produced about sex work in an effort to shed light on these imbalances. In keeping with the postmodern feminist understandings of knowledge production (Hill-Collins, 1990; Mohanty, 2003), we recognise that research is an embodied and embedded practice (Davies, 2002) and believe that it is important to step back and look critically at the field with which we all are engaged. We are especially concerned with the geopolitical locations from which information about sex work is produced, circulated, and put into practice, and in this regard, we want to clearly position our analysis in relation to our broader commitment to sex worker rights movements in the early twenty-first century.

## Regional and global trends in research about sex work

For our analysis of peer-reviewed research, we used the interdisciplinary search engine ProQuest to identify articles published between January 2006–May 2016. We searched for articles that included the key words 'sex work', 'sex workers', and 'prostitution' in their titles. These searches yielded a total of 593 results with 'sex work'; 1,237 with 'sex workers'; and 421 with 'prostitution'. When we removed all non-peer-reviewed articles (e.g., book reviews) and duplicated results, the final number considered for the analysis presented herein was: 324 articles with 'sex work' in the title; 1,168 with 'sex workers'; and 369 with 'prostitution' in the title.

The articles passed through two levels of analysis. First, they were categorised by: authors' countries of affiliation, the country the article was about, the methodology used, primary and secondary topics of focus, and if any of the authors were affiliated with a sex worker rights organisation. Then, a second more detailed examination was performed in which the abstracts – and in some cases full articles – were consulted to categorise the articles into 25 thematic categories[1] based on the chapter's primary topic. In the case of

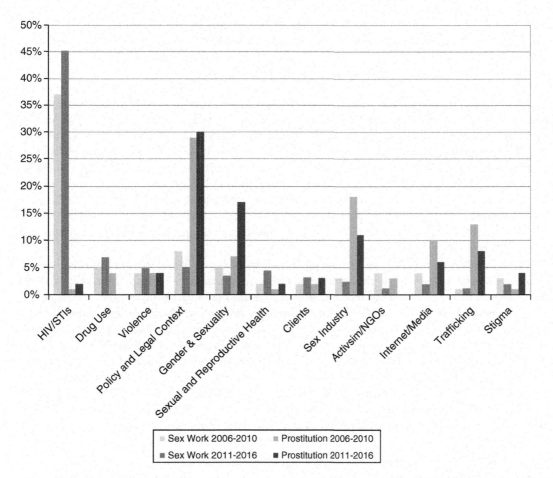

*Figure 39.1*   Primary topics of focus in peer-reviewed publications with 'sex work' or 'sex workers' in the title compared to those with 'prostitution'

papers reporting on quantitative research/analysis, the primary topic was defined as the outcome variable of interest (i.e., HIV or drug use). In qualitative analyses, the primary topic was ascertained depending on the language of the title, abstract, and key words. Figure 39.1 presents the ten most common primary topics in the academic literature in addition to the topics 'stigma' and 'trafficking'.

In the sex work literature, research on HIV/AIDS and STIs still dominates with 45 per cent of all articles from 2011–16 and 37 per cent from 2006–10. In this same block, the second most common primary topics concern 'policy' and 'legal contexts' (i.e., studies about regulation, criminalisation, decriminalisation), which represented 8 per cent of the peer-reviewed literature from 2006–10 and 5 per cent from 2011–16. Drug Use/Dependence was the third most common topic, with 5 per cent of the literature published between 2006–10 and 7 per cent between 2011–16. The fifth most common topic was 'gender and sexuality'. This literature focused on sex workers' lived experiences and intersections between gender and sex markets, i.e., male sex work, transgender sex work, and motherhood. The topic 'policy and legal context' was the most common in the literature with 'prostitution' in the title and corresponded to 29 per cent and 30 per cent of papers published in the 2006–10 and 2011–16 time periods, respectively – nearly four and six times that of the 'sex work' literature, respectively. Also different from the sex work titled literature, there are more articles about the sex industry, broadly speaking (18 per cent and 11 per cent of the total).

Although there is a difference between the sex work and prostitution literature in terms of the primary topics of focus, in both bodies of literature, there has been increased attention to policy and its impacts on sex worker health and rights. A look at the special issues published in both categories show clear tendencies towards the importance of decriminalisation for rights and health, in particular during the time period from 2010–15. For example, in 2014, *The Lancet* launched a special series on HIV and sex work (www.thelancet.com/series/HIV-and-sex-workers) that explicitly calls for decriminalisation of sex work as the most effective way to reduce sex workers' vulnerability to HIV. Also in 2014, *Criminology & Criminal Justice* published a special issue entitled, 'The Governance of Commercial Sex: Global Trends of Criminalisation, Punitive Enforcement, Protection and Rights' edited by Sanders and Campbell (2014) with articles that take a critical look at such policies. The same is true of a *Sexuality Research and Social Policy* special issue published on 'Prostitution Policies in Europe' with guest editors Crowhurst, Outshoorn, and Skilbrei (2012). Finally, in 2010, the *Journal of Law and Society* published a special issue entitled 'Regulating Sex/Work: From Crime Control to Neo-liberalism?' edited by Scoular and Sanders (2010) that features a critical analysis of regulation, criminalisation, and gentrification in diverse sex work contexts.

Given the uproar about trafficking in contemporary debates on sex work, we were surprised at the relatively few articles with trafficking as a primary topic in our preliminary findings: 28 in the sex work literature and 37 in the prostitution literature. Sensing that this could be because of the search criteria (only articles with 'sex work', 'sex workers', or 'prostitution' in the title), we conducted an additional search on literature on trafficking over the past ten years as to gain a clearer understanding of academic research trends in this particular domain. The results of this focused search are presented in Table 39.1.

There has been a large increase in the number of articles published about trafficking over the past decade; comparing the five-year time periods of 2006–10 with 2011–15, the total number of articles tripled from 117 to 362 and there was a particularly drastic increase in 2014. Three special issues published in 2014 were indicative of the contentious nature of trafficking debates. On one hand, the editors of the *Annals of the American Academy of Political and Social Science* special issue note being particularly concerned with the

*Table 39.1* Trends in the number of peer-reviewed articles published and indexed in ProQuest with 'trafficking' and 'sex' in their titles

| Year | Number of articles with 'trafficking' and 'sex' in the title |
|---|---|
| 2015 | 55 |
| 2014 | 118 |
| 2013 | 69 |
| 2012 | 50 |
| 2011 | 70 |
| SUBTOTAL | 362 |
| 2010 | 41 |
| 2009 | 14 |
| 2008 | 30 |
| 2007 | 18 |
| 2006 | 14 |
| SUBTOTAL | 117 |
| TOTAL | 479 |

'sensationalistic' nature and mischaracterisation of evidence in writing on human trafficking (Weitzer, 2014, p. 6) whereas the *Crime Law and Social Change* special issue, 'Understanding the Anti-human Trafficking Campaign' (Farrell, 2014) features pieces that are highly critical of the legalisation of sex establishments and more focused on the implementation and implication of criminal justice reform. Finally, in their introduction to the *Journal of Intercultural Studies* special issue focused on trafficking in persons, editors Chong and Clark (Chong and Clark, 2014) highlight patriarchy, gender inequality, and the feminisation of poverty as reasons that increase women's and girls' vulnerability to trafficking, yet do not engage with the literature discussing the complexities of migration, legal contexts, and women's agency. All of this literature reinforces the continued embattled nature of the field of research about trafficking over statistics, definitions, and sex workers' experiences.

Figure 39.2 illustrates the result of the analysis concerning the location of authors and subjects of research. Although the majority of articles in the sex work category (53.4 per cent) were written by multiple authors with a mix of affiliations from the global North and South, the discrepancies between which region the article is about versus where the authors are from are sharply marked. Sub-Saharan Africa and Southeast Asia, for example, make up 35.2 per cent of the foci of all of the publications, yet only 0.3 per cent of the publications are written by authors solely from these regions. This compared to North America, where this same ratio (region about/region of authors' affiliation) is 13 per cent to 9.4 per cent. It is important to note that in the mixed 'North + South' category in the sex work literature, a large number of the articles and publications pertain to public health and are signed by three or more authors, with the lead authors generally being from a North American, English, or European Union institution, and co-authors from local research centres. Finally, there is a small amount of literature that presents original research or literature reviews at a global level, including countries located both in the global North and South.

It is important not to essentialise or generalise (it is possible that there are researchers from the global South working at Northern institutions and vice versa) yet discrepancies raise important questions regarding the unequal power dynamics inherent to the geopolitical distribution of research capacities. For example, of the 220 articles in the sex work literature written exclusively by authors with affiliations in the global South, not a single one is about a country in the global North. In comparison, there are 115 articles about countries in the global South written by authors exclusively with affiliations in the global North. In fact, there is only one article in the prostitution literature with authorship exclusively from the global South about a country in the global North. The article, 'Instant Mobility, Stratified Prostitution Market: The Politics of Belonging of Korean Women Selling Sex in the U.S.' (Kim, 2016) is written by an author with an affiliation at a South Korean institution and about Korean women in the United States.

Troubling power imbalances also emerge through a combined analysis of Figures 39.1 and 39.2 in terms of thinking about primary topics and geopolitical locations. In the sex work literature, the majority of articles with authorship from Northern and Southern institutions is public health literature in which the first and last authors tend to be from a Northern based institution and the others local researchers. In other words, those who are guiding and funding the research tend to be based in the global North and the focus of their research is on the global South. For example, of the 765 articles written by authors with affiliations in Northern and Southern institutions, 405 (52.9 per cent) are about HIV/AIDS and STIs, and of these, 394 are about countries in the global South. Along these same lines, of the 228 articles in the sex work literature about sub-Saharan Africa, 123 (54 per cent) have HIV/AIDS as their primary topic and only two (0.15 per cent) about policy and legal contexts. Furthermore, of the 116 articles with policy and legal context as their primary topics in the prostitution literature, 91 (78 per cent) are about countries in the global North. Again, a similar dynamic can be found in the sex work literature, where 76 per cent (58) of the 76 articles with policy and legal contexts as their primary topic are about countries in the global North.

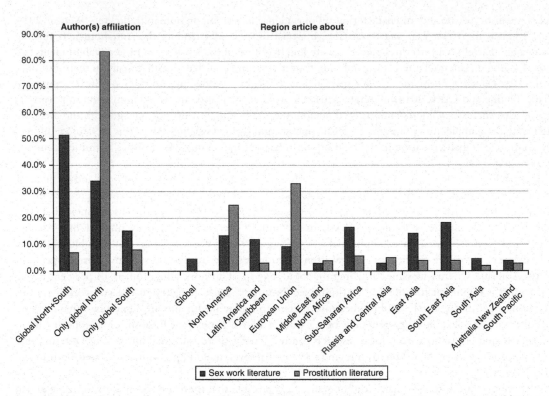

*Figure 39.2* Global regions of author affiliations and regions articles are about in peer-reviewed literature with 'sex work' and 'prostitution' in the title 2006–16

## Reflections on the trends

The data signals towards a gradual increase in the amount of sex work research across regions and trends that point towards an increasing emphasis on the importance of decriminalisation to protect and promote sex workers' health and rights. At the same time, as we noted in the beginning of our chapter, more and more countries, including our own, are (further) criminalising sex work. Such disconnects, in light of our findings, raise the following questions: What does it mean that studies on legal and policy models are conducted primarily in the global North by authors with global North affiliations? What kind of power dynamics are behind the overwhelming amount of literature about HIV/AIDS and sex work, that is primarily led and funded by Northern institutions and about the global South? What kind of bodies (political and biological) do these types of dynamics ultimately enforce? In an effort to answer these questions, in this final section, we look closely at the geopolitical, institutional, and methodological dimensions of our findings. Through our discussion, we seek to point to possible paths forward for research and activism seeking to further expand sex workers' rights at a time when they have increasingly come under attack.

We begin with the geopolitical inequalities that cross-cut all fields analysed. One of our main findings is that Northern institutional perspectives dominate the bulk of information and analyses being produced and circulated about sex work. We found a glaring lack of policy research focused on Southern contexts (especially non-BRICS countries) as compared to the repetition of studies looking at certain legal models in the global North. Questions such as whether the Swedish or New Zealand model are best might be missing other important issues such as migration or racism and how these intersect to affect how any legal model would be put in place. In Brazil, for example, we've found that the way in which the law is enacted is shaped much more by deep seeded stigma towards sex workers, sexuality politics, gender inequalities, and the whims of individual state actors than the law 'on the books' (Murray, 2014).

Although our research has not examined this aspect in depth, it is evident that the logic of funding streams is largely responsible for these dynamics. Despite positive shifts observed in recent years, research centres with easier access to funding are still predominantly located in the global North and their 'targets' or 'subjects' pertain to the global South. This dynamic is not only constraining for researchers, but also for activists. As reported by the Red Umbrella Fund (2013), while the overwhelming majority of funders are in the global North, especially the United States and Canada, followed by Europe, the bulk of the grants go to Africa, Latin America, and South and Southeast Asia – a pattern that coincides with our findings. This means that the decisions being made about what areas and projects to fund are taken thousands of miles away from where the grants are being implemented. This inevitably reinforces unequal power dynamics as the vast majority of knowledge continues to be produced without the effective involvement of sex workers and by institutional bodies that are far away and not always knowledgeable of the contexts they are speaking and writing about.

Furthermore, historical legacies also must be taken into account as they add additional layers to the complexities and tensions of local and global politics and the distortion deriving from funding trends. Within the countries where we work, the layered legacies of colonialism that remain in post-colonial structures continue to have a devastating effect on sex workers' lives. We don't have space to expand on all of these intersections here, but the current ban on sex work in South Africa for example is a remnant of the country's 1927 Immorality Act under colonial rule and 1957 Sexual Offenses Act under apartheid. The continued deep tensions between movements for decriminalisation with the anti-human trafficking abolitionist movement in South Africa are remnant of colonial discourses at the turn of the twentieth century. In fact, our findings suggest that trafficking is one of the fields where statistics, definitions, and even sex workers' experiences remain a field of contestation, despite the existence of extensive research documenting the harms of conflating sex work with human trafficking (Kempado, 2005; GAATW, 2007; NSWP, n.d.; VAMP and SANGRAM, 2018). In this context, it is not surprising that the Coalition Against Trafficking in Women (CAATW) led an aggressive opposition campaign in 2016 when they found out about Amnesty International's plans to develop a policy endorsing the decriminalisation of sex work.[2]

The longstanding imprints of colonial practices of racial segregation are also manifested in contemporary discourses on health and disease control that intersect with sex work. India's prostitution laws have roots in the English *Contagious Diseases Act* passed at the end of the nineteenth century which stipulated incarceration if prostitutes were found to have venereal diseases (Dutta, forthcoming). Similar to Brazil, sex workers were understood as a population that needed to be subjected to the guiding hand of the state in the form of the police and in the name of 'public health'. The overwhelming focus on HIV/AIDS must be read within this historical relationship between public health concerns and state control of sex workers' bodies. While we recognise that sex workers often experience heightened levels of vulnerability to HIV/AIDS, as many activists and researchers have stated before (Pheterson, 1990; de Zalduondo, 1991; Leite, et al., 2015), the pathologisation of sex workers as vectors of disease reinforces stigma around sex work and infantilises them by placing prostitution under the tutelary power of a wide variety of institutions (from biomedicine to security forces). It also ignores the plethora of human experiences, needs, and issues that encompass being a person who also happens to sell sex, creating obstacles for shifting research attention to the structural issues that time and time again have been found to be critical to protecting rights *and* health.

Indeed, our analysis of the academic literature found that the topics 'Stigma' and 'Gender and Sexuality' represented a smaller percentage of the articles with 'sex work' in the title (in particular in comparison to the literature with prostitution in the title), even decreasing during the 2011–16 timeframe as research on HIV/AIDS and on 'Gender and Sexuality' with prostitution in the title increased. A recent report published by Elsevier (2017) on gender and global research trends indicates an increase in research published with 'gender' in the title during the 2011–15 time period. They also note that published papers were split between biomedical and social science research, similar as well to our results. Although this wasn't our focus here, we see connections between sex work and gender research trends on various levels that would be worth further comparative analysis in the future.

An additional problem is that conventional methodological approaches that are undertaken on, rather than with, sex workers often result in the (re)production of superficial, sometimes inaccurate, and potentially unethical, portrayals of those who are being researched and written about. As emphasised in activist critiques of researchers, sex workers are often excluded from direct engagement in setting research agendas, implementation of the research projects, and from participating in policy discussions and public debates on the issues that directly impact their lives. Innovative research approaches that draw on visual means such as photography and drawing facilitate the inclusion of under-represented groups in research. They not only offer those involved with a unique opportunity to challenge and contend conventional depictions often associated with their lives; they can unlock improved understandings, revealing important nuances that shape how sex workers thrive, survive, and negotiate their lives (Oliveira and Vearey, 2015).

Inspired by Paulo Freire (1993 [1969]), Cornwall and Jewkes (1995) describe participatory research as a process of '[…]sequential reflection and action carried out with and by local people rather than on them' (p. 1667). For them, the decision to include a participatory approach to research reflects, 'a choice, which is both personal and inherently political' (p. 1667). Our experience has been that participatory methods and activist organisation/academic institution partnerships contribute greatly to reducing the power imbalances, yet it is not correct to assume that the mere participation of sex workers in research processes can eliminate the power differentials between those who are sex workers and those who are not (Dutta, forthcoming). Even when participatory research methods are used, the rules that govern research design and implementation often remain the preserve of researchers. The use of participatory research methods must be regarded as an ongoing practice of creating channels of communication and trust between sex workers and non-sex worker researchers for a co-production of knowledge that is nuanced and reflects the realities of lived experiences. No research method is completely neutral in scope, and researchers like us must use them critically and be mindful of their political implications every step of the way.

The central question thus becomes, in our perspective, to recognise the political nature of all knowledge production. Indeed, research is a political process and activism a form of knowledge production. We agree with Michal Osterweil when she suggests that we should not treat 'activism or political action as constitutively distinct from academic or knowledge work', but rather to conceptualise research processes as political practices, and activism as a form of knowledge production in and of itself (2013, pp. 599–600). There is a very real need to create more direct, participatory, and horizontal channels of learning. Research and participatory approaches are about long-term engagement, where data is collected using a range of techniques and where research not only strives to gain new understandings of issues and lives that can feed 'the Academy' and change policy, but where the process of making, doing, and telling is critically reflected upon and challenged. In addition to the potential impacts on the individual lives of people we work with when doing research, what we produce feeds the public narratives about sex work and funding agencies making decisions about what to research and where to invest time and resources. Failure to readily engage or recognise that the processes of making knowledge are infused in messy power fluctuations not only implicitly negates and discounts the importance of local knowledge(s) and processes, it reasserts institutional elitism and contributes to the disconnectedness between sex workers' lives and policies designed to intervene in their work contexts.

## Acknowledgements

This chapter comes from a more extensive invited paper written for the research-advocacy forum Sexuality Policy Watch as part of an exercise to map global trends in sexual politics and sexuality research during the first decade and a half of the twenty-first century. In our full paper, we conduct a critical review of global and regional trends of information produced by sex worker activists and networks, peer-reviewed literature, and international organisations during the 2006–16 time period. For this chapter, we are focusing on our analysis of the peer-reviewed literature component of our analysis, referring to the other analyses as relevant in our discussion. We would like to acknowledge Roxana Rodriguez for her vital role as a research assistant, Sonia Correa for her critical engagement and comments on the full paper, Daughtie Ogutu for her careful review and valuable insights and criticisms on the first full draft, and Richard Parker and Jonathan Garcia for their thoughtful comments and suggestions that greatly improved this chapter.

## Notes

1   Activism/NGOs, Sexual Exploitation of Minors, Clients, Drug Use/Dependence, Gender & Sexuality, Exit, HIV/AIDS, Initiation, Media/Internet/Film, Megaevents, Mental Health, Migration, Sexual and Reproductive Health, Policy and Legal Contexts, Sex Markets/Industry, Services and Interventions, Sex Practices, Stigma, STIs, Trafficking, Violence.
2   www.amnesty.org/en/latest/news/2015/08/sex-workers-rights-are-human-rights/. The news sparked a heated global controversy involving everyone from Kate Winslet to Gloria Steinem and a large campaign led by CAATW against the policy-in-formation. As part of Amnesty's institutional policy development process, they conducted consultations with sex worker rights organisations and networks, and authored a series of reports and case studies published in 2016 on sex work and human rights. They all point to the harms of criminalisation, and were perhaps the most visible reports on the sex work information landscape released by an international agency in 2016.

## References

Carrara, S. (1996) *Tributo a Vênus: A luta contra a sífilis no Brasil, da passagem do século aos anos 40*, Rio de Janeiro: Editora FIOCRUZ.
Chateauvert, M. (2013) *Sex Workers Unite: A history of the movement from Stonewall to Slutwalk*, Boston: Beacon Press.
Chong, N.G. and Clarck, J.B. (2014) 'Introduction: Trafficking in persons', *Journal of Intercultural Studies*, 35(2): 123–7.
Cornwall, A. and Jewkes, R. (1995) 'What is participatory research?', *Social Science and Medicine*, 41: 1667–76.
Crowhurst, I., Outshoorn, J., and Skilbrei, M. (2012) 'Introduction: Prostitution Policies in Europe.' *Sexuality Research and Social Policy*, 9(3): 187–91.
Csete, J. (2013) 'Victimhood and vulnerability: sex work and the rhetoric and reality of the global response to HIV/AIDS', In: L. Murthy (Ed.) *The Business of Sex*, New Delhi: Zubaan, pp. 45–80.
Das, P. and Horton, R. (2014) 'Bringing sex workers to the centre of the HIV response', *The Lancet*, 385(9962): 3–4.
Davies, M. (2002) 'Ethics and methodology in legal theory: a (personal) research anti-manifesto', *Law, Text, Culture*, 6.
de Zalduondo, B. (1991) 'Prostitution viewed cross-culturally: toward recontextualizing sex work in AIDS intervention research', *The Journal of Sex Research*, 22: 223–48.
Delacoste, F. and Alexander, P. (Eds.) (1998) *Sex Work: Writings by women in the sex industry*, San Francisco: Cleis Press.
Dutta, D. (forthcoming) 'Of festivals and rights: a story of an affirmative sabotage', In: S. Juss (Ed.) *Human Rights in India*.
Elsevier. (2017) 'Gender in the global research landscape', available at www.elsevier.com/research-intelligence/campaigns/gender-17 (accessed on 12 March 2018).
Farrell, A. (Ed.) (2014) 'Special issue: understanding the anti-human trafficking campaign', *Crime, Law and Social Change*, 61(2).
Freire, P. (1993) *The Pedagogy of the Oppressed*. New York: Continuum.
GAATW. (2007) *Collateral Damages: The impact of anti-trafficking measures on human rights around the world*, Bangkok: GAATW.
Gira-Grant, M. (2014) *Playing the Whore*, New York: Verso.
Guy, D. (1991) *Sex and Danger in Buenos Aires*, Lincoln, NE: University of Nebraska Press.
Hill-Collins, P. (1990) *Black Feminist Thought: Knowledge, consciousness and the politics of empowerment*, New York: Routledge.
Kempado, K. (2005) *Trafficking and Prostitution Considered: New perspectives on migration, sex work, and human rights*, Boulder, CO: Paradigm Publishers.
Kerrigan, D., Wirtz, A., Baral, S., Decker, M., Murray, L., Poteat, T., Pretorius, C., Sherman, S., and Sweat, M. (2012) *The Global Epidemics Among Sex Workers*, Washington, DC: World Bank.
Kim, J. (2016) 'Instant mobility, stratified prostitution market: the politics of belonging of Korean women selling sex in the U.S.', *Asian Journal of Women's Studies*, 22: 48–64.

Leite, G., Murray, L.R., and Lenz, F. (2015) 'The peer and non-peer: the potential of risk management for HIV prevention in contexts of prostitution', *Revista Brasileira de Epidemiologia*, 15: 7–25.

Mancioti, P. and Geymonat, G. (Eds.) (2016) *Sex Workers Speak, Who Listens?*, London: COST.

Mohanty, C. (2003) *Feminism Without Borders: Decolonizing theory, practicing solidarity*, Chapel Hill, NC: Duke University Press.

Murray, L. (2014) 'Victim management and the politics of protection: between "Fazer direito" and "direitinho"', *Revista Artemis*, XVIII: 28–41.

NSWP. (n.d.) 'Sex work is not trafficking', available at www.nswp.org/sites/nswp.org/files/SW%20is%20Not%20 Trafficking.pdf (accessed on 10 June 2016).

Nyangairi, B. and Ingrid P. (2015) 'Watching each others' back, coping with precarity in sex work', Healing and Change in the City of Gold, Cham: Springer, pp. 121–34.

Oliveira, E. and Vearey, J. (2015) 'Images of place: visuals from migrant women sex workers in South Africa', *Medical Anthropology*, 34: 305–18.

Osterweil, M. (2013) 'Rethinking public anthropology through epistemic politics and theoretical practice', *Cultural Anthropology*, 28: 598–620.

Pheterson, G. (1989) *A Vindication of the Rights of Whores*, Seattle: Seal Press.

Pheterson, G. (1990) 'The category "Prostitute" in scientific inquiry', *Jornal of Sex Research*, 27: 397–407.

Red Umbrella Fund. (2013) *Funding for Sex Worker Rights*, Amsterdam: Red Umbrella Fund.

Sanders, T. and Campbell, R. (Eds.) (2014) 'Special issue: the governance of commercial sex: global trends of criminalisation, punitive enforcement, protection and rights', *Criminology & Criminal Justice*, 14(5).

ScarletAlliance. (2014) 'Stepping up to the evidence on HIV and sex work: decriminalize sex work now!: sex workers at AIDS 2014', available at www.scarletalliance.org.au/library/aids2014report (accessed on 30 January 2018).

Scoular, J. and Sanders, T., (Eds.) (2010) 'Regulating sex/work: from crime control to neoliberalism?', *Journal of Law and Society*, 37(1).

UNAIDS. (2011) 'The report of the UNAIDS Advisory Group on HIV and sex work', available at www.hst.org.za/ publications/NonHST%20Publications/20111215_Report-UNAIDS-Advisory-group-HIV-Sex-Work_en.pdf (accessed on 18 September 2018).

VAMP and SANGRAM. (2018) 'RAIDED!: how anti-trafficking strategies increase sex workers' vulnerability to exploitative practices', available at www.sangram.org/resources/RAIDED-E-Book.pdf (accessed on 10 March 2018).

Walker, R. and Oliveira, E. (2015) 'Contested spaces: exploring the intersections of migration, sex work and trafficking in South Africa', *Graduate Journal of Social Science*, 11: 129–53.

Walkowitz, J. (1992) *City of Dreadful Delight: Narratives of sexual danger in late-Victorian London*, London: Viagro Press.

Weitzer, R. (2014) 'New directions in research on human trafficking', *The Annals of the American Academy of Political and Social Science*, 653: 6–24.

WHO. (2012) 'Prevention and treatment of HIV and other sexually transmitted diseases for sex workers in low and middle income countries', available at http://apps.who.int/iris/bitstream/10665/77745/1/9789241504744_eng. pdf (accessed on 30 January 2018).

# 40

# In pursuit of genomic justice
## Sovereignty, inclusion, and innovation in Mexico

*Emily E. Vasquez and Vivette García-Deister*

At the turn of the millennium as the mapping of the human genome came to fruition and the potential of genomic science for improving health drew increasing optimism, global health policymakers and scientists voiced concern that the rise of genomics might ultimately deepen inequalities in global health (Pang, 2002; Singer and Daar, 2001; *The Lancet*, 2002; WHO, 2002). When he announced the completion of the first draft of the map of the human genome in June of 2000, US President Bill Clinton remarked that 'humankind is on the verge of gaining immense new power to heal', but at the same time, he cautioned, 'we must ensure that new genome science and its benefits will be directed toward making life better for all citizens of the world, never just a privileged few' (The White House, 2000). A year later, WHO released a report entitled *Genomics and World Health* in which it acknowledged that most advances in genomics were occurring in the world's wealthiest nations and often in the private domain (WHO, 2002). That report pointed to a long history of neglect by northern pharmaceutical companies of the diseases most heavily burdening low- and middle-income countries. Would developing regions be left behind again by the 'genomic revolution'? Beyond its applications for high-cost clinical care envisioned in the Euro-American West (i.e., 'personalised medicine'), could genomic technology also be used to more broadly improve public health in the developing world?

While access to genomics-based advances and the imperative to address the needs of developing world populations were often at the fore of these discussions, additional concerns about genomics emerged from nations across the global South (Jiménez Sanchez, et al., 2008; Séguin and Hardy, 2008; Benjamin, 2009). If, in the genomic era, DNA was becoming a significant natural resource, some wondered, how might developing countries best protect this resource from foreign exploitation – a new form of bioprospecting – and, perhaps, reap its benefits themselves? Could middle- and even low-income countries carve out a place for themselves in a genomics-driven 'bioeconomy'? How might countries establish some control over the economic and biomedical potential of the DNA found in the blood, tissues, and saliva of their citizens? These concerns struck at the intersection of health and science and technology policy. At issue was not just health in the developing world, but also the economic well-being of developing nations in an increasingly tech-based global market.

Actions in response to these concerns began to take shape in several countries including Mexico, South Africa, India, and Thailand. By 2010, Mexico's approach, in particular, had emerged as a key model for how these issues might be addressed (Hinterberger and Porter, 2015; Séguin, et al., 2008; Tekola-Ayele and Rotimi, 2015). In Mexico, policymakers, national health authorities, scientific entrepreneurs, and one of

Latin America's most powerful health philanthropies, the Carlos Slim Foundation, saw in genomics the potential to improve public health outcomes and reduce health care costs. Beyond just access to genomic medicine, over time they have argued that public and private investments in genomics would promote the public good in ways that articulate with national sovereignty, promote inclusive anti-racist science, and transform care. Their claims thus linked genomic pursuits to broader struggles for justice in the domains of health and development. In this chapter, we track these claims in the Mexican context from the early 2000s to the present to better understand the implications of mobilising high-cost technoscience, like genomics, as a justice tool in the arena of global health.

In so doing, we join a number of science and technology scholars examining increasingly commonplace claims that link science and issues of justice (Bliss, 2012; Mamo and Fishman, 2013; Nelson, 2016; Reardon, 2013, 2017). Like these scholars, we distinguish justice claims as transcending the institutionalised ethics infrastructure within science and biomedicine intended to protect the rights of human subjects. Justice claims speak instead to collective interests, engage the 'equitable distribution of social goods, resources, and opportunities' (Mamo and Fishman, 2013, p. 161), and – as we will show in this chapter – can ultimately influence what the 'public good' is understood to be.

## Sovereignty

Justice claims in the arena of genomics initially emerged in Mexico in the early 2000s among lobbyists – an elite group of scientists, politicians, and entrepreneurs – who urged federal investment in the emergent field of genomic medicine (Jiménez Sanchez, 2003). These lobbyists argued that genomic medicine had the potential to transform the prevention and treatment of disease, including the diseases most burdening the Mexican health system and the national economy. But foreign researchers and biotech firms, they argued, could not be trusted to attend to Mexico's particular health concerns or to ensure the inclusion of knowledge specific to Mexican bodies – to the 'Mexican genome', in their words – in research and in the development of new treatments and diagnostic tools. Nor should foreign scientists and entrepreneurs solely profit from the discoveries made with Mexican genetic material, they argued. Genomic medicine, they contended, should be 'made in Mexico, by Mexicans, for Mexicans' (López Beltrán, et al., 2014, p. 99).

With this argument, this group successfully persuaded the Mexican Congress to commit an initial investment of US$120 million to establish a medical genomics research programme and to construct a National Institute for Genomic Medicine. Known as the 'INMEGEN' for its abbreviation in Spanish, the institute would be inaugurated in 2004 as Mexico's 12th National Institute of Health, complete with a business incubator and its own intellectual profit unit to foster private sector growth in the area of genomic medicine. With this physical infrastructure in place, these proponents (several of whom had assumed key posts within the INMEGEN's administration) next moved to secure a series of legal provisions that they argued were necessary to ensure the institute's mission could be accomplished: This policy, they claimed, would protect against scientific colonialism – where foreign researchers would obtain biological samples in Mexico and then carry them back to foreign institutions for analysis, consolidating elsewhere both the intellectual and material profits derived (Frenk, 2001; Schwartz Marín, 2011).

This provocative legal framework came to be known as Mexico's policy on 'genomic sovereignty' (Secretaría de Gobernación, 2008). Instituted as a set of amendments to the nation's General Health Law, its provisions made it illegal to transport human tissue from which DNA may be derived outside the country, without prior approval from Mexico's Secretariat of Health. Moreover, it asserted, Mexican genetic material transported to foreign territory could only be utilised for secretariat-approved purposes. The legal framework underpinning this reform, documented in official congressional records, further recognises the obligation of the Mexican state to provide citizens access to the health services that would be derived from knowledge about the genomic structure of the Mexican people. However, it explicitly acknowledges that this must be realised 'without discouraging the generation of new goods and businesses based on the development of this new technology' (Cámara de Diputados, 2008, p. 8).

The establishment of the INMEGEN and the creation of Mexico's genomic sovereignty policy thus set forth a vision of a more just world, in which public and private actors in Mexico would collectively ensure that Mexicans and their needs were not 'left behind' in the genomic era (and that Mexico would not be left out of a genomics-driven bioeconomy). But with time the meaning of these actions, taken in the name of health and social well-being in Mexico, have come to merit further consideration.

First, we turn to the centrality of the notion of the 'Mexican genome' – the idea of a genetically unique and delineable Mexican population – put forth in rhetoric and policy by lobbyists and later by INMEGEN scientists themselves as the institute's work commenced, centred on its mapping (Silva-Zolezzi, et al., 2009). Crucial to the initial lobby and then to INMEGEN's mission, was the idea that genomic medicine made elsewhere would not only fail to address the health problems most heavily burdening Mexico, but would also fail to be appropriate for Mexican bodies at the molecular level (Jiménez Sanchez, 2003). Establishing Mexican genetic uniqueness was critical. To make this argument, they invoked the notion of the Mexican *Mestizo*, a social identity and ideological cornerstone of Mexican nationalism that emerged in the country's post-revolutionary moment as a tool for national unification (Kent, et al., 2015; López Beltrán, et al., 2014). Originally a progressive defence of the country's mixture in the context of global racial mythologies in which whiteness reigned, *Mestizaje* ideology contended that in Mexico there had arisen a unique and superior blend of European, Amerindian, and African ancestry – a 'cosmic race' according to Mexican philosopher José Vasconcelos (1966). By conflating the idea of Mexican DNA with *Mestizaje* ideology, lobbyists and later INMEGEN scientists communicated why the Mexican population was sufficiently unique at the molecular level to require its very own genomics programme, all via a historically familiar narrative evoking national pride.

Yet despite its nationalist currency, *Mestizaje* ideology is deeply marked by important tensions. Alongside its power to unify much of the vast and diverse Mexican population under a single identity, *Mestizaje* also carries with it a fundamental and historically rooted 'othering' of the allegedly 'un-mixed' (specifically, indigenous populations). In the context of genomics, the hegemonic notion of the *Mestizo* discursively flattens Mexican heterogeneity into a single group, rendering peripheral to the dominant national genomic endeavour (and the related project for public health) non-*Mestizo* sectors of Mexican society, the allegedly 'pure' indigenous groups, as well as afro-descendants (Benjamin, 2009; García Deister, 2018). Moreover, given the highly publicised genetic re-inscription of the Mexican *Mestizo*, critics have argued that proponents of genomic medicine 'by Mexicans and for Mexicans' have re-awakened, and with modern scientific imprimatur, a racialised othering of indigenous communities – re-animating public endorsement of their essential difference and separateness from the core body politic (García Deister, 2018; Wade, et al., 2014). This took place just as a multiculturalist political mobilisation in Mexico seemed to have established a non-biologistical language through which indigeneity might be newly valued and celebrated (López Beltrán and García Deister, 2013; López Caballero, 2017; Moreno Figueroa and Saldívar Tanaka, 2015).

Further, as contemporary genomics provides a framework within which genomic ancestry, geographical origin, and social identity tend to align, numerous scholars have warned that a re-authorisation of race as a biological reality appears to be underway globally (Abu El-Haj, 2007; Koenig, et al., 2008; Whitmarsh and Jones, 2010); some have raised deep and warranted concerns about the consequent naturalisation of racial inequalities in contexts like the United States and, ultimately, a shift towards the biomedicalisation of solutions put forth to address them (Duster, 2015; Montoya, 2011; Roberts, 2011). As Bliss (2013) has explained, referring to the US experience, 'with differential medical care as the solution to racial injustice, the state is relieved of addressing broader sociological inequities, such as subpar living conditions and institutionalized racism' (p. 1021). That *Mestizo* identity is legitimised in publicly funded Mexican genomics in the name of health and social progress thus raises concern on this second register: globally, in contexts where Mexican identity and Mexican diaspora communities have long suffered and continue to suffer racial discrimination (Chavez, 2008; Molina, 2006; Stern, 2005), old ways of essentialising and pathologising Mexican difference appear to find new traction in the genomic instantiation of the Mexican *Mestizo* (Montoya, 2011).

Despite these problematic dimensions, the idea of the 'Mexican genome', so central to early prospects for 'genomic sovereignty' in Mexico, reflected a highly strategic approach designed in response to this field's particular financial and institutional organisation in a specific historical moment. As lobbyists sought popular approval for massive federal investment in genomic science infrastructure, the promise of a nation-specific genetic map and a pathway for the nation's independence from foreign genomic research and pharmaceutical companies served them well (Benjamin, 2009; Kent, et al., 2015). Importantly, however, as the INMEGEN's work progressed, the idea of the 'Mexican genome' would become increasingly less strategic, both in a technical sense and with regard to the entrepreneurial prospects of private investors in the field.

On a technical level, by 2010 advances in high-throughput technology for sequencing genomes and computational tools for their analysis were driving increasingly large-scale collaborations and the circulation of unprecedented quantities of genetic data around the globe in order to build ever larger data sets. With these shifts in the demands of the science itself, leaders at the INMEGEN found increasingly untenable the 'go it alone' mentality on which the institute, as well as the ideal of 'genomic sovereignty', originally had been constructed (García Deister, 2014). Scientists found and took advantage of leeway in Mexico's 'genomic sovereignty' policy, skirting the legal provisions, which regulated only the circulation abroad of tissue and blood samples, but not the data extracted from them. And so, *Mestizo* blood samples were processed, their DNA extracted, sequenced, and finally transformed into cloud-stored, digital data, increasingly, to be sent abroad (García Deister, 2014). And with this digitisation and mobility abroad, many of the benefits of holding fast to these samples' unique Mexican identity began to unravel. The question became, instead, with whom could these samples be grouped to create a larger data set?

On the entrepreneurial level, these trends would intensify as private investment in genomics in Mexico accelerated. By 2010, none other than Mexico's most powerful entrepreneur and health philanthropist, Carlos Slim, had come to see genomics as a worthy investment, with potential both for improving health and for commercial success. Yet, as we will show later, in the context of this kind of private investment and Slim's interest in broader commercial markets, the notion of genomics 'made in Mexico, by Mexicans, for Mexicans' and the core principles of Mexico's 'genomic sovereignty' would be less attractive. New justice claims, unmoored from the bindings of the nation, would next come to the fore.

## Inclusion

The Carlos Slim Institute of Health, the health sector of the Carlos Slim Foundation, created the Slim Initiative for Genomic Medicine (SIGMA) with an initial investment of US$64 million in 2010 and a second of US$75 million in 2013 – an investment surpassing the Mexican state's initial funding to build the INMEGEN. At a press conference celebrating SIGMA's launch, leaders of the philanthropy – which is based in Mexico City and tied to one of the world's largest commercial empires – announced that the initiative was intended to benefit not only Mexicans but also Latin Americans by 'supporting discovery programmes that focus on health problems with particular relevance to the region', especially type 2 diabetes and cancer, and that these programmes would leverage the region's 'unique population genetics' (CarlosSlim.com, 2010, n.p.).

SIGMA's reach would extend beyond Mexico in a second sense: the initiative would encompass the INMEGEN and other Mexico-based research centres, but the Eli and Edyth L. Broad Institute of MIT and Harvard, located in Cambridge, Massachusetts, would serve as the power-centre of the venture. As part of SIGMA's strategy, early-career scientists from INMEGEN and other Mexican institutions would travel to the Broad for advanced training residencies, and although research would include DNA samples drawn in

Mexico, the brunt of their processing and data analysis would take place at the Broad. As Dr. Eric Lander, President and Executive Director of the Broad Institute explained,

> Carlos Slim Helu is adopting a visionary engagement with America's public health … Firstly, he has recognized that progress in public health must be based on the thorough understanding of the genetic fundamentals of diseases and, secondly, he has recognized the importance of establishing solid partnerships between the scientific communities of the United States and Mexico, around a common cause.
>
> *CarlosSlim.com, 2010, para. 6, n.p.*

True to its mission, in 2013 SIGMA announced its discovery of 'the first identified common genetic variant shown to predispose Latin American populations' to type 2 diabetes (SIGMA, n.d., para. 3, n.p.). Quoted in both US and Mexican news outlets, Dr. Lander acknowledged that 'because this genetic variant is absent in Europeans, it had been previously overlooked' (Broad Institute, 2013, para. 9, n.p.). 'Most genomic research has focused on European or European-derived populations', he explained, 'It's like doing science with one eye closed. There are many discoveries that can only be made by studying non-European populations' (Broad Institute, 2013, para. 5). News reports that followed characterised SIGMA's work as an effort to 'correct a bias' in genomic studies of human disease. For example, a Forbes.com article entitled, 'Carlos Slim Gives US$74 Million to Make Genomic Research Less Ethnically-Biased', reported that by 'expanding scientific knowledge about genetics specific to Latin Americans' SIGMA was correcting a kind of 'scientific racism' (Carlyle, 2013, para. 6, n.p.).

In this way, a new and revised claim to genomic justice in the arena of Mexican genomic medicine emerged with Carlos Slim's investments. No longer an issue of national politics, SIGMA's representatives moved away from INMEGEN's earlier, strict focus on the 'Mexican genome', invoking instead a broader justice-linked theme of genomic 'inclusion' at the level of the region, which underscored the need to account for and attend to Latin Americans' genetic difference.[1] Beyond the initiative's public statements, a close review of SIGMA's research brings to the fore the strategic population 'lumping' (Benjamin, 2009) this science involved and, as we explore later, highlights the value to SIGMA's scientific enterprise of flexible, broad social identities that reach beyond nations to span continents.[2]

For its research on diabetes, SIGMA would compile a data set, drawing on samples collected from four cohort studies in Mexico City and from a large study that sampled 'Latinos' in Los Angeles (The Sigma Type 2 Diabetes Consortium, 2014a, 2014b). The Los Angeles-based cohort powered SIGMA's analyses, contributing more samples to the data set than those drawn from all four Mexican cohorts combined. The Los Angeles cohort would also open opportunities for the data's interpretation. As one scientist involved in SIGMA explained to us, the cohort of 'Latinos' from Los Angeles, 'were place of birth Mexico, South or Central America.' Given the Los Angeles cohort's broad geographical extraction, she explained, 'we decided that the study could be extended to different Latin American populations'.

Thus, SIGMA's first publication on the genetics of type 2 diabetes (2014b), which appeared in the journal *Nature*, reports that the study team discovered a variant associated with the disease that is common in 'Mexicans and other Latin Americans'. However, as several SIGMA scientists we interviewed noted, the researchers widely suspected that the variant they had identified was associated specifically with samples from Mexico or samples from people of Mexican descent. 'When the other groups [from the Los Angeles cohort] were aggregated, the association remained and became a little bit stronger', our informant explained, 'yet we know that the main contribution to [this] finding is given by Mexican mestizos'. The precise relevance of this variant throughout Latin America still 'has to be studied deeply', she cautioned, but the *Nature* paper had more value to the extent that their finding reached beyond 'just Mexico'. While the Mexican *mestizo* would remain valuable as an object of genomic currency in the transnational enterprise of genomic medicine, its lumping with the Latino/a was all the more valuable in the context of international science.

SIGMA's second paper (2014a), published in the *Journal of the American Medical Association (JAMA)*, draws on a subset taken from the same data set described previously, but turns even further away from the notion of the 'Mexican genome'. Its authors describe their sample as consisting of '3756 Mexican and US Latino individuals', but ultimately report the discovery of a variant associated with diabetes among 'Latinos'. The authors present their own definition for this 'Latino' population – a statistical creation, super-imposed on this primarily US ethno-racial identity: Latinos, they explain, 'defined as persons who trace their origin to Central and South America, and other Spanish cultures, fall on a continuum of Native American and European genetic ancestry' (p. 2306). To determine an individual sample's place on this continuum, they explain, each participant's DNA, once sequenced, was submitted to a bioinformatic assessment in order to generate its unique ancestry profile, expressed as a percentage of Native American and European ancestry. Still, while SIGMA scientists offered this technical definition, the invocation of this powerful identifier signalled the relevance of SIGMA's findings beyond Central and South America, firmly tying them to the entire US Latino population (albeit one in which African heritage is erased). Between the two variants, SIGMA's findings now had relevance throughout the hemisphere.

As in these publications, in conversations with our informants, the genetic variants that SIGMA discovered consistently shift identities – in a single conversation they are sometimes 'Mexican', sometimes 'Latin American', and sometimes 'Latino'. Far from a technical error, SIGMA's published research and our interviews with participating scientists suggest that this categorical flexibility is strategic and part and parcel of the scientific process in this arena. Broad, fluid ethno-racial categories of difference like 'Latinos' and 'Latin Americans' are powerful tools that permit the construction of large data sets and, then, the extrapolation of findings from 'statistical identities' back again to living people and their communities.

Our research suggests that these categories also serve a related commercial purpose: SIGMA Consortium members and collaborators that we interviewed acknowledged that Slim's donations to SIGMA and the Broad Institute came with a timeline and the understanding that SIGMA's research could be rapidly 'translated' into marketable technologies. 'He's an entrepreneur', one of our informants observed, 'He said, "Okay I'm going to put this amount of money, but after three years I am going to get something out of it with potential commercial value"'. Accordingly, just as the Carlos Slim Institute of Health announced its second donation to the Broad Institute to fund SIGMA 2 in 2013, Slim also launched in Mexico City a bio-tech start-up, Patia Biopharma, to develop and market medical genomic technologies. Later in interviews with a representative of that company, she would clarify that Slim's goal was always to go regional, if not global. The discovery of genetic variants tied only to Mexico was never ideal – 'Slim couldn't segment his market to that extent', she confirmed.

While SIGMA's research is not the first example (nor the last) of this kind of regional approach to genomic identity, it offers critical insight with regard to how and why genomic identity shifts – even in settings, like Mexico, where a rigid nationalised view of genomic uniqueness once seemed so central. In this case, the inclusion paradigm espoused by SIGMA was entangled with Slim's commercial interests, a condition from SIGMA's start, which aligned an understanding of genetic populations with a market-based vision of regional cohesion – an example of 'genomic branding' (Tupasela, 2017). Scholars have pointed to how commercial forces in large part have historically driven the expansion of Latino identity in the United States (Dávila, 2001; Mora, 2014) and, likewise, contributed to the cohesion of Latin America – itself an imagined community with heterogeneous origins and uncertain delineations (Rivera, 2014; Tenorio-Trillo, 2017). The Carlos Slim Institute for Health with SIGMA remind us that biomedicine is a key commercial arena where such processes are ongoing in the region. Moreover, with the shift to the more fluid, regional identities of 'Latin American' and 'Latino', genomics and its benefits are unmoored from the previous state-based social contract originally put forth by Mexico's policy on 'genomic sovereignty'. In this process of genomic branding, those Mexican citizens previously cast with a right to benefit from genomic medicine are re-articulated as members of a broad Latino/a transcontinental market, their 'right' to benefit becoming a philanthropic, but also deeply commercial, concern.

## Innovation

At a University of California-Irvine conference in 2010 focused on 'Major Trends in Global Health', the Carlos Slim Institute of Health's director general explained in his keynote address that the Institute distinguishes itself from traditional philanthropy (Tapia-Conyer, 2011). Philanthropy, he said, connotes 'an expression of love', while the Institute is committed instead to 'social investment', an approach that leverages business savvy – a perspective characteristic of today's new class of philanthrocapitalists (Birn, 2014; Fejerskov, 2017; McGoey, 2015).[3] The 'social investment' approach, he explained, involves a commitment to measurable returns in terms of social impact, risk-taking where necessary, and the promotion of innovation, efficiency, and technological solutions. Moreover, like Microsoft-billionaire Bill Gates, whose foundation has affirmed the power of technology to address global health challenges (Fejerskov, 2017), Carlos Slim's commercial empire, while widely diversified, was built on telecommunications. Fittingly, the Internet, connectivity, and digital data tracking are often central to the solutions the Carlos Slim Institute of Health promotes. The Institute also seeks widespread adoption of these innovations by public institutions at the national level. As the UC Irvine address clarified with regard to the Institute's investments in genomic science,

> [I]t's not that it's there for a high-tech laboratory. We have to make sure that it's in the hands of those in the primary healthcare contact, in public health programmes … Otherwise we are going to have, one more time, innovation [going] to those who can pay for it, not where it is most needed.
>
> *Tapia-Conyer, 2011, n.p.*

Guided by these principles, the research conducted by SIGMA on type 2 diabetes would be rapidly transformed, just as Slim had originally stipulated, into a genomic technology intended for broad uptake – a test for genetic predisposition called DIABETES*Prevent*. Launched in Mexico in 2016, the test would screen for the genetic variants that SIGMA discovered among 'Mexicans and Latin Americans' and 'Latinos', along with 14 other known variants believed to increase the risk of developing the disease. Patia Biopharma, Slim's biotech start-up established in 2013, would lead the test's marketing (first in Mexico, but then more broadly in Latin America and in Spain) – its representatives nonetheless affirming in press conferences and in promotional talks with physicians in Mexico, where the test's Mexican-ness is once again most valuable, that the test was developed 'especially for the Mexican population' (see, for example, Toche, 2017).

First available as a direct-to-consumer product online, Patia's homepage launched DIABETES*Prevent*, under the tagline 'You Can Prevent Type 2 Diabetes', at a cost of about US$50. Its cost is subsidised, Patia's representatives noted in a press conference, out of Slim's desire to make genomic medicine broadly afford-able (Miranda, 2017). The test involves a cheek swab to collect a DNA sample and a short questionnaire where users report their family history of diabetes, their ancestry (i.e., 'Western European', 'Latin America/Caribbean', 'African', 'Asian'), height, weight, and age. Initially, Patia set-up home delivery of the test via a private courier service, followed by the return of the results – a type 2 diabetes risk score – delivered by email or to a smart-phone app. This app also doubles as a health management portal where, going forward, customers are encouraged to input and track data about their health, diet, and exercise to assist them in managing their genetic risk.

With online sales somewhat slow to pick-up, Patia turned its focus to physicians, who could recommend testing to the patients they considered to be at risk (and their family members), interpret their results, and discuss options for dealing with genetic risk – principally through lifestyle changes. Most recently the firm has begun to target corporations in Mexico, promoting employee screening campaigns for gen-etic diabetes risk as a way to encourage health maintenance and, ultimately, limit diabetes-related medical expenses down the line, for which employers are in-part responsible. However, perhaps the most substantial deployment of DIABETES*Prevent* has come about via the Carlos Slim Institute for Health's connections within Mexico's secretariat of health.

One of its multiple projects in partnership with the secretariat of health (at federal and state levels) the Institute initiated in 2010 a technology-centred programme in primary health care centres nationwide, to promote early detection of chronic disease, especially diabetes, which identifies and targets patients 'at risk' of developing the illness. The programme, known as MIDO (Integrated Measurement for Early Detection), was operating in 27 of the country's 32 states by 2016 and involves the instalment of 'all-in-one tools' for screening and counselling and an online, electronic information system to enable patient monitoring over time, as well as health system planning (Tapia-Conyer, et al., 2017). As Patia's genetic test DIABETES*Prevent* went to market, the Institute amplified this existing programme, launching MIDOPlus which incorporated the genetic test into the MIDO model through a pilot campaign that would test approximately 2,000 patients (Betancourt, 2018). A second, metabolomics-based, diagnostic test marketed by Patia in Mexico was also applied through MIDOPlus to detect early signs of insulin resistance. While the Institute would subsidise the cost of the pilot initiative, this philanthropic donation would also potentially represent an investment towards future commercial returns for Patia: data from the initiative would grow the company's database substantially – which could potentially help to refine the company's proprietary algorithm. This data would also constitute the evidence base on which to demonstrate the tests' utility to the secretariat of health and other health institutions, potentially justifying a broader scale-up in Mexico and beyond.

According to the Institute's staff, in the context of a programme like MIDOPlus, the genetic test and its potential application at the national level represent a new 'paradigm' not just for medicine, but for public health more broadly. In a talk delivered to public health students in the Mexican state of Puebla in early 2018, the Institute's Director of Global Solutions presented the preliminary results of the MIDOPlus pilot campaign and explained that a new era is at hand, the era of 'personalised' public health (Betancourt, 2018). Recognising the contradictions the term implies, he explained:

> What I am going to tell you goes totally against what our public health professors have taught us since our first engagement with this discipline, that public health is about population dynamics. Here we're going to the other extreme, to the most intimate, most individual aspect of each human being. You're all going to raise your hands and say, 'no, public health is by definition a population-level approach.' But no, genomics and a few of the other fields we'll see at work today are enabling us to individualize risk, create profiles, and better characterize our population.
>
> *Betancourt, 2018, n.p.*

According to the Institute's staff, DIABETES*Prevent* is not intended just as a direct-to-consumer product. DIABETES *Prevent* is the kind of technological innovation that proves possible a re-articulation of what public health can and likely should be (Tapia-Conyer, 2014). Reflecting the Institute's values of technological innovation, efficiency, and attention to the most vulnerable sectors, this new 'paradigm' in public health will entail population stratification, with resources directed for 'active prevention' among those predicted to be most at risk for developing disease. Further, within this paradigm, risk will be surfaced – made visible through high-tech intervention – from the biological (in this case molecular) depths of each individual's body.

While representatives of the Institute have clarified publicly that they do not consider genomics a panacea for Mexico's type 2 diabetes crisis, or the only solution possible (Betancourt, 2018), the Carlos Slim Institute for Health's considerable resources and wide-reaching interventions (including the MIDO programme described earlier) are powerfully promoting the stratification of the population in order to target public health resources towards those predicted to be most 'at risk' (genetically or by other clinical measures). Indeed, afforded a prime seat at the drafting table, the Institute's vision for a more 'personalised' public health response, in 'treatment as prevention', and in detecting genetic predisposition were also written into the National Strategy for the Prevention and Control of Overweight, Obesity, and Diabetes (Secretaría de Salud, 2013).

Importantly, the Institute's promotion of 'personalised' public health comes at a time of public health crisis. Type 2 diabetes was declared a national sanitary emergency in November 2016 – the first non-infectious disease ever to achieve emergency status in Mexico – and observers have since widely critiqued the failure of the state to take action beyond this declaration, denouncing Mexico's obesogenic environment and the absence of structural policies to seriously address it (Alianza por la Salud Alimentaria, 2018; Contra Peso, 2018). In this context, the Institute's promotion of 'personalised' public health is indeed a noteworthy choice. The structural role of the processed food and soda industries as drivers of the nation's metabolic crisis, for example, are not implicated. Instead, under the Institute's model, public health attention is focused on changing lifestyle choices and promoting medicalised prevention among those predicted most likely to develop disease.

As *The New York Times* pointed out in 2006, 'when Mr. Slim speaks, Mexico listens' (Thompson, 2006, para. 7, n.p.). The significance of the Institute's vision for public health lies not only in the material investments tied up in its tech-forward public–private projects, but also in the Carlos Slim Foundation's far reaching epistemic power. Ultimately, while the potential for genomics to contribute to public health is fostering interest and also debate globally (Bayer and Galea, 2015; Brand, 2011; Evangelatos, et al., 2017), the case of DIABETES *Prevent* foregrounds lessons about how genomic innovation – not divorced from the commercial interests entangled with it – may be implicated, more fundamentally, in what both experts and publics are coming to expect public health to be, and how the state's responsibility to provide equitable health to its population is brought about.

## Justice claims

In this chapter we have highlighted three kinds of justice claims that have been linked to action in the arena of genomics in Mexico – a context widely considered a key model for how actors in the developing world might confront this new field of technoscientific possibility (Hinterberger and Porter, 2015; Séguin, et al., 2008; Tekola-Ayele and Rotimi, 2015). These shifting claims have implicated genomic science in the possibility of a more just world achieved through fortified national sovereignty, increased scientific inclusion, and the technological re-making of public health. They have also rationalised immense investment in new technological possibilities, despite their uncertain social and political consequences. By tracking who these justice claims empower and the assumptions they reinforce we have offered insight into this field's stakes for both health and social progress.

Our ethnographic attention to these claims in Mexico foregrounds a complex entanglement of philanthropy and commercial interests, sanctioned by the Mexican state. This case also highlights the largely unchecked power of today's technology-driven philanthrocapitalist engagement with global health concerns (Birn, 2014; Fejerskov, 2017; McGoey, 2015). With Carlos Slim and, of course, Bill & Melinda Gates, a class of tech-forward donors, many with fortunes linked to Silicon Valley, is spearheading solutions 'shaped by logics of the individual, the market, and of societal progress through technological innovation and experimentation' (Fejerskov, 2017, p. 948). Under their purview, global health challenges, including Mexico's metabolic crisis, are often positioned as technological problems, and justice is posited as an issue of whether and how technoscience is deployed to address them. Yet the science and justice formation put forward through this ethos of technological innovation can also trump equity, averting health interventions grounded in structural change while fuelling the dynamics of global capital accumulation.

## Acknowledgements

This research was supported by the National Science Foundation, Science, Technology and Society Division (Grant: SES-1656224) and by a PAPIIT-DGAPA-UNAM Grant: #IA401416.

## Notes

1  Epstein has traced the rise of the 'inclusion-and-difference paradigm' in contemporary medical research in the United States, which he defines as a 'research and policy focus on including diverse groups as participants in medical studies and in measuring differences across those groups' (2007, p. 17). Although this paradigm arose in part in response to social justice activists who demanded more recognition of diversity in medical research, implicit in the logic underpinning this approach to medicine is the problematic notion that particular 'social identities correspond to relatively distinct kinds of bodies … and that these various embodied states are medically incommensurable' (Epstein, 2007, p. 2).

2  We discuss SIGMA's scientific process and the representations of genomic difference in SIGMA's publications in more detail in Vasquez & García Deister (forthcoming).

3  This new breed of philanthropist approaches the operation of philanthropic foundations more like for-profit business. As McGoey (2015) writes, 'the new philanthrocapitalists claim to be more results-oriented and more efficient than earlier philanthropic donors. They want to revolutionize the last realm untouched by the hyper-competitive, profit-oriented world of financial capitalism: the world of charitable giving' (pp. 6–7).

## References

Abu El-Haj, N. (2007) 'The genetic reinscription of race', *Annual Review of Anthropology*, 36(1): 283–300.

Alianza por la Salud Alimentaria. (2018) 'Manifiesto a la nación por un sistema alimentario nutricional justo y sustentable', available at http://elpoderdelconsumidor.org/wp-content/uploads/2018/02/manifiesto-sistema-alimentario-justo-sustentable.pdf (accessed on 28 February 2018).

Bayer, R. and Galea, S. (2015) 'Public health in the precision-medicine era', *New England Journal of Medicine*, 373(6): 499–501.

Benjamin, R. (2009) 'A lab of their own: genomic sovereignty as postcolonial science policy', *Policy and Society*, 28(4): 341–55.

Betancourt, M. (2018) 'Genómica y enfermedades crónicas', paper presented at the Primera Sesión Académica de la Maestría en Salud Pública, Universidad Popular Autónoma del Estado de Puebla, Puebla, México.

Birn, A.-E. (2014) 'Philanthrocapitalism, past and present: the Rockefeller Foundation, the Gates Foundation, and the setting(s) of the international/global health agenda', *Hypothesis*, 12(1): e8.

Bliss, C. (2012) *Race Decoded: The genomic fight for social justice*, Stanford, California: Stanford University Press.

Bliss, C. (2013) 'The marketization of identity politics', *Sociology*, 47(5): 1011–25.

Brand, A. (2011) 'Public health genomics– public health goes personalized?', *European Journal of Public Health*, 21(1): 2–3.

Broad Institute. (2013) 'Mexico-US genomics partnership launches second phase', available at www.broadinstitute.org/news/mexico-us-genomics-partnership-launches-second-phase (accessed on 28 February 2018).

Cámara de Diputados. (2008) 'Proceso Legislativo – Decreto por el que se reforma la fracción V del artículo 100 y el artículo 461, y se adicionan los artículos 317 Bis y 317 Bis 1, todos de la Ley General de Salud', available at www.diputados.gob.mx/LeyesBiblio/proceso/lx/101_DOF_14jul08.pdf (accessed on 28 February 2018).

CarlosSlim.com. (2010) 'Boletín informativo', available at www.carlosslim.com/preg_resp_slim_genoma_ing.html (accessed on 28 February 2018).

Carlyle, E. (2013) 'Carlos Slim gives $74 million to make genomic research less ethnically-biased', available at www.forbes.com/sites/erincarlyle/2013/10/30/carlos-slim-gives-another-74-million-to-make-genomic-research-less-ethnically-biased/#78722fd24a82 (accessed on 28 February 2018).

Chavez, L.R. (2008) *The Latino Threat: Constructing immigrants, citizens, and the nation*, Stanford: Stanford University Press.

Contra Peso. (2018) 'Prevención del Sobrepeso, la Obesidad y las ENTs en México: Documento de Postura de la Coalición CONTRAPESO', available at http://coalicioncontrapeso.org/project/cartasecretariafuncionpublica-copy/ (accessed on 28 February 2018).

Dávila, A.M. (2001) *Latinos, Inc.: The marketing and making of a people*, Berkeley: University of California Press.

Duster, T. (2015) 'A post-genomic surprise. The molecular reinscription of race in science, law and medicine', *The British Journal of Sociology*, 66(1): 1–27.

Epstein, S. (2007) Inclusion: The politics of difference in medical research, Chicago: The University of Chicago Press.

Evangelatos, N., Satyamoorthy, K., and Brand, A. (2017) 'Personalized health in a public health perspective', *International Journal of Public Health*, n.p.

Fejerskov, A.M. (2017) 'The new technopolitics of development and the global South as a laboratory of technological experimentation', *Science, Technology, & Human Values*, 42(5): 947–68.

Frenk, J. (2001) 'México en el umbral de la era genómica: impacto en la salud pública', paper presented at the 'México en el umbral de la era genómica' symposium, Ciudad de México, México.

García Deister, V. (2014) 'Laboratory life of the Mexican Mestizo', In: P. Wade, C. L. Beltrán, E. Restrepo, and R.V. Santos (Eds.) *Mestizo Genomics: Race mixture, nation, and science in Latin America*, Durham, NC: Duke University Press, pp. 161–82.

García Deister, V. (2018) 'In sickness and in myth: genetic avatars of indigenous alterity and the Mexican Nation', In: P. López Caballero and A. Acevedo-Rodrigo (Eds.) *Beyond Alterity: Destabilizing the indigenous other in Mexico*, Tucson: The University of Arizona Press, pp. 263–83.

Hinterberger, A. and Porter, N. (2015) 'Genomic and viral sovereignty: tethering the materials of global biomedicine', *Public Culture*, 27(276): 361–86.

Jiménez Sanchez, G. (2003) 'Developing a platform for genomic medicine in Mexico', *Science*, 300(5617): 295–6.

Jiménez Sanchez, G., Silva-Zolezzi, I., Hidalgo, A., and March, S. (2008) 'Genomic medicine in Mexico: initial steps and the road ahead', *Genome Research*, 18(8): 1191–8.

Kent, M., García-Deister, V., López-Beltrán, C., Santos, R.V., Schwartz-Marín, E., and Wade, P. (2015) 'Building the genomic nation: 'Homo Brasilis' and the 'Genoma Mexicano' in comparative cultural perspective', *Social Studies of Science*, 45(6): 839–61.

Koenig, B.A., Soo-Jin Lee, S., and Richardson, S.S. (Eds.) (2008) *Revisiting Race in a Genomic Age*, New Brunswick, NJ: Rutgers University Press.

López Beltran, C. and García Deister, V.G. (2013) 'Scientific approaches to the Mexican mestizo', *Hist Cienc Saude Manguinhos*, 20(2): 391–410.

López Beltrán, C., García Deister, V., and Rios Sandoval, M. (2014) 'Negotiating the Mexican Mestizo: on the possibility of a national genomics', In: P. Wade, C. L. Beltrán, E. Restrepo, and R.V. Santos (Eds.) *Mestizo Genomics: Race mixture, nation, and science in Latin America*, Durham, NC: Duke University Press, pp. 85–106.

López Caballero, P. (2017) *Indígenas de la Nación: Etnografía histórica de la alteridad en México (Milpa Alta, siglos XVII-XXI)*, Ciudad de México: Fondo de Cultura Económica.

Mamo, L. and Fishman, J.R. (2013) 'Why Justice?: Introduction to the special issue on entanglements of science, ethics, and justice', *Science, Technology & Human Values*, 38(2): 159–75.

McGoey, L. (2015) *No such Thing as a Free Gift: The Gates Foundation and the price of philanthropy*, London: Verso.

Miranda, P. (2017) 'Lanzan prueba ue evalúa riesgo de diabetes', available at www.eluniversal.com.mx/articulo/nacion/seguridad/2017/01/26/lanzan-prueba-que-evalua-riesgo-de-diabetes (accessed on 28 February 2018).

Molina, N. (2006) *Fit to be Citizens? Public health and race in Los Angeles, 1879–1939*, Berkeley, CA: University of California Press.

Montoya, M.J. (2011) *Making the Mexican Diabetic: Race, science, and the genetics of inequality*, Berkeley, CA: University of California Press.

Mora, G.C. (2014) *Making Hispanics: How activists, bureaucrats, and media constructed a new American*, Chicago, IL: University of Chicago Press.

Moreno Figueroa, M.G. and Saldívar Tanaka, E. (2015) 'We are not racists, we are Mexicans': privilege, nationalism and post-race ideology in Mexico', *Critical Sociology*, 42(4–5): 515–33.

Nelson, A. (2016) *The Social Life of DNA: Race, reparations, and reconciliation after the genome*, Boston, MA: Beacon Press.

Pang, T. (2002) 'The impact of genomics on global health', *American Journal of Public Health*, 92(7): 1077–9.

Reardon, J. (2013) 'On the emergence of science and justice', *Science, Technology, & Human Values*, 38(2): 176–200.

Reardon, J. (2017) *The Postgenomic Condition: Ethics, justice, and knowledge after the genome*, Chicago, IL: The University of Chicago Press.

Rivera, S. (2014) *Latin American Unification: A history of political and economic integration Efforts*, Jefferson, NC: McFarland & Company, Inc.

Roberts, D. (2011) *Fatal Invention: How science, politics, and big business re-create race in the twenty-first century*, New York, NY: New Press.

Schwartz Marín, E. (2011) 'Genomic sovereignty and the "Mexican genome"', dissertation, available at https://ore.exeter.ac.uk/repository/handle/10036/3500 (accessed on 28 February 2018).

Secretaría de Gobernación. (2008) 'Decreto por el que se reforma la fracción V del artículo 100 y el artículo 461, y se adicionan los artículos 317 Bis y 317 Bis 1, todos de la Ley General de Salud', available at www.dof.gob.mx/nota_detalle.php?codigo=5053006&fecha=14/07/2008 (accessed on 28 February 2018).

Secretaría de Salud. (2013) 'Estrategia nacional para la prevención y el control del sobrepeso, la obesidad y la diabetes', available at http://promocion.salud.gob.mx/dgps/descargas1/estrategia/Estrategia_con_portada.pdf (accessed on 28 February 2018).

Séguin, B. and Hardy, B.-J. (2008) 'Genomic medicine and developing countries: creating a room of their own', *Nature Reviews Genetics*, 9(6): 487–93.

Séguin, B., Hardy, B.-J., Singer, P.A., and Daar, A.S. (2008) 'Genomics, public health and developing countries: the case of the Mexican National Institute of Genomic Medicine (INMEGEN)' *Nature Reviews Genetics*, 9: S5–9.

SIGMA. (n.d.) 'SIGMAT2D', available at www.type2diabetesgenetics.org/projects/sigma (accessed on 28 February 2018).

Silva-Zolezzi, I., Hidalgo-Miranda, A., Estrada-Gil, J., Fernandez-Lopez, J.C., Uribe-Figueroa, L., Contreras, A., … Jimenez-Sanchez, G. (2009) 'Analysis of genomic diversity in Mexican Mestizo populations to develop genomic medicine in Mexico', *Proceedings of the National Academy of Sciences*, 106(21): 8611–6.

Singer, P.A. and Daar, A.S. (2001) 'Harnessing genomics and biotechnology to improve global health equity', *Science*, 294(5540): 87–9.

Stern, A. (2005) *Eugenic Nation: Faults and frontiers of better breeding in modern America*, Berkeley, CA: University of California Press.

Tapia-Conyer, R. [University of California Television] (2011) 'Trends in global health: a social investment perspective' [Video File], available at www.youtube.com/watch?v=-NqGnGMmVSE (accessed on 28 February 2018).

Tapia-Conyer, R. [Academia Nacional de Medicina de México] (2014) 'La revolución digital y genómica para una mejor salud pública' [Video File], available at www.youtube.com/watch?v=ZGIieFA1GCU (accessed on 28 February 2018).

Tapia-Conyer, R., Saucedo-Martínez, R., Mújica-Rosales, R., Gallardo-Rincón, H., Lee, E., Waugh, C., … Atkinson, E.R. (2017) 'A policy analysis on the proactive prevention of chronic disease: learnings from the initial implementation of Integrated Measurement for Early Detection (MIDO)', *International Journal of Health Policy and Management*, 6(6): 339–44.

Tekola-Ayele, F. and Rotimi, C.N. (2015) 'Translational genomics in low- and middle-income countries: opportunities and challenges', *Public Health Genomics*, 18(4): 242–7.

Tenorio-Trillo, M. (2017) *Latin America: The allure and power of an idea*, Chicago, IL: University of Chicago Press.

*The Lancet*. (2002) 'Genomics and health inequalities', *The Lancet*, 359(9317): 1535.

The Sigma Type 2 Diabetes Consortium. (2014a) 'Association of a low-frequency variant in HNF1A with type 2 diabetes in a Latino population', *JAMA*, 311(22): 2305–14.

The Sigma Type 2 Diabetes Consortium. (2014b) 'Sequence variants in SLC16A11 are a common risk factor for type 2 diabetes in Mexico', *Nature*, 506(7486): 97–101.

The White House. (2000) 'June 2000 White House event', available at www.genome.gov/10001356/ (accessed on 28 February 2018).

Thompson, G. (2006) 'Prodded by the Left, Mexico's Richest Man Talks Equity', available at www.nytimes.com/2006/06/03/world/americas/03slim.html (accessed on 28 February 2018).

Toche, N. (2017) 'Prueba genómica para evaluar diabetes', available at www.eleconomista.com.mx/arteseideas/Prueba-genomica-para-evaluar-diabetes-20170126-0075.html (accessed on 28 February 2018).

Tupasela, A. (2017) 'Populations as brands in medical research: placing genes on the global genetic atlas', *BioSocieties*, 12(1): 47–65.

Vasconcelos, J. (1966) La Raza Cosmica: Mision de la Raza Iberoamericana, Argentina y Brasil (3 ed.), Mexico: Espasa-Calpe.

Vasquez, E.E. and García Deister, V. (forthcoming) 'Mexican samples, Latino DNA: On the Neoliberal Search for Type 2 Diabetes in the Genome', *Engaging Science, Technology, and Society*.

Wade, P., Deister, V.G., Kent, M., Sierra, M.F.O., and Hernández, A.D.d.C. (2014) 'Nation and the absent presence of race in Latin American genomics', *Current Anthropology*, 55(5): 497–522.

Whitmarsh, I. and Jones, D.S. (Eds.) (2010) *What's the Use of Race? Modern Governance and the Biology of Difference*, Cambridge, MA: MIT Press.

WHO. (2002) 'Genomics and world health: report of the advisory committee on health research', available at www.who.int/rpc/genomics_report.pdf (accessed on 28 February 2018).

# Index